500

of the most important
HEALTH TIPS
YOU'LL EVER NEED

An A–Z of alternative health hints
to help over 250 conditions

Hazel Courteney

with Stephen Langley and Gareth Zeal

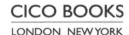

CICO BOOKS
LONDON NEW YORK

First published in Great Britain by CICO Books
an imprint of Ryland Peters and Small
20–21 Jockey's Fields
London WC1R 4BW
www.cicobooks.com

Copyright © CICO Books 2001, 2006, 2009, 2011
First edition published 2001
Revised editions printed 2006, 2009, 2011
This edition published 2013 for Index Books

Text copyright © Hazel Courteney 2001, 2006, 2009, 2011
The right of Hazel Courteney to be identified as the author of this work
has been asserted by her in accordance with the Copyright, Designs and
Patents Act 1988.

10 9 8 7 6 5 4

A CIP catalogue record for this book is available from the British Library.

ISBN: 978 1 907030 80 2

Jacket design by Jerry Goldie Graphic Design
Designed by Jerry Goldie Graphic Design

Printed in the UK by CPI Group (UK) Ltd, Croydon, CR0 4YY

PUBLISHERS' NOTE:
Always consult a doctor before undertaking any of the advice,
exercise plans, or supplements suggested in this book. Whilst every
attempt has been made to ensure the medical information in this
book is entirely safe and correct and up to date at the time of
publication, the Publishers accept no responsibility for consequences
of the advice given herein. If in any doubt as to the nature of your
condition, consult a qualified medical practitioner.

The Publishers also accept no responsibility for changes in prices,
stockist arrangements and locations mentioned herein.

Hazel Courteney is an award-winning, respected health and metaphysical writer and speaker based in the UK. In 1997 she was voted Health Journalist of the Year for her column in *The Sunday Times*. This is her fourth health book. Hazel has also written three highly acclaimed spiritual metaphysical books. For more information on Hazel's work, log on to her website: www.hazelcourteney.com.

Other books by Hazel Courteney:
500 of the Healthiest Recipes and Health Tips You'll Ever Need
500 of the Most Important Ways to Stay Younger Longer
Divine Intervention
The Evidence for the Sixth Sense
Countdown to Coherence
Mind and Mood Foods
Body and Beauty Foods

Stephen Langley MSc, ND, DipHom, DBM, DipAc, DCH, OMD is a registered naturopath, homeopath, acupuncturist, doctor of Chinese medicine, and medical herbalist. He lectures in naturopathic medicine at the College of Naturopathic Medicine (CNM) in London, Bristol, Manchester, Dublin, Galway and Belfast, as well as running a busy health practice in London and lecturing globally. Stephen has studied Holistic Medicine in China, India, America, Australia, Tibet and Japan. He can be reached via the Hale Clinic in London on 020 7631 0156.

Gareth Zeal BSc is a nutritionist and health writer with 25 years' experience. He runs a busy health practice in North Yorkshire and regularly lectures around the UK. You can reach him via his office on 01287 280733.

Author's note

Throughout the book, we have in many instances suggested specific amounts of nutrients. This is to ensure that sufficient amounts of the nutrient are taken to benefit a specific condition. In places where no specific amounts are suggested, take the supplements daily, according to the instructions on the label or from your health professional.

We have mentioned books that we have found useful, but whatever you are suffering from, believe me, there is a specialist book on it. Remember, you will fail only if you give up.

This book is not intended as a substitute for conventional medical counselling. Never stop taking prescribed medicine without first consulting your doctor. Always inform your doctor of any supplements or herbs you are taking in case these are contra-indicated with your drugs.

During the last 25 years I have read hundreds of books and many phrases and facts have remained in my mind. Wherever it has been possible, I have acknowledged the source of these phrases and facts, and to those whose names I have forgotten, my apologies for any unintentional oversights.

I also want to clarify that I personally am not paid in **any** way whatsoever to mention specific companies, nutrients or products. I mention supplements that have good research behind them, or those recommended by highly qualified professionals, that have been shown to help heal or prevent various conditions.

For the latest update on EC rulings regarding which supplements may or may not be available in the future, see page 9.

Acknowledgements

Revising and greatly updating this latest edition has been an intensive seven-month labour of love. Several wonderful people have contributed to make this book truly special. To my co-authors, Stephen Langley and Gareth Zeal – thanks for spending several days each with me to keep me up to date on the latest health news and research. And Steve, thanks for reading the proofs; your patience and integrity has been much appreciated.

Thanks also to nutritional physician Dr Shamin Daya from the Wholistic Medical Centre in London. Also my dear friend Bob Jacobs, naturopath, homeopath and nutritional scientist, for your specialist help with the Breast Cancer, Cancer, Menopause, Osteoporosis and Thyroid sections. Thank you both for your time and advice and for sharing your cutting-edge knowledge.

My gratitude also goes to bio-electromagnetics scientist Dr Roger Coghill for your help on Electrical Pollution, Jet Lag and Insomnia. My gratitude also to Sue Croft, at Consumers for Health Choice, for your update on European legislation.

This section would not be complete without also sending a big hug to my ex-PA, Lindsay Ross-Jarrett, who checked hundreds of contact details.

Finally, thanks as always to my wonderful husband Stuart – who has the patience of a saint.

DEDICATION

This book is dedicated to Sue Croft, who for more than
thirty years has devoted her life, often without reward,
to ensuring that our freedom to purchase higher-dose
vitamins, minerals and herbs is retained.
Thank you, Sue, for always being so positive, professional,
cheerful and helpful. You are a very special lady.

INTRODUCTION

WHY THERE IS STILL AN URGENT NEED FOR THIS BOOK

Einstein's definition of insanity was 'to keep doing the same thing over and over again – and expect different results'. He was right.

If I told you that 85% of your health problems, including chronic degenerative diseases associated with ageing, could be prevented, cured or greatly alleviated by simply changing your diet and taking the right supplements – would you believe me? Yet it's true.

For example, the World Cancer Research Fund now states that as many as 40% of cases of breast cancer, around 18,000 a year in the UK alone, could be avoided by following a healthier lifestyle, drinking less alcohol, keeping to a sensible weight by eating more healthily, and taking regular exercise. Published studies carried out at the School of Medicine in Puerto Rico by Professor Jaime Matta have found definitive evidence that women who take long-term multi-vitamins and mineral supplements reduce their risk for developing breast cancer by almost 30%. Another study from the Institute of Brain Chemistry and Human Nutrition at London's Metropolitan University found that women who take multi-vitamins and minerals, including vitamin D, folic acid, B vitamins, antioxidants and iron, give birth to bigger and generally healthier babies.

With more than 500,000 positive research papers regarding diet and supplements, plus freely available health information through the internet and media, you would think that our overall health would be improving – yet sadly, in many cases the opposite is happening. Without doubt some people are living longer, but not necessarily healthier, lives. Most people may be aware of what constitutes a healthy diet, yet they continue to prefer junk foods and lifestyles, without taking responsibility, or caring about the long-term consequences of their actions. We are still talking about being healthy, yet the statistics demonstrate that we are becoming one of the 'sickest' nations on earth.

When the NHS was launched in 1948 it had a budget of £437 million. In 2010 this figure reached over £100 billion – approximately equating to a contribution of £1980 for every man, woman and child in the UK.

Cardiovascular disease remains the largest killer in the West. It kills 200,000 people annually in the UK alone and costs the NHS £15 billion annually. One in every three people will develop cancer at some point in their lives; 50 years ago, this was 1 in 27.

Obesity is reaching epidemic proportions and if it continues at this rate will cost the NHS £6.3 billion by 2015. One in every five children in the UK is overweight or obese when they start school and this climbs to one in three by the time they finish primary school. Furthermore, more than eight million men and women in the UK are obese – that's one in five adults. With many adults and children ingesting as many as 40 teaspoons of refined sugars daily, from refined cereals, pre-packaged meals, cereals and fizzy drinks – is it any wonder we are piling on the pounds?

Such habits have triggered an explosion of 'late-onset' diabetes, which affects around three million people in the UK and 246 million globally. And late-onset diabetes, which 25 years ago was unheard of in anyone under 50, is now affecting children as young as 15.

All the above, plus an ever-escalating increase in people suffering from age-related conditions, such as late-onset dementia, are creating an enormous burden on the NHS.

The continuing tragedy is that virtually all these conditions are, in the majority of cases, totally preventable.

Thanks to high-profile celebrities, such as Jamie Oliver, Jenny Seagrove and Carole Caplin, thousands of adults and children are more aware of what constitutes a healthier diet. Many supermarkets and food manufacturers are gradually eliminating hydrogenated trans-fats, which raise LDL, the 'bad' cholesterol, thus contributing to heart disease, strokes, obesity, dementia and cancers. Sodium-based salts and refined sugars are also coming under fire as public awareness grows of their negative effects on health.

However, we still have some way to go: binge drinking among young people is on the rise and the consequences of New Year's Eve over-indulgence alone cost the NHS £23 million.

Even though smoking has thankfully been banned in public places, around nine million people in the UK still smoke. And two-thirds of all smokers tend to take up this dreadful habit before the age of 18.

Human nature is perverse: we may know what's healthy, but too many of us are still not acting on the information available! Why? Because most of us tend to think that it's never going to happen to us... until it does.

How much better it would be if we could take not only a lot more responsibility for our own health, but also learn more about our bodies with the aim of preventing them becoming sick in the first place. Unfortunately, too many people still hand total responsibility for their health to their overworked doctor. Most GPs are caring, hard-working people – but unless they have a specific interest in how diet and supplements can prevent or heal many conditions, they are often lacking on this type of information. During their six years' training at medical school, very few receive even a day's training in how diet, lifestyle and taking the right supplements can greatly improve and prevent many illnesses. Most of their courses are still sponsored by drugs companies, which is why prescribing a pill for our illnesses remains their usual response. But this practice rarely addresses the root cause of the condition.

Almost everyone is looking for a single magic bullet to help alleviate their health problems. Most of us are in a hurry and yet happy to react to misleading and often incorrect or misquoted health information that appears in the media with alarming regularity. But help is at hand. Certified organic food sales remain popular and, contrary to press reports, organic fruit and vegetables have been proven to contain more vitamins and minerals than their non-organic counterparts.

The more we eat organic, the less hormone-disrupting chemicals we swallow. As an example of this, a non-organic lettuce may have been sprayed 11 or more times during its brief growing cycle and the average Cox's apple will be sprayed 18 times with a cocktail of chemicals.

In addition, in 2000 I also wrote about how the 31 million mobile phones in use were linked with depression and various cancers. By 2010 around 75 million mobile phones had been connected in the UK, many for use by children – even though the Government has issued warnings that children of 12 and under should not use mobile phones. If you add the cumulative negative effects of mobile phones, microwaves, computers and all electrical equipment which pulse us with harmful electromagnetic radiation to the effects of a negative diet and lifestyle, you soon realize that all these factors combine to trigger the tidal wave of illnesses we are experiencing today. Our bodies were never designed to eat so much rubbish and ingest so many chemicals and they are telling us that they have simply had enough. We have caused most of the problems we face today – but the good news is that we can change or reverse many of them.

MRSA and *C.difficile* have been triggered by our overuse of antibiotics, but many doctors don't know that manuka honey, as well as herbs such as pau d'arco, Beta Glucans and essential oils of oregano and thyme, are known to help destroy MRSA and other superbugs. They are also unlikely to know that a leaky gut is often the root cause for many ailments, including eczema, and most autoimmune problems, such as Lupus, which are now on the rise.

With so many diseases on the increase, and with various bacteria mutating into deadlier strains faster than doctors can kill them, the time has come to discover new ways to protect ourselves.

For this reason I, and my co-authors Stephen Langley and Gareth Zeal, have **completely** revised and updated this book to give you access to the latest developments in the alternative health field. We have included several new headings, including adrenal exhaustion, a multi-factorial and misunderstood problem that has now, as a result of our high-octane, 24/7 lifestyles, reached epidemic proportions.

Also included in this edition is atherosclerosis (hardening of the arteries), which contributes to high blood pressure, heart disease, strokes and erectile dysfunction, plus conditions such as lupus, as these types of conditions are on the rise.

Throughout this book I and my colleagues have given numerous, often little-known but well-researched solutions to many health problems plus a host of proven remedies, nutrients and ideas to improve your health on a day-to-day basis. We also offer alternative answers to many common symptoms that even your doctor may not recognize – to help you become your own health detective. Remember: the body is perfectly capable of healing itself, when and if it is given the right tools for the job.

May our work give you good health – today and all days.

Hazel Courteney

IS OUR RIGHT TO TAKE SUPPLEMENTS UNDER THREAT?

Sue Croft, a director of CHC, Consumers for Health Choice, continues to spend her life lobbying MPs, MEPs and regulators, both in the UK and in Europe, to help us retain our freedom to choose higher dose supplements. She says: 'The risks remain the same today as they were in 2010. We could still lose our right to buy high-dose specialist nutrients – even a one-gram tablet of vitamin C is under threat, as are many others. The dose levels of vitamins and minerals they will allow us to buy in the UK and Europe were to be set by the 31 December 2010. To date (summer 2012) the arguments continue and we have still no idea which way it will go. What we do know is many non-supporters of natural healthcare want a decision now. They don't care what that decision is as long as they can tick the box, a view now being actively promoted in Brussels even by UK MEPs.

'Most of the people in the Member States of the EU are not used to taking higher-dose nutrients – and unfortunately the majority view that wants low dosages could prevail. For instance, the current RDI (Recommended Daily Intake) for vitamin C, needed for more than 40 functions in the body, is 60mg, but this is only just sufficient to prevent scurvy and deficiency diseases – even a goat can manufacture 4 grams daily. Yet the smaller doses are mostly available in Europe – and those countries with the largest number of votes, France and Germany, want to keep it that way. If the EU get their way, this would obviously destroy the UK vitamin and mineral market as we know it. Europe sadly considers this a price worth paying. This is horrendous. Even though there are thousands of published and verified scientific studies showing that appropriate higher dosages are both safe and beneficial, we still have a fight on our hands. This is why we are using all our influence to push the British Government to vigorously defend consumer choice on our behalf. The emerging signs remain positive.

'What most people don't understand is that here, our nutritional products are sold under Food Law: they have to be 100% safe – as safe as a loaf of bread or a tomato. And just because a medicine has a product licence (which allows the makers to make specific beneficial claims, and can cost millions of pounds that vitamin companies simply don't have), it doesn't make it safe. Vioxx, the arthritis drug, was granted a medicinal licence and has been taken by 20 million people. Unfortunately, many are now dead and others have brought massive law suits against the makers of this drug. Negative side effects from statins are also emerging on a large scale.

'Conversely, there have only been two recorded incidents of death from anyone taking supplements, and these were young children who swallowed a bottle of prescribed high-dose prescription iron tablets. In the past 18 years, there have been only eleven reported cases of people claiming symptoms, such as tingling fingers and toes, from taking certain nutrients to excess, which rapidly recede once those supplements are stopped. Vitamin B6 is vital for combating stress and regulating hormone levels – and if high doses over 250mg daily are taken for a long period of time then tingling can result – yet 50mg is essential to health. If the EU have their way, this vitamin could be banned, because it has a minor reversible effect in some people. This is ridiculous when you consider that over 60,000 people are hospitalized annually in the UK because of adverse reactions to their prescription drugs and 1200 people die annually as a direct consequence of taking prescription drugs.'

Like Sue, I feel very strongly about this subject, and I hope you will write to your MP and MEP to tell them of the health benefits you have experienced thanks to taking supplements, and to ask them to push ministers to allow us to keep our market and our right to take higher-dose nutrients intact.

For the latest news regarding this unwelcome legislation and how you can help, log onto CHC's website: www.consumersforhealthchoice.com

WHY YOU NEED NUTRITIONAL SUPPLEMENTS

How many times have you heard people say, 'Surely if I eat a healthy balanced diet, I will not need to take vitamins and minerals?' 'Expensive pee!' others exclaim.

In a perfect unpolluted world, if we could all eat plenty of fresh locally grown fruits, vegetables and grains, then indeed we should not need extra vitamins and minerals. But as we don't live on a desert island with a pure water supply, fresh fruits and vegetables and little stress, we need to give our bodies some extra protection.

The Government's campaign encouraging everyone to eat five portions of fruit and vegetables a day has fallen mainly on deaf ears: one of my co-authors, nutritionist Gareth Zeal, is often asked, 'Does ketchup count as a vegetable?' I'm afraid the answer is an emphatic NO!

A few people have changed, but the fact remains that as little as 5% of the Western population eats a truly healthy, balanced diet. The majority talk about healthy eating, but in reality continue to eat far too much pre-packaged, refined junk foods that are often packed with salt, sugar, additives and saturated fats. A few people still do not comprehend that the human body is literally made of food molecules, so your body is largely made up from what you have eaten during the last year.

Also, many commercial growers – especially from overseas – continue to harvest their fruit and vegetables long before they are ripe. Research in Spain and at Oregon State University in America have found that when, for example, cherries are picked before being ripe, the vitamin C content is halved. When blackberries were picked early, the green ones contained 74mg of anthocyanins (the blue pigment that is great for your eyes and immune system) compared with 317mg in the naturally ripened fruits. Add to this the fact that most fresh produce is flown halfway round the world and is then stored for long periods, which itself hugely depletes nutrient levels, and the message is obvious: as much as possible, buy more fresh, ripe, locally grown foods.

To survive, the human body needs 50 factors; these are 13 vitamins, 21 minerals, 9 amino acids, 2 essential fatty acids, plus carbohydrate, fibre, air, water and light. As our bodies cannot manufacture most of these substances, we must take them in from external sources – through our diet and by taking the right supplements. If the body becomes deficient in nutrients, negative symptoms will eventually result.

We can all have treats and really enjoy them – but we must stop living on them. Many times I have watched people fill their supermarket trolleys with white bread, pre-packaged meals, cakes, chocolate bars and fizzy drinks. Almost all this refined, pre-packaged and processed food contains virtually no vitamins, essential fats, minerals or fibre. We are bombarded with food advertisements claiming that products are 'packed with added vitamins'. Have you ever asked yourself why the manufacturers need to add vitamins, if the food is supposed to be nutritious in the first place?

White flour and mass-produced oils are the same. Tinned foods are sterilized at high temperatures to kill any bacteria. How many nutrients do you think are left after these processes have taken place?

Without doubt, I advocate organic farming – and the more farmers who switch to organic methods, the fewer pesticides and herbicides (known to deplete even more nutrients from our food) will be in our food, water and air. And organic food has been proven to contain more nutrients than non-organic produce. Also, the use of fewer chemicals means less acid rain, less pollution and less sickness. Natural mineral levels in soil in many countries, including the UK, are dropping, and if vital nutrients such as selenium, known to reduce the incidence of cancer and heart disease, are not in our soil, they are never going to make it into our fruits and vegetables.

Our eating habits have changed drastically during recent years. As little as 50 years ago, it was routine for the family to sit and eat home-cooked meals with freshly picked vegetables and fruits from a local farm or allotment. Today, this tradition seems to have all but disappeared and some children are not eating even one piece of fresh fruit a week. This is shocking. The longer fresh food is stored and cooked, the more nutrients are lost. If you leave an orange in a fridge for more than three days, up to 50% of the vitamin C content disappears. And, because the modern diet is less than perfect, we need to come to a compromise – which is why I take nutritional supplements and recommend specific nutrients in this book.

Unfortunately, some people still compare vitamins, minerals and essential fats in capsule forms, to prescription drugs – but remember that essential nutrients are essential to life.

On the drugs front, the trend to take statins to lower cholesterol is growing exponentially and people believe that once taking statins, they can eat all manner of high-fat food without risk. Yet statins are known to weaken all muscles, including the heart muscle, and they greatly inhibit natural production of Co Enzyme Q 10, a vitamin-like substance needed by the body to protect the heart and produce energy. Statins also deplete the mineral selenium from the body, which is vital for heart health, cancer prevention, healthy sperm and for removing toxic metals such as mercury from the body. Statins are also linked to memory loss, muscle pain and nerve damage. But LDL cholesterol levels can also be controlled by taking supplements, such as lecithin granules, garlic, B-group vitamins, vitamin C and pine bark extract known as pycnogenol, among others.

Many governments suggest minimum amounts of nutrients, called RDIs – Recommended Daily Intakes. In Europe there are RDIs for 26 nutrients and yet there are 45 essential nutrients required for health. Confusion is rife, as RDIs vary from country to country – so whom do we believe? Initially, the idea of RDIs was to prevent obvious signs of deficiency, such as scurvy (vitamin-C deficiency) in soldiers in the trenches in 1941. However, they do not in any way represent the quantities of nutrients we require for optimum health today. Nor do they represent the levels of vitamins and minerals we need to protect our bodies from the pollutants and toxins in our modern environment. What is more, RDIs take no account of individual requirements, such as age, gender or the health status of the person. For example, the current RDI for vitamin C is 60mg in the UK – but to ingest this amount from your diet, you would need to eat eight apples, three kiwi fruits or two oranges.

Currently, there is no RDI for vitamin D3, a deficiency of which is now linked to seventeen varieties of cancer, as well as to heart disease, diabetes, depression, osteoporosis and more. A growing body of research from highly accredited medical centres now states that this vitamin should be termed essential to life and every one of us needs to take an absolute minimum of 800iu of D3 daily.

In the US, the RDI for the mineral chromium, which has been proven to halve the incidence of late-onset diabetes, is 120mcg; yet in the UK or Europe no RDI exists. This is lunacy.

But there is hope. A few years ago, I met a man aged 73 who had been refused heart surgery as his arteries were so blocked. He was deemed a lost cause; totally breathless, he could not even walk across the room. A nutritional physician friend took him on. First, she completely changed his diet, then gave him supplements proven to thin blood naturally, lower cholesterol levels and to help clear some of the plaque that had built up in his arteries. Under medical supervision, he was also taught yoga. After several months he slowly but surely regained his health. Today he climbs Alpine slopes as a hobby. It's never too late to change. And as Western doctors are now seeing plaque in the arteries of children as young as 10, change is imperative.

We all need to start eating food that is as unprocessed and unrefined as possible. Natural, locally grown organic food, without pesticides and additives, plus taking the right supplements, is the way forward. There are now more than half a million clinical research papers showing that, when taken in the right amounts, nutritional supplements can, and do, work.

IMPORTANT HINTS TO NOTE BEFORE TAKING SUPPLEMENTS

If you are taking any prescription drugs you **must** advise your doctor of any supplements or herbs you wish to take in case of contra-indications. For example, the drug Warfarin thins the blood, but so does full-spectrum vitamin E and the herb ginkgo biloba. Anyone with HIV, or who is taking immuno-suppresive drugs or the contraceptive pill, should avoid St John's wort, which can reduce the effects of the medication. If you decide to begin taking supplements you must check with your GP so that you can have regular blood tests. Then, in time and with your doctor's permission, hopefully you can reduce your intake of drugs for conditions such as high blood pressure, high cholesterol and late-onset diabetes.

■ It is important to note that vitamins, minerals and essential fatty acids are nutrients essential to life. However, herbs are powerful medicines. Many prescription drugs are based on herbs. Herbs themselves are not essential to life, but, (like good food) when taken in the appropriate amounts and for the appropriate time, have proven to be of great benefit for many conditions. For instance, rosemary has been shown to protect against a host of cancers. Generally, take herbs for no more than three months at a time, have a month or so without them and then, if you feel the need, begin taking them again. Generally, look for whole herbal preparations in powder form, rather than herbal extracts that have been standardized for one particular 'active' ingredient. 'Whole herb' preparations can also be safer. For help with any herbs suggested in this book, call a qualified herbalist or health professional. Alternatively, contact The Specialist Herbal Supplies on 0870 774 4494 or log on to their website: www.shs100.com.

■ Supplements taken regularly in the long term almost always produce beneficial effects, but don't expect miracles in a week. Supplements are not magic bullets, but stimulate the body's natural healing processes, giving long-term health benefits. Generally speaking, supplementation with nutrients produces improvements in health more slowly than prescription medication, which normally just suppresses symptoms. If you start a course of vitamins, minerals or any supplements, take them regularly for at least two months in order to see the benefits. Any changes in your health may be very subtle.

■ Some supplements currently on the market have less than optimum quantities of beneficial ingredients. In general, you get what you pay for. Some low-priced supplements contain relatively small amounts of nutrients or forms of nutrients. The better quality and usually more expensive supplements generally provide better value for money in the long term.

■ Most vitamins have a good shelf life, but cease to be effective if you keep them for too long. Be aware of sell-by dates and always keep your vitamins in a cool, **dry** place – never expose them to direct sunlight.

- If you find that vitamin C irritates your gut, take it with food or try Esther C, or vitamin C in an ascorbate form. Vitamin C is more effective when taken in repeated small doses throughout the day with food.
- Take supplements with food, because this ensures better absorption, unless otherwise stated on the label. Generally, amino acids such as glutamine are best taken on an empty stomach – check instructions.
- Avoid taking supplements with hot drinks, such as tea and coffee, or with alcohol, as these can block absorption of certain nutrients.
- Some people have reactions to certain supplements, but this is quite rare. This is usually caused not by the nutrients themselves but by a reaction to one or more of the other ingredients contained in the supplement. In general, better quality supplements containing hypoallergenic ingredients are less likely to give rise to adverse reactions. If you suffer a negative reaction to any supplement or herb, stop taking it immediately. For example, most glucosamine supplements tend to be derived from crushed crab shells – so, if you are highly sensitive to shellfish, ask for the vegetarian version derived from corn, which is available from health shops.
- Products derived from bees, in extremely rare cases, may cause a reaction in anyone who suffers a severe sensitivity to bee stings. Obviously, if you know this is a problem avoid products related to bees! In the case of bee propolis, this would also apply to tree resins, including pycnogenol, which is obtained from tree bark.
- The supplements suggested in this book can be taken by anyone over the age of 16 unless otherwise stated. For children's dosages, seek professional guidance.
- Probiotics (friendly bacteria) should also contain bifidus strain bacteria. Probiotic preparations in general keep better in glass bottles and should be kept either in a fridge or freezer. There are various probiotics available that do not need to be kept refrigerated and can survive stomach acid – but in general these are best taken immediately after food unless otherwise directed.
- Natural-source, full-spectrum vitamin E is better absorbed and retained by the body than synthetic forms.
- If you are pregnant, or planning a pregnancy, do not take any supplement containing more than 3000iu of vitamin A per day. Most manufacturers state whether supplements are unsuitable to be taken during pregnancy. Pregnant women should consume no more than one portion of liver a week, as liver is high in Vitamin A – and too much vitamin A is linked to foetal damage. One portion of liver may contain 30,000 to 40,000iu of vitamin A. However, as vitamin A is vital for a healthy immune function, eye health, healthy lungs and bowels, a healthy once-a-day safe level would be 7500iu. To overdose on vitamin A you would need to take something like 85,000iu a day. **However, taking a natural-source carotene complex daily is safe, as carotenes will convert naturally in the body to Vitamin A.**
- Do not take separate iron supplements if you are over 50, unless you have been diagnosed with a medical condition that requires extra supplementation, as iron accumulates in the body and too high a level is linked with heart disease and strokes – especially in men. **Never leave iron tablets near children.**
- Keep all supplements away from young children. Any substance taken in excess can cause harm – even water. Follow the manufacturer's instructions unless your health professional advises otherwise.
- If you have any problem taking pills and cannot find liquid formulas at your health shop, use an inexpensive tablet crusher. To order, call **Health Plus** on 01323 872277 or visit their

website: www.healthplus.co.uk; or call **Lemon Burst** on 01273 872 277 or visit their
website: www.lemonburst.co.uk

- The supplements we suggest in this book should be taken in most instances until the condition is alleviated.
- If you are in any doubt about the amount of supplements you or your children should be taking, always consult a qualified health practitioner.
- Throughout this book Steve and I sometimes suggest using agave syrup as a natural alternative to refined sugars – but please note that because of agave syrup's high fructose content, which is processed in the liver, **it is not suitable for people with fructose intolerance or malabsorption problems**. Good alternatives would be blackstrap molasses, raw organic manuka honey or a little xylitol (a plant based sugar).

HOW TO USE THIS BOOK AND KEY TO CODES

Throughout this book we have suggested numerous formulas – and given the names of the companies that make them. All their details are here if you choose to contact them. If we have not mentioned a specific company, shop or brand name, then the listed supplements should be readily available from good health food stores worldwide.

No one is more aware than myself of the thousands of alternative supplements now available. In this book we have suggested many specific brands, which we have used, and/or come to trust over many years. If we tried to mention every brand by name, this book would not be an easy-to-read book of hints, but a lengthy encyclopaedia. Our choices of specific brands in **no way** infers that they are better or more beneficial than others on the market. If you have specific brands that you know and trust, check with your own suppliers or health shop who, I am sure, will stock similar supplements to those that we recommend. It is well worth noting that virtually every reputable supplement company has its own in-house qualified nutritionists who are happy to help you. Don't be afraid to call them. Most of these suppliers are happy to post orders anywhere worldwide.

BC
BioCare Ltd
Lakeside,
180 Lifford Lane,
Kings Norton,
Birmingham B30 3NU
Tel: 0121 433 3727
Email: biocare@biocare.co.uk
www.biocare.co.uk

BLK
Blackmores, based in Australia, make excellent mineral formula supplements. They are available in the UK through the Nutri Centre in London – see Nutri Centre details, right.

FSC
FSC vitamins are now called Bee Bio
Lancaster Road,
Carnaby Industrial Estate,
Bridlington,
East Yorkshire YO15 3QY
Tel: 01262 607890
Email: sales@beehealth.com
www.beehealth.co.uk

HN
Higher Nature Ltd
The Nutrition Centre,
Burwash Common,
East Sussex TN19 7LX
Tel: 01435 883484
Orders: 0800 458 4747
Nutritionist: 0870 066 4478
Email: info@higher-nature.co.uk
www.highernature.co.uk

NP
Nature's Plus (based in the USA but make a great range for children which is available through Nutrigroup Ltd in the UK)
Nutrigroup Ltd,
Waterloo House,
1 Waterloo Road,
Epsom,
Surrey KT19 8AY
Tel: 01273 573804 or 0845 2961070
Email: sales@nutriglow.com
www.nutriglow.com

NC
The Nutri Centre
The Hale Clinic,
7 Park Crescent,
London W1B 1PF
Tel: 0845 602 6744
   or (freephone) 0800 587 2290
Bookshop tel: 020 7323 2382;
Fax: 020 7636 0276
Email: admin@nutricentre.com
www.nutricentre.com

OP
The Organic Pharmacy
396 Kings Road,
London SW10 0LN
Tel: 0844 800 8399 or 020 7351 2232
Email: info@theorganicpharmacy.com
www.theorganicpharmacy.com

PN
Pharma Nord (UK) Ltd
Telford Court,
Morpeth,
Northumberland NE61 2DB
Tel: 01670 534900 or 0800 591 756
Email: info@multivits.co.uk
www.multivits.co.uk

PW
Pharm West Inc.
PO Box 9387,
Marina Del Rey,
CA 90295, USA
Tel US: 001 310 301 4015
Fax US: 001 310 577 0296
Email: infodesk@pharmwest.com
www.pharmwest.com

SVHC
Solgar Vitamin and Herb Company
Beggars Lane,
Aldbury,
Tring,
Herts HP23 5PT
Tel: 01442 890 355
For technical support or to speak to a
    nutritionist, tel: 01442 890355
Email: solgarinfo@solgar.com
www.solgar.com

SHS
Specialist Herbal Supplies
This company uses 'whole herbs' and is run
    by Malcolm Simmonds BAc, MH, MBRI
Portslade Hall,
18 Station Road,
Portslade,
Brighton,
East Sussex BN41 1GB
Tel: 0845 053 5433
Email: sales@shs100.com
www.shs100.com

VN
Viridian Nutrition Ltd
31 Alvis Way,
Daventry,
Northamptonshire NN11 8PG
Tel: 01327 878050 (call for nearest stockist
    or visit website)
Email: info@viridian-nutrition.com
www.viridian-nutrition.com

WMC
Wholistic Medical Centre
57 Harley Street,
London W1G 8QS
Tel: 020 7580 7537
Email: info@wholisticmedical.co.uk
www.wholisticmedical.co.uk

A

ABSORPTION

*(see also Coeliac Disease, Colitis, Crohn's Disease, Irritable Bowel Syndrome,
Indigestion, Leaky Gut, Low Stomach Acid and Stress)*

Many people presume that the nutrients within every item of food they swallow are auto-matically absorbed into their system, yet there are numerous health conditions, including IBS mentioned above, that greatly affect absorption within the gut. These can trigger deficiencies in most nutrients vital for health. There is also a vital intermediate stage: you swallow food, and if chewed thoroughly, then a form of amylase, an enzyme in your saliva, begins breaking down your food. But when we are stressed, and as we age, levels of amylase fall causing more absorption problems. Amylase is 30 times more abundant in the average 25-year-old than in the average 80-year-old.

The chewing process also alerts the stomach that food is on its way, which triggers stomach-acid production, ready to begin the digestion process. Chewing is the first and very important stage of digestion and most carbohydrates are partially digested in the mouth if chewed properly, as your stomach does not have any teeth! With ageing, and problems such as gastritis, stomach-acid production is also reduced. Without these natural digestive aids, absorption of nutrients through our gut walls and into the bloodstream is greatly diminished. Therefore, vital nutrients needed for tissue repair and cellular regeneration can sometimes pass through the body and out the other end undigested, thus contributing to conditions such as eczema, autoimmune conditions such as lupus, fibromyalgia and rheumatoid arthritis.

A

Absorption mostly takes place in the small intestine, but as we age enzymes produced by the pancreas (which helps to further break down sugars, proteins and fats) are also reduced. As the pace of modern life is increasing, more and more people are suffering varying degrees of absorption problems. Dr Shamin Daya says: 'The most likely cause today for malabsorption is a leaky gut, a state in which the small intestine becomes inflamed, affecting its ability to absorb nutrients.'

Stress also has a negative effect on the digestive process as it reduces absorption by shutting down enzyme production.

Symptoms of malabsorption include hair loss, low energy levels, chronic fatigue, weight loss or gain, poor bone density, dry and wrinkled skin, and dry hair and nails. Naturopath Steve Langley says, 'Almost all disease is linked to a deficiency of nutrients and/or toxicity within the body, therefore if you get your digestive system in good working order, a huge amount of health problems could be avoided.'

Foods to Avoid

- Avoid too much chewing gum, because it triggers production of stomach acid, when no food may actually be following.
- Reduce your intake of red meats and heavy, rich meals. Concentrated proteins and fats, such as red meat and cheese, are harder to digest as they require more work as well as oxygen to break them down completely. We need to maintain a high oxygen level in our tissues to keep our bodies healthy. And all junk foods reduce oxygen levels and accelerate loss of enzyme reserves in the body.

- Avoid croissants, burgers, fried foods, excessive high-sugar foods and full-fat dairy produce. The more unnatural your diet, the more the body has to produce enzymes to digest your food, and over time negative symptoms can arise.
- Cooked cheese is really hard on your digestive system.
- Modern refined wheat and related products are often hard to digest since we lack the necessary enzymes.
- Avoid drinking too much fluid with meals, as this dilutes the stomach acid – the very substance you need for digesting your meal.

Friendly Foods

- Bitter foods such as watercress, spinach or oak leaf lettuce taken in small amounts at the start of a meal will stimulate digestion.
- Aloe Vera also qualifies as a bitter food and stimulates digestion as well as soothing the gut.
- Raw, steamed or lightly cooked foods retain more enzymes, which aid digestion.
- Papaya is rich in papain, which aids in the breakdown of foods in the stomach and small intestine. It is best eaten before a main meal.
- Pineapple is rich in the enzyme bromelain, which again aids digestion. Eat a small amount before main meals or even as a dessert, as pineapple aids digestion of proteins.
- Generally increase your intake of fresh raw foods. Eat a salad at least once daily in summer. Light stir-fries and steamed vegetables are also fine.
- If you have a problem with wheat, try millet, buckwheat, barley, amaranth or quinoa-based breads, which are available in most supermarkets and health stores.

- Try rice, corn, buckwheat or millet-based pastas, which are also easier to digest.
- If you have a problem with cow's milk, try rice, almond, oat or goat's milk, which are gentler on the stomach.
- A glass of red wine can help to stimulate stomach-acid production.

Useful Remedies

- Take a digestive enzyme capsule with all main meals. These are available from health stores.
- You can also take a hydrochloric acid (HCl) with pepsin capsule with main meals, but only if you have been diagnosed as suffering from low stomach acid (see under *Low Stomach Acid*). Do not use if you suffer from ulcers or inflammatory bowel problems.
- Bitter herbs such as gentian, in tincture form, can be taken 15 minutes before each meal to stimulate production of stomach acid and digestive enzymes.
- A teaspoon of apple cider vinegar (preferably organic) in a little water taken before main meals can also help increase stomach-acid production.
- I have found the Life Extension's Agave Digestive Immune Support, which contains prebiotics, excellent for staying regular and aiding good gut health. Order from www.lef.org or the Nutri Centre (NC). Take one scoop daily with or before breakfast.

Helpful Hints

- Try not to eat late at night as this places an extra burden on the digestive system.
- Chew food thoroughly, and as much as possible eat sitting down in a relaxed frame of mind. Not always easy, but this simple act really aids digestion.
- Avoid eating for about an hour after rigorous exercise.
- Don't attempt to eat a large meal if you are under stress. Keep them small and light.
- If your digestive system is playing up or you have symptoms of irritable bowel such as bloating, wind, constipation and/or diarrhoea, then for a day or so eat soups (without bread), brown rice, vegetables, grilled fish – in other words 'easy-to-digest' foods. Also, you could try 'food combining'. Basically, this means separating concentrated proteins, such as meat, fish, eggs and cheese, from concentrated carbohydrates, such as potatoes, rice, bread and pasta.

So if, for example, you are eating fish, eat it with vegetables rather than potatoes. And if you have pasta, then also eat this with vegetables but not with meat or fish. Eat fruit in between meals or 15–20 minutes before a meal, rather than after a main meal. Fruit likes a quick passage through the gut and if it gets 'stuck' behind a main meal, gas and bloating can result. This is especially true of melon. Some nutritionists now state that food combining is old fashioned, but naturopath Stephen Langley says: 'There is no doubt that anyone with digestion and absorption problems would find, let's say, pasta and meat together pretty hard to digest. I have seen thousands of patients who have been helped by this method of eating – especially those who want to lose weight.' For this reason eat melon on its own as a starter, and don't combine it with other fruits, as melon has an even quicker transit time than other fruits, which again can trigger fermentation and bloating in the gut.

ACID–ALKALINE BALANCE

(see also Arthritis, Indigestion and Low Stomach Acid)

Practically every major degenerative disease, including some cancers, is triggered by an over-acid system. When the pH of your blood is out of balance, your skin and hair become dull, the nervous system is affected and you may suffer insomnia, arthritis, rheumatism, aching joints, skin conditions, candida, fungal infections, muscle pain and gout, which are all common symptoms of an over-acid system.

Nutritionists and health professionals have long understood the importance of maintaining a healthy acid–alkaline balance. For good health the body needs to maintain a certain acid–alkaline balance and keeping this balance is one of the crucial keys to remaining healthy and also slowing the ageing process. Every cell functions more efficiently when it is predominantly alkaline.

In general, the body needs to be around 70% alkaline and 30% acid. But in the West the average person is 80% acid and 20% alkaline, which is why we are suffering so many acid conditions such as arthritis. Many people confuse the term acid forming with the term acidic, but they are entirely different. Everything we swallow, once metabolized within the body, breaks down into either an alkaline or acid mineral-based ash or residue. Whether a substance is alkaline or acid is determined by its pH (potential Hydrogen). Stomach acid can be as low as pH 1.5, very acid, whereas saliva after eating could be as high as pH 8, which is very alkaline. Your blood has a pH, which is slightly alkaline – between 7.35 and 7.45 – and this level needs to be maintained at all costs. If the blood becomes too acid, and our buffering systems are not adequate (a common problem), then the body withdraws alkalizing minerals from anywhere it can find them; beginning with the hair, skin and nails and then moving on through the body until it begins drawing minerals from the bones, which in time contributes to conditions such as osteoporosis.

Unfortunately, most modern lifestyles and diets are almost all acid forming and if the body remains in an acid state for too long, this acidity triggers degenerative diseases. A high acid-forming diet also has a negative effect on tooth enamel – pre-packaged concentrated fruit juices are particularly at fault. Acid-forming foods deplete calcium from the body, while alkaline foods increase the body's ability to absorb calcium from the diet.

Emotions also greatly affect this balance: stress and anger trigger more acidity within the body, whereas feelings of being in control, in love, and breathing deeply through the nose re-alkalize the system. Basically, harmony alkalizes and disharmony acidifies.

A

Foods to Avoid

■ It's important to realize that just because a food is acid forming, it is not necessarily unhealthy. Proteins are acid forming, but they are also essential for good health. Therefore, if you tend to eat two, meat-based meals daily, reduce it to one. Make the other a fish-based meal, or eat pulses such as soya, aduki, butter beans, haricot beans or chickpeas (also in houmous).

■ Basically all animal produce and egg yolks are acid forming. Duck, venison, grouse and pheasant, lamb, beef and pork are all acid forming. Fish, turkey and chicken are also acid forming, but do not contain such high levels of uric acid as red meat.

■ Milk and yoghurt are alkaline before digestion but become acid forming once digested. This is why milk products are calming to an over-acid oesophagus if you suffer from an acid-type reflux after food. But in the long term this would exacerbate arthritic type conditions. It's just a case of getting a balance.

■ All nuts are acid forming, except almonds, fresh coconut, and chestnuts.

■ All grains are also acid forming, with the exception of millet, buckwheat, amaranth and quinoa. Whole grains are a healthy food and remember: these foods are not to be eliminated per se, you just need to be aware of what is acid forming.

■ All refined sugars found in cakes, biscuits, pre-packaged desserts, whips and so on are acid forming. Milk chocolate is a truly acid forming treat; it's high in oxalic acid which is linked to kidney stones – so, don't overdo it!

■ Wine, beer and spirits, coffee and tea, and fizzy drinks and sweetened fruit juices are all **highly** acid forming.

■ All drugs, prescription and social, such as cannabis, are also acidic.

■ Cranberries, plums, prunes and rhubarb are highly acid forming. But again I reiterate, these foods are healthy – in fact prunes (dried plums) are very anti-ageing. Everything in moderation.

■ Mass-produced malt vinegar, a waste product of the brewing industry, is also acid forming in the body.

Friendly Foods

■ Honey, agave and brown-rice syrup are alkalizing. But don't overdo these foods – they are still sugar! If you eat too much of them, the sugar converts to fat and lives on your hips. Again, just find a balance.

■ All vegetables are alkaline but the best are wheat grass, alfalfa, kelp, seaweed, parsley, watercress, cabbage, celery, broccoli, carrots, endives and celery. All green foods are high in chlorophyll, which is rich in magnesium, a major alkalizing mineral.

■ Cabbage, kale, broccoli, spring greens, green beans and asparagus are all great alkaline foods. Spinach contains oxalic acid, but it breaks down into an alkaline residue.

■ All fruits are healthy, and you should eat them freely, but be aware that cranberries, plums, prunes and rhubarb are highly acid forming and to a lesser degree so are blueberries, blackberries, raspberries and strawberries.

■ The most alkalizing fruits are cantaloupe melons (and all melons), papaya, dates, especially dried dates, mangoes, lemons, limes and figs. In case you are wondering, it's the alkaline mineral content and not the sugar content that determines whether a food is acid or alkaline forming in the body.

■ Pineapple, cherries, kiwi and tomatoes contain acids, but they make an alkaline ash within the body after they are digested. People who suffer indigestion immediately after a meal, and may have an over-acid stomach, often say these types of foods make their problem worse; this is because they are acid on contact and until digested. However, they make an alkaline residue once they reach the small intestine. This is why apple cider vinegar or lemon juice, with a little honey and warm water, help to re-alkalize the body and reduce symptoms of arthritis and inflammatory conditions. Take one teaspoon of each twice daily.

- Use a little organic sea salt, which is rich in alkalizing minerals.
- Drink more green and white tea, and if you prefer it sweeter, use a small amount of either manuka honey, or the plant extract xylitol which has a low glycaemic index.
- Apple cider vinegar, preferably organic, has an alkalizing effect within the body. It also helps increase stomach acid production, as it is acid on contact but alkalizing after digestion.
- If you are a chocoholic, then ask at your health shop for a raw chocolate bar. Dark, pure chocolate is usually sugar-free and is not as acid forming.

Useful Remedies

- Ask at your health shop for powdered organic formulas that contain wheat grass, spirulina, chlorella, alfalfa, broccoli and green foods and take daily.
- I take Green pH, made by Metabolics (www.metabolics.com), one small level teaspoon daily in water, preferably taken 30 minutes before a meal or in between meals. It is a mixture of green beans, garden peas, pea leaf, dry apple cider, watercress, broccoli and nettle leaf. It doesn't taste great, but is an easy and quick way to alkalize your body. Available for retail from the Wholistic Medical Centre. **WMC**
- Dr Shamin Daya suggests that taking a quarter teaspoon of soda bicarbonate in half a cup of lukewarm water twice daily between meals is an easy way to keep the body alkaline.
- Take a multi-mineral formula that contains approximately 600mg of calcium, 300–500mg of magnesium, 25mg of zinc, 90mg of potassium, in a colloidal or chelated form, which are more easily absorbed. These minerals are alkalizing.

Helpful Hints

- Stress, anger and smoking contribute to an over-acid system.
- Breathing deeply and regularly helps to re-alkalize the body. This is because when you breathe more oxygen into the body, it has an alkaline effect. When we are under stress, we tend to shallow-breathe, which leaves more carbon dioxide, more acidity, in the tissues.
- Do not brush your teeth immediately after eating or drinking high acid-forming foods and drinks, as you can lose more tooth enamel. Simply drink a little water and swill it around the mouth to help neutralize the acids.
- Meditation also re-alkalizes the body .
- Water Filter Man supply alkalizing water filters for your home. Tel: 0844 8733148; www.waterfilterman.co.uk
- Otherwise try Kangen Water – a water system that attaches to your kitchen tap that ionizes and greatly alkalizes water. It's used in Japanese hospitals with highly beneficial health results. Tel: 020 7580 7537; www.kangenmiraclewater.co.uk
- When you first wake, the body is very acid, so having fruit for breakfast helps to re-alkalize the system. A great diet for summer breakfasts – but in winter you need to keep warmer and fruit won't do the job, so try porridge sweetened with a freshly grated apple or any chopped fruit. Breakfast is also a great time to drink freshly made juices. But too much orange juice can overstimulate production of stomach acid, so go for diluted apple or pear juice as an alternative. Apple, carrot or celery juice with a little added fresh root ginger are also highly alkalizing.

A

ACID STOMACH   *(see also Indigestion and Low Stomach Acid)*

Many people complain about having an acid stomach, often mistakenly presuming that they produce too much stomach acid – hydrochloric acid, which is known as HCl. In fact, sufferers from acid stomach regularly produce inappropriate amounts of stomach acid (too much or too little) at the wrong times – which can occur through overindulgence in caffeine, alcohol or sugar, or as a reaction to stress. And as the average person eats approximately 50+ tons of food in their lifetime, which requires 300 litres of digestive juices to break it down, it's no wonder that we are suffering more and more digestive disorders. Typical symptoms are feelings of heartburn, acid reflux, indigestion, bloating and general discomfort. When you are under prolonged stress or are exhausted, your digestive system is greatly weakened. Never underestimate how long-term, negative stress and chronic exhaustion can affect the body (see also *Stress*).

Foods to Avoid

- Reduce your intake of coffee, colas, black tea, alcohol and sugar.
- Pizzas, laden with vegetable fat and cheese, are especially hard to digest as are large, rich meals and red meat.
- Full-fat cheeses and rich, creamy foods.
- Fried and very fatty foods.

- Oily, spicy foods (such as an Indian take-away with lots of sauce), which are usually packed with refined vegetable oils. These types of meals – if high in fat – are hard to digest.
- Concentrated fruit juices, especially orange, lemon and grapefruit, and raw tomato juice, which can make the problem worse. Buy non-concentrates and dilute with water.
- Reduce your intake of wheat-based foods, which can be a problem for people with acid stomach (especially croissants, which are high in butter, white bread and pre-packaged, mass-produced pies and cakes).

Friendly Foods

- A small amount of aloe vera taken just before eating can greatly aid digestion and help prevent an over-acid stomach.
- Eat more wholegrains such as brown rice, quinoa, kamut or amaranth, and try lentil, corn, buckwheat, millet or spelt-based pastas, breads and cereals. Rice cakes, amaranth or rye crackers are often easier to digest than wheat. If you adore bread, try small amounts of wholemeal varieties.
- Include plenty of lightly cooked vegetables and fruits in your diet, which are easier on the digestive system.
- Try fruit compotes or lightly grilled fruit kebabs without refined sugar. Use a little xylitol (a plant based sugar) or chopped organic dried fruits to sweeten.
- Choose low-fat meats such as venison, turkey, duck and chicken without the skin, and include plenty of fresh fish in your diet (preferably not fried).
- Replace full-fat cows' milk with organic oat, rice, soya or goats' milk.
- Experiment with caffeine-free herbal teas, such as fennel and liquorice, which reduce acidity. Camomile, meadowsweet and fresh mint teas soothe the gut.
- Fresh root ginger is very calming to the gut, as is lightly cooked cabbage, or cabbage juice made from raw cabbage. I always use water from cooking cabbage to make gravy.
- Eat more live, low-fat bio yoghurts. But if you have an intolerance to dairy from cows, then try sheep's or soya yoghurts. Please note that low-fat bio yoghurts (from cows) are usually OK as they are fermented – but if they trigger bloating, then avoid them.

Useful Remedies

- De-glycyrrhized liquorice helps to protect and heal the lining of the oesophagus and stomach. Chew 1–2 tablets 20 minutes before a meal. It can also be used as an alternative to antacids after meals. Available from health shops.
- Ask at your local health shop or pharmacy for a Peppermint Formula containing ingredients such as peppermint, gentian, fennel or camomile, which can be taken after foods.
- Slippery Elm Plus is a supplement containing slippery elm, marsh mallow and gamma oryzanol, which all help to soothe the stomach lining. **BC**
- Aloe Pura make a particularly good Digestive Aid Juice, which greatly soothes the stomach lining. Contains aloe vera, papaya, peppermint oil, camomile and slippery elm. Available from good health stores and larger chemists. www.optimah.com

Helpful Hints

- Chew all foods thoroughly and avoid drinking too much liquid with meals, as this dilutes the stomach acid, which you need to digest your meal. However, a small glass of red wine aids digestion.
- Eat little and often, avoiding large, heavy meals. The larger the meal, the greater the burden on your digestive system. Small meals are especially important if you are stressed, as stress increases stomach acid at inappropriate times.
- Take time out to eat your meals calmly – do not eat on the run. Avoid large meals if you are feeling upset.
- If you are prone to nervous conditions, join a yoga, meditation or t'ai chi class and learn to relax. Get plenty of exercise, but no strenuous exercise immediately after eating. Walking for 10–15 minutes after a meal greatly aids digestion.
- Drink peppermint, fennel, camomile or liquorice teas after a meal.
- Food combining helps relieve an acid stomach: this means separating proteins and starches to aid digestion. Basically, if you are eating a protein such as meat or fish, eat this with salad or vegetables but not potatoes, pasta or bread; conversely, when you eat bread, pasta or potatoes, eat them with vegetables or salad, not protein. Many people find that they become reliant on antacids to control their symptoms, when making a few simple changes to the diet and eating pattern can produce very significant relief in most cases. Antacids can harm the body if used excessively and many contain aluminium, which has been implicated in Alzheimer's disease.

ACNE
(see also Liver Problems and Rosacea)

Many young people, including teenagers, are notorious for eating a poor nutrient-deficient diet – and ingesting far too many fizzy drinks and too much alcohol, which will exacerbate this problem. Sugar and fat are, without doubt, the biggest offenders. Many adolescents experience acne owing to the massive increase in hormone production, which often leads to overproduction of sebum, or naturally produced oils in the skin that cause blockages in the skin's sebaceous glands. For adults, acne often results from internal toxicity, which can be caused by many factors. Constipation, candida (a yeast fungal overgrowth; see *Candida*) or food intolerances can all trigger this problem. Pre-menstrual women can also experience acne. The key factor in controlling and preventing acne is to look after your liver and ensure that toxins can be eliminated. Once the system becomes overloaded it begins dumping toxins into the skin, hence constipation and poor skin often go hand in hand.

Foods to Avoid

- Refined snacks, cola-type drinks (many of which contain as many as eight teaspoons of sugar), croissants, cakes, sweets and so on. These types of foods have to be greatly reduced if the acne is to be healed.
- Most mass-produced, pre-packed meals, cakes, biscuits and pies, which are high in sugar, salt and saturated fats, which place a great strain on the liver.
- Full-fat cheeses, pizzas, chocolates and dairy produce, fried foods and greasy burger-type foods.
- In some cases, the acne can be triggered by a food sensitivity such as cow's milk.

Friendly Foods

- Eat more beetroot, kale, celeriac and artichoke, which help to cleanse the liver.
- A glass of beetroot juice daily for a few weeks is especially useful for teenagers – which helps to control the overproduction of hormones.
- Chickpeas, soya, black-eyed, haricot and cannellini beans, as well as pulses, help the body to excrete excess hormones.
- Eat Japanese and Thai foods, such as miso and tempeh, which help to regulate hormones.
- Include more fresh vegetables and fruits such as figs in your diet – this is especially true of teenagers, who tend to eat a very poor diet. We can all do this for a certain time, but symptoms will arise once the body becomes very toxic.
- Drink 6–8 glasses of water daily.
- Add a tablespoonful of linseeds and sunflower seeds to high-fibre, low-sugar breakfast cereal.
- Snack on unsulphured dried apricots and dates as well as raw, unsalted nuts and seeds.
- Avocados are rich in vitamin E, which nourishes the skin.

- Oily fish – especially sardines, mackerel and salmon – are rich in essential fats, which regulate hormones, as are white fish such as cod, plaice, halibut, sea bass and so on. These are rich in zinc and selenium, needed for healthy skin.
- See also *General Health Hints*.

Useful Remedies

- If you take nothing else, take a good-quality multi-vitamin mineral, containing at least 15mg of zinc and 1mg of copper.
- Zinc has been shown to be as successful as taking certain antibiotics for this condition. If you are not taking a multi, take 30mg of zinc up to 3 times daily for 6 weeks, then reduce to 60mg daily. For every 15mg of zinc, you should also take 1mg of copper to maintain a healthy balance within the body.
- With acne, hormones are often an important factor. Femarone Formula contains herbs that should help, including blessed thistle, squaw vine, cramp bark and raspberry leaf. These are available as a liquid or capsules. **SHS**
- To help support the liver, try a formula based on barberry, wild yam and dandelion. Take this for 3 months. **SHS**
- Clearskin Tincture formula containing saw palmetto, red clover, agnus castus, calendula, echinacea and dandelion is a very useful formula for balancing testosterone levels in women – take 15 drops twice daily in liquids. **OP**
- Vitamin A is essential for healthy skin; if you are **not** pregnant or planning a pregnancy, take up to 10,000iu daily for two months and then switch to a high-strength, natural-source beta-carotene complex that will convert into Vitamin A within the body. **SVHC, VN**
- Natural-source, full-spectrum vitamin E 200–400iu daily reduces the tendency to scarring and helps maintain healthy skin.
- Essential fats are also important because saturated, trans- and hydrogenated fats displace EFAs in the body – take 1–3 grams of omega-3 fish oil daily.

Helpful Hints

■ *Rosa mosqueta*, a Latin American plant-based oil, can be used topically to heal scars, but don't use on active acne. Use once the acne is no longer active. Available from good health stores and chemists.

■ Taking liquid hyaluronic acid (a natural component of skin) daily in water helps to heal any scarring on the skin. For details, call Modern Herbals on 01274 889047 or log on to www.modernherbals.com.

■ Tea tree oil is highly antiseptic. Add a few drops to bath water or use cream, soap or lotion on the affected areas. As teenage boys seem to hate washing, get them to use a tea tree shower gel daily.

■ Kali Brom 6c is a homeopathic remedy that helps if the acne is on the face, chest and shoulders. Homeopathic Silica 6c is also useful twice daily. This may trigger symptoms to increase for a short time as toxins are released – but this will balance out after a couple of weeks.

■ Exercise encourages free flow of sebum and detoxification of the body through sweating.

■ Many readers have found that they've benefited from taking aloe vera juice internally and using the gel externally.

■ A thorough detox is useful for clearing acne (see *Liver*).

■ The Sher System is a skin regime especially formulated for problem skin. Contact The Sher System, PO Box 573, Staines, Middlesex Tel 01784 227805; www.sher.co.uk

ADDISON'S DISEASE

(see Adrenal Exhaustion)

ADHD – Attention Deficit Hyperactivity Disorder

(see Hyperactivity)

ADRENAL EXHAUSTION

(see also Exhaustion, Low Blood Pressure, Low Blood Sugar, ME, Stress)

Thanks to our fast-paced 24/7 open-all-hours lifestyle, adrenal problems, which are hugely multi-factorial, have reached epidemic proportions. Because symptoms vary greatly, this condition often goes undiagnosed for months or even years, and doctors urgently need to understand and diagnose this condition, which can, if left untreated, become extremely serious.

Naturopath Steve Langley says: 'It can happen at any age, but this problem is becoming more and more common in younger people, especially women. Many patients initially report having problems getting up in the morning, but say they get a "second wind" later in the evening. Other symptoms are cravings for sugar, carbohydrates, stimulants or salt, feeling tired much of the time, dark circles around the eyes and frequent urination often at night.

'Mood swings are common, or feeling dizzy or faint, which is linked to low blood sugar. In some cases, if the person remains under constant stress, then high blood pressure can arise and medical attention needs to be sought. Feeling angry or short tempered can also be common symptoms. If these symptoms are not dealt with, a sense of humour failure can occur, tears can spring up for no good reason and general malaise and depression set in.

The person knows something is wrong, but presumes he or she is just tired and keeps pushing themselves.

'Doctors often prescribe anti-depressants that simply mask symptoms and if the low blood sugar is left untreated and the person continues to eat sugar in order to function, then eventually they can collapse.'

At such a point the person may experience panic attacks. The thyroid can malfunction – becoming either under- or over-active. If the adrenals become totally exhausted Addison's disease can occur, which thankfully is pretty rare.

Many people are now suffering from burnt-out adrenals, yet clinically they do not have Addison's, which is a serious medical condition that requires long-term, life-long cortico-steroid treatment. Obviously, the secret is to recognize symptoms at an early stage and deal with them.

Your adrenal glands are two small glands no bigger than a large grape that sit on top of each kidney, like tiny pyramids. They produce the hormones: adrenaline, cortisol and DHEA among others. In everyday life, if we become stressed our age-old 'fight or flight' mode kicks in and the adrenals start pumping the stress hormones on a signal from the pituitary gland (in the brain). Basically, cortisol signals your liver to 'dump' stored sugar into your blood-stream to fuel your muscles and your brain. The problem with this drip feeding of sugar over a period of time is that it encourages insulin resistance, a common problem these days. See *Insulin Resistance*.

Years ago, this fight or flight release of stress hormones would save lives, as, once this mode kicked in, our ancestors' blood would start to thicken in case they were injured, and give them the energy to run away from any life-threatening situations. Fortunately, most of us today are not being chased by a wild animal – but our response instead of running away, which would disperse the stress hormones naturally, is to head for another caffeine or sugar fix.

The major problem today is that long-term fight or flight reactions mean that an imbalance in these stress hormones, if not dealt with adequately, can become toxic to every system in the body. High and low levels of cortisol can affect brain function. Too much cortisol can deplete calcium and other vital minerals from your bones, which in the long term can trigger osteoporosis. It also depletes vital oxygen from your blood and every organ – which is then under stress. If this continues, you may blow a fuse, be it a 'gut fuse' triggering ulcers or worse, a 'heart fuse', triggering a heart attack and so on.

An imbalance of stress hormones can trigger a cascade 'acid' reaction throughout your body. And if this situation then continues over time, then the adrenals become tired, producing ever less cortisol and therefore lower blood sugar. Depending on the person, this could eventually lead to a complete cessation of cortisol production, thus triggering Addison's disease.

Also, as the immune system is hugely disrupted, a large majority of people with adrenal problems are suffering from candida and a leaky gut. See *Candida* and *Leaky Gut*. Therefore, it's no surprise that many people suffering with adrenal exhaustion are often diagnosed as suffering from ME.

Foods to Avoid

- White flour, sugar, caffeine and alcohol all need to be avoided.
- See diet under *Insulin Resistance*.
- **It's crucial for the person to totally avoid sugar in any form** – and caffeine drinks such as Lucozade, Red Bull and so on.
- In the initial stages foods high in potassium also need to be avoided, such as figs, dates,

grapes, oranges, raisins, bananas, sultanas and mango. This is because your body will retain potassium and excrete sodium, and your blood pressure goes down.

Friendly Foods

- Protein is important as it balances blood sugar for longer, and when the body is under stress it requires more protein. Eat breakfast. Make sure you eat some protein, such as fish, eggs, quinoa, lean meats or a good-quality protein powder, with breakfast.
- Porridge and wholemeal bread (unless you are intolerant to wheat/yeast) also help to balance blood sugar.
- Use amaranth or rye crisp breads spread with humous-type spreads.
- Eat more lentils, brown rice, barley, chickpeas, experiment with wheat-free breads and rice, lentil or corn pastas.
- Fresh fish, chicken, lean meats, cooked tofu, tempeh, natto, eggs, goat's cheese, mozzarella, feta cheese would be fine.
- Vegetables such as cauliflower, broccoli, kale, spring greens, pak choi, cabbage and sprouts are all good.
- Once symptoms are more under control sweeter foods such as sweet potatoes, papaya, carrots and apples should be fine. In fact, sweet potatoes are very useful in controlling blood-sugar problems.
- Foods high in natural sodium will help replace lost sodium – samphire grass, kelp, celery, spinach, beetroot and any seaweeds (available at health food shops) are great.
- Use Himalayan crystal salt or a nori seaweed shake.
- Liquorice supports adrenal function, but tends to be high in sugar (and sometimes wheat), which will make adrenal exhaustion worse. It is usually given to Addison's sufferers but has to be a sugar-free version.
- If your symptoms are not acute, then you can use small amounts of organic agave syrup or xylitol sugar (a fruit fibre), which have a lower impact on blood-sugar levels. Available from health stores, ZyloSweet is an alternative to refined sugar. **HN**
- Green tea contains L-theanine, which helps you to stay calm. Buy organic de-caffeinated green teas.

Useful Remedies

- Take magnesium citrate. Magnesium is nature's tranquillizer and anyone who is stressed is low in this vital mineral. Take 600mg as a minimum during the day and take 200mg before you go to bed.
- Vitamin C plus Bioflavonoids – around 2–3 grams daily spread with each meal throughout the day. Bio Care make a magnesium ascorbate version. **BC**
- A high-dose vitamin B complex, 100mg of each – plus 500mg of pantothenic acid (B5) daily, as you cannot make cortisol without B5.
- Advanced Stress Formula by Holos Health contains liquorice root, gotu kola, ashwagandha, Siberian ginseng and shatavari – all of which nourish the adrenals and aid healing. Take 1½ teaspoons daily in a glass of water. See www.holoshealth.com. **NB Cannot be taken by anyone suffering high blood pressure.**
- Take Corticozyme, which contains a complex of B vitamins, magnesium and nutrients to support the adrenals. Take 2 with breakfast and 2 with lunch. Can be taken by anyone. Available from The Wholistic Medical Centre. **WMC**
- Cortisol Manager tablets contain ashwagandha, phosphatidyl serine and L-theanine (an extract of green tea). These are excellent for reducing cortisol production and calming you down. If you are a Type A person who rushes around all day, and you are stressed and need to slow down, then try taking one of these tablets when the adrenaline starts 'pumping' and

take one or two before bed. I have found them marvellous for reducing the 'fight or flight' -type symptoms and they really help me to get a good night's sleep. However, if you are at the point of total and utter exhaustion, then your body may not be producing sufficient cortisol, in which case there would be no benefit in taking this formula. To order from Integrative Therapeutics www.integrative.com (via Amazon) or for a similar product contact Hadley Wood Healthcare on 0208 441 8352 or their retail web shop at www.supersupps.com

Helpful Hints

- By now you will have realized that you need help. A saliva test via your doctor or health professional will show DHEA and cortisol levels. You may also require blood tests for thyroid function. See *Thyroid*. Once you know how severe or otherwise the problem is, then you can start to heal yourself.
- With the help of a health professional you may need DHEA supplementation.
- If you are at the stage of fainting because of low blood sugar/adrenal exhaustion, then you should avoid exercise.
- If you are simply a highly stressed person who produces the flight or flight response quickly, then get more exercise to help naturally disperse the toxic (in the long-term if not dispersed) stress hormones and watch your diet.
- Learn to meditate, which helps reduce the stress response.
- Take a deep breath more often.
- Eat every 4 hours; the worst thing you can do is to miss a meal. Some people with severe blood-sugar problems may need to eat every 2–3 hours.

- Sleep in past 8 in the morning. Cortisol production peaks at 8am.
- The more you can rest and eat sensibly, the faster you will heal. It may take 3 months to recover from total burn out.
- Go to sleep before 11pm.
- Try to have a rest at some time during the day, even a 15-minute nap.
- Read *The Low GL Diet Bible* by Patrick Holford (Piatkus Publishing) – a godsend for anyone with this problem.

AGEING

Within 25 years, 1.2 billion people – that's one in five of us – will be over 65 and more than a million people will be over 100. Within ten years for the first time in human history there will be more of us aged over 65 than children under five – and people aged over 80 are the fastest-growing portion of the total population in many countries.

Governments worry about the health-cost burden of our ageing population and yet, if you begin taking more responsibility for your health from today by eating sensibly, reducing stress and taking more exercise, you could have the capability to live a healthy, productive life until at least 100. In fact, the average child born today can expect to live to 104.

Japan, where the average life expectancy is 82, has some of the longest-living residents. Sweden, France and Italy all have life expectancies of around 80, and in the UK it's 78.8.

As we age, biological changes take place throughout our bodies. Our heart muscle becomes thinner, the capacity of our kidneys reduces and all of our organs go through some physiological change. However, these changes are not necessarily associated with illness or disease. And none of these changes causes ill health or disease on its own. The process of ageing is the breakdown of key biological functions of our mind and body and is directly related to our environment, diet, lifestyle and outlook on life.

The single most common result of the process of ageing and the leading cause of death worldwide is cardiovascular disease. Dr Michael Colgan, a renowned nutritional research scientist in the US, says that if people could eat more of the right foods and change their lifestyles, then 98% of cardiovascular disease cases and 80% of cancers would be preventable. Also that late-onset diabetes, which is reaching epidemic proportions in Western countries, is a direct consequence of over-consumption of sugar, plus stress and overuse of stimulants. It is both avoidable and manageable by good nutrition (see also *Diabetes*).

And if you eat the right foods, and take the right supplements and hormones, then a 60-year-old can have the Biological Ageing Markers – such as blood pressure, cholesterol count, lean body mass, bone density, skin thickness and so on – of a 40-year-old.

So, what causes the deterioration of our body that we call ageing?

It is now accepted that the ageing process and virtually all disease is the result of free radical damage to the cells in one form or another. This is why antioxidants such as natural-source carotenes (vitamin A) and vitamins C and E, plus minerals such as selenium hold one of the major keys to slowing down the ageing process. Free radicals are produced by our bodies when oxygen is used to create energy and during everyday processes such as breathing and eating. There is much misinformation on free radicals, which are also vital to life. They are created by the billion daily – they help to neutralize viruses and bacteria and help to kill cancer cells, so there are positive purposes for a certain amount of free radicals (also known as oxidants) in the body. But over time, as the body begins to accumulate excess free radicals, which proliferate when insufficient antioxidants are present, the system becomes overwhelmed by these unstable molecules that then break down our DNA, trigger deterioration in our blood vessels and brain, and cause damage to virtually every cell of our body. You can reduce free-radical accumulation by cutting down on burned or smoked foods, exposure to air pollution, pesticides, overuse of mobile phones, excessive sunbathing, additives and stress; and by taking more potent antioxidants, which are listed below.

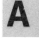

Inflammation is another major contributor to ageing. Degenerative diseases that are associated with inflammation in the tissues are arteriosclerosis, Alzheimer's, Parkinson's, diabetes, arthritis, ME, cancer, and allergies. Sources of inflammation are chronic low-level infections, and toxicity from ingesting too many foods containing additives, a deficiency in essential nutrients, foods to which we have an intolerance, and heavy metals such as mercury and aluminium.

Physical activity is crucial in helping to slow down the ageing process but severe exertion generates large amounts of free radicals and inflammation in the body. This may explain why people who spend a lot of time in the gym do not always survive longer than those who don't, and why some marathon runners and aerobics instructors age more quickly. As always, we need everything in a balance and this is the secret to slowing the ageing process.

Also, how often do you hear people say, 'It's all in my genes'? And if their parents died young, many people presume they have inherited the likelihood that they might do the same. Yes, our genes do play a huge part in the dice of life and how well or otherwise you age – but if your genes stay healthy, then your body stays healthy. If you live a healthy lifestyle, you can change which genes are expressed. In other words, if your parents and grandparents died of heart attacks, you may well have a pre-disposition for heart problems at some point. But if you live a different lifestyle and eat healthier foods, you can change the chemistry within the body and tip the scales in your favour. Genes are repairable and alterable, they adjust to our environment and state of mind. Generally, people who live to a great age are positive, adaptable and hard-working; they eat breakfast and consume plenty of freshly, locally grown fruits and vegetables.

Jeanne Calment, a French lady, lived to 122. She gave up smoking at the age of 120 in 1995, saying that 'it had become a habit', and died two years later. She was one in six billion, which shows that there are always exceptions to every rule.

Don't underestimate the extent to which your thoughts and stress levels can affect both your general health and the rate at which you age. If you repeatedly say, 'It's to be expected at my age', don't be surprised if you age faster.

In my twenties and thirties I was obsessed with ageing and spent too much time rushing around having the latest anti-ageing therapies instead of simply enjoying being young. Learn to enjoy the moment, know that you can only do your best, and have some fun.

Foods to Avoid

- Sugar triggers an inflammatory response in the body, which contributes to hardening of the arteries, which in turn contributes to heart disease and strokes, and sugar ages the skin through the process of cross linking , as much as smoking or regular sunbathing. And if you don't utilize sugar during exercise, it converts to fat in the body. Therefore, cut down on foods with a high sugar content, such as refined carbohydrates – breads, cakes, biscuits, pastries, pasta – and sweets and concentrated fruit juice. A diet of more than 40% carbohydrate intake can cause insulin resistance and trigger late-onset diabetes (see *Diabetes* and *Insulin Resistance*). Also, the body has a limited capacity to store carbohydrate in the liver and muscles and will turn excess carbohydrate into fat tissue.

- Artificial sweeteners including aspartame (Nutrasweet and Canderel), saccharin, and sucralose are synthetic forms of sugar that the body does not utilize well.
- Fried foods and all refined foods containing hydrogenated/trans-fats (see *Fats You Need To Eat*).
- Artificial preservatives and chemicals, including MSG.
- Some municipal tap water is known to contain many chemicals, hormone and antibiotic residues and in some areas also fluoride – which can accumulate in the body, causing many health problems. Fit a good water filter and make sure it's serviced regularly. Otherwise I drink Fiji, Volvic or Spa waters. Use Kangen Water – a water system that attaches to your kitchen tap that ionizes and alkalizes water. It's used in Japanese hospitals with highly beneficial health results. For full details, telephone 020 7580 7537 or log on to www.kangenmiraclewater.co.uk.
- Cut down on stimulants such as caffeine, fizzy drinks and alcohol. Alcohol taken to excess is **extremely** ageing.
- Reduce your intake of full-fat dairy products.
- Avoid shellfish, which tend to feed in polluted coastal waters.
- Avoid non-organic, preserved, smoked and cured meats (deli-type meats and bacon), as the chemicals used are carcinogenic.
- Avoid tinned, microwaved and pre-packaged foods.
- Avoid industrially produced battery eggs and chickens.
- Cut down on non-organic red meats.
- Cut down on sodium-based table salts. Use mineral-rich sea salts in moderation. I use Himalayan Crystal Salt, which is rich in organic-source minerals. Available from good health stores, or for your nearest stockists, contact Best Care Products on 01342 410303, or log on to www.bestcare-UK.com.

Friendly Foods

- Fresh fish is rich in fatty acids, especially salmon, mackerel and sardines. These days I avoid tuna, which usually has a high mercury content. White fish is rich in zinc and selenium, vital for healthy brain functioning.

- Linseeds help protect the breasts and prostate and are a good source of Omega 3. I soak a tablespoon of golden linseeds overnight in cold water, drain and use over cereals or in fruit blends for breakfast for additional fibre.
- Cook with good-quality olive or coconut oil.
- Begin adding non-GM lecithin granules to cereals and fruit blends – as lecithin is rich in phosphatidyl serine and choline, it is great nourishment for your brain and also helps to elevate the good cholesterol and metabolize fats.
- Eat more pomegranate – either the fruit or juice daily – which can help prevent atherosclerosis, a major trigger for heart disease and strokes. This fruit is also highly protective against certain cancers – especially prostate and breast cancer.
- Papaya and blueberries are 'super' fruits, which help prevent cancer; papaya also aids digestion (as does pineapple).
- All fresh fruits, fresh vegetables, salads, nuts and oatmeal (porridge) will help to reduce inflammation in the body. As much as possible, eat locally grown fresh foods.
- Sip clean water throughout the day; try to drink 6–8 glasses daily.
- Eat organic foods as much as you can because they contain lower levels of potentially dangerous pesticides and chemicals. Also, organic vegetables contain more nutrients than non-organic ones.
- A good anti-ageing diet should be composed of 50% vegetables (non-starchy, such as sweet potatoes), 20% protein (meat, cheese, fish), 20% fruits and 10% grains (brown rice, quinoa, lentils, buckwheat, millet or spelt). The vegetables should be raw or lightly cooked to preserve the nutrient content; the protein should include vegetable proteins, such as organic soya beans, haricot beans, aduki beans and so on, as well as some low-fat animal protein. Fruits should be uncooked and whole as opposed to juiced. But blended fruits remain high in nutrients that are easier for the body to absorb and utilize. The grains are best as whole grains, such as brown rice, rather than flour-based foods.
- Eat more thyme, basil and rosemary, which have powerful antioxidant properties. Rosemary is highly anti-cancerous.
- Eat more coriander, which helps remove toxic metal residues from the body.
- Prunes are highly anti-ageing as they are rich in antioxidants– but they are also acid forming. Everything in moderation.
- Eat more curries rich in curcumin, which is derived from turmeric – a highly anti-ageing spice (see below).

Anti-ageing Nutrients
- There are currently dozens of anti-ageing formulas and nutrients. But as a base line, always take a daily good-quality multi-vitamin/mineral plus an antioxidant formula, suitable for your age and gender. Always include an extra gram of vitamin C as a minimum basis to help slow the ageing process.
- Below are listed some of the most anti-ageing nutrients currently known:
  • **Vitamin C** has more than 40 functions within the body that are essential for immune function, skin repair, eye and joint health and so on. I take 2–3 grams daily as a minimum with food. Best taken in divided doses for optimum benefit.
  • **Curcumin** Much research has been done on genes and ageing. Dr Giovanni Scapagnini from The Institute of Neurological Disorders at Bethesda and his team found, when studying the long-lived people on the island of Okinawa, that because the locals eat plenty of curry, with curcumin (turmeric), their Vita Genes – which means genes of life – are 'switched on'. They also eat modestly, take regular exercise, hardly drink alcohol, nor smoke, and they keep stress at bay by regular spiritual practices such as meditation. If you

take 400mg curcumin, with 400mg bromelain and 10–20mg piperine, this helps increase the 'Okinawan effect'. Curcumin is also highly anti-inflammatory, and as most diseases of ageing are linked to inflammation and oxidation (of cells, tissues and organs), eating and taking curcumin is a great idea. It also helps support liver function. A good formula is Super Curcumin by Life Extension; log on to www.lef.org or call The Nutri Centre. **NC**

- **Omega-3 essential fats** More than 2,000 scientific studies have demonstrated the wide range of problems associated with omega3 fatty acid deficiencies. Unless you eat copious amounts of oily fish, then it's likely that you are low in omega-3 fats. Researchers believe that at least 60% of people are deficient in omega-3 fats. Essential fats keep the skin hydrated and supple, and are essential for hormone production, weight loss and controlling blood pressure. The brain cannot function properly without essential fatty acids. Fish oils are high in EPA and DHA – omega-3 fats that are not generally found in vegetable and nut sources that are vital for the brain and nervous system. The best sources are sardines, wild or organically farmed salmon, mullet, trout and mackerel. Excellent non-fish sources of omega-3 fats include flaxseeds (linseeds), walnuts, hemp and pumpkin seeds, and to a lesser extent soybeans. Include these seeds and unrefined oils in your diet; for lots more information, see *Fats You Need To Eat*. I take 3 grams daily of pure omega-3 fish oils.
- **Omega-6 essential fats** are found in sunflower, sesame and pumpkin seeds, linseeds and their unrefined oils, and evening primrose oil. Most people have plenty of omega-6 EFAs in their diet from vegetable spreads and oils.

- **Alpha-lipoic acid** is an important antioxidant that has the unique ability to pass into the brain, where it helps recycling of other antioxidants, such as vitamins C and E, plus glutathione – a vital brain nutrient. It also removes heavy metals like aluminium, mercury and lead from the brain, which helps to protect against Alzheimer's, Parkinson's and senile dementia. Because it is both water and fat soluble, it is easily absorbed in the gut. Alpha-lipoic acid also helps prevent and treat some of the complications of diabetes. Take 200mg daily with food.
- **Carnosine** is a naturally occurring antioxidant made within the body; as we age, the levels fall. High concentrations of carnosine are present in long-lived cells, such as in nerve tissues, and people who live longer have higher levels of this nutrient. Carnosine has been shown to help reverse age-related damage, especially in the skin. It also blocks amyloid production, the substance found in the brains of Alzheimer's patients. Other emerging benefits are its apparent anti-cancer effects, the removal of toxic metals from the body and it is a great immune booster. It is found in lean red meat and chicken. For optimum anti-ageing results take 50–100mg daily. Take on an empty stomach in between meals. **NC**
- **Co-enzyme Q10 (CoQ10)** is an essential factor in energy production within the cells. CoQ10 is a vitamin-like substance that is manufactured in the liver. As we age, production slows down. CoQ10 facilitates and regulates the oxidation of fats and sugars into energy. CoQ10 has profound anti-ageing effects on the brain; it also helps protect the heart. Parkinson's patients tend to be low in CoQ10, which has also been shown to inhibit cancer-cell growth and protect breast tissue, be excellent for allergy management, boost energy levels, protect from gum disease and act as an antioxidant. If you want to stay younger longer, take 100mg daily. If you are taking statin drugs to lower your LDL cholesterol levels, it is important to replenish CoQ10, which is greatly depleted by statins (see *Cholesterol*).
- **Collagen** is a vital component of healthy joints, skin, hair, nails, cartilage, ligaments and tendons, which also improves bone strength. It is the most widely distributed protein in the body and we lose about 1.5% annually after the age of 30. I take collagen powder daily in a glass of water or diluted juice 30 minutes before a main meal to help replenish this vital

protein. Super Strength Collagen Drink from Higher Nature. **HN**
- **Vitamin D3**. There is now a large body of evidence to show that a lack of Vitamin D, which is synthesized on your skin when it is exposed to sunlight, plays a part in strokes, high blood pressure, diabetes, osteoarthritis, osteoporosis, depression, muscle wasting and numerous cancers including colon and breast cancers. For anti-ageing I take 1000iu of Vitamin D3 daily. Thousands of lives could be saved annually, if we all did the same.

■ After the age of 40, If you want to help keep your skin and joints more supple, begin taking liquid hyaluronic acid (HA) daily in water. HA is a naturally occurring protein in the body. HA is what makes young skin look plump and supple. Unfortunately, as we age levels of HA in the body decline, resulting in wrinkles and joint problems. HA is used in thousands of beauty salons as an injectable to plump up lines. But it can also be taken internally in a liquid formula. Take 1ml daily in water on an empty stomach; it is very effective. For more details, ask at your health store or contact Modern Herbals – call 01274 889047 or log on to www.modernherbals.com.

■ Keep your body more alkaline, as virtually all chronic diseases associated with ageing thrive in an over-acid environment. Take a teaspoon of any organic Green Powder daily. I use Green pH, Made by Metabolics (wwwmetabolics.com), and take one small level teaspoon daily in water. A mixture of green beans, garden peas, pea leaf, dry apple cider, watercress, broccoli and nettle leaf, it doesn't taste great, but is an easy and quick way to alkalize your body. Available for retail from the Wholistic Medical Centre. **WMC**

■ After the age of 40, if you tend to eat in a hurry or have a fast-paced lifestyle, also take a digestive enzyme with main meals. There is no point taking all these great nutrients if you are suffering assimilation problems (see *Low Stomach Acid* and *Leaky Gut*).

A

■ As we age, the pineal gland in our brain produces less melatonin, which means we sleep less and sometimes have more problems getting to sleep. Melatonin is one of the most efficient antioxidants known and helps protect DNA, therefore it helps keep you younger longer. Bio-electromagnetic research scientist Roger Coghill says, 'If you take melatonin supplements that you can buy online and in the States, most synthetic tablets contain thousands of times the natural dose that your pineal gland normally produces.'

Therefore, Roger has developed a supplement called Asphalia, containing natural melatonin extracted from certain grasses which mimics the normal dose made by your pineal gland to induce sleep at night, rather than the larger doses, which are found in mass-produced tablets. Roger has permission from the MHRA (Medical Healthcare Regulatory Authority) to sell this food supplement in the UK. For more details or to find your nearest supplier, log on to www.asphalia.co.uk or call 01495 752122. Take 1 to 2 capsules 30 minutes before bed.

NB This supplement should not be taken by pregnant women in their third trimester, severe asthmatics, or children under one year.

Helpful Hints
■ People who are adaptable and have a positive outlook on life tend to live the longest.
■ Never underestimate just how much your thoughts and stress levels can affect not only your health but also the speed at which you age. If you keep saying over and over, 'It's to be expected at my age', do not be surprised if you become sicker and age faster (see *Stress*).
■ Learn to say yes to what you do want in your life and no to what you don't.
■ Have fun – laugh a lot. No one ever had engraved on their tombstone, 'I wish I had spent more time at the office.' Find a balance.
■ Stop worrying – as Dale Carnegie once said, '85% of things you worry about never happen', so stop worrying about the things you cannot change – concentrate on what you can

change. And if you really want to change things in your own life and environment, then take the steps necessary to begin the changes that you require. Be willing to act positively for the good of all, rather than just talking about it.

- Stop smoking; every cigarette you smoke can take 15 minutes off your life. Smoking ages your skin and depletes vital nutrients such as vitamin C, which are needed for healthy skin and bones, energy production, and an active immune system.
- Take regular exercise, but not to excess.
- Being overweight can shorten your life by up to 10 years (see *Weight Problems*).
- Supplementing the hormone DHEA (see *Menopause*) can help reduce inflammation and ageing in the body. Don't take extra hormones unless you need them. Never self-medicate with hormones – have a blood or saliva test. Dr Shamin Daya at the Wholistic Medical Centre at 57 Harley Street, London, is an expert on hormones in ageing. **WMC**
- Learn to meditate (see *Meditation*), for it has many proven anti-ageing benefits. Regular meditation helps you cope more effectively with stress, by reducing release of the highly toxic stress hormones adrenalin and cortisol. It also slows the ageing process.
- Reduce your exposure to mobile phones and excessive electrical equipment.
- Reduce exposure to pesticides, herbicides and toxic chemicals. Eat and drink organic foods and drinks as much as possible.
- Too much sun will age your skin, but we do need some sunshine to produce vitamin D, which helps to keep bones healthy. Sunshine makes you feel good – everything in moderation. Wear a PABA-free organic UVA/UVB sunscreen to protect the skin.

- Try using Real Sunlight lamps, available at several specialist clinics in the UK. The harmful frequencies of UVA and UVB have been filtered out, making this sunlight safe. These lamps increase levels of vitamin D3 naturally, improve collagen production and boost immune function. Call the Wholistic Medical Centre. **WMC**
- Don't overeat. Generally in the West, we tend to eat 40% more food than the body needs. Having said that, there are some people on calorie-restricted diets (proven to slow ageing) living on 1,200 calories a day, but some of them look awful! And food is meant to be a pleasure. We can all enjoy treats and not feel guilty, but we must stop living on treats.
- Get sufficient sleep – it's the easiest way to look younger longer.
- A useful website for anti-ageing research is the Life Extension Foundation at www.lef.org. They run a very efficient postal service from the US and sell supplements that can be difficult to source in the UK. You can also order hormones such as DHEA and melatonin from the Foundation. But please check if you need them first.
- Dr Nick Delgardo is a member of the American Academy of Anti-ageing and his website www.growyoungandslim.com is well worth a look.
- Always use a body lotion after bathing – there are many fabulous organic vitamin creams now widely available from health stores. Anne McDevitt offers a great range of organic and Biodynamic creams plus Glycolic Acid creams which help remove dead skin cells. For details log onto www.annemcdevitt.ie or email sales@annemcdevitt.com.
- The Life Extension Foundation offers numerous creams and serums that are based on Vitamin C, white tea, pomegranate and so on, which have demonstrated anti ageing properties. See www.lef.org for more information.

AGE SPOTS   *(see also Liver Problems and Sunburn)*

If you look at young skin, it's almost always clear with an even tone, and age spots don't normally appear until the early 40s and onwards. If you look at the buttocks of an average 60-year-old woman, they will still look young and blemish-free. The best ways to reduce and avoid age spots is to take less sun, look after your liver, and to ingest more antioxidants. Melanocytes are your melanin, or colour-producing cells, and over time, thanks to exposure to the sun, these fatty pigments or lipids begin to 'clump' together causing age spots (also known as liver spots), or uneven pigmentation of varying sizes and shapes, which begin to appear all over the body. They commonly appear on the backs of the hands, the face, the forearms, and eventually anywhere that is exposed regularly to the sun.

Foods to Avoid
- Fried and barbecued foods, saturated fats found in full-fat dairy products, meat pies, cakes, fatty meats.
- Alcohol and too many fats, which place a strain on your liver.
- Mass-produced refined foods and meals, which are often packed with hydrogenated and trans-fats, plus sugar, which all age the skin (see *Fats You Need To Eat*).
- Reduce non-organic foods, which are often high in additives and pesticides.

Friendly Foods
- To help avoid age spots it is important that the body is eliminating unwanted fatty deposits properly. Lecithin granules, available from all health stores, help emulsify and break down fats. Take 1 tablespoon daily over cereals, fruits and yoghurts. Lecithin is also found in soya products and eggs.

- Eat more antioxidant-rich foods, organic fruit and vegetables, especially red, orange or dark-green fruits and vegetables, such as pomegranates, papaya, blueberries, carrots, apricots, watercress, pumpkin, broccoli, spring greens, pak choy, red peppers, red and purple berries and tomatoes.
- Use tahini or olive oil as a spread instead of hydrogenated margarines and spreads.

Useful Remedies
- Antioxidants help to mop up or neutralize the free-radical reactions that are triggered by sunbathing. Therefore, take a high-strength antioxidant formula including 200iu of full-spectrum Vitamin E, vitamin C, zinc and selenium as a base.
- Beta-carotene helps to encourage melanin production; make sure it's a natural source carotene complex that contains all the carotenoids. Solgar Vitamins and Viridian make a good version. **SVHC, VN**
- Potassium chloride is important also for removing congestion and fatty deposits in the tissues. You need 50mg potassium chloride per tablet, three times a day. **BLK**
- Take at least 1 gram of vitamin C daily.
- Essential fatty acids, known as EFAs, help to reduce the sun's negative effects. If taken regularly they help keep your skin looking younger for longer (see *Fats You Need To Eat*). Take 2 grams of pure omega-3 fish oils daily.
- Pycnogenol – pine bark extract – has been shown to help maintain elasticity of the skin. Take 80mg daily. **PN**

Helpful Hints
- Use a factor 15 sunscreen on the backs of your hands and on your face, and take more care in the sun – you really will reap the benefits in later life.
- If you have young children, keep in mind that a huge amount of skin damage can be done

before a child reaches 16. If children are allowed to burn, then they are more likely to suffer skin cancers in later life. Some sun is healthy, but all things in moderation. Time and again, I see young children and teenagers on beaches in the midday sun with red, blistered skin and no hat! (See *Sunburn*.)

- The secret is not to let the skin burn and turn red. We all know the sensible precautions – to cover up between 11am and 3pm and to always wear a hat in hot midday sun – but a huge majority of us are simply not doing it. Start protecting the skin from an early age. If you do want to tan, do it slowly – don't burn.
- Ask at your health store for an antioxidant-rich cream; there are now dozens of creams containing grape-seed extract, and vitamins C, E and so on. Use this on the age spots daily.
- Cigarettes age your skin. Stop smoking.
- Glycolic acid derived from sugar cane is a gentle way to eliminate dead skin cells and skin discolorations, because as we age cell turnover within the skin slows down. These creams are fairly successful if used now and again, especially when combined with kojic acid. If you use these creams, then as always use an SPF antioxidant cream in tandem. To see the range of products, log on to www.annemcdevitt.ie or email sales@annemcdevitt.com.
- Modern lasers are highly successful at removing age spots, but it is important that you make sure to see a dermatologist or doctor who has experience of this work. I had mine done at The Skin Clinic, 144 Harley Street, London W1G 7LD by Dr Thomas Bozek. Tel: 020 7224 0988. For further details and to find your nearest clinic, call 0844 669 6939 or log on to: www.sknclinics.co.uk.

ALCOHOL
(see also Liver Problems)

Alcohol is responsible for at least 35,000 deaths in the UK annually, and 300 people die every week from liver disease –and 95% of these deaths are entirely preventable.

Thanks to the huge increase in binge drinking, especially among the young, specialists are now seeing more and more young people in their twenties with the liver problems usually associated with people over 50. In fact, around 37% of young men and 23% of young women regularly binge drink – and these figures are climbing. Up to one in three adults in the UK drinks enough alcohol to be at risk of developing liver disease.

Every time you drink alcohol, it acts as a diuretic and causes dehydration. It also upsets blood-sugar levels, adrenal function, irritates the gut and causes the body to excrete vital minerals and vitamins, especially the B-group vitamins, which help keep your nervous system, hormone production, hair and nails in good shape. The more you drink, the more effect it has on your behaviour.

Moderate consumption of alcohol, meaning a single unit, which is equal to half a pint of ordinary-strength beer, lager or cider, or a small measure (25ml) of spirits, or a standard pub measure (50ml) of fortified wine such as sherry or port, has been shown to be slightly protective against heart disease.

A glass of aged or organic red wine is fine. The nutrient content of alcohol is very low, but many people have a drink believing they are protecting their heart and choose to forget they are elevating their risk of hormonal cancers, particularly breast cancer. Alcohol places an enormous strain on the liver, as it reduces its ability to detoxify the body. Over-consumption of alcohol can lead to fatigue and dehydration, as well as disruptive sleep patterns, and can deplete many vital nutrients from the body. In extreme cases of bingeing, the bladder can burst.

Pregnant women risk foetal abnormalities if they consume alcohol during pregnancy and it should be avoided if you are trying to become pregnant. During pregnancy, give it up. Think of your future. When you are young, you think, 'It will never happen to me' – but believe me, it can and does.

Foods to Avoid
- Avoid eating fresh or tinned grapefruit juice if you are drinking alcohol, as this will increase the toxicity of the alcohol.
- Saturated fats place a great strain on the liver. Avoid fatty, heavy, rich meals – especially sausages, cheese (especially melted cheese as in pizzas), rich pâtés, burgers, pre-packaged meat pies, and so on.
- Never ply anyone who is drunk with coffee, as this will further dehydrate the body, which can increase the concentration of alcohol in the system. (See *General Health Hints*.)

Friendly Foods
- Eat plenty of fresh fruits and vegetables, especially broccoli, artichokes, cauliflower, beetroot, celeriac, celery, fennel and radicchio to help to detoxify the liver.
- Eat plenty of soluble fibres such as linseeds (soaked flax seeds), oat bran and low-sugar cereals such as muesli or porridge.
- Drink at least 6–8 glasses of water daily.
- Use unrefined olive, walnut or sunflower oils for salad dressings.
- See also *General Health Hints*.

Useful Remedies

A

- The herb milk thistle (silymarin) has been proven to help detoxify and regenerate the liver. Take 500mg of the whole-herb supplement twice daily with meals for one month. During this time, you need to cut down your intake of alcohol to give the liver time to repair. **SHS**
- Take a couple of capfuls of organic pure aloe vera Juice daily before foods, as aloe supports the liver and acts as a mild anti- inflammatory.
- If you drink only occasionally, take 1 high-strength milk thistle capsule before and after drinking.
- Taking 500mg twice daily of the amino acid methionine away from food helps the liver to recover. It's a great liver de-toxifier.
- Take a good quality multi-vitamin and mineral daily for your age and gender. Nature's Plus, Solgar, Lamberts, Metabolics and BioCare all make good multis. **NP, SVNC, BC, WMC**
- To avoid hangovers, take 2 grams of evening primrose oil, 1 gram of vitamin C, a B-complex, plus 500mg of milk thistle with a full glass of water before going out. Repeat this dosage the next morning upon waking.
- The herb Chinese kudzu extract contains diadzin, which has been known to be beneficial for treating alcoholism. Not only does kudzu extract help reduce the craving for alcohol, but it also acts as a muscle relaxant, which helps to overcome some of the withdrawal symptoms. Take 10–20 drops of the tincture or 2 tablets before you take a drink. **NC**

Helpful Hints
- Do not give a person coffee to sober them up as coffee is a diuretic, which depletes fluid from the body and makes the alcohol content in the body even more concentrated.
- For every alcoholic drink, make sure you have a non-alcoholic one in between. Generally drink more water, as alcohol severely dehydrates the body. Avoid alcohol when flying, because the pressurized cabins cause considerable dehydration.
- If you have a hangover, you need to raise your blood sugar quite quickly upon waking. Eat a banana or blend various fresh fruits such as figs, papaya, dates and/or raisins and low-fat, live yoghurt (or rice milk) and drink immediately, or drink some diluted fruit juice.

- Drink 3 glasses of water slowly as soon as you wake up, to rehydrate the body.
- Homeopathic Nux Vomica 30c. Take one before bed and another upon waking to help reduce a hangover. This really helps. **OP**
- Bingeing on alcohol is **extremely dangerous** – it creates too much shock in the liver. Vomiting is a clear indication that the body has reached a danger level and you must stop drinking.
- If you must drink, have a couple of drinks daily – but do not drink to excess. Better-quality red wine seems to confer the most health benefits, owing to antioxidant substances called polyphenols present in the skin of red grapes. The grapes' skins are discarded during the processing of white wine. Pinot Noir as a choice of red confers most health benefits.
- Dandelion root tea tastes bitter, but is excellent for cleansing the liver.
- The liver detoxifies most efficiently between 1 and 3am – but for it to do this you need to be lying down, so burning the midnight oil and beyond adds even greater strain on your liver.
- Remember it takes 20 minutes for alcohol to have an effect and more than one hour for the body to process each unit. If you are concerned about the amount that you (or a member of your family) are drinking, call Drinkline on 0800 917 8282 for advice and information. The line is open 24 hours a day, seven days a week. All calls are treated in the strictest confidence and Drinkline provides a full support service for people with drink problems as well as their families. Otherwise, contact Alcohol Concern on 020 7566 9800 or log on to their website, www.alcoholconcern.org.uk.

ALLERGIC RHINITIS

(see also Allergies, Candida, Hayfever and Leaky Gut)

The incidence of allergic rhinitis is without doubt increasing, as more and more people suffer toxic overload and food sensitivities. Typical symptoms include a runny nose, sneezing, sinus congestion plus itchy and watering eyes, usually immediately after being exposed to any foods or external pollutants, such as traffic fumes. Unlike hay fever, allergic rhinitis tends to affect people all year round, although symptoms can be worse at certain times of year when pollen counts are high. In some individuals it is triggered by a food intolerance, the most common being a sensitivity to cow's milk and other dairy products or wheat. This will need to be addressed for the problem to be resolved: you can take all kinds of herbs and supplements in efforts to relieve the problem, or worse still antihistamines, but this will not address the root cause of the condition. For example, when I eat a high-sugar food, my nose starts running within seconds, which is a shame as I have a sweet tooth! But this demonstrates how immediate any effect can be. This condition can also be linked to candida and/or leaky gut syndrome. See *Candida* and *Leaky Gut*.

Foods to Avoid
- Avoid sugar and high mucous-forming foods, such as full-fat dairy products, cheese and chocolate, as much as possible. Soya milk and foods can cause this problem for many people.
- Reduce white flour and pasta, orange juice, tomatoes and any other foods to which you may have an intolerance. Keep a food diary and note when symptoms are worse.
- Wheat and dairy produce from cows are known to be triggers for this condition, but it could just as easily be bananas or tomatoes.
- Wine and dried fruits, which contain sulphites, can also trigger this condition in some people.

Friendly Foods

- Eat more curries, rich in turmeric , which helps to calm the inflammatory response.
- Include plenty of garlic, onions, horseradish, root ginger and freshly squeezed fruit and vegetable juices (but not carton juice) in your diet.
- Fresh pineapple contains bromelain, which reduces inflammation. But don't drink the juice, which is high in sugar.
- If you have an intolerance to wheat, try rye, rice or amaranth crackers and oat cakes. Ask at your health shop for wheat-free bread and pasta.
- Dairy alternatives include organic rice, soya, goat's, almond or oat milk. Soya milk does, however, trigger excess mucous in some people.

Useful Remedies

- If symptoms are acute, take up to 5 grams of vitamin C in an ascorbate form daily with meals spread throughout the day, plus 500mg to 2 grams of pantothenic acid (vitamin B5).
- Take a bioflavonoid complex: 500mg to 2 grams daily when acute.
- Take 500mg of bromelain – an enzyme from pineapple, which helps to break down mucous and reduce the allergic response, therefore reducing the discomfort.
- Nettle tincture or tea three times a day helps to alleviate symptoms.
- Quercetin, another flavonoid, helps to reduce the allergic response: take 400mg x 3 times daily whilst symptoms are acute.
- Beta Glucans 1-3, 1-6, derived from yeast cell walls, are proven to strengthen the body's innate immune system (the immune system you were born with), making it more resistant to pathogens from food and air. Take 250–500 mg daily.

Helpful Hints

- Keep a food diary and note when symptoms become worse. You should also note if certain toothpastes trigger the problem or even a walk near a main road can make symptoms worse.
- During an acute attack, a homeopathic nasal spray called Euphorbium Spray is extremely effective. It helps to relieve a runny nose, congestion and headaches. **NC, SL**
- Dust and other airborne allergens can be reduced in your immediate environment by using an ionizer.
- Try New Era tissue salt Nat Mur for alleviating allergic rhinitis.
- I recommend that you try the Neil Med Sinus Rinse. It's incredibly easy to use and really helps to reduce allergic reactions linked to the sinuses and also reduces the incidence of sinus infections. Available from most good chemists. Well worth using daily. Find details via www.neilmed.com.

ALLERGIES
(see also Leaky Gut and Liver Problems)

Allergy problems, such as asthma, eczema and rhinitis, are responsible for an estimated 13 million GP consultations a year and 20 million people in the UK alone are thought to have either an allergy or a sensitivity to various substances. One in every four of us suffers some kind of sensitivity at some point in our lives. Allergies or sensitivities to various foods or substances are the most common triggers for a multitude of symptoms from coughing, itchy skin, skin rashes, joint problems, fibromyalgia, autoimmune conditions such as lupus, wheezing, runny nose, sneezing, watery eyes, chronic sore throats and so on. Many doctors still state that food intolerances are 'all in the mind' – but ask anyone who suffers chronic bloating after eating wheat or a razor-sore throat within an hour of eating chocolate if they are imagining their symptoms, which of course they aren't.

The severest form of allergy triggers anaphylactic shock – which is life threatening and needs immediate medical attention. People with severe allergies usually carry an injection of adrenaline, which would need to be injected immediately if that person were exposed to a specific allergen such as peanuts or a bee sting.

Allergies or sensitivities from external sources such as pesticides, food additives, paints, pollution, perfumes, animal hairs, grass, plant and tree pollens are also widespread. As much as 31,000 tonnes of pesticides are sprayed on crops in the UK every year and there are more than 311 licensed pesticides in use in the UK alone. If you eat a non-organic apple, it may have been sprayed up to 18 times before you eat it. An average person ingests 14kg of toxins through their skin alone each year. Therefore it's no wonder that we are suffering a variety of reactions. Allergies and sensitivities are the body's way of saying it has had enough and cannot cope with more toxins – which is why symptoms appear when the system becomes overloaded with toxins and/or stress.

Also, many people only partially digest food proteins, which can sometimes break through the gut wall. The body treats these particles as it would an infection and attacks them as an enemy, which if left untreated can cause a myriad of allergic-type symptoms and eventually contribute to autoimmune disease and severe gut problems. The secret to controlling allergies and sensitivities is to reduce your exposure to all pollutants.

Foods to Avoid

- Eggs, dairy produce from cows, wheat, oranges, tomatoes, corn and soya are common allergens.
- All food additives found in mass-produced foods and monosodium glutamate.
- Caffeine, peanuts, chocolate, beef, yeast and shellfish.
- It's worth noting that the foods you tend to crave and eat the most are usually the ones that are causing most problems. Wheat and cow's milk are the most common.

Friendly Foods

- This is a possible minefield until you know which foods are your problem, but generally eat more brown rice, pears, lamb, cabbage, lentils, papaya, leeks, green peas, aduki beans and sweet potatoes, which are usually well tolerated. Amaranth crackers, buckwheat or quinoa are also low-allergen foods.
- Include more flaxseeds (linseeds are best soaked overnight in cold water), sunflower seeds and organic sunflower and olive oil in your diet. These foods are a good starting point that very few people react to.
- Papaya is rich in digestive enzymes.
- Live, goat's and sheep's yoghurt contain friendly bacteria and are more easily digestible than cow's milk.
- Raw cabbage juice is high in L-glutamine, known to help to heal a leaky gut. Try making fresh juices daily that include a little chopped raw cabbage, a tiny piece of root ginger, carrots, apples and a tablespoon of aloe vera juice. Drink immediately after blending, while all the enzymes and nutrients are still active.
- Drink small amounts of liquorice tea, which also helps heal the gut and reduces stress. Nettle tea helps reduce the allergic response.
- Fennel tea will aid digestion if taken after meals – if wind and bloating are a problem.

Useful Remedies

- Histazyme, a complex containing calcium, vitamin C, zinc, bromelain, silica, vitamin A and manganese, acts as a natural antihistamine. **BC**
- HEP 194 contains various herbs, the enzyme lipase, the amino acid methionine, and B-vitamins, which all help to support the liver. **BC**

- Beta Glucans 1-3, 1-6, derived from yeast cell walls, are proven to strengthen the body's innate immune system, making it more resistant to pathogens from food and air. Take 250–500 mg daily. It can also be taken by children and reduces the likelihood of food intolerances triggered by a weakened innate immune system. Dr Paul Clayton, based in the UK and US, is a medical pharmacologist. His website provides information on beta glucans: www.healthdefence.com. Glucosan, developed by Dr Clayton, is available from Vitalize Health products. Call 0870 042 8423 or log on to www.vitalizeshop.co.uk.
- Betaine hydrochloride – stomach acid (HCl) – is often lacking in people suffering allergies. HCl is available from most health stores; take one capsule just as you begin eating your main meal. Not to be taken if you have active stomach ulcers, in which case try a digestive enzyme tablet (without HCl), available from all health stores.
- The amino acid L-glutamine can help heal a leaky gut. Take 1 teaspoon in a little diluted fruit juice or water – but not orange juice – 30–45 minutes before main meals twice daily until symptoms ease.
- A good-quality multi-vitamin and mineral daily.
- Once you have identified your intolerance, the above can be reduced to the multi-vitamin and mineral and the HCl or digestive enzyme daily.
- A common homeopathic remedy for runny eyes and nose is Allium 6c, or if there is swelling Apis 6c, taken 3 times daily.
- There is now good evidence showing that taking healthy bacteria (probiotics) regularly will reduce the amount of 'allergens' from food that may pass through the gut wall. Take one capsule daily after food. For details ask at your health shop or speak to the nutritionist at BioCare. **BC**
- H Metabolism tablets by Metabolics help reduce high histamine levels in the body triggered by the allergy. Take two capsules, three times daily if symptoms are acute. Available from the Wholistic Medical Centre. **WMC**
- Finnish researchers have found that when expectant mothers are given prebiotics during the final weeks of pregnancy – nutrients extracted from the agave plant, which support the growth of healthy bacteria in the gut and enhance immune function – their babies were far less likely to suffer respiratory infections or develop conditions such as asthma. For details of Agave Digestive Immune Support, see www.lef.org.

Helpful Hints

- It is important to have an allergy test to find your worst offenders. One of the best I have found is available from the York Test Laboratories. Tel: 0800 458 2052 or log on to www.yorktest.com; Genova Diagnostics do a FACT test which looks for inflammatory markers indicating that the body is reacting to certain substances. Tel: 020 8336 7750 or log on to www.gdx.uk.net.
- Another excellent method is the Bio Meridian Test for food intolerance and leaky gut, in which the practitioner measures via electrodes your reactions to a huge list of foods and substances. For practitioners see www.biomeridian.com or call Sheila Partridge on 020 7580 7537.
- Subscribe to a free E-newsletter, which is especially for allergy sufferers at www.allergyuk.org
- It is vital to chew food more thoroughly.
- Avoid large meals, which overload the digestive system and liver and can trigger an allergic response.
- Many toothpastes, shampoos, soaps, detergents and perfumes, body lotions and sunscreens contain a myriad of chemicals. Buy products in their most natural and unadulterated state. For anyone who suffers dermatitis or skin allergies, The Green People Company makes organic skin, hair and body creams and toothpastes. Tel: 01403 740350. Email: organic@greenpeople.co.uk. Website: www.greenpeople.co.uk.

- The Organic Pharmacy also makes organic creams and their team of homeopaths is always very helpful in suggesting herbal or homeopathic remedies. **OP**
- To test if you have a food sensitivity, first take your resting pulse rate. Then for at least 14 days completely avoid the food you want to test – for example, wheat. Then try eating the food you have avoided on its own – for example, Weetabix in water or plain brown toast. Take your pulse at 15, 30 and 60 minutes after eating the specific food. If your pulse has increased by more than 10 beats a minute, it is likely that you have sensitivity to the test food. Or have a blood test such as The York Test – details above.
- Many allergic and chemically sensitive people can benefit enormously by switching from tap water to mineral or filtered water. Tests in the US found that 98% of environmentally ill patients improved by eliminating tap water. For details, call The Pure H2O Company on 01784 221188. Email: roger@pureh2o.co.uk. Website: www.pureh2o.co.uk.
- Use Kangen Water – a water system that attaches to your kitchen tap that ionizes and alkalizes water. It's used in Japanese hospitals with highly beneficial health results. For full details, call 020 7580 7537 or log on to www.kangenmiraclewater.co.uk.
- Dr Jean Monro, who has worked at the Breakspear Hospital in Hertfordshire in the UK for 25 years, says, 'Before the industrial revolution conditions such as hayfever did not exist. But since then we have done a great job of polluting our atmosphere and thus our bodies. We now know that an accumulation of a variety of pollutants, such as paint sprays or pesticides (there are hundreds of others), acts as the initial trigger; these chemicals become the sensitizers – and in most cases the membranes within the nose and throat begin to react and become inflamed. Then the body treats the next thing that comes along, such as grass pollens, as a threatening foreign invader, which increases any inflammation and induces allergic type symptoms. But it's the chemicals that sensitize the body in the first place. Chemicals can have a local affect such as on the skin – and then this effect is communicated to the rest of the body by neural (nerve) pathways and a sensitivity is born.

A

'The neural pathway is extremely important because it is the body's sense of awareness, which firstly triggers the dendritic cells, which then send a message to the autonomic nervous system that controls pulse, breathing and temperature. And if someone suffering a severe reaction to, say, peanuts – reacts, even if that peanut happens to be in someone's pocket across the room – we now know that this instantaneous effect is triggered not only by particles of the peanuts but also by the frequencies emitted by the peanut, which have an instant effect. It's important for people to realize that not only do we all emit our own unique signature range of frequencies – but so does everything around us, from asbestos to our foods. And if you have a specific substance/food or whatever emitting a frequency that is incompatible with your own, then symptoms will eventually show up.

'After 20 years' research, we have developed new vaccines based on frequencies that can help to neutralize any reaction to substances found to trigger a response, and these vaccines are proving very effective. This is the medicine of the future.

'Also, the more that people stay away from synthetic chemicals and reduce the body's toxic overload, the less allergies and sensitivities will occur.'

This is fascinating research and for anyone who wants more details about allergy and environmental medicine, log on to www.breakspearmedical.com or call 01442 261333.

ALOPECIA

(see Hair Loss)

ALZHEIMER'S DISEASE (AD)   *(see also Memory)*

Alzheimer's disease (AD) affects around 700,000 people to varying degrees in the UK, and was first described and documented between 1900 and 1906 by the German neurologist, Alois Alzheimer – hence its name. The term 'dementia' is used to describe the symptoms that present themselves when the brain is affected by specific diseases. Dementia affects one in every 14 people over the age of 65, and as we are an ageing population figures are expected to rise.

Three in every 10 people over the age of 70 say they suffer with poor memory or concentration, or with confusion. The good news is that most of us have similar problems, but only about 1 in every 15 actually has Alzheimer's disease.

AD is a progressive, degenerative disease that attacks the brain, triggering symptoms such as memory loss (especially of the short-term memory), confusion, agitation and frequently forgetting names, places, appointments and recent events. Mood swings can become common place as well as a gradual withdrawing from everyday life, especially as a person's confidence and his or her ability to communicate is affected. It is the loss of memory of how to do everyday tasks that tends to make a familiar life almost impossible.

In the early stages AD sufferers have symptoms of absent-mindedness and an inability to learn new things. Judgement and intellectual and social functioning begin to go awry. Later there is loss of logic and memory and poor co-ordination. Speech deteriorates and symptoms of paranoia may appear. In the final stages, the AD sufferer completely loses touch with their surroundings and becomes unresponsive. Needless to say this is very traumatic, not only for the sufferer but also for their family. **The tragedy is that AD is, in most cases, a preventable disease and can even be reversed to some degree.**

There is no doubt that genes play a part – researchers have found that those with a variation in the gene MTHFD1L may be twice as likely to develop Alzheimer's – but, by changing our lifestyle and diet, we can in the majority of cases change which genes are expressed and load the dice more in favour of good health, even in later life. One of the most common theories for a cause of AD is metal toxicity, most likely with aluminium and mercury. A 1980 study of 647 Canadian gold miners who had routinely inhaled aluminium since the 1940s (a common practice thought to prevent silica poisoning), found that all the miners tested in the 'impaired' range for cognitive function, suggesting a clear link between aluminium and memory loss. And while aluminium is certainly harmful to the brain, there are other key factors that can lead to degeneration of the brain.

Researchers have found a significant imbalance of metals in AD patients, especially mercury, mainly deposited in areas of the brain related to memory. Mercury is known to cause the type of damage to nerves that is characteristic of AD, and researchers have found that early-onset AD patients have the highest mercury levels of all (see *Mercury Fillings*).

Another factor is homocysteine, a toxic compound produced during the metabolism of proteins; an increased homocysteine level is a strong, independent risk factor for the development of dementia. At the University of Gothenburg in Sweden, in a lengthy study of 1500 women concluded in November 2009, Alzheimer's disease was more than twice as common among women with the highest levels of homocysteine. The higher the homocysteine level, the greater the damage to the brain. Homocysteine is readily recycled or broken down within the body by vitamins B6, B12 and folic acid. Therefore, by taking a B-complex daily (or many companies now make homocysteine support formulas), homocysteine levels can be kept in check. There is also a home test kit from York Test that will give you your homocysteine level. For details, call 0800 458 2052 or log on to www.yorktest.com.

Alzheimer's is also characterized by amyloid plaques, and as beta amyloid is an inflammatory protein, inflammation is now considered to be an underlying cause of AD. The amyloid plaques build up outside nerve cells (neurons) and eventually destroy or damage the neurons – thus impairing brain function.

Cortisol, the stress hormone, can also cause great damage in the brain, as cortisol causes the connections between brain cells to shrivel up, which contributes to AD. There are good supplements to help control cortisol production. (See *Stress*.)

Free radicals and an excessive intake of refined, processed foods that are low in antioxidant vitamins such as A, C and E are also contributing factors. Basically, the more pollutants and refined foods we are exposed to, the more vital minerals and vitamins are excreted from the body and brain function deteriorates. Eating the right foods, taking supplements that nourish the brain, and taking more exercise increases circulation to the brain, and memory can often be improved. (See also *Electrical Pollution* and *Memory*.)

Foods to Avoid
- Avoid refined grains in products such as white bread, rice and pasta. These grains will have had most of their nutrients, including B-vitamins, removed in the refining process, and remember that elevated homocysteine levels can be controlled by taking more B-vitamins, B6, B12 and folate.
- Avoid foods containing traces of aluminium such as commercial chocolate, desserts, baking powder, processed cheeses, chewing gum and pickles.
- Eliminate any food containing the food additives aspartame (an artificial sweetener) or Monosodium Glutamate MSG, which are suspected neuro-toxins.
- Avoid ready-made meat pies, cakes, and pre-packaged meals that are not only cooked in aluminium containers but also packed with saturated fat, sugar and salt.
- Reduce your intake of saturated fats found in fatty meats and full-fat dairy produce.
- Reduce your intake of caffeine, sugar and alcohol, which can all deplete vital nutrients and interfere with brain function. Sugar is particularly deadly for brain function and contributes to beta-amyloid deposits, which are one of the main problems for AD patients. US President Ronald Reagan ate jelly babies by the bag every day and developed AD.

Friendly Foods
- A Japanese study found that AD patients did not eat fish, but ate more meat and rarely ate green/yellow vegetables and tended to be lacking in vitamin C, carotenes and omega-3 essential fats. A high intake of animal fats and a high cholesterol level also increases the risk for dementia in later life.
- AD patients are often lacking in the vital brain nutrient acetylcholine, which is manufactured by the body, found in oats, soya beans, eggs, cabbage and cauliflower.
- Sprinkle a tablespoon of soya lecithin granules over breakfast cereals, into yoghurt or over fresh fruit. Lecithin is rich in acetylcholine – but make sure the brand you choose contains at least 30% of this nutrient. Other foods containing this vital brain nutrient are egg yolks and fish, especially sardines.
- Essential fats are vital for proper brain functioning and reducing inflammation within the brain (and body), as brain inflammation and poor circulation is also linked to AD. Lack of omega-3 fish oils has now been demonstrated to be a factor in Alzheimer's and dementia. Eat more oily fish especially organic farmed salmon, mackerel and sardines. Use organic flax, or sunflower oil for your salad dressings, and avoid heating these oils. Foxes and many other animals instinctively will often eat only the heads of their prey – that's because the brain is rich in essential fats.

- Eat more avocado and sprinkle wheat germ over breakfast cereals, fruit dishes and salads as they are rich in vitamin E.
- Sweet potatoes are high in natural-source carotenes, and will help to nourish your brain.
- Include organic farmed salmon, herrings and mackerel in your diet, which are rich in omega-3 essential fats. Include plenty of organic linseeds, sunflower and pumpkin seeds, which are all rich in healthy fats. Sprinkle them into breakfast cereals, and toasted or raw with salads and vegetables, these seeds are delicious (see also *Fats You Need To Eat*).
- Include antioxidant-rich foods such as berries, especially blueberries, blackberries, pomegranate, prunes, plus dark green leafy vegetables, and any other brightly coloured fruits and vegetables. (See *General Health Hints*.)
- Garden sage has been found to prolong and improve memory functioning, owing to its powerful anti-inflammatory and antioxidant effects. Sage also inhibits the enzyme that breaks down acetylcholine. Use plenty of fresh sage over cooked foods or make sage teas. **Avoid sage if you are pregnant as it stimulates the uterus.**
- Use plenty of fresh coriander over salads and sprinkle over cooked dishes, as coriander helps to remove toxic metals from the body.
- Eat plenty of pomegranate, as it helps keep arteries healthier and therefore helps to keep blood flowing.
- Blueberries are rich in potent brain-protecting antioxidants.
- Use nori seaweed flakes instead of salt – as they also help eliminate heavy metals from the body.
- Adding cayenne pepper to meals aids circulation.
- Eat more fresh root ginger and fresh rosemary for their anti-inflammatory properties.

A

Useful Remedies
- Take a multi-vitamin/mineral/essential fats/antioxidant formula daily for your age and gender that also contains brain nutrients as mentioned above.
- Magnesium (300mg daily) and potassium phosphate (75mg daily) are important for nerve connections in the brain. **BC, BLK**
- Silica helps to eliminate aluminium from the body. Take 75mg per day. Fiji mineral water is especially pure and rich in silica.
- Natural-source, full-spectrum vitamin E x 600iu and vitamin C x 1 gram taken 3 times a day with meals have been shown to slow the progress of Alzheimer's and to help prevent onset of dementia. Placebo-controlled studies have shown that full-spectrum, natural-source vitamin E is more effective than drugs in reducing the symptoms of Alzheimer's.
- Ginkgo biloba is a herb from leaves of what the Chinese call the memory tree. Try 120–240mg daily, which helps to increase circulation to the brain and protects neurons. In rare cases ginkgo can cause a rash in which case you would need to stop taking it. **Do not take this herb if you are taking Warfarin or Aspirin stronger than 75mg daily.**
- B-vitamins are destroyed by stress and alcohol, but are needed for the formation of acetylcholine and for the manufacture of other neuro-transmitters within the brain and nervous system, so take a high-strength B-complex daily, especially if you're stressed.
- Curcumin, a substance found in the spice turmeric (widely used in curries), may be part of the reason AD is uncommon in India compared with Western countries. Studies in India found a less than 1% incidence of AD in the over-65s. Curcumin reduces degenerative, inflammatory responses to amyloid. Try 1 or 2 curcumin standardized extract capsules daily with food.
- Lipoic acid is a vital brain nutrient that can help to reduce heavy metals in the brain and body. As it's fat soluble, it also protects nerve cells from damage. Take 200mg twice daily for prevention.

- Take HM Chelate by Pure Encapsulations Inc, a chlorella-based formula that also contains quantities of selenium, zinc, Vitamin C, coriander, N-acetylcysteine and lipoic acid – all of which help to pull heavy metals from the body. Take 3–6 capsules daily well away from food.
- Take 2 grams of omega-3 fish oils daily plus one GLA – they are vital for brain function and also highly anti-inflammatory. **BC**
- The herb aswagandha has been found to help protect areas of the brain that are needed for memory function – it also helps modulate cortisol production.
- Cognitex from The Life Extension Foundation contains phosphatidycholine, phosphatidylserine, vinpocetine, grape seed extract, wild blueberry, ashwagandha, ginger and rosemary – all great nutrients to help keep your brain healthy. **NC**
- Research over 15 years from Dr Hirokazu Kawagishi of Shizoka University in Japan has demonstrated that pure extract of the Lion's Mane Mushroom has a remarkable ability to increase nerve growth factor (NGF) in the brain, which in turn helps make more neurons. Take daily for at least 3 months as nerves do not grow overnight! Scientist Roger Coghill, based in the UK, supplies a pure extract of the Lion's Mane. For details or to find your nearest supplier, log on to www.asphalia.co.uk or call 01495 752122.

Helpful Hints

- As a general prevention – ask your GP to measure your C reactive protein levels, which show the amount of inflammation in your body. Inflammation in the arteries triggers a host of problems, therefore if you have inflammation take steps to reduce it, as in the long term it can save your life. Markers of inflammation are redness, swelling, heat or/and pain.
- Avoid stress. Stress stimulates the adrenal glands to produce a hormone called cortisol, which can **greatly** damage your brain. Learn to relax regularly, and walk regularly which is very relaxing, or try yoga, t'ai chi, massage or meditation. (See *Stress* for more supplements that can reduce cortisol production.)
- Stop smoking – research indicates that smokers are twice as likely to develop dementia in later life. Avoid drugs such as cannabis and Ecstasy, which are associated with memory loss if used in the long term.
- Have your hormone levels checked, because lack of hormones such as oestrogen, progesterone, DHEA and testosterone are also known to affect the brain. Never self-medicate with hormones.
- Regular exercise has helped many sufferers restore some functions, especially memory. Learn ballroom dancing, which is great exercise and good for the brain! Walk daily to increase circulation and get much-needed oxygen to your brain.
- If you have mercury fillings, you are advised to have them removed. It is imperative this is done by a dentist who specializes in this procedure, as increased mercury poisoning can result if the proper precautions are not taken to protect you during the filling removal (see *Mercury Fillings*).
- Because of the link between aluminium and AD, avoid aluminium cooking utensils and pans, and food stored in aluminium containers. Do not allow food to be in direct contact with aluminium foil, don't heat foods wrapped in foil. Use stainless steel or glass cookware. Some antiperspirants contain aluminium, so use natural deodorants such as PitRok, available from all chemists and health stores.
- Simple antacids are often based on aluminium salts and should also be avoided. Aluminium is also found in toothpastes, some cosmetics, processed cheeses, baking powder, buffered aspirin and table salts often contain aluminium, which is used as a pouring agent. If our

mineral levels are low, then the body tends to absorb more aluminium, so this is another reason to include a good multi-mineral in your everyday health regimen.

- Chelation therapy helps to remove deadly metal toxins from the body. There are several clinics in the UK – for details, call Arterial Disease Clinic, 32 Bolton Road, Atherton, Greater Manchester M46 9JY on 01942 886644.

- Use it or lose it. Keep the brain working with simple exercises like doing crosswords and force your brain to work by counting down from 500 each day in multiples of various numbers; such as 500 less 7 = 493, less 7 = 486 and so on. Try writing and using regularly the opposite hand to the one you normally use. Extend your arms out at shoulder level, rotate one hand clockwise and the other anticlockwise and then change over – make your brain work. Buy a dictionary and learn to use and spell at least one new word every day. Learn Sudoku, as it stimulates the brain.

- Eat organic food as much as possible and drink filtered or bottled water. Many pesticides are now linked to neurological problems and these chemicals along with aluminium are finding their way into our drinking water, so use a good water filter that removes all of these residues. Contact The Pure Water Company on 01784 221188, or log on to www.pureh2o.co.uk.

- Use Kangen Water – a water system that attaches to your kitchen tap and ionizes and alkalizes water. It's used in Japanese hospitals with highly beneficial health results. For full details call 020 7580 7537 or log on to www.kangenmiraclewater.co.uk.

- Avoid overexposure to mobile phones and computers. Certain studies have shown that exposure to electromagnetic radiation significantly increases the risk of AD, or makes it rapidly worse. So working with or near computers, VDUs and similar equipment, may harm your brain and evidence of how mobile phones affect the brain is continuing to mount (see *Electrical Pollution*).

- Maintaining circulation to the brain is essential, as poor blood supply to the brain will starve it of oxygen and nutrients. This is why regular exercise is important.

- Certain prescription drugs including statins are known to cause side effects, which appear similar to symptoms of senile dementia. Anyone who feels that they may have the onset of dementia should immediately consult a qualified doctor, who is also a nutritionist. (See *Useful Information*.)

- For more help, visit www.alzheimers.org.uk.

- Read *The Alzheimer's Prevention Plan*, a very useful book by Patrick Holford (Piatkus), or *The Better Brain Book* by David Perlmutter and Carol Colman (Riverhead Books). **NC**

ANAEMIA

Anaemia tends to come in two forms – pernicious anaemia and iron deficiency. If you have pernicious anaemia, it is owing to a lack of intrinsic factor needed to absorb vitamin B12, which is needed for the production of red blood cells in the body. In the past it was always thought necessary to have B12 injections; however, research has now shown that 1mg (1000mcg) of B12 taken daily can rectify this deficiency. A number of disorders can create B12 malabsorption, including gastritis, Crohn's disease and coeliac disease. Smoking also inhibits absorption of iron.

If you have been diagnosed as suffering from anaemia the normal procedure is to take a large amount of iron – but it is very important to make sure that the co-factors, which are vitamin B12, folic acid and vitamin C, are taken at the same time to optimize absorption.

Iron deficiency can be brought about by a number of factors, such as losing more blood than the body can replace naturally, common among women who suffer very heavy periods, and which should always be investigated by a GP or a gynaecologist. An underactive thyroid is also linked to low iron levels (see *Thyroid*).

Over-consumption of tea and coffee can somewhat inhibit iron absorption from your food. Many people take an iron supplement when they are feeling tired, but it is always worthwhile having blood levels of iron checked before you begin supplementing iron, which accumulates in the body. Too much iron in older people, especially men, is linked to heart disease. Therefore no one over 50 should take iron supplements unless they have a medical condition that requires iron. Common symptoms of low iron levels are fatigue, headaches, increased heart rate, shortness of breath, bleeding gums, confusion, feeling faint and pale skin. If you are found to have low iron levels, it's important that your doctor should find the root cause for the anaemia. Orthodox cancer treatments such as chemotherapy and radiation are known to induce anaemia in some patients. Alcoholics are also often found to be low in folic acid and B12. Lack of testosterone in older men can also trigger anaemia. Generally, vegetarians eat less iron than non-vegetarians. However, in Israel they found that blood iron levels were actually higher in vegetarians, which is probably owing to their high consumption of fruit and vegetables. Vegetarians who do not eat sufficient fruit and vegetables can be low in iron. Vegans most definitely would need to take B12 supplements – 50–100mcg daily.

Foods to Avoid
- Excess amounts of black tea and coffee, which can reduce absorption of iron from food. It's the tannins in the tea that reduce absorption of iron from the diet.
- Excessive intake of high-fibre foods will have a similar effect, but they are needed for good bowel health, so if you need iron supplements, take them in between eating high-fibre foods.

Friendly Foods
- Liver and most meats are rich in iron – especially lean steak and venison. Chicken, pheasant, partridge, grouse, pigeon, kidneys, hare and cockles are also good sources.
- Wheat bran and wholewheat flour and wheat germ contain good amounts and most breakfast cereals contain added iron.
- Dried fruits such as apricots, raisins and prunes are also a good source of iron. As dried fruits are high in sugar, soak them for a few minutes in warm water to reduce the sugar content. Drain before serving. Buy dried fruits with no added sulphites.
- Almonds, cocoa and curry powder and raw parsley contain moderate amounts of iron.
- Leafy green vegetables such as watercress, sprouted foods such as alfalfa, broccoli, spinach, pea sprouts, kale, cabbage and organic tomatoes are also rich in iron.
- Blackstrap molasses is rich in iron, as is brewer's yeast.
- Prune juice is rich in iron.

Useful Remedies
- Take 1g of vitamin C daily with food, plus 400mcg of folic acid and 1mg (1000mcg) of B12 daily, as these help to increase absorption of the iron.
- As B-vitamins work together within the body, take a B-complex with the above.
- If you are very anaemic then you can also take iron ascorbate for one week every month, 15–45mg, as it is an easily absorbed form of iron. **Avoid iron sulphate, which may damage mucous membranes in the digestive tract and can cause constipation. Always keep iron supplements away from children.**

- Vitamin A and iron together are more effective than taking iron on its own. Take 5000iu. But if you are pregnant only 3000iu of vitamin A can be taken daily and only while symptoms of anaemia last.
- Trace minerals such as zinc, copper and selenium are also needed to aid increased utilization of iron, so also take a multi-mineral daily.

Helpful Hints

- When taking an iron supplement it is generally best to take it with a small glass of pure fruit juice, which seems to aid absorption owing to the vitamin-C content in fruit juice.
- Iron is so vital for health that we store it in our bodies, but if taken in excessive amounts, it can become toxic and is known to cause constipation in some cases. The exception to this is women who suffer from heavy periods and are feeling exhausted. Pregnant women can benefit from liquid formulas, such as Floradix or Spatone, available from health stores.
- Many scientists now state that no one over 50 should take a separate iron supplement unless they have a medical condition that requires it, as high levels of iron are linked to an increased risk of heart disease, especially in men. If large amounts of iron are recommended because of anaemia, then it is best to see a qualified nutritionist who can re-balance your diet and supplements (see *Useful Information* at the back of this book).
- As we age our stomach-acid levels fall, which means that nutrients are often poorly absorbed from the foods we eat. Taking a digestive enzyme with meals improves absorption.
- There is a genetic disorder called haemochromatosis, which affects 1 in every 200 women, in which iron and large amounts of vitamin C should not be taken. A simple blood test can detect this condition.

A

ANGINA

(see also Atherosclerosis, Cholesterol, Circulation, Heart Disease and High Blood Pressure)

Angina affects about 1 in every 50 people, and in the UK there are an estimated 1.4 million people suffering from this condition. Around 10–15% of women and 10–20% of men over 65 suffer from angina. Angina is often experienced as a pain in the chest, most frequently after exertion such as running up a flight of stairs, but in extreme cases after getting out of a chair. Stress over long periods thickens the blood – see *Stress*. Angina, meanwhile, is brought on by an inadequate supply of oxygen via the blood to the heart muscle. Over many years arteries begin laying down sticky deposits, which harden and eventually cause a narrowing within the blood vessels. See *Atherosclerosis* for prevention and self help for hardening of the arteries.

Typical symptoms include pain in the centre of the chest, which sometimes spreads to the neck/jaw area and down the left arm. The pain can be accompanied by breathlessness, feeling faint, sweating and/or nausea. If you have any of these symptoms, please seek medical attention as a matter of urgency. Cocaine use increases oxidation within the heart, and it damages the heart in a very short time – people who use such drugs are potentially inviting heart disease.

If you are diagnosed as suffering from angina, it's time to make lifestyle changes. For example, if you smoke and are overweight but are willing to change your diet, start exercising and quit smoking – you can reduce your risk of a heart attack or stroke by 400%.

Foods to Avoid

- Cut down on alcohol, which in the long term depletes the body of B-vitamins. When you ingest alcohol, levels of homocysteine (see under *High Blood Pressure* and *Alzheimer's*

Disease), a toxic amino acid linked to heart disease, are raised. Beer contains folate and vitamin B6 – so try an occasional beer instead of spirits and wines.

- Reduce your intake of animal fats, including full-fat dairy produce, pre-packaged cakes, and meat pies, sausages and milk chocolates.
- Avoid sodium-based salt – use magnesium, potassium-based sea salts such as Solo Salt, available from health stores. Or buy some powdered kelp, which is rich in iodine and minerals, and use as a salt substitute.
- Reduce your intake of refined sugars found in cakes, biscuits, fizzy drinks and desserts, which convert to hard fats inside the body if not used up during exercise and contribute to hardening of the arteries.
- Avoid all foods containing hydrogenated or trans fats and fried foods. At all costs, avoid mass-produced, highly refined cooking oils. You can see rows of them in plastic bottles at every supermarket and they are usually bright yellow. (See *Fats You Need To Eat*.)

Friendly Foods

- Pomegranate has been shown to help reverse atherosclerosis (hardening of the arteries) within a year by up to 25% if taken daily, either as a juice or as fresh fruit.
- Oily fish such as salmon, tuna or mackerel are rich in omega-3 fats, which help to thin the blood naturally, as do onions and garlic.
- Cocoa – found in pure dark chocolate – is rich in flavonoids, which helps improve endothelial (smooth muscle) function and improves blood flow. This does not mean that you should be eating lots of dark chocolate! But one or two squares a day of organic dark chocolate are good for you. Milk chocolate does not have the same benefits as it's higher in fat and sugar and lower in cocoa.
- Use a little extra virgin olive oil, pumpkin seed, linseed or walnut oils on salad dressings.
- Eat an avocado a week – rich in vitamin E.
- Include plenty of fresh root ginger in your diet, which improves circulation.
- To help lower LDL cholesterol, often a contributing factor of angina, eat plenty of soluble fibre either from fruit, vegetables, oats or flax seeds (also known as linseeds). See all dietary advice under *Cholesterol*.
- Dried beans such as haricot, kidney, chick peas, soya beans and whole grains such as brown rice, buckwheat, quinoa, millet and barley are all rich in fibre and help to control cholesterol.
- Margarines such as Benecol or Vitaquell are somewhat healthier or use an olive oil-based spread.
- Use non-dairy, organic rice, oat or soya milks, or try low-fat goat's milk.
- If you can follow a vegan diet with the addition of fish (preferably oily), this would be the ideal solution.
- Sprinkle a dessertspoon of high-potency lecithin granules over cereals and salads to help lower LDL cholesterol levels.

Useful Remedies

- There are several formulas that offer pomegranate, blueberry and cocoa in one capsule – available from the Life Extension Foundation (www.lef.org). Currently called Endothelial Defense, with full-spectrum pomegranate. Take 2 capsules daily.
- Taking 1–3 grams of the amino acid L-carnitine daily helps improve functioning of the heart and reduces symptoms associated with angina.
- Taking 100mg twice daily of Co-enzyme Q10 has helped angina patients manage more exercise with fewer symptoms. High-potency CoQ10 is made by Pharma Nord. **PN**
- Natural-source, full-spectrum vitamin E – 400–500iu taken a day – for at least 1 or 2 years thins the blood naturally.

- Fish oils supply EPA and DHA, essential fats that thin the blood naturally. Take 3 grams daily to help reduce chest pain.
- To help reduce angina pain, it is known that high doses of vitamin C and the amino acid lysine, work together to help reverse atherosclerosis. Many companies now make these in a duo formula. To be effective you would need to take 4–5 grams of vitamin C spread throughout the day with food, along with 3 grams of lysine daily in between meals.
- Magnesium helps regulate the heartbeat. Begin on 200mg daily and increase to 400mg.
- Include a good-quality multi-vitamin and mineral in this regimen.
- As many heart conditions are linked to stress, take a good B complex daily, which will support your nerves.
- See supplements under *Atherosclerosis*.

Helpful Hints

- Smoking tends to constrict arterial blood flow – so give it up.
- Remember that negative stress in the long term thickens the blood and constricts arterial flow. See *Stress*.
- If you are overweight, then it is wise to lose weight. Rather than going on a strict diet, this is best achieved by eating healthily. See *General Health Hints* and *Weight Problems*.
- With your doctor's permission, embark on a programme of gentle exercise. Start by walking or swimming for 15 minutes daily, gradually building up to 30 minutes, and then an hour. Tai chi and qiqong are excellent forms of gentle exercise.
- Intravenous antioxidant therapy (chelation) helps to clear blocked arteries and with your doctor's permission is well worth a try. For details, call the Arterial Disease Clinic on 01942 886644.

A

ANTIBIOTICS   *(see also Candida, Immune Function, MRSA and Thrush)*

Doctors and public alike are now becoming aware of the dangers of over-consumption of antibiotics. Nevertheless, around 38 million prescriptions are still written annually in the UK, costing the NHS £175 million. Because of the overuse of antibiotics, bacteria are mutating and many are becoming resistant to increasing numbers of antibiotics, which has in turn triggered an increase in MRSA, C difficile and Acinetobacter, mainly in hospitals. Some people still resort to the use of antibiotics whether they really need them or not. Antibiotics kill the friendly bacteria in the gut, which have an essential role to play in gut and general health. In the long term, antibiotics suppress our immune system, and along with the loss of healthy bacteria in the gut they often allow fungal infections such as candida to flourish. Whenever you have taken an antibiotic, you need a probiotic. Antibiotics mean anti-life and probiotics the opposite – pro-life. Probiotics are supplements containing friendly bacteria called acidophilus or bifidus.

Many doctors report that patients continue to demand antibiotics for colds and flu – which are caused by viruses – but it's only if you contract a secondary infection such as bronchitis, which is bacterial, that antibiotics may be valid.

Taken in the long term, antibiotics can have a very negative effect not only on your immune system, but also on your gut. Eventually this can reduce absorption of nutrients from your food (see also *Absorption* and *Leaky Gut*). Antibiotics can also trigger Athlete's Foot – see *Athlete's Foot*.

Foods to Avoid

- If you have taken antibiotics, avoid foods such as alcohol, sugar and too much sweet fruit (especially bananas, grapes, dates, mangoes, apples, melons and kiwi), which ferment easily within the gut, for one month. Fermentation tends to lead to an overgrowth of unfriendly bacteria, which can trigger conditions such as thrush and candida.

- Avoid mouldy cheeses, which also cause fermentation in the gut.
- Avoid yeast-based breads and foods, such as Marmite and Bovril.

Friendly Foods

- Fruits that don't ferment are OK to eat in moderation – these include berries, blueberries, blackberries, raspberries, as well as cherries plus tropical fruits such as papaya. Eat fruit 30 minutes before a main meal or in between meals to avoid more fermentation
- Pineapple contains the enzyme bromelain, which increases the effectiveness of many antibiotics. Additionally, it acts as a digestive aid, so eat a couple of fresh pineapple chunks before meals.
- Eat plenty of sugar-free, live, low-fat yoghurt, containing acidophilus and bifidus. Read labels, as many so-called 'live' yoghurts are extremely high in sugar, including those that claim to lower LDL cholesterol.
- Artichokes and beetroots contain inulin, which is a substance that encourages the growth of friendly bacteria.
- Garlic encourages the growth of friendly bacteria and also kills bad bacteria as well as helping to fight infections.
- Yeast-free breads and the odd scone are fine, but no jam and cream, please!

Useful Remedies

- Acidophilus and bifidus are healthy bacteria. Take two capsules daily after food for four weeks after completing the antibiotics. Keep these sensitive, live, healthy bacteria in the fridge. Bio Care also make Replete powder, which can be dissolved in water, which will help the gut to rebalance quickly. You can also buy enteric-coated probiotics which do not need to be kept in the fridge. **BC**
- prebiotics, nutrients derived from the agave plant have been shown to increase the natural production of beneficial bacteria in the gut and enhance immune function. I take one scoop of Agave Digestive Immune Support daily in my morning fruit/nut, breakfast blend. For details, log on to www.lef.org or call The Nutri Centre in London on 0845 602 6744.
- Take a B-complex vitamin that includes 0.5–5mg of biotin daily. Biotin is greatly depleted by antibiotics. Lack of biotin affects your skin, hair and nails.
- Goldenseal tincture (1ml) or capsules taken twice a day for up to 2 weeks, or grapefruit seed extract, act like natural antibiotics, and can also be taken to avoid infections in the first place.
- Olive leaf extract is an anti-bacterial, anti-viral and anti-parasitic plant extract that helps to dissolve the coating of bacteria and prevent viral replication. Take up to 4 tablets daily.
- Beta Glucans 1-3, 1-6, derived from yeast cell walls, are proven to strengthen the body's innate immune system, making it more resistant to pathogens from food and air. Take 250–500mg daily. It's a case of one type of yeast killing an altogether more pathogenic type of yeast –
the candida.
- Vitamin D3 helps antibiotics to work more efficiently, and in its own right has anti-bacterial properties. Take 800iu daily.
- Bee propolis is a natural antibiotic used by bees to sterilize their hives. Many therapists and doctors find that two propolis capsules taken every day with at least 1g of vitamin C can lead to a general improvement in health and enhanced resistance to infections.
- A herbal formula containing echinacea, wild indigo, myrrh and low-odour garlic called echinacea compound – take 3–6 capsules daily – helps to boost the immune system. **SHS**

Helpful Hints

- Some plastic, mass-produced chopping boards – advertised as being anti-bacterial – are helping to make people even more resistant to antibiotics, therefore use natural wood chopping boards and simply wash thoroughly in warm, soapy water.
- A little dirt never hurt anyone, and our obsession with bleaching and using anti-bacterial cleansers is not only damaging the environment – but is also in the long term weakening our immune systems.
- If you feel low when taking antibiotics, rather than waiting until you have finished the course, with your doctor's permission, start taking the acidophilus as soon as you begin to feel below par. Also take a high-strength, B-complex vitamin.
- A naturopath or nutritionist can help you restore your immune system (see *Useful Information* at the back of this book).

APHRODISIACS – Male and Female   *(see Libido Problems)*

ARTHRITIS – OSTEO AND RHEUMATOID

(see also Acid–Alkaline Balance, Gout and Lupus)

Osteoarthritis

There are more than 200 types of arthritis, and one in every five adults in the UK suffers from various types of arthritis. Sadly around 12,000 children in the UK suffer juvenile arthritis. By the age of 65, as many as 75% of the Western population are arthritic. It seems that women suffer with arthritis far more than men and it costs the NHS around £6 billion annually to treat.

Over time the cartilage, which cushions and surrounds the joints, breaks down and the bones can become thickened and distorted, which restricts joint movement. In most cases it affects the load-bearing joints – hips, knees, spine and hands. There is a popular misconception that exercise makes you more prone to developing osteoarthritis. In reality, exercise helps to keep your bones healthier and joints more supple.

Primary osteoarthritis develops when our natural cartilage repair process can no longer keep pace with the degenerative wear and tear we can suffer with age. Secondary arthritis is usually triggered by a trauma, such as a broken joint or a fall, or any underlying joint disease. Arthritis has now reached epidemic proportions in the West.

Weight-bearing exercise such as walking, weight-lifting and so on help prevent bone loss (see *Osteoporosis*). Yoga keeps you supple, but if you play contact sports, such as rugby, football or hockey, then the joints are more likely to be damaged.

The majority of people who suffer from osteoarthritis eat too many acid-forming foods (see *Acid–Alkaline Balance*). Basically, proteins such as meat and dairy produce from cows, plus refined carbohydrates like white bread and pizzas are acid forming, whereas fresh vegetables and most fruits plus millet are alkalizing. And if we could all eat less acid-forming foods, many illnesses could be eradicated.

People who develop osteoarthritis are frequently told that they should avoid the nightshade family, which includes tomatoes, potatoes, peppers and aubergines. Out of these tomatoes seem to be the worst offender, as tomatoes contain an alkaloid that can trigger inflammation in the joints, but any foods to which a person is sensitive would need to be avoided. It has been shown that 60–70% of people who avoid these foods for at least 6 months or more see benefits. Being overweight places more stress on joints, which will add to the problem in later life. In cultures such as Okinawa, near Japan, where people eat a mainly wholefood, wholegrain or vegetarian diet, arthritis is virtually unknown.

Foods to Avoid

- Reduce your intake of coffee, alcohol, fizzy drinks and shop-bought cakes, pies, pastries, bread, and pastas that are made with refined white flour and white sugar, which are all highly acid forming.
- Avoid known triggers such as tomatoes, potatoes, aubergines and peppers.
- Gluten, contained in wheat, rye, oats and barley, is a problem for many people.
- Oranges and orange juice can make symptoms worse in some individuals.
- Greatly reduce cow's milk, red meat, high-fat cheeses (especially Stilton), fried foods, sausages, meat pies and chocolate (which is highly acid forming).
- Avoid all white and malt vinegars, which are highly acid forming.
- For anyone suffering gout-type problems, also eliminate foods containing large amounts of purines, which break down into uric acid in the body, as excess uric acid can trigger severe inflammation in small joints, especially the toes. High purine foods are red meats, alcohol, lentils, shellfish, anchovies, mackerel, herrings, sardines and organ meats.

Friendly Foods

- Cherries, plums and blackberries are acid forming, but they help to mobilize uric acid out of the joints, to be excreted in our urine. Cherries and cherry juice are best for gout.
- Pineapple contains bromelain, which is highly anti-inflammatory.
- If you do not suffer from gout, then eat fresh oily fish such as mackerel, organic farmed salmon or sardines three times a week. Mackerel and sardines, along with herrings, are high in purines.
- Sweet potatoes, pumpkin, apricots, papaya and carrots are rich in carotenes and fibre, and the sweet potatoes are a good alternative to ordinary potatoes.
- Grains such as millet, brown rice, amaranth, barley, quinoa, buckwheat and so on are all preferable to refined wheat products. Choose wholemeal breads and try pastas made from corn, buckwheat, rice and lentil flours. Try amaranth crisp breads, sugar-free oatcakes and low-sugar gluten-free muesli or porridge.
- Ask for gluten-free variety breads.
- Eat more fresh green vegetables to re-alkalize your system. One of the quickest ways to do this is to buy a juicer and juice raw cabbage, watercress, celery, parsley and a little root ginger, and drink immediately. You can also make delicious fruit blends (remember we are blending here, not juicing, so you also get the peel which contains all the fibre). My favourite is half a cup of fresh blueberries, a chopped pear, a chopped apple and a sliced banana, a heaped teaspoon of any organic-source, 'green'-based powder from your health store (see *Useful Remedies*), a tablespoon of soaked linseeds (flax seeds) and aloe vera juice, all blended with a cup of organic rice or almond milk. Fabulous!
- Fresh root ginger can be made into a wonderful pain-relieving tea. Add a small cube of fresh root ginger to a mug of boiling water, add half a teaspoon of honey and apple cider vinegar and sip when warm.
- Blackstrap molasses is rich in calcium, potassium and magnesium, which all help the joints. Try adding a teaspoon of the molasses and a tablespoon of organic apple cider vinegar or a little lemon juice into a cup of warm water, which helps you to absorb more minerals from your diet and helps to re-alkalize your system. For those who prefer honey, buy organic,

preferably locally produced, and if at all possible unrefined, which contains more natural minerals. If your symptoms are severe, drink this cocktail up to three times daily.

- Use organic, unrefined olive, sunflower, walnut or sesame oils for your salad dressings.
- Eat at least one tablespoon of linseeds (flax seeds soaked overnight), or sunflower, pumpkin or sesame seeds daily, as they are rich in essential fats that are vital for healthy joints. Hazelnuts, cashew, almonds and walnuts are all rich in essential fats to nourish the joints. An easy way to eat more of them is to place 2 tablespoons of each in a blender, whizz for 1 minute and store in an air-tight jar in the fridge. Sprinkle over breakfast cereal, fruit salads or into low-fat, bio yoghurts daily.
- Try herbal teas such as devil's claw and nettle and use dandelion coffee.
- Add more turmeric and cayenne pepper to your cooking, because they help to reduce inflammation.

Useful Remedies

- One of the best nutritional supplements known to help this condition is the amino sugar, glucosamine sulphate. A number of studies have found that taking 1500mg daily can substantially reduce pain and improve mobility. Initially take 1500mg of glucosamine a day until symptoms improve and then lower the dose to 500mg daily. This may take several months. **NB Glucosamine is usually derived from crab shells, so if you have a severe intolerance to shellfish avoid this supplement. But, it is also available in a vegetarian formula derived from corn.** For more details contact Health Perception on 0800 046 1846, or log on to www.health-perception.co.uk. The Glucosamine combined with MSM, methylsulfonylmethane, a form of sulphur, seems to be even more effective.

A

- To help quickly re-alkalize your system, take Green pH, made by Metabolics (www.metabolics.com) – one small level teaspoon daily in water. A mixture of green beans, garden peas, pea leaf, dry apple cider, watercress, broccoli and nettle leaf, it doesn't taste great, but is an easy and quick way to alkalize your body. Available from the Wholistic Medical Centre. **WMC**
- Niacinamide (no-flush vitamin B3) is a great alternative to glucosamine, which helps to reduce joint pain. Take 500mg 3 times a day. Some people reap the benefits in as little as 4 to 5 weeks, but ideally 3 months to a year is a good time scale to take this vitamin. **NB Be sure to ask for the 'no-flush' variety, as common niacin can cause a flushing effect that can be quite shocking if you are unprepared.**
- As all the B-group vitamins work together, add a B-complex to your daily regimen.
- To help reduce the pain, take a couple of teaspoons of cod liver oil daily, which also includes pain-relieving vitamin D. Or take 3 cod liver oil capsules daily. Many fish oils are now high in toxins that have been pumped into the world's oceans, most notably dioxins (deadly chemicals formed during incineration of plastic) and PCBs (persistent industrial chemicals used in electrical equipment), and many fish oils contain far too many toxins that can adversely affect hormones. Try Seven Seas' One a Day pure cod liver oil, available at all health stores. You can take either cod liver oil or pure omega-3 fish oils, such as Eskimo 3 or Pharma Nord. If the pain is especially bad, you can take up to 3 grams of fish oil daily. **PN**
- Natural-source, full-spectrum vitamin E 400iu daily helps to reduce pain.
- Take 1–3 grams of vitamin C daily in an ascorbate form with meals, which does not irritate the gut and has anti-inflammatory properties. Vitamin C is vital for healthy synovial fluid that surrounds the joints.
- Ginger, curcumin and boswellia are herbs with highly anti-inflammatory properties, take 3–4 tablets a day.
- The formula Ligazyme Plus, made by BioCare, contains vital minerals such as calcium, boron,

magnesium, rutin, silica plus vitamins A and D and digestive enzymes, which all support connective tissue and encourage healthier bones. **BC**

- Include a good-quality antioxidant formula in your regimen, which helps stabilize cartilage membranes.
- Curcumin capsules are really useful for reducing inflammation and increasing circulation. Take 2–3 capsules daily in the middle of main meals.
- Homeopathic Rhus Tox 6x helps to relieve stiffness when you first move around. It is especially good for people whose symptoms are worse when it's cold and wet.
- Homeopathic Ruta Graveolens 30c often helps if tendons are sore and if spine and joints feel sore and feel worse when it's cold and wet.
- Use liquid hyaluronic acid (HA). HA is a naturally occurring protein found in all bone and cartilage structures in the body. HA provides the cushioning affect in all joints and it's the high content of HA in young people that keeps their joints (especially the knees) so supple. As we age, levels fall. By taking 1ml daily in water you can help restore some of the elasticity in connective tissue and joints. It is also useful for rheumatoid arthritis. For more details ask at your health store, or call Modern Herbals on 01274 889047 or log on to www.modernherbals.com

Rheumatoid Arthritis (RA)   *(see also Leaky Gut and Lupus)*

Rheumatoid arthritis is primarily an inflammatory disease of the smaller joints, such as wrists, ankles, fingers and knees. It is an autoimmune disorder whereby the body's own immune system starts attacking joint tissue and is very much linked to leaky gut syndrome (see *Leaky Gut*). RA is linked to conditions such as lupus. It is a chronic disease and tends to progress with time but many people find the pain and stiffness comes and goes for varying periods of time. RA affects three times as many women as men and most often occurs between the ages of 25 to 50. Over-acidity in the body and uric acid deposits in the joints is a contributing factor (see *Acid–Alkaline Balance*).

The pain and stiffness are usually worse upon rising, and tend to wear off as the day progresses. The joints can become warm, tender and swollen. Fatigue, low-grade fever, loss of appetite, and vague muscular pains can all accompany RA. Researchers have found that at least one-third of people can completely control their rheumatoid arthritis by eliminating foods to which they have an intolerance. The most common culprits are any foods and drinks from cows, plus the nightshade group (see Foods to Avoid under *Osteoarthritis*). Gluten is a problem for many sufferers of RA. Some people even react to various beans, including kidney, mung and aduki.

Other triggers are a leaky gut, which is when food molecules pass through the gut wall, thus triggering an allergic response. Many RA sufferers also have parasites and candida, a yeast fungal overgrowth. There can also be a genetic susceptibility (see *Candida* and *Leaky Gut*).

Heavy exercise may cause RA to progress faster, but gentle exercise such as swimming, t'ai chi, yoga, stretching and walking are more helpful. Researchers have found that many rheumatoid arthritis sufferers are deficient in the major antioxidant nutrients, vitamins A, C and E, plus the mineral selenium – but particularly vitamin E. The majority of RA sufferers also appear to be low in stomach acid and supplementing with betaine hydrochloride (stomach acid) can help. (See also *Low Stomach Acid*.) Betaine helps to digest the proteins and most people who have allergies have a problem digesting certain proteins. If you have active stomach ulcers, do not take the betaine and use a papaya- or pineapple-based digestive enzyme capsule instead.

RA is virtually unknown in primitive cultures where the diet is mainly alkaline-forming foods, nor do these people have antibiotics or refined foods, which also contribute to RA.

Autoimmune disease for the most part takes years to develop; years of eating too many foods that don't agree with your physiology, plus stress, lifestyle and so on all contribute to the condition. However, if you change these actions, then over time your body is perfectly capable of healing itself.

Foods to Avoid
- Animal fats eaten to excess tend to aggravate RA. Avoiding all dairy produce from cows, plus meat (especially red meat), sugar and eggs helps some people.
- Avoid or greatly reduce known triggers such as tomatoes, potatoes, aubergines, peppers and gluten.
- Oranges and orange juice can be a problem for most people with RA.
- Coffee, chocolate in general, peanuts, spinach, strawberries, rhubarb and beetroot are all high in oxalic acid, which seems to further aggravate RA in some people.
- Greatly reduce your intake of refined sugary foods and drinks.
- Avoid wheat and any foods containing gluten, citrus (especially oranges and grapefruit), corn, food additives, colourings and flavourings. Keep a food diary and note when symptoms are more acute. Eliminate these foods for a week or so and see if this helps.
- Beans such as aduki, mung and haricot contain a lectin, a protein that is hard to digest; if you like these foods, be sure to take a digestive enzyme.

Friendly Foods
- Eat more curries made with curcumin (derived from the spice turmeric), which has powerful anti-inflammatory properties.
- Eat more pineapple – it is a rich source of bromelain, which is known to have highly anti-inflammatory properties.
- Cherries mobilize uric acid out of the body – eat them regularly when in season or use frozen cherries.
- Eat oily fish, such as organic farmed salmon or mackerel, at least 3 times a week or take a couple of teaspoons of fish oil daily. These omega-3 essential fats reduce uric acid levels. (See also *Fats You Need To Eat*.)
- Use linseed (flax seed) oil plus unrefined olive or hemp seed oil in salad dressings.
- A vegan diet has been shown to help some individuals.
- Root ginger, plus the spices turmeric and boswellia, have anti-inflammatory properties. These will not alleviate the problem, but they can substantially reduce the pain and give people more mobility.
- Make a tea using fresh ginger and lemon juice.
- Eat plenty of garlic and use rice, oat or almond organic milks as alternatives to dairy produce from cows.
- Avocado and raw wheat germ is rich in vitamin E and essential fats.
- Eat lots more green vegetables, especially raw green cabbage, kale, spring greens, watercress, parsley and endives. Alternatively, add an organic green food powder based on wheat grass, spirulina, alfalfa, chlorella and green foods, available from health food stores, to cereals, juices and desserts.
- Under professional guidance, juice fasts can greatly reduce symptoms.
- Modest amounts of aloe vera are helpful, as aloe is anti-inflammatory, aids gut health and improves the production of digestive enzymes.

Useful Remedies

- For those who don't like fresh pineapple, bromelain is available as a supplement. Take one capsule – 500mg – of bromelain on an empty stomach to increase its effectiveness.
- The herbs curcumin and boswellia are also available in tablet and capsule formulas, 1200–1600mg of any one.
- Evening primrose oil can help, but you would need very high amounts and the reason people take EPO is for the GLA (gamma linolenic acid) content. GLA is highly anti-inflammatory and is available as a supplement. Take 1–4 grams daily. **BC**
- Vitamin C, 1–3 grams daily spread throughout the day taken with meals, plus 400–800iu of natural-source, full-spectrum vitamin E.
- A multi-mineral containing 30mg of zinc, 100–150mcg of selenium plus traces of copper is known to help reduce pain.
- EPA-DHA pure fish oil 1–4 grams daily
- Many sufferers of RA benefit from taking vitamin B5 pantothenic acid; 500mg can be taken 4 times a day. Pure Royal Jelly has a high B5 content.
- As B-vitamins work together, include a B-complex.
- L-glutamine is an amino acid found in cabbage; 500mg x 3 times daily can help heal a leaky gut. Take 30 minutes prior to a meal.
- Sufferers of RA are often lacking in healthy bacteria within their guts, therefore a daily prebiotic powder with breakfast such as Agave Digestive Immune Support helps the gut to naturally produce more friendly bacteria. Log on to www.lef.org or call the Nutri Centre. **NC**

- A multi-mineral formula taken daily helps to re-alkalize the body.
- Vitamin K2 has been found to reduce inflammation in RA sufferers and is vital for bone and arterial health, as K2 keeps calcium out of the arteries and in the bones. **If you are taking blood-thinning drugs such as Warfarin, you need to avoid vitamin K.** Otherwise, try 100mcg daily.
- Vitamin D3 is useful for slowing progression of RA and has a protective effect against autoimmune conditions – take 3000iu daily for one month, then stop for a month, then take a maintenance dose of 1000iu daily.
- A fermented wheat germ extract known as Avemar has demonstrated remarkable immune-modulating effects and helps restore balance in immune systems that are over-stimulated. Avemar has been shown in numerous trials to reduce the symptoms of autoimmune disease, including RA. Take one sachet daily in water at least one hour before breakfast. Also available in capsules. Must be kept refrigerated. Details on www.avemar.com. **NC**
- Olive leaf extract has been proven to reduce inflammation and some people derive great pain relief by taking 500mg, 3 times daily before meals. Available from all good health stores.

Helpful Hints for All Types of Arthritis

- A short fast under professional guidance almost always alleviates symptoms, as it reduces the toxic load within the body. And once you look after your liver and heal any gut problems, symptoms are greatly reduced.
- If you are overweight this places more strain on the load-bearing joints, so lose weight.
- Hot and cold compresses applied alternately will help reduce swelling and pain for 20 minutes at a time. Cold compresses are especially good if the affected joints feel hot to the touch. Moist hot packs help reduce pain and stiffness.
- Joint cartilage needs plenty of fluids, so drink six glasses of water daily, which also helps eliminate uric acid. Hard water can sometimes exacerbate arthritic-type symptoms, because it is packed with minerals, but in an inorganic form that is hard to absorb. However, fruits and vegetables are able to absorb the inorganic minerals and, aided by sunlight, convert

them to an organic form – and when minerals are in an organic form, they become more bio-available to us.

- To ingest the 21 minerals that are essential for life, it makes sense to eat far more fresh fruits and vegetables. But unfortunately thanks to pollution, over-farming and acid rain, most soils (especially in the UK) no longer contain sufficient minerals needed for good health. And if the minerals are not in the soil, they are never going to make it into our vegetables (although organic foods generally contain more minerals). This is why we all need to begin taking a daily multi-mineral.
- Numerous people have experienced benefits after taking pure aloe vera juice daily for several months.
- Nettle tea taken regularly has helped reduce the pain and swelling for many people.
- To re-alkalize your system, take a good-quality green powder such as Green pH, made by Metabolics (www.metabolics.com) – one small level teaspoon daily in water, preferably taken 30 minutes before a meal or in between meals. A mixture of green beans, garden peas, pea leaf, dry apple cider, watercress, broccoli and nettle Leaf, it doesn't taste great, but is an easy and quick way to alkalize your body. Available for retail from the Wholistic Medical Centre. **WMC**
- Use Alkabath salts, which are more powerful than Epsom salts and help to eliminate toxins from the joints. For your nearest stockists, call Best Care Products on 01342 410303 or log on to www.bestcare-uk.com. They also supply water distillers. See also *Acid–Alkaline Balance*.
- Use Kangen Water – a water system that attaches to your kitchen tap that ionizes and alkalizes water. It's used in Japanese hospitals with highly beneficial health results. For full details, call 020 7580 7537 or log on to www.kangenmiraclewater.co.uk.
- Topically applied oil of wintergreen can help ease the pain and inflammation.
- Homeopathic Apis 30c helps in rheumatoid arthritis when there is swelling and rheumatic pains that are worse for heat.
- If the RA is in the small joints, ask at your homeopathic pharmacy for Actea Spicata-3c, taken 3 times daily between meals helps reduce the pain.
- The Chinese exercise regimes of t'ai chi or qigong have helped many sufferers, as these exercises are easy to practise, even with severely impaired mobility. RA can be greatly affected by stress, so make sure you stay as calm as possible (see *Stress*).
- Call the Arthritic Association on Freephone 0800 652 3188 or 01323 416550 between 10am and 1pm or 2 and 4pm on weekdays, or log on to their website: www.arthriticassociation.org.uk. This charity provides very good dietary advice and has a great website. Annual membership costs £6.

ASTHMA

(see also Allergies and Leaky Gut)

Over 5.5 million people in the UK now suffer from asthma, 1.2 million are children and the problem is escalating. The cost to the NHS is over £1billion annually.

Asthma affects the bronchial tubes leading to our lungs, resulting in periods of wheezing and shortness of breath. Pollution from traffic fumes, especially diesel and overuse of pesticides, is without doubt a huge contributing factor, and during school holidays incidents of attacks are reduced as there is less traffic.

Other atmospheric pollutants such as pollen, cigarette smoke and car exhaust fumes can all be triggers, as can house dust mites and moulds. Stressful situations and chronic exhaustion can also trigger an attack, as can eating foods to which you have a sensitivity (such as sulphur dioxide, used as a preservative in many dried fruits and salt). You can also suffer exercise-induced asthma. There is also a link between parasites and asthma

People who take paracetamol every day are twice as likely to suffer asthma, and if you take it twice weekly you are 80% more likely to be affected.

Several studies have also demonstrated that expectant mothers given prebiotics, which enhance immune function by encouraging healthy bacteria to be produced in the gut, are less likely to have babies who suffer asthma. And, infants given prebiotics and probiotics suffer far less incidences of asthma.

Foods to Avoid

- There is a strong association between asthma and dairy products, especially cow's milk in children.
- Any foods to which you have an intolerance will make you more susceptible to attacks. The most common are wheat, mass-produced cereals, nuts, chocolate or tomatoes. For details of good tests, see *Allergies*.
- Reduce intake of all meats, eggs and full-fat dairy produce from any source (cow's, sheep's, goats and soya), which can increase mucous production.
- A recent study in Taiwan showed that people who eat a lot of meat, especially liver and high-fat foods, were more likely to develop asthma.
- Sodium-based salt in any foods (some people can have an attack after eating too many crisps).
- Some mass-produced, ready-prepared salads, dried fruits, wines and beers contain sulphur dioxide, which is known to trigger problems in sensitive individuals.
- Avoid sodium benzoate, which is frequently found in soft drinks and MSG.
- Generally avoid all mass-produced, pre-packaged foods.
- Avoid aspirin.

Friendly Foods

- Depending on your level of sensitivity, if you have a problem with dairy products, then try rice, almond, hemp, quinoa or oat milks. Be aware that some people react to almonds, so try the other milks first.
- Green leafy vegetables, fresh fruits and organic honey are rich in magnesium, which helps the airways to relax. A lack of magnesium is linked to breathing problems. Brown rice, avocados, spinach, haddock, watercress, oatmeal, porridge, baked potatoes, navy beans, lima beans, broccoli, bananas, soya beans and unrefined nuts are all rich in magnesium.
- Include more lentils, garlic and onions in your diet, which help to fight infection and clear the lungs.
- As asthma is often linked by nutritional physicians to a 'leaky gut', include plenty of fresh ginger in your diet, which is very soothing. Cabbage and aloe vera juice also help heal the gut (see *Leaky Gut*).
- Eat oily fish three times a week, which is rich in vitamin A and is said to reduce the severity and frequency of asthma attacks. Sweet potatoes, apricots, papaya, watermelon and pumpkin are also high in natural-source carotenes, which naturally convert to vitamin A in the body.
- Use extra-virgin, unrefined olive and sunflower oils in salad dressings and include plenty of linseeds (flax seeds), pumpkin, sunflower and sesame seeds in your diet.
- Cauliflower, apples, papaya, pears, cherries, grapes, pineapple, kale, and green tea are all great foods for the lungs.
- Buy a juicer and make yourself a carrot, ginger, cabbage, radish, apple and celery mix – drink

immediately. Try different mixes daily, which is a great way to get health-giving nutrients into the body.

- Vine-ripened tomatoes are rich in lycopene, which is beneficial for the lungs (and prostate). Cooking in a little olive oil helps release the lycopene.
- Sprinkle turmeric on your meals or add to cooking, as this herb has anti-inflammatory properties and supports the immune system.
- After an attack, drink plenty of fluids to help break up mucous so that it can be expelled.
- Children who eat more fresh fruits and vegetables are known to suffer fewer attacks.
- Eat more edible white membranes in lemons – they contain limonene, which is great for the lungs.

Useful Remedies
- Do not give large doses of supplements to young children – take advice from a nutritionist. See *Useful Information* at the back of book.
- Take a good-quality, multi-vitamin daily; plus a multi-mineral containing 400–800mg of magnesium; plus 200mcg of selenium, as low levels leave you more at risk from an attack.
- Vitamin C in the form of magnesium ascorbate. Take 1 gram, 3 times a day with meals to help open the airways. **BC**
- Take vitamin B6, 150mg a day; B12, 1,000–2,000mcg a day; plus a B-complex. Asthma medication depletes B vitamins, especially in people who are sensitive to sulphates.
- The enzyme bromelain extracted from pineapples. Taking 400–500mg once or twice daily helps to reduce mucous production and ease breathing.
- Take 60mg a day of natural-source beta-carotene complex if you suffer from exercise-induced asthma.
- The herb ginkgo biloba – 120–240mg standardized extract, or 3–4ml of tincture, taken daily – has been shown to improve circulation and decrease asthma symptoms. **SHS**
- Trials in America found that people with low levels of Vitamin D suffered more attacks. Take a minimum of 800–1000iu daily.
- Quercetin, a polyphenol compound found in red wine and garlic, acts as an anti-inflammatory – and has been found to greatly reduce the incidence of asthma attacks in which chemicals are involved. Take 500mg daily with food.
- Specialist Herbal Supplies 'Lung Formula' contains bronchial-dilating herbs, which help open the airways. **SHS**
- Try Respiratory De-Tox formula made from ginger, myrrh, garlic, echinacea and lobelia – 15 drops a day. This helps expand the airways and keep the respiratory tract clearer. **OP**
- Pine bark extract, known as pycnogenol, has been shown to ease breathing in asthma patients. Take as directed. **PN**
- Take a prebiotic, probiotic formula daily.
- As many people who suffer asthma have a 'leaky gut', see *Leaky Gut* – and if you think the symptoms apply to you, then take a digestive enzyme with all main meals.
- As low levels of omega-3 essential fats, plus GLA (gamma linolenic acid) also tend to be low in asthma sufferers, take a one gram fish oil daily plus 2 grams of Mega GLA. **BC**
- Colostrum, which is found in breast milk, helps support the immune system and aids healing of a leaky gut; it's very helpful for babies and children suffering from asthma. Up to the age of two, take a quarter of a teaspoon twice daily on an empty stomach. Over 2 years – half a teaspoon twice daily. Take this for just one month. **NC**

Helpful Hints
- People who are overweight tend to suffer more breathing and inflammatory problems.
- The steroidal inhalers deplete magnesium from the body, which can mean a sufferer becomes

ever-more dependent on their inhaler – which is why a daily intake of magnesium is absolutely crucial.

■ Avoid chlorinated pools as exposure to chlorine can constrict the airways.

■ Use an ionizer in any room in which you are going to spend any length of time, as it can reduce the amount of pollen and dust in the air.

■ Use Ultra Breathe, a very handy, inexpensive device that does a great job of exercising the lungs. It costs £16.95 plus £2.95 for postage and packaging. For details log on to www.ultrabreathe.com.

■ Try to avoid antibiotics during the infant years, as they have been linked to an increased risk of developing asthma in later life.

■ Acupuncture has proved useful for many sufferers.

■ Check for food and environmental allergens – see details of good tests under *Allergies*.

■ It is incredible how many people suffer breathing problems simply because they are not using their lungs properly. Most asthmatics benefit from tuition in proper breathing techniques. Every 20 minutes or so, remember to take a deep breath down into your lower-abdomen area. Buteyko is a breathing technique that has been known to help with asthma. For further information and to find a local practitioner, call the Buteyko Breathing Association on 01277 366 906 or log on to www.buteykobreathing.org.

■ Shallow breathing is associated with being stressed. Learn relaxation techniques or consult a hypnotherapist who can teach you how to relax (see *Useful Information*).

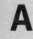

■ Take gentle exercise such as yoga, t'ai chi, swimming or walking. Exercise reduces stress and helps you to breathe, which should help to reduce the incidence of asthma attacks.

■ Consult a nutritionist (see *Useful Information*).

■ Homeopathy has proved especially helpful for children, but be sure to consult a qualified homeopath. Call the Organic Pharmacy in London on 020 7351 2232 during office hours and have a word with the on-duty pharmacist; or call any homeopathic local pharmacy that you trust.

■ Have a regular massage using essential oils of camomile and lavender.

■ A company specializing in indoor, air-quality equipment is the JS Air and Water Centre. Tel: 01903 858657 or log on to www.airandwatercentre.com.

■ Stress is a major factor in asthma – so try and stay calm. (See *Stress*.)

■ It may be worth consulting a chiropractor or cranial osteopath as blocked airways may link back to nerve compression in the spine.

■ For a further range of asthma information, contact Asthma UK on 0800 121 6244 or log on to www.asthma.org.uk.

ATHEROSCLEROSIS – Hardening and narrowing of the arteries

(See also Angina, Cholesterol, Circulation and Heart Disease)

Atherosclerosis is technically narrowing of the arteries and arteriosclerosis is hardening of the arteries, but most people describe both as hardening of the arteries. The most common cause of atherosclerosis is based upon damaged LDL cholesterol, oxidized fatty deposits, which over the years adhere to our artery walls. In addition a high homocysteine level, a marker for heart disease, causes inflammation of the inner arterial lining. To try to repair the damage, the body produces collagen to form a cap over the damaged tissue, which can then attract calcium deposits, which is why this condition is most commonly referred to as hardening of the arteries.

Atherosclerosis is the leading cause of disability and death in the Western world and is the major trigger for most heart conditions including angina, coronary heart disease, plus strokes, circulation and memory problems and complications in diabetics. My father, although thin like me, died of a heart attack at just 50 and his death certificate read atherosclerosis. He had spent a lifetime smoking, eating the wrong foods and not taking sufficient exercise. He was also exposed to considerable amounts of stress.

Genetic factors are believed to play a role in hardening of the arteries, but without doubt, our diet has a huge part to play. And because of the increase in junk food intake and little exercise, cardiologists are now seeing this condition in teenagers – which is shocking.

Foods to Avoid
- The days of people eating lard as my father did regularly are long gone – however, lard has been replaced by hydrogenated, trans fats found in mass-produced pies, cakes, sweets, cheap milk chocolates, ice cream, biscuits, sausages, fried foods and most take-aways. Some supermarkets, such as Marks and Spencer, have now sensibly banned these fats in their foods; hopefully, others will follow suit.
- Greatly cut down on sodium-based salts, found in virtually all pre-packaged meals, pies, pizzas and so on.
- Avoid cheese in general, although a small of amount of goat's or cottage cheese is fine. Or ask for low-fat cheeses. Have cheese as an occasional treat.
- Reduce your intake of red meat, but if you do have meat, try to make it organic and cut the fat off. Venison, turkey, chicken breast, rabbit, guinea fowl, pheasant – all of these are fine in moderation.
- Reduce your intake of all full-fat dairy products – this includes butter.

Friendly Foods
- Pomegranate has been proven during trials in Israel to disrupt formation of plaque, and has also shown some benefit in reducing blood pressure. Practically every supermarket now sells pomegranate seeds ready to eat and I take at least a tablespoon daily. Otherwise, drink the juice daily: trials in America found that when patients drank the juice daily for a year, atherosclerosis was reduced by as much as 25%.
- Include garlic in your diet, as it protects against the oxidation of LDL cholesterol.
- Curcumin, extracted from the spice turmeric, used in curries, lowers LDL.
- Eat more oily fish, especially organic farmed salmon, pilchards, sardines and mackerel.
- Pure, dark chocolate is low in fat, dairy and sugar and high in flavonoids, which also protect LDL against oxidation and improve blood flow. You can eat two small squares daily, of high-quality, dark chocolate.
- Eat more fresh root ginger and artichokes.
- Drink more organic green and white tea, which helps to lower LDL.
- Red wine contains polyphenols, such as resveratrol and quercetin, which help to protect LDL against oxidation – one of the main triggers for atherosclerosis.
- For a larger list, see Friendly Foods under *Heart Disease*.

Useful Remedies
- There are several formulas that contain pure cocoa, concentrated pomegranate, and either blueberry extract or superoxide dismutase, an enzyme known to defend the body against oxidative stress. The Life Extension Foundation make a good one called Endothelial Defence, with full-spectrum pomegranate. Details can be found at www.lef.org. NC

- Otherwise, take a full-spectrum pomegranate formula. **NC**.
- Take a garlic capsule such as Allimax daily. It contains a good level of allicin, the active ingredient in garlic, which helps thin the blood naturally.
- The spice turmeric contains curcumin, which has highly anti-inflammatory properties – and as atherosclerosis is basically inflammation of the arteries, taking this spice daily in a concentrated form with meals can greatly reduce plaque forming. Take around 1 gram daily in divided doses with food. See www.lef.org.
- Omega-3 essential fats are vital for healthy arteries – take 2 grams daily.
- Vitamin C helps protect the artery walls – take 2–3 grams daily in divided doses with food.
- Carnitine is an amino acid that helps remove fat deposited in the arteries. Take 500mg three times daily, 30 minutes or so before food.
- Full-spectrum, natural-source Vitamin E (400iu daily) protects against oxidation of LDL, as does lipoic acid (200mg daily).
- Take a high-strength B complex or take Homocysteine Formula by Metabolics – one three times daily. To order, log on to www.metabolics.com or contact the Wholistic Medical Centre. **WMC**
- If you are taking statins, you need to take the nutrient Co-enzyme Q10, which protects the heart muscle as statins reduce production of this essential nutrient. Take 100mg daily.
- Several studies have demonstrated that a lack of vitamin K2 *accelerates* arterial calcification, whereas taking K2 daily (approx 100mcg) can help keep excess calcium in the bones and out of your arteries. **NB Vitamin K cannot be taken by people on Warfarin.**

- Niacin – Vitamin B3 – is known to help reduce arterial plaque, raise levels of HDL (the 'good' cholesterol), which in turn helps remove cholesterol deposits from artery walls. But niacin can trigger a flushing for about 45 minutes after taking it, especially in women. No-flush niacin does not have this plaque reducing effect. For plaque reduction, you would need to take 500–1000mg of B3 daily for several weeks. Begin by taking 500mg of the flavonoid quercetin with breakfast, which greatly reduces the flushing sensations, then at lunch try 100mg of niacin and again another 100mg with supper. Be sensible – work on increasing the dose that you can manage and take at appropriate times to suit your schedule. Niacin is more effective if taken with 100mcg of chromium daily.
- **NB In rare cases, regular intake of niacin can have a negative effect on the liver, therefore if you have ever suffered from any liver disease do not take niacin. It can also in some people upset a sensitive gut.**

Helpful Hints
- Hormones play an important role in this condition – thyroid, DHEA, progesterone and testosterone and oestrogen levels need to be checked and balanced as required.
- See Helpful Hints under *Cholesterol*, *Circulation* and *Heart Disease*.
- Having an animal to stroke regularly helps to lower cholesterol and blood pressure naturally!
- Have a carotid artery doppler ultrasound, which gives a good indication as to how much plaque you are laying down in your arteries. It costs approximately £300. For details, contact the European Scanning Centre, 68 Harley Street, London W1G 7HE. Tel 020 7436 5755. Alternatively, speak to your GP.
- Several studies have confirmed a link between gum disease and atherosclerosis – therefore have regular dental check-ups and practise good oral hygiene.

ATHLETE'S FOOT   *(see also Antibiotics and Candida)*

Athlete's foot is caused by a fungal infection of the skin and is characterized by itchy, flaking and cracked skin, especially between the toes and on the soles of the feet. This problem can be transmitted in public places such as swimming baths, where people walk barefoot, and in moist atmospheres. Wear socks made from natural fibres, such as cotton, silk or bamboo, which allow the skin to breathe, and change footwear regularly. It is important that feet are dried properly after bathing or exercise. Persistent athlete's foot is often associated with an overgrowth of candida in the gut (see also *Candida*).

Foods to Avoid
- Avoid sugar when symptoms are acute. Sugars ferment and feed yeasts in the body.
- Avoid foods containing yeast such as cheese, wine, yeasty breads, beer, mushrooms, vinegar, soy sauce and yeast-based drinks such as Bovril and Marmite.
- Grapes are high in sugar and may have moulds on the skin. Blueberries should also be avoided for a short time as they, too, often have moulds on their skin.
- Peanuts should also be avoided.

Friendly Foods
- Shitake mushrooms are the exception, as they naturally contain beta glucans, which help reduce fungal infections.
- Eat plenty of garlic and onions, which are anti-bacterial and anti-fungal.
- Live, low-fat yoghurt contains acidophlius and bifidus – eat at least 250 grams a day.
- See also diet under *Candida*.

Useful Remedies
- If you have sore open patches, chiropodist Margaret Dabbs suggests applying salt water to aid healing and then using pure emu oil, which is a good anti-fungal with anti-inflammatory properties to aid healing. For details, log on to www.margaretdabbs.co.uk.
- Apply some liquid grapefruit seed extract (known as citricidal) externally. **NC**
- Black walnut and calendula tincture, applied topically and taken internally twice a day, can be effective.
- Try tea tree, manuka and neem cream. Apply twice daily. **OP**
- Pierce a low-odour garlic capsule in powder form and sprinkle on the affected area.
- Beta Glucans 1-3, 1-6, although derived from yeast cell walls, are proven to strengthen the body's innate immune system and kill pathogenic yeasts. Pharma Nord make a version that is free from yeast protein. Take 250–500mg daily. **PN**

Helpful Hints
- Pau d'arco is the bark from a South American tree and boosts immune function and helps fight fungal infections. It makes a very pleasant tasting tea and is also easily available in capsules. Take six capsules daily or drink several cups as tea. It can also be added to a foot wash made with tea tree oil.
- Add 5–10 drops of citricidal liquid to a footbath and soak feet twice daily.
- You may not want to try this! Dip an old cloth in fresh urine and wrap around the affected area – urine is a natural anti-fungal. Change the 'bandage cloth' daily.
- Most sports shops now sell socks made from bamboo, a sustainable material that has anti-bacterial properties.

A

AUTISM

(see also Allergies and Leaky Gut)

According to the National Autistic Society, approximately 500,000 people, mainly children in the UK, have autism, with 40% of those waiting at least three years for a clear diagnosis. Four times as many boys are affected as girls, with symptoms generally beginning in early childhood. Its numerous symptoms include an inability to communicate and concentrate, impaired language and learning, disturbed sleep patterns, hyperactivity, abnormal social relationships, rituals and compulsive behaviour.

Autism is linked to a lack of essential fat (EFA) intake during pregnancy, as 60% of our brains are made from EFAs. Low vitamin D levels during pregnancy and in infants are also linked to debilitating brain dysfunction. It also now appears that genetic and environmental factors contribute to autism.

Meanwhile, reports are ongoing linking the increase in autism to toxic overload. This could either be from vaccines – I believe that the MMR (measles, mumps and rubella) vaccine could trigger delayed responses in some cases, which could either be generated by the mercury content of vaccines or the vaccine itself. Other causes are exposure to pesticides, PCBs and heavy metals such as mercury, lead and aluminium, plus chemicals in foods such as phenolic compounds and salicylates (see below).

Research also shows that incompletely digested particles of wheat and dairy were found in higher amounts in children with behavioural problems and a link is widely acknowledged between neurotoxins such as mercury in the brain and autism. Problems with digestion, absorption and elimination are often seen and most children with autism have a leaky gut. Reduced breakdown of proteins in milk and gluten (wheat, rye, oats and barley) leads to 'neurotoxins' entering the brain and disrupting brain chemistry. Many autistic children have also been given large doses of antibiotics, which in the long term can trigger more gut problems – these in turn can initiate intolerances and sensitivities to many foods (see also *Allergies*, *Candida* and *Leaky Gut*).

Poor immune function and sluggish liver function (see under *Liver Problems*) can contribute to this condition, as can fungal overgrowth (see *Candida*). I have heard of several cases where autistic children have been referred to psychiatrists, and when given mind-altering drugs the children's symptoms worsened considerably.

Foods to Avoid

- Remove all gluten from the child's diet. This is in most breads, biscuits and cereals. Remember that rye, barley and oats also contain gluten. Many doctors are now happy to prescribe gluten-free products on the NHS. Some children suffered withdrawal-type symptoms and became worse before their parents noticed improvements.
- Dairy produce from cows should also be avoided.
- Soya foods and products are potentially high risk for a negative reaction in autism. Eggs, citrus fruits, chocolate, peanuts, or any nuts to which there is an intolerance. Shellfish have been found to cause many problems associated with food intolerance/allergy and leaky gut.
- Avoid all pre-packaged, junk-type foods and drinks that are packed with salt, sugar and animal fats. Keep a food diary and note when symptoms become worse.
- Avoiding additives found in packaged and processed foods is a must, as they may contain compounds that can be toxic to the brain when the body fails to break them down properly.
- For some children avoiding excitotoxins – chemicals that stimulate the brain – is helpful. Foods rich in salicylates (a form of excitotoxins) are oranges, almonds, apples, apricots, tomatoes, cherries, cranberries, cucumbers, grapes, nectarines, tangerines, peaches, plums,

peppers, prunes and raisins. For the full list, check out www.feingold.org. **Before removing all these foods from a child's diet, have an intolerance test done first and only remove foods to which there is an intolerance. Such foods may well be able to be reintroduced at a later date.** One of the easiest is The York Test – for details, log on to www.yorktest.com, email customercare@yorktest.com or call 0800 458 2052.

- To make sure that your child does not suffer nutritional deficiencies when avoiding foods, work with a qualified nutritionist or a nutritional physician (see *Useful Information* at the back of this book).

Friendly Foods

- As far as possible, give your child only organic, whole foods that are free from pesticides and rich in magnesium, vitamin B6 and folic acid; especially green leafy vegetables such as cabbage, watercress, kale, broccoli and string or kidney beans.
- Gluten-free cereals plus carrots, broccoli, baked beans, parsley, spinach, watercress and sesame seeds are all high in calcium, which will hopefully reduce the incidence of self-injury and have a calming effect. Some supermarkets sell Genius gluten-free breads – developed by Lucinda Bruce-Gardyne, whose children suffer from gluten intolerances. For more details, stockists and their products plus some good recipes, log on to www.geniusglutenfree.com.
- Most supermarkets and health food stores now offer good gluten-free ranges.
- Essential fats are vital for healthy brain functioning. Recent research shows that autistic children have lower levels of the omega-3 fats in the brain – these are found in oily fish, nuts and seeds. Give your child oily fish (organic farmed salmon, unsmoked mackerel or sardines) at least twice a week, and use unrefined, organic pumpkin, sunflower, sesame, flaxseeds (linseeds) and walnuts daily if the children do not have a sensitivity to these seeds. Add cold-pressed organic seed oils to cooked foods and use in salad dressings. See also *Fats You Need To Eat*.
- Avocado is rich in mono-unsaturated healthy fats.
- Papaya, bananas, pears, blueberries, mango, pomegranate and other fruits should be fine.
- Make sure they eat plenty of fresh fruits and vegetables plus buckwheat-, potato- or rice-based pastas, fresh fish, lean meats, pulses, brown rice or quinoa.

Useful Remedies

- If you are pregnant, **speak to your doctor** about taking optimum doses of Vitamin D, which stimulates proper brain development. The Canadian Pediatric Society recommends that pregnant women should take 2000iu of Vitamin D daily. Formula-fed infants need 400iu daily and breast-fed infants can be given 600-800 iu of vitamin D daily. Toddlers who do not get regular sun exposure can take 800–1000 iu daily.
- Magnesium is needed to support nerves and autistic children tend to be low in magnesium, known as nature's tranquilliser. Give them 15mg per kilo of body weight daily.
- Also vitamin B6 – 25–100mg daily for a child of 2–6 years. Many children with autism have also been found to be low in folic acid, one of the B-group of vitamins, so try to include a B-complex daily. As children tend to not like tablets, try adding liquid B-vitamins to their food. BioCare make a liquid formula called Vitasorb B. (Nature's Plus also make great vitamin and mineral ranges for Children.) **BC, NP**
- Zinc deficiency is also associated with this problem, especially with boys, so try adding liquid multi-minerals into fruit desserts as an easy way for your child to ingest sufficient minerals. BioCare and Nature's Plus make liquid minerals. They need around 30mg daily.
- Many parents have found that including an essential fatty acid formula has helped their children enormously. Try Efamol's Efalex capsules or Eskimo Omega-3 fats for kids. **NC**
- Dissolve an additive-free vitamin C tablet into water daily to boost immune function; take

with meals. One gram daily for a child aged 2–6 years. After the age of 7 the dosage can be increased to 2 grams daily, taken throughout the day with meals.

■ A good probiotic, taken daily for a month, will help build up the good bacteria in the gut, thus supporting digestion. BioCare do a powdered one that is easily sprinkled onto foods. They contain only the probiotic and either freeze-dried strawberry or banana. **BC**

■ www.positivehealthshop.com stock Nutri's low-allergy, cherry-and-banana flavoured multi, Ultra Care for Kids. It has added digestive support and good fats for brain health. Add a scoop to juice and shake, or add to a fruit smoothie.

■ Beta glucans derived from yeast cell walls are safe for children to take and improve their innate immune system functioning, which can help reduce the severity of reaction to foods. Dr Paul Clayton, a former scientific advisor to the Government's committee on the safety of medicines, says, 'Thanks to our modern over-sanitized environment and intensive farming methods that have removed virtually all beta glucans from our diet, our ability to resist infections has become compromised.' You can break a capsule of the Beta Glucans 1-3, 1-6 daily into cold foods – and children can safely take 250–500mg daily. Most parents report that when their children are given beta glucans regularly, they suffer from less infections.

■ The Pasteur Institute in Paris studied 250 autistic children and found that their brains synthesized less than half the normal amounts of melatonin – the hormone produced in the pineal gland to encourage sleep. And when they gave these children tiny doses of melatonin their conditions improved, in some cases radically.

■ Scientist Roger Coghill, based in the UK, has developed a supplement called Asphalia, which contains natural melatonin extracted from certain grasses to maintain melatonin levels. Roger has permission from the MHRA (Medical Healthcare Regulatory Authority) to sell this natural food extract supplement in the UK. For more details or to find your nearest supplier, log on to www.asphalia.co.uk or call 01495 752122.

Helpful Hints

■ For a healthy mayonnaise full of healthier fats, add 4 tablespoons of live, sugar-free soya yoghurt to 2 tablespoons of cold-pressed linseed oil. Stir in a teaspoon of lecithin granules, available in health food stores. Leave to stand for half an hour and stir again before serving.

■ Try to remove all chemicals from the child's environment such as perfumes, chemical cleaning products and toiletries – look out for unnatural flavourings in toothpastes. Green People, Jason, Kingfisher and Waleda all make safer toothpastes and toiletries.

■ Aspirin has salicylate-like qualities so is best avoided in those that are sensitive to salicylates.

■ Beware of colourings and flavourings in cheaper vitamin supplements, as even these may cause a reaction.

■ Many parents have had some success in using homeopathy to minimize vaccine damage. Call The Organic Pharmacy on 020 7351 2232 and ask for a remedy to suit your child's specific symptoms.

■ Dr Ben Feingold researched the link between diet and behavioural problems. He is the creator of the very successful Feingold diet, which includes avoiding salicylates. Check out his website, which is full of helpful information and tips, at www.feingold.org.

■ A great book called *New Optimum Nutrition for the Mind* by Patrick Holford (Piatkus), the founder of the Brain Bio Centre, is full of a huge amount of useful information and tips on dealing with autism, as is *Dietary Interventions in Autism Spectrum Disorders* by Kenneth J Aitken (Jessica Kingsley Publishers), which is available from the National Autistic Society (www.nas.org.uk).

■ For further help, the National Autistic Society can be contacted on www.nas.org.uk. They also have an autism helpline on 0845 070 4004.

- Because each case of autism is so unique, I suggest that before embarking on this programme you consult a nutritional therapist. Search for one at www.autismfile.com. You can also contact the Brain Bio Centre (Food for the Brain), which can be reached on 020 8788 3801, or log on to their website at www.foodforthebrain.org.

AUTOIMMUNE DISEASE

(See Coeliac's Disease, Crohn's Disease, Lupus, Rheumatoid Arthritis and Sjogren's Syndrome)

BACK PAIN

In 2010 over 400,000 people in the UK went to their doctor for back pain, resulting in 5 million lost working days. For years I have suffered chronic back pain after a bad fall onto concrete that affected my spine and resulted in three herniated discs. If you are a fellow sufferer, you have my utmost sympathy. Yet there is so much we can and should do to support ourselves.

Some companies sensibly train their staff how to lift properly and, as with most health conditions, prevention is better than cure. Until recently, most people thought that bed rest was the most sensible option, but we now know that 'right and light' exercise under the supervision of a professional is definitely preferable.

The centre of the back can be thought of as a column made up of 33 pieces of bone called vertebrae. The spinal column is strengthened by ligaments, which run the length of the spine, and is supported by muscles, which attach to the vertebrae through tendons. It is important to have back pain diagnosed and, in an ideal world, you should see a chiropractor or an osteopath on a regular basis.

I have seen people with ME and chronic fatigue who have received huge benefits by having their back and necks manipulated back into place. I have also seen people who have ended up on crutches or even in a wheelchair, when all they needed was a good chiropractor. One lady I knew well was given such strong painkillers after continually complaining of back pain that she ended up wandering the streets suffering from memory loss. Yet when her desperate husband finally paid and took her to a chiropractor, she was able to hugely reduce the painkillers and live a normal life!

Doctors need to refer more patients with back pain to an osteopath, chiropractor or a cranial osteopath. And if they won't, I suggest you find your nearest practitioner and pay privately.

Chronic low-level back or loin pain can also be linked to a kidney infection. Also the heavier a person tends to be, the more likely they are to experience back pain.

Foods to Avoid
- If you are in pain, it is worth avoiding or reducing foods and drinks containing caffeine, which reduces our ability to make endorphins – the body's natural pain-killing chemicals.
- Reduce your intake of meat and sugar, which will exacerbate any inflammation. (Stress can also exacerbate inflammation.)

Friendly Foods

- Eat oily fish at least twice a week for its anti-inflammatory properties. Anchovies, farmed organic salmon, herring, mackerel and sardines are all good.
- Add fresh rosemary to meals to improve circulation and aid healing.
- Ginger, turmeric and cayenne pepper can all improve circulation and have anti-inflammatory properties.
- Adding a teaspoon of turmeric to cooked foods, soups, stews, curries and risottos can help to reduce pain.
- Cauliflower, berries, sweet potatoes, fresh fruits (especially cherries and papaya) and green leafy vegetables are all rich in vitamin C, which helps to produce collagen, which in turn makes up 90% of the bone matrix and also acts as a mild anti-inflammatory.

Useful Remedies

- Collagen is a vital component of healthy joints, cartilage, ligaments and tendons; it also improves bone strength. It is the most widely distributed protein in the body and we lose about 1.5% annually after the age of 30. I take collagen powder once daily in a glass of water or diluted juice 30 minutes before a main meal to support my back. Super Strength Collagen Drink from Higher Nature. **HN**.
- Blackcurrant seed oil is high in gamma linolenic acid (GLA), which is highly anti-inflammatory. Take 3–4 grams daily while inflammation is acute, plus 2 grams of omega-3 fish oils. **NC**
- While symptoms are acute, take 1500mg of glucosamine plus MSM daily. This amino sugar, plus the MSM, helps to restore the thick gelatinous nature of the fluids and tissues around the joints and in between the vertebrae. Glucosamine with the MSM, an organic form of sulphur, has been found to be more effective against pain. This takes time! Once the pain is eased, lower the dose to a maintenance intake of 500mg daily. **If you suffer a severe sensitivity to shellfish do not take this supplement, which is usually made from crushed crab shells.** Instead look for vegetarian glucosamine, derived from corn. For more details, call Health Perception on 0800 046 1846 or log on to www.health-perception.co.uk.
- Taking 3–4 tablets a day of a combination formula containing ginger, curcumin and boswellia can also help to reduce the pain and inflammation. Pukka Herbs make a good formula (www.pukkaherbs.com).
- Calcium 500–1000mg, with 500–800 mg of magnesium daily – many companies make them in one tablet. These minerals are known as nature's tranquillizers and help to reduce muscle spasm.
- Take 3 grams of vitamin C over the course of the day, in an ascorbate form – this vitamin helps to produce collagen.
- Try Ligazyme Plus, a supplement devised by a chiropractor that contains calcium, vitamin C, bromelain, magnesium and rutin, which all help support the skeletal system. **BC**
- Cayenne pepper capsules can help to reduce the inflammation and increase circulation to the affected area. Take 3–4 capsules daily with food. **SHS**

Helpful Hints

- As soon as possible after any injury, consult a chiropractor or osteopath. To help reduce the immediate pain and muscle spasm, wrap some ice cubes or a bag of frozen peas in a towel and place on the painful area for 10 minutes every hour.
- Most towns now have alternative health centres that include chiropractic, acupuncture and/or physiotherapy. Go along and see if they can help.
- You can buy from any chemist gels that feel cold when applied that can help reduce the pain – plus creams, such as Deep Heat, which help reduce the muscle spasms.

- Back pain often has its root in poor posture. This is compounded by the fact that we now tend to lead very sedentary lives, which weakens the supporting structures of the spine and makes them much more prone to injury. Much severe back pain is caused by muscle spasm.
- Work on holding in your core tummy muscles; this really helps to support your lower back.
- If you have a helpful boss and you sit at a desk all day, ask for an ergonomic chair. I literally cannot work without mine and find it almost impossible to sit in a normal chair. See www.online-ergonomics.co.uk.
- Take regular breaks, stand up, walk around, have a stretch and roll your shoulders.
- If you have chronic lower back pain, try using a special back seat. I carry mine everywhere – in the car, on planes, in restaurants and so on – and cannot sit for more than two minutes without it. Available from John Bell and Croydon in London on Tel: 020 7935 5555 or log on to www.medesign.co.uk.
- Before agreeing to any surgery, always consult a chiropractor or osteopath for a second opinion (see *Useful Information*). However, always report severe and persistent back pain to your doctor.
- Make sure you have a good bed mattress such as Tempur, which supports your spine, but is neither too hard, nor too soft. Better-quality orthopaedic mattresses are expensive, but worth the long-term investment.
- If you are extremely tired and under stress, not only does your immune system begin to suffer, but also your body in general. In other words, when you stop supporting your body, it stops supporting you. If this is the case, then you need to take a long, hard look at your lifestyle and get more rest.
- Acupuncture is known to help in many cases and is great for reducing inflammation and pain.
- For general back maintenance, yoga can be very beneficial as it improves flexibility, strengthens the spine and improves posture, protecting it from injury in the long term.
- Alexander Technique and Pilates teach individuals how to maintain their back and general health through better posture and exercises. With my ongoing chronic back problem, Pilates has been my saviour. (See *Useful Information*.)
- Walk more – this helps to tighten the abdominal muscles, which in turn supports the back. Treat yourself to a pair of MBT (Masai Barefoot Technology) shoes, which are made using state-of-the-art technology to support the feet. They are used by orthopaedic therapists and physiotherapists the world over. For more details, log on to www.swissmasai.com.
- Swimming is a great exercise because, although the back muscles are worked, they are protected from jarring by the support given by the water. But obviously do not swim if your symptoms are acute.
- Use good bath salts such as Epsom salts or Alkabath to help reduce muscle spasm. Alkabath salts are more powerful than Epsom salts and help eliminate toxins from the joints and re-alkalize the body. For your nearest stockists, call Best Care Products. Tel: 01342 410 303 or log on to www.bestcare-uk.com.
- Have a weekly aromatherapy massage – the essential oils penetrate into the bloodstream and really help calm the muscle spasms, which can leave you doubled up in pain. Roman camomile, lavender and eucalyptus oils can all help reduce pain.
- Use a 'wheat or lavender bag' – these bags are available in most health shops. You heat them in the microwave and apply to painful muscles. Alternate with the ice packs for more relief.
- For further help, contact BackCare, the charity devoted to helping you relieve your back pain, 16 Elmtree Road, Teddington, Middlesex TW11 8ST; or call their helpline on 0845 130 2704. Website: www.backcare.org.uk

BAD BREATH *(see Halitosis)*

BEREAVEMENT

(see also Adrenal Exhaustion, Depression, Immune Function and Stress)

Losing a loved one at any age can be a devastating blow to your life and wellbeing at every level. Therefore, after a loved one's passing, it is vital for you to express your feelings and let your emotions out. Grief, anger and guilt have a tremendous impact on the physical body.

Tears shed in trauma contain high levels of stress chemicals – let them out and don't be afraid to break down. When my mother died in my arms I was inconsolable and, like millions of others, I turned to good mediums, who could give me specific messages that only the two of us knew.

During the past 17 years, I have written regularly about life after death and have received hundreds of letters from people of all ages who have lost a loved one. Their sense of loss and grief is often overwhelming. But how different we might all feel if we knew that our loved ones live on. During the late nineties I went through a near-death experience with a medical doctor present and my story is well documented in my book *Divine Intervention* (CICO Books).

These days I write from a totally different perspective as I have an absolute personal 'knowing' that we all go on. I and many scientists now believe that our unique energy field, which contains all the information about us, simply moves to another frequency level, which cannot be seen by our physical eyes. When you turn on your radio or TV you can tune into hundreds of different channels or stations and receive or see huge amounts of information. And just because you cannot see these signals, it does not mean they are not there!

The spirit realms exist on various frequencies, but more sensitive people can hear and see them. I have interviewed and met dozens of people who, by learning to meditate and stilling their minds into a more receptive alpha state, have heard messages, after time, from departed loved ones for themselves. Obviously, some people are better at this than others, but we all have the capability to hear other realms. When some people suddenly begin hearing voices they are labelled as being mentally ill; some are – but others have simply begun hearing the spirit world and it is vital that the medical world begins to recognize this possibility. See also *Spiritual Emergency*. I have listed much of the science in my books *The Evidence for the Sixth Sense* (CICO Books) and *Countdown to Coherence* (Watkins).

Foods to Avoid
- Although at times of stress we tend to crave far more comfort foods, as much as possible keep junk, sugary, pre-packaged meals, which place a strain on your immune system, to a minimum. But then again, at times of extreme stress, the brain burns more sugar. Therefore, if you don't mind putting on a few pounds, enjoy your treats – but don't go overboard.
- Caffeine, alcohol and sugar place a great strain on your adrenal glands, which further increase the feelings of total exhaustion. See *Stress* and *Thyroid*.

Friendly Foods
- At times of extreme emotional stress, it is easy to forget our own health. It is important to eat as healthily as possible, which will not only help your nervous system to cope but also boost your immune system. You help no one by allowing yourself to become ill. Try to eat one meal daily containing quality protein such as fish or chicken with fresh vegetables and fruit.
- Make a fruit smoothie. Place one scoop of hemp seed protein or whey protein, half a cup of blueberries, one banana, a spoon of linseeds that have been soaked overnight in water (or

ready-ground Linwood flax seeds) and sunflowers seeds, a few raisins (if you like drinks sweet), and a chopped apple into a blender. Blend with some rice milk, and drink. This mixture will give you energy and good nutrients. Add any fruits you love and experiment.
- See also *General Health Hints*.

Useful Remedies
- Take homeopathic Ignatia 30c and the Bach Flower Remedy Star of Bethlehem, which help to reduce the feelings of shock and grief.
- Take a high strength B-complex daily to support the nerves.
- Take a good-quality multi-vitamin and mineral.
- Kali Phos New Era Tissue Salts are excellent for reducing stress. Take 4 tablets under the tongue in between meals twice daily.
- Try L-theanine and Lemon Balm formula to help keep you calmer. L-theanine is extracted from green tea and it helps to reduce production of the stress hormones cortisol and adrenalin. You can also use this at night to aid sleep. See also *Stress*. **NC**

Helpful Hints
- If you have a friend, colleague or relative who is dealing with the death of a loved one, take time out to shop and prepare the odd meal for them. This will help to support not only their physical needs but also, by having someone to talk to, their emotional needs.
- Cruse Bereavement Care, a charity founded in 1959, has 180 branches in the UK. For their helpline call 0844 477 9400 (9.30am–5pm weekdays) or log on to their website, which is at www.crusebereavementcare.org.uk.
- The Compassionate Friends is a nationwide organization of bereaved parents offering understanding, support and encouragement after the death of a child or children. Members of TCF receive regular issues of TCF News and a quarterly newsletter. For further information, contact The Compassionate Friends' helpline on 08451 232304 (10–4pm and 6–10pm). Email: helpline@tcf.org.uk or log on to www.tcf.org.uk.
- To find a medium in your area, contact the Spiritualist National Union, Redwoods, Stansted Hall, Stansted, Essex CM24 8UD. Tel: 01279 816363. Website: www.snu.org.uk. If they are unable to locate a medium, they are happy to give details of your nearest spiritualist church.

B

BLADDER PROBLEMS   *(see Cystitis, Incontinence and Prostate Problems)*

BLEEDING GUMS   *(see also Fluoride)*

Bleeding gums can be triggered by over-enthusiastic brushing or by gum disease, and they can also indicate a lack of vitamin C or bioflavonoids. Bleeding gums may also denote a lack of the vitamin-like substance Co-enzyme Q10.

Bacteria in the mouth and bleeding gums are also being linked to heart disease – but this could well be linked back to a lack of CoQ10.

To make sure you are not suffering from anything more serious, go along and see your dentist and make sure you see an oral hygienist at least twice a year for a proper scale and polish. When plaque builds up gum disease, such as gingivitis, can take hold. If left unchecked, you can lose your teeth. Believe me, after all the problems I have suffered with my teeth during the last decade, I know your own teeth are very precious and should be taken care of at all costs.

And if you tend to suffer with a constantly dry mouth – you should investigate potential problems such as Sjogren's syndrome (see *Sjogren's Syndrome*) an autoimmune condition that can affect the mouth and gums.

Foods to Avoid

- The plaque-forming bacteria that cause chronic gum disease thrive on sugar. Young children especially should be allowed only small amounts of fizzy drinks, sweets and puddings that are high in sugar.
- Keep refined carbohydrates including biscuits, cakes and sweets to a minimum. Or make your own biscuits using oats, raisins, seeds and agar or brown rice syrup.
- Avoid all foods and water containing fluoride, which is a by-product of the plant fertilizer industry. Calcium fluoride may have reduced the number of cavities, but sodium fluoride is a poison and in my opinion should not be allowed into our drinking water. This is mass medication without consent.

Friendly Foods

- Foods containing plenty of fibre, such as leafy green vegetables, brown rice and fresh fruits like apples, papaya, figs and cherries, are all rich in vitamin C, which supports healthy teeth and gums.
- Garden sage makes a great mouthwash for inflamed or bleeding gums, an inflamed tongue, mouth ulcers or a sore throat. Simply add 1–2 teaspoons of chopped leaves to a cup of boiling water. Allow to cool. Place in a screw-top jar and use twice daily as a mouthwash. You can also gargle with this mixture while it is still warm. **NB As sage stimulates the muscles of the uterus, DO NOT use sage during pregnancy.**
- Agave syrup and xylitol can be used as more natural alternatives to refined sugar. Higher Nature make a product called Zylosweet. **HN**
- Chew liquorice sticks regularly to keep teeth and gums clean and to reduce bacteria in the mouth.
- Drink at least 6–8 glasses of filtered water daily.
- Dilute concentrated fruit juices at a ratio of 1 part juice to 4 parts water.
- Thai foods such as lemon grass, coriander and garlic help keep teeth healthy and the coriander helps eliminate heavy metals from the body.

Useful Remedies

- Co-enzyme Q10 is well known to improve gum health. Take 60–100 mg a day.
- Vitamin C with bioflavonoids, 1–2 grams a day in divided doses with food.
- A good-quality multi-vitamin and mineral for your age and gender

Helpful Hints

- Do not clean your teeth directly after eating fruit, as you can brush away weakened enamel and cause erosion.
- Mercury from amalgam fillings is also known to cause swollen, bleeding gums (see *Mercury*).
- Eat a piece of fruit after main meals. This increases saliva production, which is alkaline and neutralizes the acid produced by the bacteria, which is responsible for dental decay. Apples are excellent, but if you eat sweet or highly acid fruits after a meal, such as oranges, then simply swill your mouth with water immediately afterwards.
- Also, if you eat very sugary desserts, swill the mouth with water afterwards. Don't brush for at least an hour.
- Gengigel is a gel and mouthwash containing hyaluronic acid – a natural substance that forms an important part of gum formation. This gel helps to reduce inflammation. For details, call Revital on 0800 252 875, or log on to www.revital.com.

- Vitamin C supplements containing sugar when chewed will attack tooth enamel and weaken the lining of the mouth.
- Use a good electric toothbrush.
- Practise good daily dental hygiene by using floss and a natural tea tree mouthwash. Clean your teeth and gums daily using a water pick appliance, adding a few drops of tea tree oil and 1 drop of clove oil, which is an excellent antiseptic, to the warm water. Water Tooth Cleaners are available from large chemists including John, Bell and Croydon in London. Tel: 020 7935 5555.
- Toothpaste containing sodium lauryl sulfate (SLS) can thin the lining of the cheeks and may weaken gum tissue. Ask at your health shop or at good chemists for toothpastes that are SLS free.
- Avoid toothpastes containing fluoride.
- There are also numerous herbal toothpastes containing everything from Co-enzyme Q10 and vitamin K to support your gums, to red clover and herbs known to help ladies through the menopause! Find one that suits your needs. Green People, Pharma Nord, Optima and Jason all make healthier toothpastes.

BLOATING   *(see Candida, Constipation and Flatulence)*

BODY HAIR, EXCESSIVE (Hirsutism)   **B**

Many women suffer this problem after going through the menopause; some can be affected when they are much younger. This problem usually begins with extra hairs on the face and sometimes hair begins growing in-between the breast area. It is normally owing to an excess of male hormones called androgens, which are produced by the ovaries or the adrenal glands. It is important to consult your doctor if you have unexplained excess body hair. But this condition can often be helped if you can balance your hormones naturally (see *Menopause*). The condition is often related to polycystic ovarian syndrome (see *PCOS*).

Foods to Avoid
- Cut down on alcohol and excess caffeine, which can affect hormone levels – as can stress.
- Reduce animal fats from dairy and red meat.
- If you cook food in plastic containers, and if you also buy food wrapped in cling film or use cling film at home, then chemicals within the cling film can leach into your food, especially if it is heated in a microwave. The chemicals that are released from the cling film can have an oestrogen-building effect within the body, which in turn can trigger a whole host of hormone-related problems.
- If PCOS is a factor, reduce refined sugar to a minimum as this leads to surges of insulin, which is needed to balance sugar levels in the body. As far back as 1980, researchers found that an excess of insulin is linked to higher testosterone levels – and higher testosterone levels trigger hair growth.

Friendly Foods
- Include more hormone-regulating foods, such as tempeh, organic tofu, chickpeas and fennel.
- Eat more beans, lentils, and leafy greens including broccoli, cauliflower, cabbage, artichoke and beetroot, all of which help cleanse the liver of toxins and help to balance hormones.
- Eat more linseeds (flax seeds should be pre-cracked or soaked overnight in cold water),

sunflower and pumpkin seeds, plus Brazil nuts. Brazil nuts are rich in essential fats, which also help regulate hormones.

- Avocados and oily fish are rich in essential fats needed to regulate hormones.
- Fill up on fibre, which binds to excess hormones so that they can be easily removed from the body. Oat or rice bran, fruit (especially apples), wholegrains, such as brown rice, quinoa, amaranth would be ideal.
- Fresh root ginger and fish is rich in zinc, which aids the absorption of fatty acids that regulate hormones.
- Make sure you drink plenty of fluids.

Useful Remedies
- The herbs that have proved most useful for reducing excess body hair are dong quai and agnus castus, which help to normalize hormonal levels. Take 500mg of either or both daily. Try the agnus castus in the first instance. Femarone 40 Plus contains blessed thistle, squaw vine, and black cohosh; take 2 capsules 3 times daily with food for 3 months. (Femarone 40 Plus also comes in drops.) SHS
- Black cohosh taken 500mg twice a day has been used successfully to inhibit and reverse facial hair growth in women. Many companies now sell all these herbs in one formula – try 500mg twice daily or take 1ml of a tincture.
- Herbs used for the related condition PCOS are liquorice, saw palmetto, paeonia and agnus castus. Take 5mls of each daily.
- Chromium polynicotinate – 100–150mcg taken twice daily helps balance blood sugar and reduce sugar cravings.
- Lipoic acid regulates blood sugar and liver function, which in turn helps regulate hormones. Take 200mg twice daily with food.
- Several companies now make Cruciferous Vegetable Extract Capsules that contain pure extracts of broccoli, watercress, cabbage and so on. Take as directed to help naturally balance hormones. See www.lef.org.

Helpful Hints
- A study of women with excess body hair found that acupuncture reduced both hair density and length and significantly reduced their levels of androgens – male sex hormones. See *Useful Information*.
- If you are overweight, this can add to the problem. See *Weight Problems*.
- Women with excessive body hair may be short of the hormone progesterone, which helps balance the male hormones that women also produce in small quantities. Many women don't ovulate regularly (but still have periods), often triggered by stress, excess pollution in the environment or foods containing herbicides, which have an oestrogen-like building effect. As progesterone is produced only after ovulation or during pregnancy, progesterone deficiency is becoming more common; hairier legs and chins are one sign.
- Natural progesterone, made from yams in a cream, can reduce hairiness when used for some time. It is available on prescription in the UK (but freely available in the US). The natural progesterone information service has more details about the use of progesterone and contacts for doctors who will prescribe it in the UK. Check out www.npis.info or call them on 07000 784849. You can order natural progesterone creams for your own use by calling Pharm West. Log on to www.pharmwest.com or, if you are calling from the UK, dial 001 310 301 4015.

BODY ODOUR

We are all covered in bacteria and in certain parts of the body such as under the arms and between our legs bacteria can accumulate. Unpleasant body odour is usually associated with poor hygiene habits, but it can also indicate internal toxicity. The skin is a route of elimination that is used by the body when other routes – such as the liver, bowels and kidneys – are struggling to cope and become overloaded. Also if you eat too much garlic, the smell begins to ooze through your pores. It's very healthy for the person who has eaten it, but not so pleasant for those around you!

Foods to Avoid
- Reduce the amount of low-fibre foods you eat such as jelly, ice cream, white breads and pastas, cakes, biscuits and so on.
- Avoid full-fat dairy produce, which triggers mucous production and can exacerbate constipation.
- Any foods that ferment in the gut, such as mouldy cheeses or high-sugar fruits such as mango, banana, dates and grapes, can eventually trigger body odour. Eat such fruits in between meals rather than after a meal, as they are more likely to ferment.
- Cut down on sugar and alcohol.
- Red meat and heavy fatty meals such as melted cheeses are hard to digest and slow your digestion and elimination.
- Avoid any foods to which you are intolerant – especially wheat and cow's milk, which trigger constipation in many people. See *Constipation*.

Friendly Foods
- Drink 6–8 glasses of filtered water daily to help flush toxins from the body and reduce constipation.
- Add a tablespoon of soluble fibre to your breakfast cereals such as linseeds (flax seeds need to be soaked overnight in cold water or use ready cracked linseeds such as Linwood), plus hemp seeds, or oat or rice bran – all available from health stores.
- Treat yourself to a blender and a juicer. To help cleanse your system blend any selection of fruits you like with a tablespoon of added soaked linseeds (flax seeds), a dessertspoon of oat or rice bran, plus a teaspoon of a good-quality green food powder or hemp seed protein with a cup of organic rice milk. If you drink this cocktail instead of having an evening meal or for breakfast, it really helps to clear you out! If you add half a teaspoon of powdered essential fats, it helps even more. Omega Plex EFA formula is available from BioCare. **BC**
- On alternate days, juice any green foods, plus artichoke, celery, apple, raw beetroot, a little fresh root ginger and aloe vera juice, which will all help to detoxify your system.
- Generally, eat more artichokes, chicory, beetroot, watercress, alfalfa sprouts, broccoli, cabbage, kale, fennel, leeks and onions – which all aid detoxification.
- Adding fresh coriander to these juices and meals helps keep the bacteria that can cause unpleasant body odour under control.
- Eat more pineapple and papaya, which are rich in digestive enzymes.
- Kelp, almonds, buckwheat, millet, brown rice, and figs are all rich in magnesium – often lacking in constipated people.

Useful Remedies
- Healthy bacteria acidophilus/bifidus help improve gut functioning – take 2 capsules daily after meals.
- A deficiency of the mineral zinc is related to excess perspiration – take a multi-vitamin and mineral daily, which usually contains 15mg of zinc, and then take a further 15mg before bed.

- Any organic green food supplement powder containing chlorella and/or wheat grass is a great way to increase elimination.
- The mineral silica really helps to reduce body odour. Take 75mg daily. **BLK**

Helpful Hints

- When the bowels are moving frequently, the body doesn't have to try to eliminate toxins through the skin.
- Fresh, live yoghurt with acidophilus and bifidus eaten on a regular basis keeps gut flora in good shape.
- Take a shower every day and change underwear regularly.
- Dry-skin brushing will help to break up and remove toxins stored under the skin, so that the body can eliminate them. Combine this with an Epsom salt bath to really help flush out toxins that may cause odour. Use 1 cup per 60lbs of body weight and add to a warm bath. Soak for 15–20 minutes and rub your skin all over with a wash cloth. Don't rinse off before getting out of the bath tub. Just dry off and retire for the evening. Keep some water handy by the tub as a warm bath can make you thirsty.
- Dab milk of magnesia under the arms. Because of its high pH, it helps to prevent bacteria from proliferating.
- Wear cotton or silk next to the skin, which enables the skin to breathe.
- If persistent, body odour may indicate liver dysfunction, digestive problems and/or yeast infections, which are probably best investigated by a qualified nutritionist or a doctor who is also a nutritionist (see *Useful Information*).
- Try PitRok – the natural, odourless mineral salt deodorant, which prevents bacterial growth without the use of harsh chemicals or aluminium. Just wet the crystal and glide it over the skin. It is also available in a spray. For your nearest stockist call Sevendelta Limited on 01278 428200 or contact info@sevendelta.co.uk.

BOILS
(see also Immune Function and Liver Problems)

Boils are normally triggered by an acute bacterial infection of a hair follicle caused by the bacteria *Staphylococcus aureus*. If you suffer from boils on a regular basis, it's the body's way of telling you that your immune system is very run down, you're most probably consuming a poor diet, and you are full of toxins. Boils are more common in diabetics and AIDS patients and may be accompanied by a slight fever. The secret to controlling boils is to keep your liver clean, as once the liver is overloaded, or you become constipated, then toxins are dumped into the skin, which is your largest organ. See also *Constipation*.

Foods to Avoid

- Any foods and drinks high in sugar, which will lower immune function.
- Reduce your intake of red meats and full-fat dairy produce, especially cheese, chocolates, double cream and so on.
- Avoid all pre-packaged meals, and mass-produced cakes, biscuits and snacks containing hydrogenated or trans-fats.
- Eliminate mass-produced burgers, fried foods and oily take-away meals.

Friendly Foods

- Eat more soluble fibres such as linseeds (flax seeds soaked overnight in water and drained or use the ready cracked types), or oat or rice bran to encourage faster elimination of toxins from the bowel.

- Use small amounts of xylitol sugar and agave syrup instead of refined sugars, as they have a lower glycaemic index and the xylitol also helps reduce constipation.
- Include more garlic and onions, which have antiseptic properties that help cleanse the gut.
- Eat more fresh beetroot, fennel, celeriac and artichokes, which help to cleanse the liver.
- Eat plenty of fibre in the form of lightly steamed vegetables, jacket potatoes, brown rice and fruits with the peel left on where practical. Apples are great for the skin – but make them organic.
- Eat low-fat, live yoghurt, which contains healthy bacteria acidophilus and bifidus.
- Drink at least 6–8 glasses of water daily.
- See *General Health Hints*.

Useful Remedies
- Zinc is a vital mineral for healing the skin and stimulating the immune system. Take 30mg a day. While symptoms are acute, take 30mg three times daily and then reduce to 30mg daily.
- Vitamin C: take 1 gram in an ascorbate form 3 times a day with meals for one month and then reduce to 500mg daily.
- Vitamin A is also great for healing the skin. **If you are not pregnant or planning a pregnancy**, take up to 20,000iu daily for 7 days. Then switch to natural-source carotenes daily, which convert naturally to Vitamin A in the body until the boil has gone.
- Solgar make an excellent carotene complex. Take one daily.
- Place some goldenseal tincture on a cotton swab and apply it directly to the boil. Goldenseal helps to kill off the bacteria *Staphylococcus aureus*.
- prebiotics – nutrients extracted from the agave plant, chicory, onions and so on – support the growth of healthy bacteria in the gut and enhance immune function. They are really useful for hugely reducing constipation. Take one scoop each morning. For details of Agave Digestive Immune Support, see www.lef.org or call the Nutri Centre. **NC**.
- See also Supplements under *Acid–Alkaline Balance*, as an over-acid system can be linked to problems such as boils.

Helpful Hints
- Apply a little tea tree oil on a cotton swab to the boil once it has burst.
- Goldenseal can also be used as a poultice. The boils do not normally rupture if you use this herb.
- If you do want the boils to come to a head and possibly rupture, 2 dessertspoons of Epsom salts in half a pint of hot water can be applied directly to the boil to enhance draining.
- Try a mixture of homeopathic silica, arnica and belladonna 30, which will help to reduce pain and help the boil pop. Once it has popped, clean it with tea tree oil and Goldenseal. **OP**
- After the boil has come to a head and suppuration has finished, take a mixture of hypericum and calendula 30 twice a day to help it heal.
- Recurrent boils would benefit from a detox.
- Get plenty of exercise, which helps detoxify the skin, and wash as soon as possible after exercise.
- Saunas, particularly infra-red, help to clear blocked pores and drain toxins from the body.
- Try reading *The Holistic Beauty Book* by Star Khechara (Green Books), available from the Nutri Centre. **NC**

BREAST CANCER (see also Cancer)

Although breast cancer remains the most common cancer in women in the UK (126 cases are reported daily in the UK alone), there are plenty of measures that we can take to help prevent and heal breast cancer. The World Cancer Research Fund now states that as many as 40% of cases – around 18,000 a year in the UK alone – could be avoided by following a healthier lifestyle: drinking less alcohol, keeping to a sensible weight and taking regular exercise. Women who are overweight are at a far greater risk of developing oestrogen-dependent cancers. Meanwhile, the incidence of breast cancer in women over 50 has fallen significantly in countries where less women take orthodox HRT, which has been shown to increase the risk for breast cancer by over 60%, compared to those who do not use it. Bio Identical Hormone therapy, especially when creams are used, have been shown to be safer. (For more details, see *Menopause*).

A few women are so frightened of contracting breast cancer, as their mother, sometimes their grandmother and other relatives died of this disease, that they have their breasts removed as a precaution. My mother died from breast cancer, but I would not undergo such radical surgery unless I actually had cancer. Scientists have now identified that a faulty gene (the NRG1), which is not inherited, is involved in more than 50% of breast cancer cases.

Our inherited genes control the structure and function of our body, but if our genes stay healthy then our body can stay healthy. If you live a healthy lifestyle you can mostly change which genes are expressed. In other words, if your parents and grandparents died of heart attacks, or cancers, you may well have a pre-disposition for heart problems and cancer. But if you live a different lifestyle and eat healthier foods, you can help change the chemistry within the body and stack the odds more in your favour.

Meanwhile, risk factors for breast cancer include orthodox HRT, the contraceptive pill, excessive intake of saturated animal fats, dairy products, alcohol, pesticides, herbicides, and a low intake of protective fruit and vegetables, which are rich in antioxidants. Research from Montreal has also found a link between breast cancer and women who work with synthetic fibres and petroleum products.

Also, many young women overproduce oestrogen and this is one of the reasons they suffer with symptoms of pre-menstrual syndrome. If you eat a healthy diet the body excretes these hormones via the liver. However, if the diet is high in saturated animal fats or alcohol, not only is it harder for the body to excrete these oestrogens, it tends to recycle them into an aggressive form, which begins attacking tissue.

Residues of pesticides and herbicides, known to trigger various cancers, are now in our food chain and drinking water and these toxins are deposited in fatty tissue within the body, so the more you avoid contact with such substances, the more you reduce your chance of contracting cancer.

Foods to Avoid
- Reduce your intake of alcohol to no more than 3–5 units a week. See *Alcohol*.
- Animal fats should be kept to sensible levels; eat lean organic meats.
- Reduce your intake of dairy, especially from cows, sheep and goats, and if you do eat dairy make sure it's low fat.
- Pesticides and plastics act like strong oestrogens within the body, which are known to trigger certain cancers; this is why you need to eat organic food as much as possible. Never re-heat a pre-packaged meal in its plastic container as the chemicals leach into your food. Transfer them to glass or stainless steel cookware before heating.
- There has been much misinformation in the media about soya, saying that it causes hormone activity that is non-beneficial to health. Although this argument is ongoing, it is generally accepted that fermented soya in the form of miso or tempeh is beneficial. Cooked tofu is fine, but if in doubt avoid unfermented soya products such as soya yoghurt or milk. Soya

isoflavones act like a weak oestrogen, which helps block stronger negative oestrogens in our environment, so therefore soya isoflavones in capsule or tablet form are fine.

■ Avoid fried foods.

Friendly Foods

■ As a **preventative** measure eat cooked soya beans, chick peas, lentils, beans (dried beans are best), and fermented soya products, such as tempeh. Japanese and Thai women, who do not eat a Western diet, have a much lower incidence of breast cancer and this appears to be due to their regular consumption of fermented soya-based foods, which are rich in phyto-oestrogens and isoflavones, which contain genistein. And genistein helps inhibit the growth of cancer cells. Eat organic and/or GM-free soya in its traditional form – tofu, miso, soy sauce and tempeh.

■ Broccoli, cabbage, Brussels sprouts, alfalfa sprouts and especially watercress and papaya all contain substances that are protective against breast cancer.

■ Raw linseeds (flax seeds soaked overnight in water and drained or use the ready-cracked versions) sprinkled regularly onto meals contain a fibre called lignan, which helps to protect breast tissue.

■ Eat more essential fats – see *Fats You Need to Eat*.

■ My favourite way to ingest a lot of nutrients quickly is by juicing. Juice some organic raw carrots, cabbage, apple, fresh root ginger, raw beetroot, radish and celery, add to this a teaspoon of any organic green food supplement and some organic aloe vera juice.

■ In cancer the only problem with juicing is that some of the live enzymes and nutrients and almost all of the fibre is left in the juicer, so scrape them out and add them to your juice; it makes the mix thicker, but you then receive far more nutrients. For this reason I use my blender quite a lot as then you get the whole fruit including the peel. A great meal replacement is to chop a banana, an organic apple (remove the pips), a small box of blueberries, a teaspoon of *non*-GM soya lecithin granules and some green food powder (I use organic hemp seed powder for its high protein content). I also add some sunflower seeds and soaked linseeds (flax seeds), a cup of low-fat organic rice milk and blend this for 30 seconds; it makes the most deliciously healthy and filling shake.

■ Replace margarines containing hydrogenated and trans fats with healthier spreads such as Biona or Vitaquell. Or use olive oil or organic coconut oil.

■ Many patients with cancer have low levels of the carotenes. Apricots, papaya, sweet potatoes, asparagus, French beans, broccoli, carrots, mustard and cress, red peppers, spinach, watercress, mangoes, parsley, tomatoes are all rich in carotenes. Fresh, organic carrot juice is a great source, but don't overdo the carrot juice as your skin may turn orange!

■ Pomegranate has been found at City of Hope Hospital in Duarte, California, to suppress proliferation of breast cancer cells. Eat this superfood daily or take a pomegranate concentrate capsule daily.

■ Take extra fibre daily, which keeps toxic wastes and old hormones from being absorbed from the colon into the bloodstream. The colon must be kept clean and bowels emptied regularly for healing to occur in the body. Add a tablespoon of oat or rice bran (or soaked flax/linseeds) to the fruit blends and drink daily – and remember to include more water in your regimen.

■ Drink plenty of water to aid elimination.

■ Iodine is stored in breast tissue and low iodine can encourage excess oestrogen production and increase sensitivity of breast tissue to oestrogen, therefore use nori kelp shakes or iodized Celtic sea salt instead of sodium-based salts to naturally increase iodine levels.

■ Add more curcumin found in turmeric to your foods. It is highly anti-cancerous. **NB If you are undergoing chemotherapy, then check with your GP before taking large amounts of this spice.**

B

- Drink more organic green or white teas, because these have been shown to have certain anti-cancer properties.

Useful Remedies to Prevent and Heal Breast Cancer

- For prevention, if you don't like soya-based foods, take a one-a-day isoflavone supplement. HN
- If you have cancer, you can take 5–7 grams of vitamin C daily in an ascorbate form with food for a few weeks. In such doses you may experience loose bowels, in which case cut the dose by 500mg a time until your bowels normalize. For maintenance and cancer prevention take 2 grams daily in divided doses with food.
- Vitamin D3 is crucial in preventing cancer of all types. Take a minimum of 1500iu daily for prevention. If you have breast cancer, take 2000–3000iu daily as this vital vitamin has been shown by scientists at the University of Toronto to prolong survival. A day exposing your skin to sunlight can create 20,000iu of Vitamin D.
- Take a high-strength antioxidant formula that contains vitamins C and E, plus zinc and selenium.
- Natural-source carotenes are vital as an antioxidant. Take one capsule daily for prevention and two daily if you have breast cancer. Solgar and Viridian make an excellent carotene complex.
- **If you have breast cancer,** take Co-enzyme Q10 x 100mg, three times daily. This important co-enzyme has been shown to inhibit cancer-cell growth and protect breast tissue. **To aid prevention,** take 100mg daily.
- Beta Glucans 1-3, 1-6 are proven to strengthen the body's innate immune system. Pharma Nord make a version that is free from yeast protein. Take 250–500 mg daily. **PN**
- A good quality multi-vitamin/mineral.
- Indole-3-carbinol (I3C) is a phytochemical supplement isolated from cruciferous vegetables (broccoli, cauliflower, Brussels sprouts, turnips, kale, green cabbage, mustard, pak choy and so on), which has been shown to inhibit the growth of oestrogen-receptor-positive cells. This supplement has well researched anti-cancer and healing potential. To ingest therapeutic quantities of indole would require eating enormous amounts of raw vegetables, as cooking tends to destroy these phytochemicals. Take one tablet daily or as directed. From the Nutri Centre. **NB Pregnant women should not take this supplement as oestrogen is needed for healthy foetus growth.**
- With your doctor's permission, start taking the hormone melatonin. A high percentage of women with oestrogen-receptor-positive breast cancer have low plasma levels of melatonin, the hormone produced in the pineal gland at night that helps induce sleep. Begin by taking 1mg nightly before bed. This can trigger vivid dreaming in some cases. Your GP can give you a prescription for melatonin, or it can be bought freely in the US. Call Pharm West on 00 353 46 943 7317 or email: infodesk@pharmwest.com. Otherwise, it can be ordered via the Life Extension Foundation at www.lef.org.
- Bio Electromagnetics scientist Roger Coghill has developed a supplement called Asphalia, containing natural melatonin extracted from certain grasses. Take 1 to 2 capsules 30 minutes before going to bed. Roger has permission from the MHRA (Medical Healthcare Regulatory Authority) to sell this food supplement in the UK. For more details or to find your nearest supplier, log on to www.asphalia.co.uk or call 01495 752122. **NB This should not be taken by severe asthmatics, pregnant women or children under one.**
- For prevention of breast cancer, the methylating B Vitamins help switch 'bad' oestrogens back to 'good' oestrogens. Either take a high-strength B-complex daily or use a Homocysteine Lowering Formula.
- **If you have breast cancer,** Avemar, an extract of wheat germ, has been proven to modulate immune function and improve the effectiveness of conventional treatments, if taken daily one

hour before food. For details and to view its large body of independent research, log on to www.avemar.com. For further information on Avemar. see *Cancer*.

■ Take 3 Pomegranate Concentrate capsules daily to help suppress breast cancer cells proliferating. **NC**

Helpful Hints

■ Ask your specialist about cryotherapy, a minimally invasive 'freezing' therapy that involves destroying cancer cells using a cold gas. Results to date have been very positive.

■ If you are going to have chemotherapy, see details of the CTC test in the *Cancer* section. This test will help your specialist to find out which specific chemotherapy will suit your unique physiology.

■ Examine your breasts once a month. If you find even the hint of anything unusual or any type of lump, see your doctor immediately. Remember the earlier any problems are detected, the greater your chance of a complete cure. Many lumps are simply benign cysts, so the sooner you see your doctor, the better.

■ Several studies have linked excessive use of mammogram X-rays to an increased risk of developing breast cancer.

■ Antiperspirants often contain chemicals that are absorbed into the body; they stop you from sweating, but this is nature's way of getting rid of many unwanted toxins. The majority of breast cancers occur in the part of the breast nearest the armpit. Use natural tea-tree-based antiperspirants or ones that are free from aluminium such as Pit Rok Crystal.

■ Avoid wearing a bra for too much of the day. Women who wore a tight fitting bra for 14 hours or longer a day were 50% more likely to develop breast cancer. At the very least, find yourself a comfortable, loose-fitting bra that doesn't block lymph drainage.

■ Some women who have had their breasts removed find that any remaining lymph glands, especially under the arms, can be really painful. Manual lymph drainage can often relieve the discomfort (see *Useful Information*).

■ Keep your stress levels to a minimum (see *Stress*).

■ As much as possible take regular exercise, but not to excess.

■ Breast cancer is more common in people who are overweight and obese. Take steps to control your weight (see *Weight Problems*).

■ Read Patrick Holford's book *Say No to Cancer* (Piatkus). If you have specific queries that you need help with, log on to www.patrickholford.com.

■ I also recommend Dr John Lee's book, *What Your Doctor May Not Tell You About Breast Cancer* (Warner Books).

■ Another wonderful book is *Your Life in Your Hands; Understanding Preventing and Overcoming Breast Cancer* by Jane Plant (Virgin Books).

■ Contact Penny Brohn at Cancer Care (formerly the Bristol Cancer Help Centre), Chapel Pill Lane, Pill, Bristol BS20 0HH. Helpline: 0845 123 2310 (9.30am–5pm weekdays). Email: helpline@pennybrohn.org; website: www.pennybrohncancercare.org.

BREAST PAIN and TENDERNESS

(see also Breast Cancer and Pre-menstrual Tension)

Tender breasts are a common symptom of pre-menstrual tension (PMT – also known as pre-menstrual syndrome or PMS) when they can become increasingly swollen and tender prior to menstruation. Breast pain is often associated with other symptoms such as fluid retention, abdominal bloating and an excess of the hormone oestrogen. Tender breasts during the first few months of pregnancy are quite common. But if breasts are tender the whole month or if the discomfort becomes severe, it is important to see a doctor. If you find any lumps of any size or shape in your breasts, seek medical attention immediately. Exercise is one way of reducing the symptoms of PMT as this encourages lymphatic drainage. On the other hand, wearing a bra for more than 12 hours a day can reduce the body's ability to drain the lymph nodes.

Also, women who take oestrogen-only HRT or use oestrogen bio-identical hormone creams may find their breasts swell and become tender; if so, you may need to reduce dosage and see your health professional.

Foods to Avoid
- Caffeine – complete avoidance can reduce the symptoms of breast pain. Moderate reduction doesn't always work; it does need to be complete elimination. Remember that caffeine is not just in tea and coffee but also in cola, many energy drinks, chocolate and some over-the-counter cold remedies.
- Alcohol should be kept to a minimum, as it can increase breast pain.
- Sodium-based salt tends to aggravate fluid retention, which can exacerbate breast tenderness. Ask at your health shop for a magnesium-based sea salt and use sparingly. Nori seaweed flakes from health shops or via www.clearspring.co.uk can be used instead of salt and are rich in iodine.

Friendly Foods
- Eat plenty of sunflower and sesame seeds and linseeds (flax seeds preferably soaked overnight in cold water), which all contain essential fatty acids, which should help reduce breast tenderness. See *Fats You Need To Eat*.
- Eating organic, fermented soya-based foods such as tempeh, miso, natto, edamame (fresh green soya beans, which you cook like peas) on a regular basis can also reduce the tendency to painful breasts and help to balance hormones.
- Drink herbal teas, such as red clover, plus dandelion coffee.
- Add kombu or nori seaweed to bean dishes. They contain iodine, which helps reduce mastitis-type pains. Iodine is stored in breast tissue and low iodine can encourage excess oestrogen production and increase sensitivity of breast tissue to oestrogen, therefore use nori, kelp shakes or iodized Celtic sea salt instead of sodium-based salts to naturally increase Iodine levels. Anyone suffering breast cysts may be lacking in iodine.
- Eat more broccoli, cauliflower, kale and cabbage, which help to balance hormones naturally.
- Beetroot, artichokes and chicory support the liver, which has to metabolize hormones.

Useful Remedies
- Take 400mg of magnesium for its muscle-relaxing qualities.
- Take full-spectrum vitamin E, 200–600iu a day, for 3–4 months.
- Take a good-quality B-complex that contains 50mg of B6 – take another 50mg of B6 separately. The dose should total 100mg daily.
- Evening primrose oil is useful for this problem, but you would need around 2–3 grams daily.
- Take the herb agnus castus – 500–2000mg a day or 2ml of tincture should help regulate hormone levels more naturally.
- Take a good-quality multi-vitamin and mineral for women.
- For those of you who do not eat appreciable amounts of broccoli, cauliflower and cabbage, several companies now make Cruciferous Extract capsules and you can take one or two of these daily. **NC**

Helpful Hints

- In Chinese medicine breast pain is often caused by liver congestion; see *Liver Problems*.
- Regular exercise (running or walking 1–3 miles a day) can relieve tenderness. Many women find it uncomfortable to run when their breasts are tender, but if you exercise on a regular basis tenderness should not be so much of an issue for the 7–10 days prior to a period. Wear a sports bra.
- Exercise improves circulation and aids drainage of the lymph system. Mini-trampolines are wonderful, as is any vigorous exercise such as fast walking, swimming or dancing.
- Lymphatic drainage massage is well known for improving drainage, thereby reducing swelling and pain (see MLD [manual lymphatic drainage] in *Useful Information*).
- Sometimes breast pain is due to an imbalance of oestrogen and progesterone, which causes tender breasts and breast cysts, known as fibrocystic breast disease. It is becoming increasingly common because of the high levels of oestrogen pollutants we are exposed to from excess pesticides and herbicides. Using a natural progesterone formula found in creams and capsules may reduce the cysts and tenderness in a few months. You can order natural progesterone from Pharm West. **PW**
- If, after three months on the above regimen, there is no improvement, see a qualified nutritionist who is also a doctor (see *Useful Information*).

BRITTLE NAILS   *(see Nail Problems)*

BRONCHITIS   *(see also Immune Function)*

This common problem is triggered when the bronchial tubes – your airways – become infected. Older people with compromised immune systems are more likely to be affected.

Bronchitis can have a viral or bacterial origin, and symptoms normally occur when you have an upper respiratory tract infection. Bronchitis is more common during winter months. If you contract a cold or flu, immune function can become very low indeed – thus allowing any infection to take hold and spread down towards the lungs. For some sensitive individuals, tobacco smoke is enough to set them off, but with other people exposure to pollens and other toxins they inhale can lead to an attack of bronchitis. The effects of prolonged negative stress and/or insufficient sleep can greatly deplete immune function; and nutrient deficiencies and lack exercise can also make you more prone to bronchitis. This is because at such times you rarely take deep breaths. Having said this, if your immune system is low and you over-exercise, then you can become more susceptible. Do everything in moderation.

Some cases can be managed without the use of antibiotics, but if you find it painful to take a deep breath, have a temperature for more than 48 hours, or can hear a rattle in your chest when you breathe or cough, you absolutely **must** consult a doctor. If the infection reaches your lungs it can develop into pneumonia.

Having suffered bronchitis a couple of times in the past that resulted from colds caught on long plane journeys, I can assure you this condition is no laughing matter. Once you have the weakness you really need to look after yourself. If my immune system had been in better shape I would have been more able to fight off these infections. See also *Immune Function*.

From experience, the secret I have found to avoiding bronchitis in the first place is at the first sign of a sore throat to eliminate all sugar, chocolate and any 'white' foods such as biscuits and cakes, and by taking the homeopathic remedy Streptococcus 10M. I also use a sinus rinse called Neil Med Sinus Rinse daily – by doing this I can stop infections developing. In fact, since I have used the sinus rinse daily, I have not suffered a single sinus infection. See www.neilmed.com. (And no, they don't pay me to say this!)

Foods to Avoid

- Greatly reduce your intake of any foods containing sugar – this includes concentrated fruit juices, as sugar greatly reduces your immune system's ability to fight infections.
- While symptoms are acute, avoid all dairy products from cows and also soya milk. (Rice milk should be OK.) Especially avoid chocolate, cheese, refined carbohydrates such as cakes, pastries, biscuits and, for some people, all other soya products – all of which can create more mucous.
- Avoid any foods and oils containing hydrogenated or trans-fats, as they trigger inflammation in the body and are linked to asthma.
- Reduce fried foods, which can trigger inflammation in the body.

Friendly Foods

- Eat plenty of fresh fruits and vegetables. When you feel this poorly, your digestive system can labour under the strain. Therefore eat fresh vegetable soups, which are an easy way to ingest nutrient-dense foods. Thickening them with sweet potatoes, pumpkin, carrots and squash – all rich in vitamin A – also helps boost your immune system.
- Barley, brown rice and miso can also be added as well.
- Papaya, mango, pineapple and apricots are also great lung foods.

- Apples are great for lung health but can be sprayed with many different pesticides – go organic and eat two apples daily to support your lungs.
- Garlic, leeks and onions are really cleansing and have antiseptic properties.
- Horseradish, which has antibiotic properties, can be used in small amounts to destroy the bacteria in the throat that can cause bronchitis. Take a small amount 10 minutes away from other foods. This also helps clear the sinuses.
- Vine-ripened tomatoes are rich in lycopene, which is great for your lungs. The lycopene is released when the tomatoes are cooked in a little oil.
- Guavas and pink grapefruits are also rich in lycopene.
- Eating fish regularly helps to reduce the frequency and severity of bronchial attacks, and if you are undergoing one, the oils in fish can provide a strong anti-inflammatory effect.
- Quercetin – a protective flavonoid – helps defend you from the harmful effects of pollution and smoke. Found in apples, pears, cherries, grapes, onions, kale, broccoli, garlic, green tea, and red wine.
- Limonene found in the rind and edible white membrane of citrus fruits – oranges, lemons, limes, tangerines and grapefruit – may help to protect the lungs.
- Increasing vitamin B1 (thiamine), found in peas, wholegrain rice, sunflower seeds and pine nuts, is essential for maintaining the health of the lungs.
- Brown rice, avocados, spinach, haddock, oatmeal, baked potatoes, navy beans, lima beans, broccoli, yoghurt, bananas and unsalted nuts are all rich in the mineral magnesium, which is also vital for healthy lungs.
- As zinc has anti-viral properties that fight colds and flu, eat more oysters, pumpkin seeds, fresh root ginger and unrefined nuts.
- As you are likely to be running a temperature, drink at least 6–8 glasses of water or fluids daily.
- Make teas with fresh lemon juice, a small piece of root ginger and a little manuka honey which has anti-viral properties. Also, drink lots of herbal teas, such as liquorice, fenugreek and elderberry.

Useful Remedies

■ Include a high-strength multi-vitamin and mineral suited to your age and gender as part of your daily regimen.

■ Whichever multi you take, make sure it contains 400mg of magnesium, as studies have found that people who take more vitamin C (up to 4–5 grams with meals in divided doses whilst acute) and magnesium tend to have healthier lungs.

■ Bromelain, extracted from pineapples, is extremely effective for bronchial conditions, as it improves lung functions and helps loosen any mucous. While symptoms are acute, take 500mg of bromelain three times daily, plus 4–5 grams of vitamin C in an ascorbate form with meals divided throughout the day.

■ N-acetyl cysteine (NAC) helps to break up mucous and reduces the bacterial count for people suffering with bronchitis. Take 500mg twice a day 30 minutes before food. Studies have shown that people who take NAC on a regular basis suffer fewer incidences of bronchitis, colds and flu. NAC helps to support the liver and has been shown to reduce the frequency and duration of attacks of chronic obstructive pulmonary disease.

■ For 7 days, you can also take 25,000iu of vitamin A (if you are pregnant, only take 3000iu). And from then on for prevention, take 15mg of natural source carotene daily – as it converts naturally in the body to Vitamin A.

■ Useful herbs for boosting immune function and reducing bacteria are echinacea, ashwagandha, goldenseal and elderberry.

■ Liquorice is anti-inflammatory, anti-viral and can be very useful with bronchial conditions. Buy whole liquorice from health stores.

■ Zinc gluconate lozenges really help to reduce the coughing and sore throat.

■ Beta Glucans 1-3, 1-6 are proven to strengthen the body's innate immune system (the immune system you are born with). Pharma Nord make a version that is free from yeast protein. Take 250-500mg daily. **PN**

■ Expectorant herbs that help to clear any 'gunk' in your lungs are garlic, white horehound and euphorbia. They can be taken either in capsules or as a tincture. **OP**

Helpful Hints

■ Inhaling steam is really helpful for opening up the lungs. Add a few drops of Olbas oil or any pure eucalyptus oil into a bowl of boiling water. Place a towel over your head and really inhale the steam through your nose. If you do this 4–5 times daily, it helps to loosen your chest.

■ If you have a tendency to suffer bronchitis, take a 3-month programme in the autumn to boost the lungs and clear any mucous out of the lungs. The herbs in the programme include elecampane, goldenrod, thyme and pau d'arco. **SHS**

■ Echinacea taken regularly helps prevent viral bronchitis from progressing into a more dangerous bacterial infection. A good formula is Ultimate Echinacea Complex, which includes astragalus and wild indigo, which boost the immune system. To order, log on to www.holoshealth.com.

■ If the infection becomes serious, and you are prescribed antibiotics, as soon as you finish the course begin taking the healthy bacteria acidophilus and bifidus for at least 6 weeks to replenish healthy bacteria in the gut, which in turn helps immune function. **BC**

■ Don't exercise near main roads, where pollution levels can be lethally high. Learn to exercise your lungs. Professional singers rarely catch a cold – they use their lungs more. Sing along to your radio and give your lungs a workout!

■ In general terms, whenever you are suffering from a bronchial infection, you should stay in bed and rest for at least 2 days. The more you try to struggle on, the slower your recovery.

■ Use an Ultra Breathe, a very handy, inexpensive device that does a great job of exercising the lungs. £16.95 plus £2.95 p&p. For details, visit www.ultrabreathe.com.

BRUISING

The discolouration of the skin is caused by blood leaking from damaged blood vessels into the tissues of the skin. It is a normal process but some people bruise excessively, especially older people. Excessive bruising is often due to a deficiency of vitamin C and/or bioflavonoids, the water-soluble pigment in fruits. People who take blood-thinning drugs, such as Warfarin, are also more likely to bruise easily. But if you suffer regular bruising not associated with a hard knock or injury, it can indicate rarer underlying problems such as leukaemia, so if in *any* doubt check with your GP.

Foods to Avoid
■ Avoid all highly processed foods such as mass-produced cakes, biscuits and pre-packaged meals, which are generally lacking in any nutrients.
■ Don't cook foods for too long, as cooking greatly reduces nutrient levels.
■ See *General Health Hints*.

Friendly Foods

■ Eat plenty of foods high in vitamin C such as kiwi, cherries, peppers, blueberries, blackberries, plums, pineapple and papaya.
■ Include more leafy green vegetables in your diet, in particular, kale, cabbage, spinach and pak choy.
■ Buckwheat is very high in rutin, therefore try buckwheat pasta and make pancakes.
■ See also *General Health Hints*.

Useful Remedies
■ Take 1–3 grams of vitamin C in an ascorbate form daily with food spread throughout the day plus 500–2,000mg of bioflavonoids, to help strengthen capillaries.
■ Pycnogenol – pine bark extract – has been shown to help protect vein walls and reduce the risk of bruising. Take 80mg daily. **PN**
■ Rutin Complex includes bromelain, a flavonoid extracted from pineapple. It has an anti-inflammatory effect. Take 500mg of bromelain daily until bruising disappears.
■ The herb horse chestnut is excellent for bruises. Take 500mg daily until symptoms disappear.

Helpful Hints
■ For bruising after a trauma, such as surgery, homeopathic arnica is a wonderful remedy. If you have had surgery of any kind, you can take Arnica 30c every 4 hours until the bruising fades. Arnica cream or witch hazel gels used topically are also really helpful for reducing the swelling.
■ For deeper tissue damage use Ledum 30c 3 times daily for 4–5 days.
■ Comfrey ointment speeds up soft-tissue healing. **OP**.
■ For sprains and injury-type swellings, use an ice pack to help reduce the immediate swelling. In an emergency, I use a bag of frozen peas, wrapped in a towel and placed directly over the swelling for 10 minutes every hour.

BURNS, MINOR

First-degree burns affect the very top layer of the skin. Second-degree burns leave blisters but usually heal without scarring or infection. Third-degree burns are far more serious and affect the full thickness of the skin, leaving it charred or white. These burns need urgent medical attention to reduce the risk of infection and scarring. Also, if you come into contact with acid, solvents or chemicals that burn the skin, as quickly as possible dowse the area with running cool water to lessen the damage. If a child drinks any chemical such as bleach that burns the oesophagus, do not encourage vomiting as it will also burn on its way back up. If possible, allow the patient to drink milk and seek immediate medical help.

Foods to Avoid
- Avoid too many foods and drinks containing sugar or alcohol, because they will slow the healing process.
- Generally, avoid highly processed, refined foods, which contain almost no nutrients.

Friendly Foods
- High-quality protein is vital in the initial stages for tissue healing. Include plenty of organic free-range chicken, fresh fish, beans and lentils or even a good-quality whey protein powder, such as Solgar's Whey To Go or Hemp Seed Protein Powder, in your diet. These are very digestible forms of protein that will help to speed skin healing. Or ask for a whey powder that includes extra L-glutamine, an amino acid that will also help with tissue healing.
- Unprocessed, preferably organic nuts and seeds, such as sunflower and pumpkin seeds, are rich in essential fats and zinc, which are vital for healing the skin.
- Wheat germ and wheat germ oil are rich in vitamin E, which aids the process of skin-healing and reduces scarring.
- Eat plenty of fresh fruits and vegetables high in natural carotenes, such as apricots, sweet potatoes and spinach, to help heal the skin. Cantaloupe melons, carrots and green leafy vegetables are good, too. Papaya and pineapple are especially healing.

B

Useful Remedies
- The herb gotu kola has been used to aid healing of burns for centuries. You can either take 500mg daily or take 1–2ml of tincture.
- Take natural-source vitamin E; 500iu twice a day until the wound heals.
- Vitamin C is vital for the production of collagen, take up to 3 grams daily with food – buy a formula that also contains bioflavonoids.
- Collagen is the most widely distributed protein in the body and as we age levels fall. Sufficient collagen is vital for healthy skin – therefore to aid healing take one scoop of marine extract Collagen Powder daily 30 minutes before your main meal **HN**.
- Also take a good-quality vitamin and mineral supplement that contains 30–60mg of zinc, which aids skin-healing and boosts immune function.
- MSM (organic sulphur) encourages wound healing and is anti-inflammatory – take 1000mg twice daily until the burn heals.
- Pure aloe vera can be applied either topically as a gel or drunk internally as a liquid (these are two separate products). Aloe Pura make an excellent range. Take daily until healed.

Helpful Hints
- You can bathe the burn in cold water for up to 30 minutes, if necessary. Dry with a clean, sterile dressing and smother with sterile aloe vera gel.
- Try Dr Christopher's Burn Paste. This consists of a mixture of runny honey, preferably manuka, and wheat germ oil (which you buy and mix for yourself), to which you add

comfrey root powder. When you spread it on the skin, this really helps to speed the healing process. **SHS** (for the comfrey powder)

■ Take Bach Homeopathic Rescue Remedy every few hours to reduce the feelings of shock.

■ Cover the affected area with a thin layer of manuka honey and then cover with a sterile gauze. Honey is a very effective antiseptic, is anti-bacterial and can also speed the healing process. You can now buy manuka honey dressings from large pharmacies – they are made by Comvita.

■ In India, fresh potato peelings are placed on burns. The wounds heal more quickly and infection is reduced.

■ Papaya pulp has been shown to be effective in sloughing off dead tissue, preventing wound infection. Papaya is rich in enzymes that aid healing.

■ Calendula cream helps to soothe the pain and promote tissue repair.

■ Lavender oil helps to aid burn healing.

■ Homeopathic Cantharis 6x, taken two or three times daily, will help to reduce the blisters.

■ MSM cream (organic sulphur cream) containing vitamin A and E, B5, aloe vera and comfrey extract, can be applied topically to aid healing of minor burns. **HN**

BURSITIS

This is also commonly known as tennis elbow or housemaid's knee and is an inflammation of the bursa, the sac-like membrane containing the fluids responsible for lubricating the joints. It is most common in the shoulder, elbow, hip and knees and can cause severe pain or tenderness, particularly when the person places any weight on that joint. Orthodox medicine offers anti-inflammatory drugs and sometimes cortisone injections. My husband has suffered tennis elbow, which was triggered by too much weight lifting, and after the injections he found great relief – but within 3–4 months, the pain and tenderness returned and was even worse than before. He has found some relief by resting his elbow completely and when he is under less stress or on holiday the pain recedes.

Foods to Avoid

■ Reduce your intake of caffeine, alcohol and sugar, which can increase inflammation within the body – and thus increase pain.

■ Cut down on animal-based foods and junk-type meals, which are very acid forming (see *Acid–Alkaline Balance*).

■ Avoid plums, rhubarb, prunes and orange juice, which are acid forming.

Friendly Foods

■ Eat more foods such as kale, watercress and spring cabbage that re-alkalize the body – the greener the better. See *Acid–Alkaline Balance*.

■ Include plenty of fresh fruits in the diet.

■ Millet, quinoa and buckwheat are alkaline foods – sprinkle the fine grains over a low-sugar breakfast cereal or use for baking.

■ Eat more fresh ginger, oily fish, pineapple and papaya, which have anti-inflammatory properties.

■ Use turmeric and cayenne pepper in meals as they have anti-inflammatory properties.

■ See also *General Health Hints*.

Useful Remedies

■ Take 1–3 grams of vitamin C with bioflavonoids daily in divided doses with meals until symptoms ease.

- Omega-3 fish oils have anti-inflammatory properties: take 1–3 grams a day of fish oils that contain EPA and DHA, which are key essential omega-3 fatty acids.
- Take 1,000–4,000mcu of the enzyme bromelain, extracted from pineapple, for its anti-inflammatory properties.
- Turmeric and Boswellia Complex contains the herbs ginger, boswellia, turmeric and ashwagandha, which all have anti-inflammatory properties. Take up to 4 tablets daily. Available from Pukka Herbs – log on to www.pukkaherbs.com or call 0845 375 1744.
- Collagen is a vital component of healthy joints, cartilage, ligaments and tendons. It is the most widely distributed protein in the body and we lose about 1.5% annually after the age of 30. Take one scoop daily in diluted apple juice 30 minutes before eating. Super Strength Collagen Drink from Higher Nature. **HN**.
- Glucosamine sulphate, an amino sugar with MSM (an organic form of sulphur), helps to restore the gelatinous fluids around the joints. Take 1500–2000mg daily, and once symptoms are alleviated reduce to 500mg daily. If you are allergic to shellfish, ask for the vegetarian version by Health Perception, available from all health stores.
- Manganese; 10mg daily helps to speed up tendon repair and ease pain.
- Liquid hyaluronic acid (HA) taken daily in water on an empty stomach aids tissue repair. HA is a naturally occurring protein in the body but as we age levels fall. For more details, ask at your health store or contact Modern Herbals – call them on 01274 889047 or log on to www.modernherbals.com.

Helpful Hints

- Glucosamine gel with horse chestnut extract applied locally can help ease the inflammation. From Health Perception – their website is www.health-perception-store.co.uk.
- Apply a bag of frozen peas wrapped in a tea towel to ice the painful area for 10 minutes every few hours. This really does help to reduce inflammation and pain. You can alternate the cold compress with a warm ginger compress – simply add a piece of root ginger to boiling water. Let it steep for 10 minutes, soak a cloth in this mixture and press on the painful area for 10 minutes. Make the compress as warm as possible without burning yourself! Otherwise use a warmed wheat or lavender bag.
- Use an elasticated bandage during the day to limit swelling. Elevate the affected area above the level of the heart to encourage drainage of fluids out of the injured area.
- Avoid weight training when pain is acute, as this will further aggravate the problem.
- Acupuncture works really well for this condition.
- Gentle aromatherapy massage using oils such as Roman camomile, ginger, marjoram and geranium can also help to relieve the pain.
- Check out www.repetitiveusetherapy.com – this site gives some great tips plus a list of therapists who specialize in treating this condition.

B

C

CANCER
(see also Breast Cancer)

One in three people die of cancer – yet Professor Martin Wiseman, medical and scientific advisor to the World Cancer Research Fund, states that 39% of the 12 major cancers are preventable through better diet, drinking and exercise habits. In the UK this means that almost 80,000 cases, out of the 210,000 cases diagnosed annually, could be prevented.

There are more than 200 types of cancer, each with their own name and treatment; the four most common cancers – breast, lung, colon and prostate – account for nearly half the deaths in the UK. Although cancer can strike at any age, the great majority of cancer patients are 60 and over. Yet whatever your age, there are plenty of things you can do to reduce your risk, or, if you contract cancer, to help yourself.

Newer screening methods, such as the CTC (Circulating Tumour Cell Test), shown to be highly effective in tests by the Department of Internal Medicine at the University Hospital in Essen in Germany, help to give your doctors an exact picture of which treatment and type of chemotherapy will be more effective in your unique case. You can send a small blood sample by post. More details can be found at www.adnagen.com.

At University College Hospital in London, a light treatment known as PDT is being used to easily kill cancer tumours in a host of cancers and has proven hugely successful. Prince Charles supports www.killingcancer.co.uk, the charity raising funds for further research and to help make this treatment more widely available.

Meanwhile, the earlier any cancer is diagnosed, the more likely the patient is to survive. Thousands of people recover every year and there is always hope.

It is now known that many cancers are triggered by environmental factors including excessive free radicals, radiation, viral infections and chemicals. Diet is a huge factor. Other possible triggers are parasites and fungi. The bacterium *Helicobacter pylori* – the trigger for most stomach ulcers – is also linked to gastric-type cancers.

Free radicals are unstable molecules formed within the body during normal metabolic processes, or are produced by stress, excessive exercise, pollution, fried food, radiation and so on. Known risk factors for cancer are diets that are high in saturated fats, sunbathing to excess, exposure to toxic chemicals found in burnt food, petrol fumes, pesticides, preservatives, excessive hormones, multiple nutrient deficiencies, and over-exposure to certain electromagnetic fields (see *Electrical Pollution*).

You can inherit a tendency towards certain cancers, yet you can change gene expression and stack the odds more in your favour by eating a better diet and living a different lifestyle. Eating healthily, staying physically active and maintaining a healthy weight can cut your cancer risk.

Various cancers have been linked to over-consumption of specific foods, for example, people who regularly consume overly processed foods such as hot dogs, smoked and preserved meats, fried foods, bacon and mass-produced burgers are more likely to develop bowel cancer. And excessive intake of dietary animal-based fats results in higher levels of oestrogens, a known risk factor for cancers especially of the breast and ovaries. Emotions affect our health, too, and tragic stories of people who suffer a major shock in life, such as the loss of a partner through death or divorce, and then develop cancer within a few years, are common. My mother was angry and bitter after my father died aged only 50 from a heart attack. In later life she developed a cancer that killed her, and I firmly believe it was her overall attitude to life, plus her high-sugar diet, that contributed to her contracting cancer. This is why I believe that healing emotional scars, as well as physical ones, is crucial to our long-term health.

There has also been research showing that if you work in an environment with negative people or a boss who tends to be very domineering and controlling, then you are more likely to become ill.

There are always exceptions. Some people eat healthily, exercise and really take care of themselves, but still develop cancer. Others smoke until they are almost 100 and are fine. We all carry within us our own genetic strengths and weaknesses, and if our genetic ability to adapt is overwhelmed by a poor diet, stressful lifestyle, pollution overload and so on, then naturally occurring genetic errors can accumulate and overpower our body's ability to correct the damage.

The orthodox approaches to cancer treatment rely mainly on surgery, chemotherapy and radiotherapy. Unfortunately, these approaches place a considerable additional burden on our bodies and often have negative side effects.

However, the picture has begun to improve. Naturopath and nutritional scientist Bob Jacobs says: 'Natural extracts such as Avemar (see *Useful Remedies*, below) have been found to enhance orthodox treatments and patients who, for instance, take Avemar and Tamoxifen together fare better than those who just take the Tamoxifen.

'There are many steps that you can take if you are to have the best chance of surviving the crisis and going on to enjoy a happy, productive life. Make no mistake, all cancers are a challenge, and surviving and thriving after cancer can mean that healing yourself becomes a full-time occupation. So a holistic strategy should include elements such as detoxification, an optimum diet, nutritional supplements, specific anti-cancer remedies, and mental, emotional and spiritual healing.'

Bob Jacobs adds: 'One of the most important things you can do that offers you the best chance of avoiding or beating cancer is to eat a very low animal protein, low sugar, healthier diet – starting NOW.'

According to The World Cancer Research Fund (WCRF), eating at least five portions of vegetables and fruits each day could, in itself, reduce cancer rates by 20%. The WCRF asserts that half of all breast cancer cases, three out of four cases of stomach cancer and three out of four cases of colon cancer could be prevented by dietary measures alone. It must be your choice whether you go the natural route, the conventional route, or try a combination of both. There are no guaranteed results, but the more right actions you take, the more positive reactions you are likely to see.

Foods to Avoid to Help Prevent or Heal Cancer
- All non-organic meat. If you want to eat red meat, then have no more than 75–100g (3–4oz) twice weekly. If you have cancer, avoid all red meat.
- Eliminate processed meats, sausages and bacon from your diet.
- Reduce or eliminate all dairy produce, especially from cows. If you do eat dairy produce, make it organic and low-fat. Replace cow's milk with organic rice, oat or almond milks.
- Eliminate white flour, rice and pasta-based foods.
- Limit your alcohol intake to, say, one glass of organic red wine a day. Eliminate alcohol if you have been diagnosed with cancer.
- Eliminate sugar, coffee, sodium-based salt, and any pre-packaged, tinned and mass-produced foods, such as burgers or take-aways. Especially reduce sugar, as cancer cells feed on sugar.

- Avoid re-heating pre-prepared foods in plastic containers, as the plastics they release into your food can increase your risk for more aggressive hormonal-type cancers.
- When food is fried, burnt or smoked, cancer-causing chemicals are created – therefore avoid these types of cooking methods. This is why crisps, sausages, smoked meats and fish and barbecued foods should be kept to a minimum.
- Reduce your use of sodium-based table salts; instead use an organic sea salt and add a little to the food on your plate.
- You could also use powdered kelp instead of salt.
- Use nori flakes, a seaweed that helps eliminate heavy metals such as aluminium and mercury from the body, as these metals are also linked to cancer. Available from www.clearspring.co.uk.

Friendly Foods to Help Prevent and Heal Cancers

- Eat more papaya. Dr Nam Dang at the University of Florida says: 'Papaya has a dramatic anti-cancer effect against a broad range of lab-grown tumours, including cancers of the cervix, breast, liver, lung and pancreas'. Papaya, and also pineapple, contain the enzymes bromelain and papain. These enzymes help dissolve away the protective protein coating that surrounds most cancer cells. Eating a small amount of papaya before a meal also aids digestion.
- Fresh mango, high in polyphenols, has also been found to kill colon and breast cancer cells in the lab. Eat more mango!

- Eat more organic foods and if you have cancer, only eat organic. This is because many non-organic foods contain the residues of up to 311 pesticides that are either known carcinogens or hormone disrupters. They are allowed on food only because the levels are very low – and no negative effect is expected. This might seem reasonable, except we do not know of their accumulative cocktail effect.
- Use more fresh or dried rosemary in cooking. Use rosemary seasonings to reduce production of HCAs (heterocyclic amines) – the cancer-causing compounds created when food is fried or barbecued.
- Eat more rhubarb and strawberries – but not if you suffer kidney stones, as they are high in oxalic acid, but great against cancers.
- Most anti-cancer diets recommend juicing, but the pulp contains healthy phospholipids, which are essential for healthy tissues. Therefore, chop all the ingredients and blend, or if you have a juicer, then scrape out the pulp and add this to your juice mix; it will be thicker, but healthier. Avoid shop-bought fruit juices.
- Eat more garlic and onions.
- For cancer prevention, eat soya in its traditional, fermented form – such as tempeh, natto or miso. The soya is best cooked. Soya contains anti-cancer compounds. A healthy amount is around 50–100g (2–4oz) of fermented soya in total a day. Soya is without doubt beneficial to adults, but it should not be given to small infants and children. Infant soya milk formulas give the infant a daily dose of phytoestrogens, which helps to protect adults against cancer; for infants, however, the levels may be too high. The obvious first choice is to breast-feed infants for the first year.
- Non-GM soya lecithin granules are also a great food for adults, as lecithin lowers LDL (the bad cholesterol), improves memory and helps protect against many cancers.
- Eat more organic Brussels sprouts, watercress, cauliflower, cabbage, spring greens, kale, shitake mushrooms and garlic, which all help to fight cancer. Why not make this a great, quick anti-cancer soup? Put two carrots, two heads of broccoli, half a pack of tempeh, a tablespoon of vegetable stock and some water in a blender for a delicious immune-boosting soup. Add almond milk if you want it creamy, and spices such as curcumin if you like it hot. Heat and serve.

- Generally, eat more curries or dishes containing curcumin, which can diminish the risk for many cancers, especially gastric and pancreatic cancers.
- Drink plenty of filtered water, which helps to wash out toxins from the kidneys. Try Kangen Water – a water system unit that attaches to your kitchen tap and ionizes and alkalizes the water. It's used in Japanese hospitals with highly beneficial health results. For full details, call 020 7580 7537 or visit www.kangenmiraclewater.co.uk.
- Boil, steam or bake, eating most of your food raw or lightly cooked. Try 'steam-frying' food using a watered down soya sauce, plus herbs or spices for taste.
- Non-organic carrots, lettuce, apples and many other healthy foods are overloaded with pesticides and herbicides that are associated with an increased risk of cancer. Throw away the outer leaves when preparing non-organic vegetables, such as cabbage or lettuce, and always wash these vegetables thoroughly.
- Just one serving of crisp or raw organic cabbage each week can help reduce the risk of colon cancer by as much as 50%. Make more coleslaw: grate raw cabbage, carrot, apple, and add a few raisins, pumpkin seeds and a small amount of low-fat mayonnaise.
- Eat at least five pieces of fresh whole fruit a day. Vitamin C and natural beta-carotene and lycopene are potent anti-cancer nutrients. Lycopene is a carotenoid found in tomatoes, which has been shown to reduce the risk of many cancers, especially prostate cancer but also reduced the risk of cancers in the colon, rectum, pancreas, throat, mouth, breast and cervix. If you are not allergic to tomatoes, eat 6–10 servings weekly. When the tomatoes are heated in a little olive oil, more lycopene is released. Otherwise, guava or pink grapefruit contain plenty of lycopene.

- All foods that are rich in carotenes help reduce the risk of cancer. These include carrots, apricots, papaya, cantaloupe melons, asparagus, sweet potatoes, pumpkin, parsley, mustard and cress, red peppers, spinach, spring greens, watercress, raw mangoes, tomatoes and French beans.
- To ingest highly absorbable nutrients quickly, place a selection of your favourite fruits in a blender with a tablespoon of organic green food powder, such as Viridian 100% Organic Green Food Blend Powder, and a dessertspoon each of mixed seeds, such as sunflower, sesame, linseed (one tablespoon flax seeds soaked overnight in a cup of cold water) and pumpkin – adjust the amount for your personal choice. Blend with a cup of organic rice or almond milk. If you are undergoing chemotherapy or radiotherapy, add at least a tablespoon of pure whey powder to this mix. Whey is a highly absorbable form of protein containing the amino acid L-glutamine, which helps to soothe an irritated gut. As weight loss is often a problem with cancer, whey is a very useful food as long as it's GM-free. Alternatively, you can use organic hemp seed (or whey) protein (available at all good health stores), a vegetarian protein that's easy for the body to absorb and utilize. This can be used as a meal replacement. My favourite blend is papaya, blueberries, apple, a slice of pineapple and a banana, plus the seeds and sometimes organic aloe juice with the hemp seed protein. To ring the changes, I add a pear or strawberries and varying seeds to the blend. It's delicious and highly nutritious.
- Vegetarians seem to develop fewer cancers than non-vegetarians, as animal proteins feed cancer cells. People who live in Thailand and Japan have much lower incidence of most cancers, so adopting a Far Eastern diet – fewer refined foods, less meat and more fish – may well be a good way of staying healthy.
- Drink more organic green and white tea; it contains powerful antioxidant polyphenols that have been investigated for their cancer-protective effects and found to be even more powerful than vitamins C and E. It is believed green tea consumption, on average 3 cups a

day, may be another reason behind the relatively low rate of cancer in Japan. Otherwise try white tea, a variant of green tea from the plant, *Camellia sinensis*.

- Eat whole foods, unprocessed nuts, beans and seeds. Anything in its whole form, such as oats, brown rice, barley, quinoa, lentils, almonds or sunflower seeds, is high in the anti-cancer minerals zinc and selenium. Buy a pack each of organic sunflower seeds, pumpkin seeds, sesame seeds and, if you do not have a sensitivity to nuts, hazelnuts, Brazil nuts, almonds, walnuts and linseeds (flax seeds that have been soaked overnight in water or use ready cracked linseeds – and keep them in the fridge once opened). Mix a tablespoon of each in a blender and keep in a jar in the fridge. Sprinkle daily over fruits, cereals, soups and desserts.
- If you eat bran to keep your bowels regular, avoid wheat bran, which can irritate the gut. Try oat or rice bran instead.
- Minimize alcohol. Alcohol is associated with an increased risk of cancer. Red wine does, however, contain antioxidant nutrients called polyphenols, which are associated with a reduced risk of heart disease. One glass a day is the recommended maximum. Red grape juice contains the same antioxidants without the alcohol.
- Animal fats are a major contributing factor in cancers; greatly reduce your intake of saturated fats from meat, full-fat dairy produce, chocolates, cheeses, sausages, meat pies, cakes and so on. Avoid any foods containing hydrogenated or trans-fats. Once you start reading labels you will be appalled at how much saturated fat you are ingesting. Never fry with mass-produced, highly refined oils. Use only organic sunflower, sesame, walnut or olive oils for salad dressings. Eat more oily fish, which are rich in omega-3 fats, especially sardines, farmed, organic salmon, fresh anchovies, mackerel, herring and fresh tuna (see *Fats You Need To Eat*).
- Cut down on stimulants, such as sugar and caffeine. Sugar has been shown to lower your immune function for up to five hours after consuming it.
- The World Cancer Research Fund offers an online library of healthy recipes. Find them at www.wcrf-uk.org.
- Take vitamin D – 1000iu daily.

Useful Remedies If You Have Any Type of Cancer

- A fermented wheat germ extract known as Avemar, sold in more than ten countries, has demonstrated in numerous studies from the US, Hungary, Israel and Russia remarkably beneficial immune-modulating effects. In over 100 published research papers based on independent research, this extract has been shown to increase life expectancy without side effects. Most crucially, it reduces the toxic effects of chemotherapy and radiotherapy, while at the same time enhancing the effectiveness of orthodox oncology treatments. Avemar can be taken by anyone suffering solid tumours and malignant haematological diseases, regardless of the stage of the disease. It improves overall health, helps most patients gain weight and aids recovery from surgery. Take one sachet daily in water at least one hour before breakfast. Must be kept refrigerated. Also available in capsules, but you would need quite a few, therefore powder is easier to take once a day. Details can be found at www.avemar.com and it is available to buy in the UK and Europe from the Nutri Centre. **NC**
- Some cancer specialists fear that vitamins and minerals can prevent the orthodox treatments from working. However, numerous studies show that the right nutrients support your immune system and help fight the cancer. A research paper has been published in the UK stating that even taking a multi-vitamin/mineral can extend a cancer patients life by two years.

- Vitamin C, 3 or more grams a day in an ascorbate (non-acidic) form in divided doses with foods. Can take up to bowel tolerance, which would be around 8 grams daily.
- Selenium 200mcg daily – especially if you have any type of skin cancer.
- A high-potency multi-vitamin/mineral without iron, as excess iron has been linked to cancer cell growth.
- Take 1200mcg of folic acid plus a daily B-complex, which helps to stabilize genes.
- Indole 3 Carbinol (I3C) is a phytochemical isolated from cruciferous vegetables (broccoli, cauliflower, Brussels sprouts, green cabbage) that has been shown to inhibit the growth of oestrogen-receptor-positive cells, which are linked to hormonal-type cancers. The Life Extension Foundation makes Triple Action Cruciferous Vegetable Extract that contains I3C, watercress and rosemary, plus apigenin – a powerful plant extract that has been found to block the development of cancer. Find out more at www.lef.org. **NC**
- If you weigh under 160 pounds, you need only one capsule daily; over this weight you could take two. **NB Pregnant women should not take this supplement as oestrogen is needed for healthy foetus growth. Do not take this supplement if you use antacids.**
- If you have cancer, take 2000iu of Vitamin D 3 daily, as a lack of this vital nutrient is now linked to 17 cancers. In fact, many nutritional physicians now state 4000iu would be preferable. Keep in mind that during a day in the sun your body can produce 20,000iu daily.
- Curcumin helps to fight the cancer and support the Phase 2 detoxification pathway of the liver. Take 1–3 grams daily with food (see below).
- Natural-source beta-carotenes, which convert naturally to vitamin A in the body, can boost immune function and are a powerful antioxidant. Take one capsule daily. **PN, SVHC, VN**

Supplements to Help Prevent Cancer

- Take a good-quality, high-strength multi-vitamin/mineral every day.
- Additionally, take a good, high-strength, antioxidant complex daily that includes natural-source carotenes.
- Curcumin, found in turmeric, used in most curries and Eastern dishes, is a great anti-cancer spice. It enhances immune function and helps inhibit new blood vessel growth that occurs as tumours grow. It is especially useful for skin, liver and colon cancers. It also helps remove toxic metals from the body and helps block pesticide-type pollutants from entering cells. Add to your diet. It can be found in capsule form in most health shops. If you are undergoing chemotherapy, make sure that you check with your GP before taking high dosages of this spice. Available from Pukka Herbs – call 0845 375 1744 or visit www.pukkaherbs.com. Nature's Plus, The Life Extension Foundation and Lamberts all make excellent formulas, too. **NC, NP**
- Co-enzyme Q10 – 100mg daily helps protect cells against abnormalities.
- Take 1 gram of vitamin C daily, more if you're stressed or ill.
- Take 200mcg selenium daily.
- Take 400iu of natural-source, full-spectrum vitamin E daily.
- Take 200mg daily of alpha-lipoic acid, which helps protect the liver and detoxifies heavy metals from the body.
- Vitamin D3 is now known to be a vital anti-cancerous nutrient. For everyday protection, take a minimum of 1000iu daily.
- Calcium and magnesium have been shown to reduce the side effects of chemotherapy. With your specialist's permission, take a duo formula, such as Solgar's Cal/Mag, twice daily, before and during chemotherapy sessions.
- Essential fats help block cancer cell division, so take at least 1 gram of pure omega-3 fish oils daily

Helpful Hints

- See *Acid–Alkaline Balance* – as keeping your body more alkaline improves health and retards cancer.
- With professional help, detox your body. To find a qualified nutritionist, see *Useful Information* at the back of the book.
- If at all possible, begin taking regular saunas (the best are far infra-red saunas) as heat helps to eliminate toxins from the body. You can buy these for home use. Don't use public saunas if they are busy, as you may pick up other people's toxins. Ask if you can have the sauna on a lower heat (120–140°C/248–284°F) and then you can stay in for a few minutes longer.
- Minimize your exposure to pollution. Remember, anything that is combusted produces free radicals, so reduce your exposure to car exhaust fumes. Electrical pollutants can also cause problems; only use mobile phones for 10–15 minutes at a time, at most. Reduce your exposure to other electrical pollutants – microwaves, TVs and so on – and don't sleep with an electric clock by your bed (see *Electrical Pollution*).
- Avoid having too many X-rays, most especially CAT scans which put you at a higher risk (a 1 in 80 chance) of developing cancers. Reduce the number of mammograms, which have been shown to increase the risk of breast cancer.
- Never use chemical pesticides and herbicides in your garden and home. Ask for environmentally friendly natural products. Greatly reduce or eliminate your exposure to non-organic foods, cleaning fluids, garden sprays, insect sprays.

- If you smoke, give it up and stay away from smoke-filled rooms, as passive smoking has now been shown to trigger cancer.
- There is specialist help available at the International Center for Cell Therapy and Cancer Immunotherapy, based at the Weizmann Centre in Tel Aviv, Israel, where they treat cancer patients from all over the world using the patients' stem cells and/or vaccines made from their relatives' donated blood. www.CTCIcenter.com Tel: +972 77 777 9255.
- If you are already undergoing any type of cancer therapy, Dr Rosy Daniel (the former Medical Director of the Bristol Cancer Help Centre) says that nutrition is vital to help bring back up the white blood cell count. She advises patients to eat plenty of organic fresh fruit and vegetables along with wholefoods such as brown rice and brown bread. All animal fats should be avoided. She also recommends that cancer patients take a good antioxidant formula, which contains vitamins A, C and E, plus natural beta-carotene complex, and zinc and selenium. Dr Daniel stresses that fear drains energy levels and advocates any therapy that can reduce anxiety, such as spiritual healing, Reiki, relaxation exercises, visualization, acupuncture or homeopathy. Dr Daniel has written a wonderful book called *The Bristol Approach to Living with Cancer* (Constable Robinson), available from the Centre for £7.99 – call 01275 370112.
- Contact the charity Killing Cancer, run by David Longman, which focuses on informing cancer patients about the alternative to chemotherapy and radiotherapy – using Photo Dynamic Therapy (PDT), which eliminates the need in some cases for any radical intervention and drugs. Prince Charles supports their work at University College Hospital in London. It's well worth looking at their website – www.killingcancer.co.uk.
- Laugh a lot. Watch films and programmes that make you laugh; laughter boosts your immune system. Stay as positive as possible: without doubt, the patients with the more positive outlook heal and recover more quickly. This does not mean that you cannot shed tears, as tears release stress chemicals, and you are not meant to be a positive saint all the time! An inspiring book that uses this theme is *Love, Medicine and Healing* by Bernie Siegal (Rider).
- Oxygen Therapies are worth looking into. Dr Otto Warburg in the US won a Nobel Prize for Medical Research for discovering that if the body has sufficient oxygen, then cancer cells

cannot proliferate. For further information, I suggest you read *The Oxygen Prescription* by Nathanial Altman (Healing Arts Press), or *Flood Your Body* with Oxygen by Ed McCabe (Energy Publications).

- At the Hospital Santa Monica in Mexico, Dr Kurt Donsbach has used intravenous hydrogen peroxide for years. For details, log on to www.donsbach.com.
- In the UK some of these therapies are available (as well as high-dose intravenous nutrients such as vitamin C). For further details, contact Dr Wendy Denning in London on 020 7224 2423.
- Many associations offer help, counselling and advice. One of the best is The Penny Brohn Cancer Care (formerly the Bristol Cancer Help Centre), Chapel Pill Lane, Pill, Bristol BS20 0HH. Call 0845 123 2310, email helpline@pennybrohn.org or visit the website at www.pennybrohncancercare.org.
- Read Patrick Holford's *Say No to Cancer* (Piatkus). If you've realized you need to fully educate yourself about cancer and how to avoid it, this book is a great place to start. Or log on to www.patrickholford.com.
- Another useful book is *Anticancer: A New Way of Life* by David Servan-Schreiber (Penguin).
- There are hundreds of excellent books on cancer; for more details, call the Nutri Centre Bookshop on 020 7323 2382.

CANDIDA   *(see also Allergies, Antibiotics, Leaky Gut and Thrush)*

Candida albicans is a yeast that is responsible for the condition known as thrush. Common symptoms include itching in the vagina, anus or penis areas. Doctors estimate that at least 75% of women will experience it at some time in their lives. Although commonly found in the vagina, candida can also occur in the throat, mouth and gut.

Normally, relatively low levels of candida are present in the gut as they are balanced by large amounts of healthy bacteria, which helps to keep the yeast in check. Problems arise when the yeast begins to overgrow in the gut. This ultimately triggers a variety of symptoms including bloating, wind, constipation/and or diarrhoea, food cravings (especially for sugar and wheat-based foods), headaches, mental confusion, memory problems, impotence, inability to concentrate, spots in front of the eyes, mood swings, skin rashes, persistent coughing, regular bouts of thrush, arthritis-type aching joints and chronic fatigue. Candida can change its form and burrow through and irritate the gut lining, which increases the risk of food sensitivities and an exacerbation of the symptoms above (if you suffer recurrent bouts of candida, see *Leaky Gut*).

It is crucial to keep the candida under control by using herbs, supplements and, most importantly, dietary changes. One of the primary triggers for candida is overuse of antibiotics plus eating too much refined sugar. Others are long-term use of the Pill, and steroids, chemotherapy, diabetes, HIV and pregnancy. Many women believe that you cannot have candida if you don't have thrush, but the majority of women with candida do not have thrush. Men are also sufferers. Naturopath Steve Langley says: 'Thanks to our over-processed, high-sugar diets and stressful lifestyles, candida imbalances now affect up to 75% of the population, both men and women. It can become a serious condition if left untreated and remains little understood by many doctors.' He is right.

During my teens I was given dozens of antibiotics for my acne, thrush and ear infections. Every time the thrush returned, I would be given more antibiotics, which in the long run only made the vicious cycle worse. I strongly advise that anyone testing positive, via stool or saliva tests, for high levels of candida, should consult a doctor who is also a nutritionist (see *Useful Information*).

Foods to Avoid
- Initially, remove all yeast and fermented food from the diet – this includes breads, all aged or mouldy cheeses including Stilton, Brie, Camembert and so on. Alcoholic drinks – especially beer and wine – ginger beer, vinegar and foods containing vinegar (ketchups, pickles, salad cream, baked beans), soya sauce, gravy mixes (many contain brewer's yeast), miso, tempeh and mushrooms.
- I know it's hard, but try to avoid all white-flour products containing yeast/and or refined sugar for at least two weeks, including crackers, pizza and pasta.
- Sugar feeds the yeast – so for a month avoid sugar in any form including honey, maltose, dextrose or sucrose and really sweet fruits such as grapes, peaches, kiwi and melon. Blueberries/ blackberries and strawberries can also harbour moulds. Avoid these fruits until the candida has been brought under control. I know it will be hard as sugar is highly addictive but you also need to avoid dried fruits, fruit juices and canned drinks for this period as they are high in sugar. Artificial sugars such as aspartame should also be eliminated. Sugar is the biggest problem with candida and we cannot overstate just how much refined sugar needs to be avoided.
- Avoid malted products – found in some breakfast cereals, brown Ryvita and malted drinks, such as Ovaltine and Horlicks.
- Avoid peanuts, peanut butter and pistachio nuts, which tend to harbour moulds.
- Avoid cow's milk for one month.
- If you have really severe candida, for the first two weeks also avoid courgettes, carrots, corn, and any of the squash family, as they quickly convert to sugars in the gut.
- Avoid any foods you know you are intolerant to.

Friendly Foods
- Garlic has potent anti-fungal action; raw is best. If you're worried about your breath, chew on some parsley.
- Eat fresh fish and shellfish, chicken, turkey and lean meats, eggs, cooked tofu and pulses.
- Research shows that a candida infection leads to inflammation. To help combat this, eat more oily fish – salmon, mackerel, herring, anchovies and sardines – along with nuts (unsalted and not peanuts) and lots of organic, unrefined seeds, which are also rich in essential fats.
- Include more artichokes, asparagus, aubergine, avocado, broccoli, cabbage, cauliflower, Brussels sprouts, celery, green beans, leeks, lettuce, garlic, onion, parsnips, spinach, tomatoes and watercress in your diet. These types of vegetables encourage healthy bacteria to proliferate.
- Fruits that are OK are apples, pears (not over-ripe), a little pineapple and cherries. Papaya and pomegranate are OK if not too over-ripe.
- Use organic rice, oat, coconut or almond milk instead of cow's milk.
- Eat live, plain unsweetened yoghurt, which contains the healthy bacteria acidophilus and bifidus. Yoghurt is fermented, which means it's easier to digest than milk.
- Brown rice, lentils, corn, millet, buckwheat or rice pasta, oat cakes, soda bread, scones made with a little butter or organic raw walnut butter are all OK. **HN**
- As a wheat substitute, try yeast-free rye bread. It can take some getting used to but for a month it's acceptable. Most supermarkets and health shops now offer wheat- and/or yeast-free breads.
- Coriander and thyme are great herbs for helping to control this infection, so use liberally in soups and stews.

Useful Remedies

- Prebiotics are certain foods that encourage healthy bacteria in the gut to multiply, thereby enhancing immune function. I have found a great one based on the agave plant called Agave Digestive Immune Support, which I take every morning in my breakfast whiz. Or just dissolve one scoop of this powder in water. It really helps keep you regular! See www.lef.org. **NC**
- Probiotics are the actual healthy bacteria, which help keep the candida under control. Jarro-dophilus EPS, made by Jarrow, will help replenish gut flora; take one daily after food. It is enteric coated, which means it can pass through stomach lining, and does not need to be kept in the fridge. **NC**
- Take one yeast-free B-complex.
- Take a multi-vitamin and mineral for your age and gender.
- AD 206, containing ginseng and pantothenic acid, supports adrenal function, which is often exhausted in candida patients. **BC**
- To help cleanse the liver, take 1 HEP 194 and 1 gram of vitamin C. **BC**
- Take a good digestive enzyme, such as Polyzyme Forte, with main meals. **BC**
- Floraguard is a duo-pill that combines anti-fungals such as oil of oregano, which is effective against many yeasts and parasites. However, do not use this formula if you suffer from active stomach ulcers. **BC**
- Take 1 Pau D'arco Plus, a potent anti-fungal formula made specially to help eliminate the fungus. **BC**
- Otherwise, try a formula containing black walnut, pau d'arco and calendula tincture; take 2–4ml twice a day. **FSC**
- Glutamine is great for healing and calming an irritated and inflamed gut. Take up to 5 grams twice a day, half an hour before food. **HN**
- I realize I have suggested numerous supplements here – there is certainly no need to take them all, I am simply giving you plenty of choices!

Helpful Hints

- Follow the yeast/sugar-free diet for 2–4 weeks before you add in any anti-fungal supplements or you may kill off the candida quicker than your body can dispose of it. This could lead to a general feeling of malaise. Should this happen at any time, drink more fluids, up your vitamin C and reduce your anti-fungals for a day or two.
- If indigestion and bloating are a problem and digestive enzymes do not help, you may still be low in stomach acid. See *Low Stomach Acid*.
- As candida is usually linked to multiple food intolerances (especially to wheat, sugar and dairy), consider a food-intolerance test. Contact Genova Diagnostics on 020 8336 7750 or check out www.gdx.uk.net.
- A comprehensive stool test and parasitology can also check for evidence of candida (plus other yeasts) in your body in addition to parasites and your levels of good bacteria. Contact Smart Nutrition on 01273 775480 or visit www.smartnutrition.co.uk for details.
- Many women who suffer candida are very stressed and exhausted. The best thing you can do to help boost immune function is to go away for at least a week. Get more sleep. Identify and deal with stress (see *Stress*).
- Avoid compost heaps, cut grass and staying too long in moist, humid atmospheres where moulds can thrive.
- Women who wear nylon underwear are twice as likely to suffer from thrush as those who wear cotton underwear.
- Any types of perfumed bubble bath products can aggravate thrush, so are best avoided. A better choice is to add a few drops of tea tree essential oil to your bathwater. It has powerful

anti-fungal and antiseptic properties. **NB Do not use neat directly on areas of delicate skin such as the vagina or penis.**

- For further help, contact the National Candida Society, PO Box 151, Orpington, Kent BR5 1UJ. Email info@candida-society.org or visit their website at www.candida-society.org.uk, which is full of heaps of information. Membership is £15 annually, and includes a helpline on Thursdays along with lots of extra support.
- Recent research indicates that people who have persistent and chronic candida may have intestinal parasites. Herbal combinations containing wormwood, tincture of black walnut hull and cloves, plus the amino acids ornithine and arginine, help eliminate parasites. For details of candida cleansing formulas, contact G&G Food Supplies – call 01342 312811, email sales@gandgvitamins.com or visit www.gandgvitamins.com.
- Read Erica White's *Beat Candida Cookbook* (Thorsons), which has more than 250 recipes, many of which are quick and easy to prepare.

CARPAL TUNNEL SYNDROME (CTS)

(see also Sjogren's Syndrome)

Carpal tunnel syndrome (CTS) is caused by the compression of the median nerve that runs under tissues in the wrist. People who use keyboards and other machinery on an everyday basis are the most frequent sufferers. Symptoms range from pain to numbness or tingling in the fingers. CTS is relatively common in pregnancy and more women suffer than men. It is also linked to an underactive thyroid, weight gain, arthritis and Sjogren's Syndrome. The single most successful supplement for this condition is vitamin B6.

If CTS becomes severe, then the protective covering of the median nerve known as the myelin sheath can be damaged by the long-term inflammation resulting in permanent nerve damage.

Foods to Avoid
- Because this problem is often associated with fluid retention, avoid adding too much sodium-based salt to food. Use a little magnesium-based sea salt for cooking.
- Reduce your intake of salty foods such as crisps, pre-packaged meals, pies, soy sauce and so on.
- Foods containing monosodium glutamate (MSG), often found in high amounts in Chinese take-aways and used in many Japanese restaurants, dehydrate the body. MSG depletes vitamin B6 from the body, as does the contraceptive pill.
- In some people, foods such as oranges, tomatoes and wheat further exacerbate the problem.
- Avoid all foods containing trans- and hydrogenated fats and animal fats, which increase inflammation.
- Greatly reduce your intake of sugary foods, as sugar also increases inflammation.

Friendly Foods
- Eat foods rich in vitamin B6: liver, cereals, lean meat, green vegetables, unrefined organic nuts – especially walnuts and Brazil nuts – and fresh and dried fruits.
- Eat more brown rice, beans, lentils, pulses, wholemeal pasta and breads.
- Eat oily fish such as organic-farmed salmon, tuna, mackerel, herrings, anchovies and sardines, which are rich in omega-3 fats that have anti-inflammatory properties.
- Use organic extra-virgin olive oil for salad dressings and cooking.
- Eat pineapple before meals, which contains bromelain that helps to reduce inflammation.

- Bilberries, cherries and blueberries are all rich in bioflavonoids, which have anti-inflammatory properties.
- Cook with more ginger, turmeric (curcumin) and cayenne, as they are highly anti-inflammatory. Eat more curries.
- Drink at least 6–8 glasses of water a day.
- Drink more organic nettle, green and white tea.

Useful Remedies
- Take B6, 100–400mg, plus a B-complex daily while symptoms are acute.
- Take magnesium, 200–600mg daily, in divided doses, which nourishes nerve endings and relaxes muscles.
- Take a multi-vitamin and mineral for your age and gender.
- Take 1–2 grams of evening primrose oil or 500mg of Mega GLA, as gamma-linolenic acid (GLA) from evening primrose oil is highly anti-inflammatory. **BC**
- Alpha-lipoic acid helps protect against nerve damage; take 150-200mg daily.
- Omega-3 fish oils help protect the myelin sheath. Take 2 grams daily.
- The herbs white willow bark and devil's claw are highly anti-inflammatory; take 1–2 grams daily whilst symptoms are acute. **NB If you are allergic to aspirin or taking blood-thinning drugs, such as Warfarin, do not take this supplement.**

Helpful Hints
- Glucosamine gel applied topically can help reduce the inflammation.
- If you are a regular computer user, try to find an ergonomic keyboard, which will be easier to use.
- If symptoms are severe, buy a wrist splint containing magnets, available from good pharmacies and health stores.
- Sleeping heavily on your side, with your wrists under you, can also cause CTS. If you wake up with numb hands, immediately shake them and give them a massage to restore circulation.
- Acupuncture and daily massage with homeopathic Rhus tox ointment are also helpful. **OP**
- Log on to www.repetitiveusetherapy.com, a really useful site that lists therapists who specialize in helping treat this condition.

CATARACTS

(see also Eye Problems)

Poor or 'foggy' vision affects more than 80% of people aged 75 or over. As we age, the normally clear and transparent lens of the eye oxidizes to become cloudy, which can severely impair vision and changes the way we see colours. Other symptoms include pain in the eyes on exposure to any glaring lights and problems driving at night. Many people who live in the Tropics develop cataracts, and they are a major cause of blindness in developing countries. Cataracts are becoming more common in the West in people who tend to take too much sun. A poor diet lacking in antioxidant nutrients, smoking, diabetes and overuse of steroids and other prescription drugs can all cause cataracts. As with so many other conditions, cataracts are much easier to prevent than to cure. Once you have cataracts, the normal approach is laser treatment; however, some individuals claim to have reversed their cataracts with a combination of herbs and nutrients.

Foods to Avoid
- Smoking, fried foods and sugar speed up the oxidation process and make cataracts more likely to develop.

- Sugar increases cross linking in the skin and within the blood vessels. The more sugar you eat, the more inflammation you will have in the body.
- Cut down or reduce animal-based fats, and avoid hydrogenated and trans-fats.

Friendly Foods

- Bilberries, cherries and blueberries are very rich in bioflavonoids, which help protect the eyes. Any blue, red or orange fruits and vegetables will nourish the eyes.
- Leafy green vegetables, in particular spinach and watercress, contain lutein, the powerful antioxidant, found in most green vegetables, that has specific properties for protection of the eyes.
- Sweet potatoes and butternut squash have high levels of carotenes, which convert naturally to vitamin A within the body. Other good sources of carotenoids are carrots, green vegetables, mango, papaya, tomatoes, apricots, cantaloupe melons and pumpkin.
- Include plenty of oily fish in your diet, which is rich in vitamin A.
- All foods high in vitamin C, vitamin E and selenium help to support the eyes. These include wheat germ, avocado, sprouting seeds such as alfalfa, sunflower, pumpkin and linseeds, eggs, nuts, lean meats, wholegrain cereals and fresh fruits, especially cherries, kiwi fruit and green peppers.

Useful Remedies

- People who take vitamin C on a regular basis over a number of years are at a much lower risk of developing cataracts. The eyes require a high concentration of vitamin C. Take 2 grams daily in an ascorbate form with food.
- People with low levels of vitamin E are nearly four times more likely to form cataracts, so take 400iu of natural-source full-spectrum vitamin E daily included in a good-quality multi-vitamin mineral.
- Take 1–2 capsules of Bilberry Eye Formula each day. People who consume bilberry on a regular basis have a much lower risk of forming cataracts. **FSC**
- Ultraviolet light destroys vitamin B2 (riboflavin), so take a B-complex daily.
- Carnosine, an amino acid, greatly reduces cross linking in the body and brain. Take 100mg daily in between meals.
- Lipoic acid helps prevent cataracts forming as it helps protects against loss of vitamins C and E. Take 150mg daily with food.

Helpful Hints

- Anyone concerned about developing cataracts should protect their eyes from bright sunlight with sunglasses that have been verified for UV-filtering ability. Wrap-around sunglasses are the most effective. If you work outside, wear a hat to protect your eyes. UV-filtering contact lenses are also available; ask your optician for details.

CATARRH   *(see also Allergic Rhinitis, Allergies and Sinus Problems)*

Catarrh, or chronic congestion in the nasal passages and sinuses, can be caused by an inflammatory response to airborne pollutants (from pesticides, paints, insect sprays, chemical-based air fresheners etc) – and the inflammation can then be further aggravated by other substances such as grass pollens, house dust mites or cat fur. However, in most cases it is triggered by foods that you eat (or crave and eat) on an everyday basis, such as cow's milk and related products – cheese or chocolate. Wheat-based foods, such as croissants, are often high in sugar and fats, which can also trigger symptoms in some people.

Many people assume that dairy products cause catarrh, but in reality this is only the case if you have an intolerance to these foods. Catarrh can just as easily be caused by wheat, eggs, citrus or any foods to which you have an intolerance. It is important to get to the root cause of the problem, so if you are suffering with a lot of catarrh, look at the foods you eat daily. Cut out one food at a time and keep a diary of the results. After a few weeks it is usually easy to find the culprit (see also *Leaky Gut*).

Catarrh is the body's response to some sensitivity, whether it is a food or other substance that does not agree with your physiology.

Foods to Avoid
- Avoid any foods to which you have a sensitivity or intolerance. Typically these might include cow's milk and produce, especially full-fat cheeses, yoghurts and chocolate, plus caffeine, citrus fruits and juices, peanuts, wheat, and foods from the nightshade family, which includes tomatoes, potatoes, aubergines and peppers.
- I personally also find that goat's cheese and soya milk or yoghurts tend to leave me feeling very 'bunged up'. Also avoid rich, creamy sauces.
- Avoid foods containing too much refined sugar, which weakens the immune system making you more susceptible to food intolerances. And most foods high in sugar are also high in saturated fats.

Friendly Foods
- Garlic, ginger, horseradish, onion, cayenne pepper, pineapple and pears can help the body fight an infection if there is one and loosen up mucous so the body can expel it more easily
- The herbs thyme, rosemary and fenugreek make great expectorants, which help relieve congestion. Either make a strong tea and drink, or add these herbs to foods.
- Be sure to eat plenty of wholegrains, such as brown rice, quinoa, barley, lentils, fruits and fresh vegetables.
- When people go on a cleansing diet, the catarrh almost always disappears. In the initial stages of a de-tox, the body can produce more mucous for a short time as it cleanses itself.

Useful Remedies
- New Era make tissue salts specifically for catarrh.
- Try Napiers Sage and Garlic Catarrh Remedy. To order from Napiers Wholesale, call 0131 202 0960.
- Take Mucolixir by Neutrocology. **NC**
- Take 1 gram of vitamin C with added bioflavonoids twice daily with meals.
- Sinus and cattarh pills containing a homeopathic mixture of Kali Bich, Pulsatilla, Merc Sol, Thuja, Chamomilla and Hydrastis Canadensis 30 can help address infected green or yellow mucous, and are suitable and safe for babies and adults. Cough and mucous tincture contains elecampane, coltsfoot, pulmonaria, liquorice and mullein and helps clear coughs and mucous (even stubborn ones). **OP**
- An excellent nasal spray is Weleda's rhinodoron spray with aloe.
- Quercetin, a flavonoid found in red wine, tea, apples and red grapes, taken in supplement form helps to reduce the inflammatory response. Take 250mg twice daily.

Helpful Hints
- Ask at your health store for a nasal spray such as Salcura – which really helps to clear the sinuses.
- Neil Med Sinus Rinse, a saline nasal rinse, has given me huge relief from chronic nasal problems. It is incredibly easy to use – to order, call 0800 032 6073, or log on to www.neilmed.com.

- Make a soup from 6 onions, a whole bulb of garlic, a small spoon of honey, 2.5cm (1in) of fresh root ginger and, if you're brave, a bit of cayenne pepper, in a vegetable or chicken stock. This will fight most infections and help clear catarrh.
- Invest in a humidifier/air filter or ionizer to help keep the air free of potential allergens.
- Many people have found that lime flower tea is useful for reducing catarrh.
- If your ears are blocked due to excess mucous, use warm 'hopi' ear candles, which gently remove excess wax and congestion. For details, contact Revital – call 0800 252 875 or log on to www.revital.co.uk.

CELLULITE

(see also Circulation)

Cellulite is suffered by nearly nine times as many women as men. This is partly due to the different structure of the skin, and the fact that women have more underlying fat cells. Cellulite is mainly due to water retention plus an accumulation of toxins in the body, which have weakened the connective tissue just below the surface of the skin. It is much less common in female athletes who have very low body fat. Cellulite could be greatly avoided if you look after your liver and your lymphatic system.

Foods to Avoid

- High saturated fat foods, such as chocolate, clog up the lymphatic system, which will contribute to more cellulite.
- Refined carbohydrates such as mass-produced cakes and biscuits plus meat pies and pastries.
- Foods with a high salt content such as tinned foods, pre-packaged foods and take-aways, which also tend to contain a lot of saturated fats. Salt retains more fluid in the tissues, which means you are storing more toxins.
- Also avoid too much coffee and alcohol, which place a strain on the liver, which is already struggling to deal with the toxins from your diet. The more you take care of your liver, the more your skin will improve. (See *Liver Problems*.)

Friendly Foods

- Eat plenty of complex carbohydrates like beans, lentils, fruits, vegetables, and brown rice. These foods are fibrous, which aids faster elimination of toxins, making fat deposits less likely.
- Make sure you drink plenty of water and add organic seeds, such as sunflower, pumpkin and linseeds, to fruits, salads and cereals.
- Pectin in apples helps to eliminate toxins – eat an organic apple or two daily.

Useful Remedies

- The herb gotu kola is by far the best-researched and most successful remedy for cellulite when taken orally. Try 500mg, 3 times a day for 2–3 months.
- Take a multi-vitamin and mineral daily for your age and gender.
- Horse chestnut cream, gel or lotion applied twice a day reduces some of the swelling and discomfort and helps to strengthen the connective tissues, which tend to be damaged when you have cellulite. Available from all good health stores.
- Cellulite tincture contains bladderwrack, alfalfa, horse chestnut, dandelion and gotu kola to improve microcirculation, elimination and oxygenation, as well as speeding up the metabolism. **OP**
- A formula that helps to clean the lymph is Essential Detox Combination, which contains clivers, blue flag, burdock and yellow dock. Take one teaspoon in a glass of water, three times daily. For details, log on to www.holoshealth.com.

Helpful Hints

- Massage in any form is beneficial, as it increases circulation and lymph drainage. If you are not able to treat yourself to a massage on a weekly basis, invest in a skin brush, which increases circulation and helps eliminate toxins from the body. Skin brushes are available from all health shops and the Body Shop.
- Detox body oil (juniper, rosemary, grapefruit and fennel) helps detoxify and firm the body by improving microcirculation, oxygenation and elimination. Juniper and fennel are natural diuretics. Use with a skin brush every morning. **OP**
- Begin taking more exercise to encourage circulation and elimination of toxins. Rebounding on a mini-trampoline and yoga are great for reducing cellulite.
- Walk regularly. Stretching aids detoxification from soft tissues.
- If you need to lose weight, do it gradually, as losing weight too quickly can make the appearance of cellulite much worse

CHILBLAINS *(see also Circulation and Raynaud's Disease)*

Chilblains are triggered by poor circulation and are characterized by red inflamed areas that affect the extremities. Chilblains can cause intense itching, swollen toes and sensitivity to heat and cold. Some unfortunate individuals suffer in both hands and feet. It is more common in cold weather, because the small blood vessels in the skin naturally constrict when it is cold. If you tend to suffer from chilblains every winter then you need to improve your circulation

C

Foods to Avoid

- Anything that worsens circulation – this inevitably means foods that tend to encourage hardening of the arteries such as animal fats, full-fat dairy produce, low-fibre foods, such as ice cream, jelly, fatty puddings, chocolates and cakes. See dietary advice in *Atherosclerosis* and *Circulation*.

Friendly Foods

- Oily fish, cayenne pepper, garlic, onion, ginger, soluble fibre, such as linseeds (flax seeds that have been soaked overnight in cold water and drained), plus oat and/or rice bran. All of these foods can help either to improve circulation or help reduce levels of LDL (the 'bad' cholesterol), which in the long-term will help your circulation. (See *Fats You Need to Eat* and *General Health Hints*.)
- Eat more pineapple, which is a natural blood thinner and acts as an anti-inflammatory.

Useful Remedies

- The herb gotu kola really helps increase circulation to the extremities. Take 500mg twice daily with food.
- Natural-source, full-spectrum vitamin E, 400iu a day, helps to thin the blood naturally.
- Take niacin (vitamin B3), 30mg–100mg daily, which pumps blood into the minor capillaries. **NB If you are taking niacin for the first time, only take 50mg and slowly increase to 100mg or more daily, as niacin causes a flushing sensation in the skin. This is simply blood moving into the small capillaries, but it can make you look like a freshly cooked lobster for a while. As all the B-vitamins work together, also take a B-complex.**
- Omega-3 fish oils help to reduce stickiness in the blood. Take one gram daily with main meal.
- Include a multi-vitamin and mineral in this regimen plus 1 gram of vitamin C with bioflavonoids, which helps to strengthen small capillaries.
- Bromelain, extracted from pineapple, is a natural blood thinner. Take 250mg daily.

- Add a few drops of ginger tincture to water and sip throughout the day – it really helps warm you. This is made by Metabolics – call them on 01380 812799 or visit www.metabolics.com.

Helpful Hints

- Smoking restricts circulation – so give it up.
- Have a regular massage or reflexology. Essential oils such as black pepper or rosemary (do not use black pepper undiluted) can be rubbed into your feet every morning to improve blood circulation.
- Regular exercise, such as walking, rebounding and skipping, all increase microcirculation.
- I used to suffer chilblains every winter, after having varicose veins removed years ago. The surgeon told me that I would still have plenty of veins left, but the legacy has been poor circulation. Obviously, the key would have been for me to have avoided varicose veins in my youth! Keep this in mind and wear bed socks during winter months.
- **Never** wear tight-fitting shoes, especially when it is bitterly cold, as this really aggravates chilblains by restricting circulation to the toes. Invest in fur-lined boots during cold weather.
- Try massaging homeopathic *Tamus communis* cream into the chilblains. This cream is made from wild black bryony root, and has helped many people.
- Homeopathic Agaricus 3x or 6x can be taken two or three times daily. This is a classic homeopathic remedy for chilblains.

CHOLESTEROL, HIGH AND LOW

(see also Heart Disease and Strokes)

Around two in every three people have high cholesterol and the problem is escalating. Every year in Britain alone, more than 200,000 people die as the results of a heart attack or stroke, and a high cholesterol count increases your chances of becoming one of these statistics by more than 60%.

Cholesterol is a fatty substance manufactured by the liver and is a vital component of every cell. There are two types of cholesterol: HDL (high density lipoproteins) and LDL (low density lipoproteins). The HDLs are good for us – the easy way to remember this is H is for healthy. The LDLs are generally bad for us – L stands for lethal. Then there are Triglycerides – another type of fat, which are carried in the blood primarily by the LDL, and we generally find high levels of triglycerides associated with high LDL.

A cholesterol blood reading above 6mmol/L is considered high. Interestingly most people who die of heart disease or stroke have normal or low cholesterol but having high cholesterol indicates imbalances.

A healthy reading should not be greater than 5mmol/L. But even within a 'healthy' range, it is the ratio of HDL to LDL that is the important part (although it is more likely to be better the lower the figure; LDL should be less than 3mmol and HDL should be higher than 1.2mmol).

It appears that the problem lies with the LDL, and specifically whether that LDL oxidises (like rust) in our blood vessels, causing damage and occlusion. The LDL will oxidize unless we have some form of insurance such as plenty of 'fat-soluble' antioxidants to 'mop it up', such as vitamin E.

Ideally, 20–40% of your total cholesterol should be HDL. There is also a type of cholesterol, VLDL (very low density lipoprotein), which is extremely bad for you.

You need cholesterol for healthy cell membrane production and the manufacture of hormones. It is also needed to help in the synthesis of bile acids for the digestion of fats and for production of vitamin D. Low cholesterol levels are linked to depression and in rare cases suicide, which is why fat-free diets are definitely not a good idea. For years we have been told to avoid certain foods, especially eggs, because they contain cholesterol. In fact, blood levels of LDL cholesterol are more affected by eating too much fat and sugar, rather than foods such as eggs, which contain cholesterol (see *Friendly Foods*).

If you do have a high cholesterol level, two of the most important supplements you can take are natural-source full-spectrum vitamin E, which helps to prevent the cholesterol oxidizing, and B-group vitamins including B12, B6, B3 and folic acid, all of which prevent the elevation of homocysteine levels (see below), which again tends to oxidize cholesterol and leads to plaque formation in the arteries. Thanks to eating too much animal fat, many children in the West now have raised cholesterol and arterial plaque by the age of 10. But while cholesterol levels have been used for many years as a possible way to predict our risk of heart attacks and strokes, that's only part of the story. Medical science is now beginning to re-think the role that cholesterol plays in heart disease and strokes.

Homocysteine levels are now also being recognized as an important indicator for heart disease and stroke. Homocysteine is a toxic amino acid produced during the metabolism of proteins and high levels are associated with an 80% increased risk of heart disease and strokes, even if you have a healthy cholesterol level. The good news is that there is now an easy way to test your own homocysteine levels (see *Helpful Hints*), and you can lower levels naturally, by simply taking more B-vitamins (see under *Useful Remedies*). If your level of homo-cysteine is high and you are taking B-vitamins to lower it, retest your levels periodically to see if you are taking sufficient dosages.

C

High plasma levels of homocysteine cause damage to artery walls, then LDL cholesterol (the bad cholesterol) can easily stick to them – which triggers the cascade of events that leads to heart disease and strokes. It is also linked to numerous other age-related conditions from Alzheimer's and diabetes, to obesity and mental health problems such as schizophrenia.

Places where high saturated fats are consumed (for example, The Netherlands and Finland) have higher elevations of LDL, whereas places, such as Japan, with relatively low saturated fat intake have lower LDL levels. But other factors are important as well. Our cho-lesterol will naturally tend to rise (as liver function decreases) up until age 65 and high cholesterol will be more common in men younger than 55 years old than in women of the same age. However, after menopause women's cholesterol rises and women over 55 will tend to have higher levels than men.

Around 20% of the body's total cholesterol is obtained from the diet, and the body man-ufactures the rest. Studies have shown that overweight people produce 20% more cholesterol than people of normal weight for their age, usually triggered by eating too much fat and sugar, stress and smoking. However, if you have a persistently raised cholesterol level but eat a healthy diet, you may have an underactive thyroid. Also, people with blood type A are more susceptible to high total cholesterol.

Optimum liver function helps you to make more good cholesterol, therefore the more you look after your liver, the more likely you are to have a healthy level (see *Liver Problems*). About one person in 100 has a genetic predisposition to high blood cholesterol levels and even this can be helped through diet and taking the right supplements.

Statins are currently being treated as magic bullets to treat high cholesterol and approxi-mately 7 million people in the UK take statins regularly. But statins have been found to have considerable negative long-term consequences for some people – including memory loss, loss of libido, muscle pain and nerve damage (possibly to the myelin sheath that coats nerve endings)

Statins mask an underlying imbalance such as a fatty liver, and although statins lower LDL and total cholesterol, they only have a modest effect on boosting the artery-cleansing HDL. Statin drugs do not, however, lower the dangerous triglycerides. Also, statins place a strain on all muscles, including the heart muscle, as they lower production of a vitamin-like substance – CoQ10, which is produced naturally in the liver. But as we age production of this vital substance slows and statins exacerbate the problem further.

Anyone taking statins **must** take a daily CoQ10 supplement. In fact, naturopath Steve Langley says: 'The average 70-year-old does not have adequate reserves of CoQ10 and if such a person is then given statins, it could reduce CoQ10 levels to a critical state and trigger heart problems.'

Several doctors are now openly linking some of the side effects of statins to lowered levels of CoQ10.

Foods to Avoid

- Eating too many barbecued or burnt foods, especially meat, hard margarines, fried foods and so on, causes cholesterol to oxidize, which makes it more dangerous, and once oxidized it begins attaching itself to artery walls. And as we age cholesterol tends to oxidize at a faster rate, therefore the more antioxidants we eat, the less cholesterol oxidizes, and the more likely you are to remain healthier for longer. Cut down on your intake of animal fats and full-fat dairy produce and eat more essential fats (for a full list, see *Fats You Need To Eat*).

- Read labels – and as much as possible, avoid mass-produced foods and oils that contain hydrogenated or trans-fats.
- Refined carbohydrates, white rice and pastas, processed white breads, cakes etc, can reduce the production of HDLs, and white bread eaters usually have higher cholesterol levels than those who eat mainly wholemeal varieties.
- Sugar, if not burnt for energy during exercise, converts to fat in the body and resides on your hips – and in the long run raises LDL cholesterol.
- Eggs contain cholesterol, but this is balanced by a high choline content (great for memory), which breaks down the cholesterol. However, some scientists say that if an egg is fried, this causes oxidative damage – and it's the frying that causes the problems, not the eggs themselves. It makes sense, then, to boil or poach eggs. Buy organic eggs or eggs containing omega-3 fats, which are now available in all major supermarkets.
- Alcohol and coffee (especially if microwaved), taken to excess, have been shown to raise cholesterol levels.
- Greatly reduce the amount of sodium-based salt you use.

Friendly Foods

- Studies have shown that two glasses of red wine for a man and one for a woman a day tend to raise HDL but won't affect LDL levels.
- Generally, you need to increase your fibre intake. Eat more oat or rice bran, rolled oats, wheat germ, and any beans and peas such as soya beans, red kidney beans, lima beans, broad beans, chick peas and lentils. Wholegrains, such as brown rice, whole wheat, barley, rye, millet and quinoa, are great for controlling cholesterol.
- Increase your intake of fresh fruit and vegetables (raw, steamed, roasted or stir fried, not deep fried or boiled). Green vegetables are especially rich in magnesium and potassium, as are cereals (also rich in B-vitamins), honey, kelp and dried fruits, such as dates.
- A couple of raw organic carrots or apples per day can lower cholesterol levels.
- Eat porridge for breakfast. Make with half low-fat milk (or even better rice/almond or oat milk) and half water. Add a chopped apple and a few raisins to sweeten, rather than sugar.

- Buckwheat is high in glycine, and has been shown to lower cholesterol levels. Buckwheat flour makes great pancakes.
- Fermented soya products, such as natto, miso and tempeh, can help to raise HDLs and lower LDLs.
- Soya lecithin granules are a great way to help lower LDL and help to control the growth of kidney and gall stones. Sprinkle a tablespoon daily over cereals, into yoghurts and onto fruit salads. Make sure it's a non-GM source.
- Increase your intake of healthier fats found in olive oil, avocados, coconut oil, sunflower, pumpkin, sesame and linseeds, plus walnuts and Brazil nuts and their unrefined oils (see *Fats You Need To Eat*).
- Oily fish such as salmon, trout, mackerel, anchovies, herring and sardines contain a fatty acid known as eicosapentaenoic acid (EPA). This helps to make the blood less sticky, so lowers the risk of coronary heart disease. Garlic and onions do the same.
- Look for spreads that are free from hydrogenated and trans-fats such as Biona or Olivio. Or blend a small amount of organic butter with a little olive oil.
- Otherwise use small amounts of walnut, almond or hemp seed butters. Available from health shops and Higher Nature. **HN**
- Vegetarians tend to have lower cholesterol levels.
- Use an organic, mineral-based sea salt, available from all health stores. I use Himalayan Crystal Salt, which is rich in organic source minerals.
- Look for eggs that are labelled as containing omega-3 essential fats. These chickens are fed on seeds that are rich in essential fats and therefore they lay healthier eggs!
- Drink dandelion root tea, which helps liver function, and green tea, which helps to lower cholesterol levels.
- Globe artichoke, celeriac, kale and fennel stimulate liver function and cell regeneration and can help lower blood cholesterol.
- Eat more live, low-fat, plain yoghurt containing lactobacillus/acidophilus, which lowers blood cholesterol levels by binding fat and cholesterol in the intestines.
- Drink plenty of water – at least 6–8 glasses daily.

Useful Remedies
- Statin drugs, which are now available over the counter from pharmacies, these drugs block the enzyme that makes cholesterol. The same enzyme also makes CoQ10 (Co-enzyme Q10), a vitamin-like substance that is needed to protect against heart disease. Therefore, if you are taking statins it is really important that you also take 150mg of CoQ10 per day. Research shows people on statins (such as lipitor, lescol, mevacor and zocor) have low levels of CoQ10, which can eventually trigger heart problems.
- As a base, take a good-quality multi-vitamin and mineral daily.
- Take 1 2 grams of fish oil daily.
- Evidence has shown that taking garlic each day could help lower overall cholesterol blood levels and increase the levels of HDL over LDL cholesterol. This is especially true if you are an A or an AB blood type.
- Include a high-strength antioxidant formula that helps prevent the cholesterol from oxidizing. **HN**
- Make sure that any multi you take includes 400iu of full-spectrum, natural-source vitamin E, which helps protect against oxidation of LDL.
- Alpha-lipoic acid also helps prevent oxidation of LDL; take 200mg daily.
- Folic acid, B12 and B6 all lower levels of homocysteine in the blood, thus reducing our risk of heart disease. A good B-complex should contain 400mcg folic acid, 10–20mg B6 and 50–100mcg B12.

- Taking 200mcg per day of the mineral chromium can help elevate HDL levels while reducing cravings for sugary foods.
- The minerals calcium and magnesium are useful for reducing cholesterol. Take 1000mg of calcium and 600mg of magnesium daily.

Helpful Hints

- There is now an easy test to discover your plasma homocysteine levels. Made by York Laboratories and backed by The British Cardiac Patients Association, it's a simple pinprick method that can be done by post. For details, call York Labs on 0800 458 2052, or log on to www.yorktest.com.
- Exercise is vital for controlling cholesterol; it can raise HDL levels and lower LDL. Try to walk for at least 30 minutes daily and do some kind of aerobic exercise 3 times a week.
- Smoking increases oxidation of LDL.
- Eating smaller meals every three to four hours, rather than three big meals per day, can help lower cholesterol.

CHRONIC FATIGUE   *(see Exhaustion and ME)*

CHRONIC OBSTRUCTIVE PULMONARY DISEASE

(see Bronchitis and Emphysema)

C

CIRCULATION   *(see also Chilblains, Cholesterol and Raynaud's Disease)*

Good circulation is fundamental for good health, as all parts of the body require sufficient oxygen and nutrients to function optimally. Good circulation also enables us to eliminate toxins more efficiently. And it's amazing how many conditions are linked to poor circulation. Common symptoms range from cold hands and feet to leg ulcers and varicose veins. Hair loss can be triggered by poor circulation to the head. More serious problems involve restricted circulation to the heart and brain as in strokes.

If you laid out your blood vessels end to end, it is estimated that they would encircle the globe twice over – that's a lot of miles. No wonder we end up with so many circulatory problems. As we age our arteries become thickened (atherosclerosis) or hardened (arteriosclerosis), and many people of all ages are exercising less, so in turn our circulation becomes less efficient.

Numerous conditions associated with ageing – leg ulcers, memory loss, atherosclerosis, cold hands and feet – are all linked to poor circulation. Our arteries make up a major part of our blood circulatory system and contain about 15% of our blood supply at any given moment. Healthy arteries have thick, muscular walls, which are necessary for the pressure of the blood moving through them. Your heart weighs just 280–310g (10–11oz) and it is about the size of a clenched fist. The left side of the heart forces blood into the arteries, which carry the bright red, nutrient-rich, oxygenated blood through the body.

The oxygen (from the lungs) and nutrients (absorbed into the arteries via the gut) are taken up by the cells, before the blood (now a darker, bluish colour) is returned to the heart via the veins, and the right chamber of the heart then pumps it through the lungs. Veins are more numerous and hold more of the body's blood (about 70%), and they transport blood laden with waste products, and partly depleted of oxygen, back to the heart.

From the lungs the re-oxygenated blood returns, purified, to the left chamber, ready for redistribution, and the whole cycle begins again. Veins are forced to move against gravity much of the time. In order to maintain normal blood pressure, an adequate supply of blood must be returned to the heart from the peripheral vessels. Two main factors are responsible for this 'uphill' flow from the legs and abdomen to the heart. Firstly, muscular contractions compress veins, thus squeezing the blood along. When a person stands still for a long time, such as soldiers on sentry duty, the blood pools in the lower limbs due to the force of gravity and in the long term, as the leg valves become weaker, can trigger varicose veins. This pooling of blood means that there is insufficient blood returning to the heart to maintain blood pressure, and less blood makes it to the brain. In extreme cases fainting can result, which forces the person into a horizontal position and alleviates the problem.

Secondly, as we get older, especially if we have a sedentary lifestyle, we tend to breathe more shallowly, which has a direct effect on our circulation. Coronary heart disease is almost always due to a condition called atherosclerosis (see *Atherosclerosis*), where fatty deposits attach themselves to the insides of the arteries. Arteries that were once smooth and elastic become rough, inflexible and narrow (see *High Blood Pressure*). With this narrowing, the volume of blood that the arteries can transport is reduced. Factors that contribute to atherosclerosis are long-term negative stress, cigarette smoking, high cholesterol, a high homocysteine level, a high-fat diet, excessive salt, and so on.

Once an area has been damaged, fats from the blood, including cholesterol, accumulate and build up a thick fatty layer called plaque. This plaque narrows the artery and a clot may detach itself and, if it causes an obstruction inside the coronary artery, a heart attack can occur. If it blocks an artery leading to the brain, it can cause a stroke.

This slow build-up of plaque and consequent narrowing of the artery can also lead to a condition called angina, which is very common after 50. The pain of angina (which can vary considerably) is generally felt when the person is under stress or more demands are put on the heart muscle during exercise. The pain of a heart attack is a more 'crushing' pain in the chest, which can radiate to the jaw or down the left arm (see *Heart Disease*).

Blood pressure tends to increase with age. Normal blood pressure depends on a number of factors including the elasticity of the arterial walls, amount and consistency of the blood, digestion, smoking, weight and stress. High blood pressure can cause heart attacks and strokes. An aneurysm can occur when there is a weak spot in an arterial wall which balloons out and releases blood into surrounding tissues, which is why looking after the integrity of your veins and arteries can help keep you healthier at any age.

Foods to Avoid
- Salt hardens your arteries (which need to be elastic) and although it is essential to life, most people consume too much inorganic salt in the form of sodium chloride. Too much salt can result in high blood pressure, because where salt goes water follows! It is found in most tinned, pre-packaged, mass-produced foods, burgers, crisps, laxatives, antacids and carbonated drinks, especially canned fizzy drinks.
- Reduce animal fats such as red meat, full-fat milk and dairy produce, cheese and chocolates.
- Pies, pastries, cakes and foods made with saturated/hydrogenated trans-fats, such as lard and margarines, should be avoided or reduced (see *Fats You Need To Eat*).
- Avoid or greatly reduce your intake of fried foods. Never fry with mass-produced vegetable oils.
- Avoid coffee, caffeine and other stimulants, which can ultimately lead to a constriction of blood vessels.
- Avoid excessive alcohol. A glass of red wine with meals, however, can be beneficial.

Friendly Foods

- Try chopping up seaweeds, such as kelp, over your food instead of salt. Kelp or nori flakes can be used instead of salt.
- Use organic mineral-rich sea salt, but only over the food that is in front of you! I use Himalayan Crystal Salt, which is rich in natural minerals. Available from the Nutri Centre, good health shops and some supermarkets. **NC**
- Vitamin C is vital for healthy circulation because as a major antioxidant it helps protect blood vessels from damage. Foods naturally high in vitamin C include blueberries, sweet potatoes, cherries, guavas, kale leaves, parsley, cantaloupe melon, broccoli, strawberries and peppers.
- Tomatoes, grapes and blackberries are high in bioflavonoids.
- Garlic and onions help to thin the blood naturally.
- Wheat germ, avocados, nuts and seeds are all rich in vitamin E, which also helps to thin the blood naturally.
- Foods rich in rutin help to strengthen the small blood vessels. So eat more buckwheat, the peel of citrus fruits, rose hips and apple peel.
- Silica-rich foods, such as lettuce, celery, millet, oats and parsnips, help to strengthen arterial and vein walls. Fiji mineral water is rich in silica.
- Linseeds (flax seeds soaked overnight in cold water then drained) and sunflower and sesame seeds, and fish oils contain essential polyunsaturated fatty acids, known as omega-3 fatty acids, that have been shown to lower the 'bad' LDL fats and thin the blood.
- Try eating at least 3 portions of fish a week, such as wild organic salmon, mackerel, sardines or anchovies. Tuna can be high in mercury.
- Unrefined Brazils, walnuts, hazelnuts, almonds, seeds and their unrefined cold oils, are excellent sources of essential fats; avocado (eat one a week) is also a rich source of mono-unsaturated fats.
- Sprinkle GM-free lecithin granules, which emulsify 'bad' fats, over your breakfast cereals, into yoghurts or over fruit to help lower LDL cholesterol.
- People on high-fibre diets are four times less likely to suffer from circulation problems and heart disease. Soluble fibre (that is, beans, lentils, brown rice) consists of compounds that bind to bile salts and this helps lower cholesterol levels.
- Use oat or rice brans in your diet.

Useful Remedies

- Pycnogenol – pine bark extract – encourages nitrous oxide production, which in turn relaxes blood vessels and arteries. Take 80mg daily. **PN**
- The herb gotu kola helps increase circulation to the extremities such as feet and hands through its vasodilatory action on peripheral blood vessels. Take 500mg twice daily.
- The herb butcher's broom is high in rutin, a bioflavonoid, which helps to tone the vein walls. It is therefore very beneficial in treating varicose veins. **NB As butcher's broom is a vasoconstrictor (the opposite to gotu kola), caution should be taken if you suffer from high blood pressure.** Take 500mg twice daily.
- The herb horse chestnut has a similar action on varicose veins as its components help strengthen the small capillaries. Take 500mg daily.
- V-Nal contains butcher's broom, horse chestnut, B-vitamins and rutin. Made by Bional and available from all health stores. All the above herbs are usually used for varicose veins, as they strengthen veins, have anti-inflammatory properties and reduce swelling, thus making venous return to the heart more efficient.
- Various studies have taken place that show that patients who are suffering from visual and hearing problems that are linked to poor circulation, such as tinnitus, have demonstrated

improvements in their condition after taking ginkgo biloba for 3 months. Take 120mg daily in one dose.

- Vitamin C with bioflavonoids helps to strengthen capillaries. Take 2 grams daily with food – spread throughout the day.
- Vitamin E helps reduce stickiness in the blood; take 200iu daily of full-spectrum, natural-source vitamin E. This is especially true for type A and AB blood types, which tend to be 'stickier' than other blood types.
- Niacin (vitamin B3) increases circulation. **NB Niacin can induce a short-term 'flushing' or reddening of the skin, so begin with 30mg and work up to 100mg daily.**
- Ginger helps to warm the body, so make a ginger tea infusion daily and add grated fresh root ginger to stir-fries and fruit salads.

Helpful Hints

- Long-term stress constricts blood vessels and causes the blood to become stickier and will impede circulation. This in turn can trigger heart attacks or strokes. Deal with stress levels.
- Exercise is a wonderful way to help increase circulation. Just taking a brisk walk every day can be very helpful, as it warms the blood, relaxing the arteries. Skipping, dancing, rebounding and power walking all help by gently pounding the feet.
- Massage and reflexology are important, especially for people who, for health reasons, cannot exercise much, or those who lead a more sedentary lifestyle. Aromatherapy massage using essential oils, such as rosemary, black pepper or ginger, can be very effective in aiding circulation.
- Skin brushing also aids circulation. Work upward from the feet and hands towards the heart, rubbing briskly; try to do this 5 times a week in the bath or shower.
- If you smoke, give it up, as it impairs breathing and hence circulation.
- Acupuncture has a long history in the treatment of poor circulation and high blood pressure. The action of the needles promotes better circulation through unblocking stagnation of both qi and blood (see *Useful Information*).

C

COELIAC DISEASE *(see also Absorption and Leaky Gut)*

Research indicates that 1 in every 100 people suffers this autoimmune condition, and up to 500,000 suffer this problem in the UK alone, which often goes undiagnosed for years. It can happen at any age and sufferers cannot break down a protein called gluten, which is present in wheat, rye, barley and oats. Some coeliacs appear to be able to tolerate small amounts of spelt, a low gluten-type of wheat, but for the majority of sufferers spelt would definitely need to be avoided.

The gluten damages the lining of the small intestine which can create a leaky gut. This is when food particles 'leak' through the gut wall triggering other health conditions. See *Leaky Gut*.

Symptoms include frequent indigestion, abdominal pain, loss of weight and depression. The stools can be pale, frothy and foul smelling. It is very important that if you suffer from any or some of these symptoms over a period of several months you see a doctor. The longer you suffer from coeliac disease, particularly if it goes undiagnosed, the more likely you are to do more damage to the gut lining. This greatly reduces the body's ability to absorb adequate levels of nutrients, which can even lead to malnutrition. Coeliacs are also at a higher risk for osteoporosis, due to mineral malabsorption.

Foods to Avoid

- Any foods containing wheat, rye, oats, barley and spelt are absolutely crucial to avoid. Quite a few people with coeliac disease also have a problem with cow's milk and dairy products or soya foods.
- You will also need to avoid cakes, desserts and any cereals containing gluten.
- Until the condition is under control, also avoid fatty meats, sausages, pies and processed meat products, as they can often contain wheat.

Friendly Foods

- Fortunately, these days, there are plenty of gluten-free foods available, most of them fairly palatable. Some will be high in sugar so be sure to read labels carefully – sugar converts to fat in the body if not burned up during exercise, and in coeliac sufferers, fat can be poorly absorbed. Look out for the gluten-free Orgran or Barkat ranges of products.
- Look for breads, instant foods, and flours made from grain alternatives, such as quinoa, amaranth, millet, corn, rice, buckwheat and lentils.
- You can also try sprouted wheat bread that is free of gluten.
- Dairy alternatives to cow's milk include rice, oat, coconut, quinoa, pea and almond – available from all good health stores.
- Eat plenty of leafy greens, which are rich sources of magnesium and calcium. Cabbage is rich in the amino acid L-glutamine, which helps to heal the gut – try making fresh vegetable juices that include raw cabbage, a little root ginger, which is very soothing, plus any vegetables you have to hand. If you cook cabbage in water, save the water and make gravy with it. Or add cabbage to stews and soups.
- Try to eat more fish to provide vitamin D, which is often deficient in coeliac sufferers.
- Eat plenty of unrefined organic nuts, seeds and fish; and free-range, low-fat meats, such as venison, pork and turkey, to keep up zinc intake often deficient in coeliacs. Try to use only organic meat.
- Essential fats are needed to heal the gut, so use a little organic sunflower, sesame, olive or walnut oil for salad dressings.
- Eat an avocado once a week, as they are rich in vitamin E.
- Papaya is very healing and pineapple breaks down gluten, so if you are borderline then eat fresh pineapple before meals to aid digestion,

Useful Remedies

- None of the supplements suggested will cure coeliac disease, it's just that the vast majority of these nutrients are often deficient in coeliac sufferers. It is very important to increase your intake of these nutrients to prevent deficiency.
- Calcium (500mg daily) and magnesium (250mg daily) are vital minerals, as many coeliac sufferers have a low bone density – take with vitamin D, which aids calcium absorption.
- Folic acid – 400–800mcg, and vitamin B6 – 50–100mg, daily. Include a B-complex as well as the extra daily folic acid and B6.
- Take a high-strength, natural-source carotene complex, which converts naturally to vitamin A in the body – needed for healing.
- Many coeliac sufferers are low in vitamin D, a deficiency of which is linked to a host of health problems, including cancers and osteoporosis. Take a minimum 1000iu of D 3 a day.
- Take a high-strength multi-vitamin and mineral (preferably in liquid form) to make up for any other nutritional deficiencies. **BC.**
- Omega-3 fats are vital; take 2 grams of omega-3 fats daily (see *Fats You Need To Eat*).
- Bromelain helps to break down gluten and is anti-inflammatory. If you are borderline, take 250mg Bromelain before each main meal.

- Take a full-spectrum digestive enzyme, such as Poly-Zyme, to aid absorption. **BC**
- Slippery elm tablets/or aloe vera can help to reduce the irritation. Take one tablet/or capful of the aloe with each meal.
- Aloe Pura make a great 'stomach formula' – available from good health stores and larger chemists, or see www.optimah.com.

Helpful Hints
- If you have any of the symptoms mentioned, then ask your doctor for a blood test.
- If you are a severe coeliac, you will need to avoid all utensils that have been in any contact with gluten.
- Breast-fed children are much less likely to develop coeliac disease than those fed on cow's or soya milk formulas. Formula milks are harder to digest and potentially can cause health problems later on.
- The Village Bakery in Cumbria make great wheat-, rye- and barley-free breads and cakes. Sold at most health stores. Call the bakery on 01768 898437 or visit their website at www.village-bakery.com.
- Research from Finland shows that small amounts (50–70g) of oat-based products can be tolerated by coeliacs without damaging intestinal absorption.
- For further information, visit www.coeliac.org.uk.

COLDS and FLU
(see also Antibiotics and Immune Function)

Colds and flu are caused by viruses, and the secret to avoiding them is to keep your immune system in great shape. See also *Immune Function*. Newer virus strains such as swine and bird flu, which are potentially a serious threat, are sadly becoming more commonplace, often triggering unnecessary panic. Yet if we could all keep our immune systems functioning optimally, we could avoid becoming sick in the first place.

Flu symptoms are usually far more severe and include a fever, aching joints and dreadful headaches. With colds there is plenty of congestion, often accompanied by a headache. With heavier bouts of flu your joints ache, and all you want is bed rest, which is one of the fastest routes to recovery. If you have a temperature, your doctor will likely suggest taking two paracetamol every four to six hours to help bring it down – yet having a temperature is nature's way of killing the invading bugs.

If an infant has a high temperature, it is important that they are taken to see a doctor. And if an adult has a high temperature for more than two days, again, he or she should seek medical assistance.

Only if you contract a secondary bacterial infection – meaning if it hurts to breathe and you are wheezing – may antibiotics be warranted; see also *Bronchitis*.

We become more susceptible to colds and flu if we overwork, over-train or consistently eat a poor diet high in saturated fats and sugars. For example, if you eat a sugar-rich pudding and a bar of chocolate, and are then immediately in contact with someone suffering from a cold or flu, you have doubled your chances of picking it up. Also, lack of sleep greatly lowers immune function, as does long-term negative stress.

Foods to Avoid
- All refined sugars and carbohydrates, such as white bread, cakes pies and biscuits plus high-fat foods, alcohol and caffeine. All of these can weaken the immune system and make us more susceptible to infection.

- Generally, while you have a cold reduce your intake of mucous-forming foods such as cheese, chocolate and full-fat dairy produce. Mucous will also form as a reaction to any foods to which you have an intolerance; see *Allergies* and *Catarrh*.

Friendly Foods

- It's crucial to keep up your fluid intake – tea and coffee dehydrate the body, so drink plenty of water and herbal teas. Pau d'arco or green tea will help boost immune function. Fluids help the lymphatic system to function efficiently.
- Garlic and onions are great foods, as they are anti-bacterial and have antiseptic properties. A traditional remedy for colds and flu is a soup made with 6 onions, a whole garlic, 2.5cm (1in) of grated fresh ginger, and some cayenne pepper mixed in a vegetable or chicken stock. You could also add lemongrass. For children, it is probably preferable to leave out the cayenne pepper – although it does make the other herbs more effective, it is often too hot for them.
- Liquorice is a pleasant-tasting food that you can make into tea and eat as confectionery if it is sugar-free. It has both anti-viral and anti-bacterial properties and will soothe the throat when it's inflamed (see *Sore Throat*).
- While you have a cold or flu, try to base your diet on fruits, vegetables, brown rice, barley and quinoa, adding in a little fish, chicken or pulses. Keep your diet clean. See *General Health Hints*.
- Drink plenty of lemon and ginger herbal tea or make your own: finely chop a 2.5cm (1in) piece of fresh ginger, stand it in boiling water for 15 minutes with a squeeze of lemon juice and freshly chopped spring onions, strain and sip.

Useful Remedies

- One of the best remedies I have found is The Wellness Formula, made by Source Naturals Inc. It contains garlic, propolis, elderberry extract, olive leaf extract, vitamin C, astragalus, zinc and grapeseed extract – a perfect combination of nutrients needed to boost immunity, as they are anti-viral and bacterial. At the first sign of a sore throat or feeling that you have something coming, take 1 or 2 capsules, three times daily. They are amazing. Available at all good health stores.
- Propolis – from bee hives – has anti-viral and anti-bacterial properties. Taking 1 to 3 grams daily can help reduce the severity of a cold and taken all year round (500mg daily) can help boost immunity.
- Echinacea and golden seal, taken either as tincture or tablets every couple of hours, help fend off a cold or flu. Echinacea has been shown in a number of studies to shorten the length of a cold from 7 days down to 3–4 if taken regularly; generally 1–4ml every 2–3 hours. A great anti-viral formula, Ultimate Echinacea Complex, is available from www.holoshealth.com. Take 1 teaspoon in a glass of water at the onset of symptoms – up to 3 doses daily while symptoms persist.
- I tend to take herbs such as echinacea in the winter when we are more susceptible to colds. It is more effective when taken cyclically. Take for a month, then stop taking for a week. Continue throughout the winter.
- Vitamin C is strongly anti-viral and research has shown that it can shorten the severity and duration of most colds and flu, if taken in sufficient amounts. During the winter, take 1 gram daily, but if you feel a cold coming on, increase your intake to 1 gram, 3 times daily. Take it with meals in an ascorbate form until the cold has gone.
- A huge percentage of people are lacking in Vitamin D, known as the sunshine vitamin – and we should all now be taking 1000iu of vitamin D3 daily to keep our immune systems in better shape.

- Take a multi-vitamin and mineral that contains at least 30–60mg of zinc to boost the immune system while fighting an infection.
- If you are suffering from a sore throat, try zinc gluconate lozenges that contain 15–25mg of zinc. Take one every three to four hours. The zinc lozenges help to kill any bacteria that is in the throat.
- Olive leaf extract acts like nature's antibiotic. I take two daily to help keep my immune system in shape when I am feeling run down.
- Sambucol is an extract of the European black elderberry plant, which has potent anti-viral properties. If taken at the onset of a cold or flu, it can help reduce the severity and length of the illness. Available from health stores.
- Beta Glucans 1-3, 1-6 are proven to strengthen the body's innate immune system and are especially useful for children. Pharma Nord make a version that is free from yeast protein. Take 250–500 mg daily. Can be taken all year round by adults and children (250mg daily) to boost immune functioning. **PN**
- N-acetyl cysteine (NAC) is an amino acid that really helps to boost levels of glutathione, one of the body's most potent antioxidant defences. In a large study of older adults who took 600mg twice daily 30 minutes before meals for six months, only 25% of those taking part experienced any flu-like symptoms. In the placebo group (those who were given a 'blank' pill), it was 79%. NAC helps to inhibit virus replication and has shown good results against the H5N1 bird flu virus.

Helpful Hints

- If I start a sore throat, I take homeopathic Streptococcus 10M immediately along with the Wellness Formula and my bad throat almost always disappears.
- Homeopathic Aconite 30c can be taken two or three times daily at the onset of a cold to help stop the cold from developing.
- Ainsworth's famous Anti-Cold and Flu Remedy is a homeopathic preventative for colds and flu symptoms, which is tailored to the current strains each year. They also supply a remedy called Anas Barb Co, which is for use at the onset of a cold or flu to prevent symptoms from developing further. Contact Ainsworth Homeopathic Pharmacy, who are based at 36 New Cavendish Street, London W1G 8UF. Call them on 020 7935 5330 or log on to www.ainsworths.com.
- Keep warm and avoid changes in the temperature of your surroundings for at least 48 hours until symptoms subside. Rest is essential if you have a temperature.
- Do not struggle into work if you have a really bad cold – all you do is make it last longer and you pass it on to your colleagues.
- Washing your hands regularly, and not shaking hands with anyone who has a cold or flu, are the best ways of avoiding giving your cold or contracting other people's colds and flu, as viruses can easily permeate the soft skin on the palms of the hands. Washing hands is especially true for kids, whose hygiene levels are often lacking!
- Use tissues when you sneeze or cough and bin immediately. Your germs can spread up to 3m (10ft) around you every time you sneeze.
- Viruses are airborne and spread quickly at large gatherings. Avoid being in stuffy, smoky rooms for too long. Get plenty of exercise and fresh air.
- Use the Neil Med sinus rinse daily: it helps remove gunk from the sinuses and reduces bacteria held in the nose and sinuses. Brilliant. Available from all good chemists.

COLD SORES

(see also Herpes)

Cold sores are caused by the herpes simplex virus. Once contracted the virus lies dormant in the body and tends to re-activate if you become run down or stressed, or after sudden exposure to very hot or cold weather. Some women suffer an attack during menstruation. Others find that if they eat large amounts of nuts or chocolate containing the amino acid arginine, on which the virus thrives, this can also trigger an attack. There have been a number of studies showing that you can reduce the frequency of attacks by taking vitamin C and the amino acid lysine on a regular basis.

Foods to Avoid
- Foods that are very rich in arginine, an amino acid found commonly in chocolate, lentils, beans and nuts.
- As sugar triggers inflammation and lowers immune function, you should greatly reduce your intake of any sugar. Also avoid refined foods made with white flour, cakes, biscuits, pre-made desserts, and high saturated-fat foods that are often high in sugar.
- Avoid trans- and hydrogenated fats (see *Fats You Need To Eat*).
- Certain people notice when they eat too much dairy produce from cows they suffer an attack.

Friendly Foods
- Eat good-quality protein, such as lean meats including turkey, chicken, duck (without any skin), lean pork, white fish, salmon, eggs, corn and soya, all of which are rich in lysine, an amino acid that has been shown to interfere with replication of the virus.
- Plain live yoghurt should be fine and is high in lysine
- Quinoa is an excellent source of protein.
- Goat's cheese should be fine as it is high in lysine.
- Garlic and onions are highly anti-viral.
- See *General Health Hints*.

Useful Remedies
- At the onset of an attack, take up to 4 grams of lysine daily. Many companies now make lysine and vitamin C together. At the onset also take 4 grams of vitamin C daily with food.
- To help prevent attacks take 1 gram of vitamin C daily. Take 3 grams of propolis capsules and use the cream topically to help shut down an attack and ease the irritation. Then take 500mg of propolis daily to help prevent further attacks. Propolis is strongly anti-viral – and in studies has been proven to be more effective than some anti-viral drugs. **NB If you suffer severe allergy to bee stings, avoid propolis.**
- Olive leaf extract is another great supplement for cold sores as it is highly anti-viral. At the onset of an attack take 500mg, 3 times daily with food, until symptoms subside.
- If you find you or your children regularly suffer cold sores you definitely need to include a good quality multi-vitamin and mineral that contains Vitamin D3 in your regimen. There are now plenty of sugar and additive-free chewable vitamins for children (Nature's Plus make great ranges for kids), or add liquid vitamins and minerals to their food. **BC**

Helpful Hints
- Make sure you change your toothbrush and face towels regularly because these can harbour the virus.
- Over-exposure to bright sunshine can also encourage replication of the virus.
- Calendula tincture can be dabbed directly onto the sores.
- Homeopathic Rhus Tox 30c helps to eliminate the eruptions. Take as soon as the tingling starts. Take twice daily for 3 days.

■ Several people have told me that when they take Bach Rescue Remedy internally and dab it externally onto the cold sores it prevents the cold sore from developing. As Rescue Remedy is also available in a cream, this is certainly worth a try.

COLITIS
(see also Crohn's Disease and Leaky Gut)

Colitis means 'inflammation of the colon', and is a chronic, non-specific inflammatory and ulcerative disease of the colitis. Most commonly it develops between the ages of 15–40, but can start at any age. Symptoms include abdominal pain, tenderness or cramping – particularly in the lower left side. There may be a change in the stools, with episodes of frequent watery bowel movements that usually contain mucous and blood. In severe cases between 5 and 20 motions can be passed daily, causing severe dehydration and/or anaemia.

Around two-thirds of sufferers experience intermittent symptoms and for about 5% of people colitis has a rapid onset. This condition tends to start in the rectum and then spreads back up into the bowel.

To make sure you get a correct diagnosis, you would need to have stool tests and have an internal examination and a barium enema X-ray. The risk for colon cancer is increased with colitis.

There is an autoimmune component similar to Crohn's and there may be parasites, too much fat in the diet, stress, a leaky gut and/or food intolerances (mainly to wheat, gluten and dairy produce from cows). Many nutritional physicians now believe that a leaky gut is the root cause for conditions such as colitis – see *Leaky Gut*.

C

Foods to Avoid
■ Any food that is an irritant to the bowel, particularly in the acute stage – this would usually be wheat, gluten, any type of bran, dairy produce from cows including all cheeses.
■ Avoid very hot or cold foods, spicy foods and vinegar.
■ Absolutely avoid processed foods, fried foods, red meats (especially pork).
■ In the acute stages also avoid raw fruits and vegetables.
■ Avoid refined sugar, which creates inflammation in the body
■ The main intolerances are dairy produce, wheat, corn, tomatoes, citrus, potato and chocolate.

Friendly Foods
■ Rice, millet, barley and quinoa are generally well tolerated.
■ Mashed pumpkin, buckwheat, sweet potato, carrots, papaya, mango are all rich in carotenes.
■ Chlorophyll heals the bowel – therefore eat more green foods such as watercress, spring greens, cabbage. Green powders, such as Viridian 100% Organic Green Food Blend, are useful for these conditions .
■ Eat more home-made soups and stews.
■ Alkaline broth can be made with cabbage juice, potato water and carrots.
■ Fresh fish is high in zinc, and zinc aids tissue healing.
■ Oily fish are great for their omega-3 content, which aids healing.
■ Once the healing process has started, then try porridge, oat or rice brans, and generally eat more fibre. Keep a food diary and note when symptoms are worse – also note your emotions.
■ If you need sugar use small amounts of organic agave syrup or ZyloSweet, which have a low glycaemic index. HN

Useful remedies
■ One of the best gut healers is aloe vera juice. Aloe Pura make a stomach formula. Take before meals three times daily.

- Slippery elm bark powder really helps to soothe the gut. Best taken on an empty stomach half an hour before meals. **SHS**
- Take a natural-source carotene complex, as vitamin A is vital for soft tissue healing.
- Take a multi-vitamin/mineral for your age and gender.
- Liquorice root – deglycerinated, sugar free, can help heal the gut.
- Good bacteria are important, especially the Bifido bacteria. Use Jarro-Dophilus EPS – take one daily with food. **NC**
- You may need DHEA, a hormone usually lacking in these types of conditions. Have a blood test to find out.
- Take vitamin B-complex, as folic acid is needed to help reduce the likelihood of colon cancer.
- 2 grams of omega-3 fish oils daily to reduce inflammation.
- Sea buckthorn (an omega-7 essential fat) helps to heal the mucosal lining – try 2 grams daily for a month, then reduce to 1 gram. **PN**

Helpful Hints
- Try Kangen Water – a water system unit that attaches to your kitchen tap and ionizes and alkalizes water. The gut heals more quickly when alkaline. This water is used in many Japanese hospitals with highly beneficial health results. For full details, call 020 7580 7537 or log on to www.kangenmiraclewater.co.uk.
- As stress is a major factor, deal with stress in your life. Learn to meditate, have counselling.
- Breathe more deeply – learn to let go of the small stuff. It's not worth dying for. See *Adrenal Exhaustion* and *Stress*.
- Try homeopathic Merc cor 6c x 3 times daily if there are hot, bloody stools with mucous and cutting pains in the colon.
- Make sure you get plenty of rest and relaxation, which is the best way to allow the body to heal itself. Be kind to yourself.

CONJUNCTIVITIS
(see also Eye Problems)

Conjunctivitis is an inflammation of the outer surface membrane that lines the eye. This can be triggered by an external allergen, such as perfume or an insect spray, in which case the eyes are usually very red, itchy and irritated. But if conjunctivitis is caused by bacteria or a virus, this can be accompanied by a yellow or white mucous-type discharge and needs to be treated by a doctor. People who suffer chronic conjunctivitis are often very run down, their immune system is under functioning and they are usually deficient in vitamins A, C and D.

Foods to Avoid
- All foods and drinks containing sugar, which reduces the body's ability to fight an infection.
- Reduce your intake of animal fats, including cheese and chocolate, plus white-flour-based cakes, breads and biscuits, all of which will weaken the immune system.
- See *General Health Hints*.

Friendly Foods
- Bilberries, blueberries, blackberries and all blue- and purple-coloured fruits are rich in antioxidant nutrients that nourish the eyes.
- Foods rich in vitamin A such as leafy green vegetables, calves' or lambs' liver, cod liver oil, carrots and fish help encourage healthy eyes.
- Natural carotenes found in tomatoes, sweet potatoes, papaya, apricots, mangoes, spinach and all greens and raw parsley are all great foods for the eyes.

- Eat more fresh pineapple – it is rich in the enzyme bromelain, which is known to have anti-inflammatory properties.

Useful Remedies
- Echinacea, eyebright and bilberry tincture; 1–4ml a day. Available from health shops.
- Bromelain – take 500mg twice daily with food.
- Take a high-strength, full-spectrum carotene complex, which converts naturally to vitamin A in the body. **SVHC, VN**
- Vitamin C (1 gram, 2–3 times per day with meals) and zinc (30–50mg per day) will help strengthen your immune system.
- A multi-vitamin/mineral for your age and gender.
- Omega-3 fish oils help reduce inflammation in the body. Take 1 gram daily.

Helpful Hints
- Do you know that many eye drops are actually made from urine? Urea is an important component that helps to break down mucous deposits and has anti-microbial actions. Bathing the eyes in fresh urine (which is a sterile liquid) on a cotton wool pad can help to alleviate most eye problems.
- Conjunctivitis is highly contagious when caused by a viral infection. Be really careful not to use the same handkerchief or tissue to wipe both eyes. Be scrupulous with hygiene and make sure no one else uses your towels, make-up or pillow.
- Eyebright tincture plus goldenseal tincture: take 2 drops of each and add to an eye bath full of purified or boiled water and use when cool. Use twice daily.
- Dilute homeopathic Euphrasia mother tincture in an egg-cup full of cooled boiled water and use as an eye bath. Alternatively, you can try Visualize Herbal Eye Wash with chamomile and blueberry (herbal eye drops also available). Available from good health stores or log on to www.dry-eyes.co.uk.
- Chamomile and calendula herbal teas can be used to make warm compresses to soothe the eye. The heat also helps kill the bacteria that cause the infection.

CONSTIPATION and BLOATING

(see also Absorption, Candida and Leaky Gut)

Even though government advisors, health magazines and doctors all advise us to eat more fibre, we are one of the most constipated nations on earth. In an ideal world we should have a bowel movement after every meal – but most people in the West are lucky if they have one a day. Having clean bowels is one of the best ways to prevent most diseases in later life.

Even if you have a daily bowel movement, you can still be constipated. Over time, we can experience a gradual build-up of matter, which adheres to the walls of the intestines and becomes compacted in certain sections. This build-up is caused by insufficient fibre and too many refined foods, which can eventually inhibit proper assimilation of nutrients from the diet and supplements. It also adds to the weight of the colon, therefore placing more stress on the lower organs like the uterus and bladder.

Millions of men and women have large, protruding abdomens. This means that all the major organs in that area, such as the liver, heart and bowels, are surrounded by a layer of deadly fat deposits. They are also likely to be carrying a lot of waste matter. Henry VIII had more than 34kg (84lb) of faeces in his bowel after his death and he had a very big abdomen indeed!

When food leaves the small intestine, which is almost 7 metres (over 20ft) long, it passes into the large intestine or colon where it is gradually compacted into semi-solid faeces. The bowel is a term for the large intestine. Most of the absorption of nutrients from our diet and supplements happens in the small intestine.

The large intestine (colon) is primarily involved with the excretion and elimination of foods. The more faeces in your bowel, the more toxic your entire system becomes. If you are not eliminating properly, these toxins are re-absorbed into the bloodstream and can be eventually dumped into the skin, resulting in conditions such as acne. People from primitive cultures tend to evacuate twice the amount of faeces that their Western counterparts do, due to their higher intake of fibre and raw foods.

Peristalsis is the rhythmic movement of the colon, which helps to move the waste material out of the body. If you tend to eat a poor diet that is low in fibre, then the muscles in the colon can become lazy, which over time can lead to chronic constipation – and food putrefies in the bowel. Basically carbohydrates (fruit, breads, pasta and so on) ferment if not broken down properly, whereas protein (meat, eggs, cheese, fish) will putrefy. Also if you over-eat, food putrefies in the bowel, triggering symptoms such as bloating, gas, constipation or diarrhoea, irritable bowel, poor skin, dull hair and so on.

Haemorrhoids or piles (similar to varicose veins of the anus) are the result of years of straining to go to the loo and straining also contributes to varicose veins in the legs. If ever you experience blood in your faeces or any noticeable changes in bowel habits, it is **vital** that you see a doctor immediately.

Foods to Avoid

- Animal products, especially red meats, have a long transit time through the bowel and should only be eaten in moderation.
- Many people do not have the enzyme needed to break down lactose, the sugar in milk, which can also lead to putrefaction in the bowel. This is especially common in Asian, African and Caribbean people.
- If you tend to be a big dairy fan, try cutting back, as all dairy-based foods are mucous forming, which adds to congestion in the small intestine. However, organic rice, oat, almond or goat's milk are generally better tolerated.
- Refined sugars found in cakes, biscuits, desserts and highly processed foods ferment in the gut, causing gas and bloating as unhealthy bacteria proliferate. Healthy bacteria, which are known as probiotics, help break down digested foods and aid in the manufacture of certain B-group vitamins. If these healthy bacteria are missing, your digestion and elimination will be impaired.
- When you mix flour and water, it makes a gooey paste; it does the same in the bowel, so cut down on pastries and flour-based foods.
- Many people are sensitive to wheat, so try cutting back and see if the bloating reduces. Keep a food diary and note when symptoms are worse.
- Low-fibre foods such as jelly, ice cream and soft desserts, all white flour products and refined breakfast cereals contain virtually no fibre and plenty of sugar, which will all 'gum up' the works!
- Also avoid foods to which you have an intolerance; for example, cow's milk has been found to be responsible for a lot of infant constipation.
- Cut down on full-fat cheeses and don't eat melted cheese over food – it sets like plastic in the intestine.

Friendly Foods

- Linseeds (flax seeds) are a blend of insoluble and soluble fibres, which bulk the stool, encouraging it to move gently through the bowel. I soak a tablespoon of linseeds every night in cold water and then drain them the next morning and add to a fruit smoothie, which breaks up the linseeds and makes them fibrous. You can buy golden linseeds or ready-cracked flax seeds (which should be kept in the fridge) from all health stores. For a healthy breakfast smoothie recipe, see *General Health Hints*.

- Bran is an insoluble fibre derived from rice, soya or oats. The insoluble fibre is needed to stimulate the bowel to work properly. Wheat bran is fine as long as you don't have an intolerance to wheat, otherwise this can actually aggravate the problem.
- Try eating more brown rice (or rice bran) plus beans, such as black-eyed beans, kidney, haricot, butter and cannelloni, which are high in fibre.
- Whole-wheat rye bread, Ryvita-type crisp breads, rough oatcakes, or amaranth crackers can be eaten as an alternative to wheat bread.
- Other high-fibre foods are fresh and dried figs, blackcurrants, ready-to-eat dried apricots and prunes, almonds, hazelnuts, fresh coconut and all mixed nuts.
- All lightly cooked or raw vegetables and salads will add more fibre to your diet.
- Eat fruit in between meals or before meals.
- Eat more live, low-fat yoghurts, which contain healthy bacteria – a lack of which can exacerbate constipation.
- Drink at least 6–8 glasses of water daily.
- Psyllium husks are a soluble fibre, which add bulk to the stools. Take a tablespoon of psyllium husks in water before breakfast to help keep things moving. Then make sure you drink plenty of water during the day. Water is essential when taking psyllium.

Useful Remedies

- Use 1–2 teaspoons a day of any good-quality organic green powder, such as Viridian 100% Organic Green Food Blend, to aid bowel function and alkalize tissues.
- Otherwise use Green Magic Powder – containing Hawaiian spirulina, chlorella, lecithin, barley and wheat grass, kamut, pectin apple fibre, kelp and wheat sprouts, CoQ10, royal jelly, artichoke powder and lactobacillus acidophilus, as it is a great all-round way to ingest good nutrients, healthy bacteria, keep the body more alkaline and help keep you regular. For details, log on to www.itsgreenmagic.com, or call Helen Cruikshank on 08453 279688.
- Acidophilus and bifidus are healthy bacteria, which can be taken after a meal, particularly if constipation has started after antibiotics. **BC** Or try Jarro-dophilus by Jarrow, which does not need to be kept in the fridge. Take one daily after food. **NC**
- Prebiotics are plant nutrients that support the growth of your existing good bacteria. They do not overly ferment and really help to keep you regular. I use Agave Digestive Immune Support. One small scoop daily with breakfast. Find out more at www.lef.org. Available in UK from The Nutri Centre. **NC**
- Another excellent prebiotic is Molkosan Vitality drink from Bioforce, proven to help improve bowel transit time. For list of stockists, call 01294 277344 or log on to www.avogel.co.uk.
- Vitamin C powder with added calcium and magnesium – 1 level teaspoon 2–3 times a day for a few days with food – can help soften the stool and increase the frequency of bowel movement; magnesium also helps to increase bowel motions, as it is a smooth muscle relaxant.
- One of the best ways I have found to eliminate constipation is to replace one meal a day with a fruit and vegetable blend, while eliminating all flour from any source for at least two days. I put a tablespoon of organic aloe vera juice, a banana, half a cup of blueberries, an organic apple, a slice of papaya and any fruit I have to hand, plus a teaspoon of any good green food mix, a tablespoon of sunflower seeds and a tablespoon of soaked linseeds (flax seeds) into a blender. To this I add half a cup of organic rice milk and blend. It's delicious

and packed with fibre. On alternate days I make a vegetable juice to which I still add the aloe vera juice but not the rice milk.

■ The Herbal Colon Programme – based on Dr Christopher's (he was a respected naturopath in the US) herbal cascara formula. For details of The Herbal Colon Programme, call Specialist Herbal Supplies. **SHS**

Helpful Hints

■ Squatting to pass faeces helps to encourage elimination, as it is a more natural position for the colon.

■ Overuse of laxatives makes the bowel lazy.

■ It is very important that you eliminate any underlying causes for your constipation. Visit your GP and make sure there is nothing more serious going on.

■ Do not bear down too much when you have a bowel movement as this places a strain on the vascular system and can, over time, lead to varicose veins and haemorrhoids or piles. Remember, rather than fall asleep after every meal, go for a leisurely walk. This will make you feel less bloated, aid digestion and encourage healthier bowels.

■ In Chinese medicine the best time to walk is between 5am and 7am, which encourages the colon to work more efficiently. I think I'll pass on this one! Walk at any time to aid elimination.

■ When you feel the need to pass a motion, be sure not to ignore the signal; take the time to read a magazine on the loo.

■ For healthy bowel movements you need about a pint of fluid in between each meal to get waste moving through successfully.

■ Stress is a **major** factor, as it slows down the peristalsis movements.

■ When you add more fibre to your diet and you're not used to it, it is essential that you drink more water. Adding fibre without more fluid can actually aggravate the problem.

■ In the elderly a lack of folic acid has sometimes been found to be the cause of constipation, so supplementing with folic acid in the form of a good-quality multi-vitamin/mineral should be helpful.

■ For severe constipation, and with your doctor's permission, consider colonic irrigation. If done properly, it can be a godsend. For details of practitioners, see *Useful Information*. You can also use a lukewarm water enema at home. Available from Best Care Products – call 01342 410303 or email info@bestcare-uk.com.

CONTRACEPTIVE PILL   *(see Infertility and Pill, Contraceptive)*

COUGHS   *(see also Bronchitis and Colds and Flu)*

Coughs are often due to an infection, such as a cold or flu and sometimes asthma. Many people who smoke develop a persistent cough. Sometimes the cough can lead to production of phlegm; if this is yellow or green in colour it indicates a bacterial infection, in which case you need to see a doctor. If you have a cough that persists longer than two weeks or produces blood at any stage, it is very important to seek medical attention and have an X-ray. Coughs that produce a lot of catarrh are often helped by mullein and other expectorant herbs. If the cough is dry and tickly, cherry bark is more useful. A persistent cough, especially after eating foods containing wheat, gluten or sugar may be linked to candida (see *Candida*), a food intolerance or leaky gut.

Foods to Avoid

- For a few days, eliminate all cow's dairy products – even skimmed milk, low-fat cheeses and milk chocolate. I also find that if I have a cold I also need to avoid soya milk, which can increase mucous production.
- Cakes, biscuits, sausage rolls, meat pies, burgers and so on should be avoided for at least 14 days to give your sinuses and throat time to clear all mucous. Also avoid white bread and pasta.
- Most foods containing sugar tend to be high in fat, and sugar lowers immune functioning.

Friendly Foods

- Manuka honey – one teaspoon before each meal helps coat the throat but also has antiseptic properties. The higher the Umf (5+ to 20+), the stronger its antiseptic properties.
- Drink plenty of water to keep the throat well lubricated.
- Pineapples help loosen up mucous and make breathing easier. Fresh pear juice is also good for easing coughs.
- If the cough is making you feel tight-chested and congested, try adding horseradish, cayenne or ginger to meals.
- Liquorice, either drunk as a tea or sucked as a pure (sugar-free) liquorice juice stick, can be very soothing.
- Tea made from fresh thyme can ease the cough and has historically been used to treat whooping cough.
- Eat plenty of fresh vegetables, chicken, fish, pulses, grains and fresh fruit.
- Drink herbal teas such as lemon and ginger and try organic rice, almond or oat milk as a dairy substitute.
- Any food to which you have an intolerance – for example, in my case, chocolate – can give you a sore throat and cough.
- Live, low-fat plain yoghurts, (including goat's milk) are usually well tolerated and they help to boost friendly bacteria in the gut.

Useful Remedies

- Comvita propolis elixir is a great remedy for coughs. It contains propolis, tea tree and manuka honey. It is antiseptic, immune boosting, and soothing. Available from all health shops.
- Bioforce Ivy–Thyme Complex Tincture, taken as directed.
- Zinc lozenges. Suck one every 3–4 hours to ease discomfort of sore throats and reduce the tickling of the cough. Ultimate Zinc-C Lozenges from Now contain vitamins A and C, zinc, echinacea, bee propolis and slippery elm.
- Olive leaf extract acts like a natural antibiotic and has been found especially useful for respiratory problems. Take 3 capsules daily while symptoms last.
- Include a multi-vitamin and mineral in your regimen.
- Ultimate Echinacea Complex by Holos Health can stop coughs developing further. Take one teaspoon in water 3 times daily until relief is obtained. Log on to www.holoshealth.com.
- Massaging a little tea tree oil onto your throat externally may help.
- Use a liquorice and glycerine throat spray called Naturalife Throat Coat – available from good chemists and health shops.

Helpful Hints

- If you begin wheezing after food or when stressed, you may have developed a touch of asthma – see *Asthma*. Consult a doctor.
- If you find you get tight-chested after exercise, 2 grams of vitamin C can often be very helpful. But also see a doctor.
- Taken at the first sign of a cough, homeopathic Aconite 6c can help prevent the cough from developing.

- Keep a food diary and note when symptoms are worse. For example, if your nose runs within a few minutes of eating certain foods, especially cow's milk, wheat and sugar-based foods, then you may be sensitive to those foods. High-sugar fruits such as grapes can be a problem for some people.
- Dilute a few drops of essential oil of sweet marjoram and frankincense in a grapeseed oil base and massage into your chest and back to encourage deeper breathing.
- Take 2 tablespoons of aloe vera juice every day to soothe your throat and help boost your immune system.
- Stop smoking.

CRADLE CAP
(see Dermatitis and Eczema)

CRAMPS
(see also Circulation)

Most people will experience cramp at some time or other and it's a painful muscular spasm or contraction, often caused by a poor blood supply to the muscles. It can also be triggered by extreme exercise and certain prescription drugs such as Protelos, the osteoporosis drug.

Unless you live in a very hot country where you are sweating profusely, it is unlikely to be due to a lack of sodium (salt) – that is, dehydration. Chronic depletion of body fluids from diuretics and poor fluid intake predispose seniors to cramps. Cramp is most commonly caused by poor circulation and lack of magnesium, calcium or potassium. Low levels of calcium and magnesium are common in a normal pregnancy unless these minerals are supplemented to the diet. Magnesium deficiency is very common in the West and cramps are often the first sign of magnesium deficiency.

Foods to Avoid
- Cut down on white-flour-based foods such as white rice, biscuits, cakes, pizza and pasta, and all forms of sugar and coffee.
- Avoid carbonated drinks; they contain phosphoric acid, which increases calcium loss from the bones.
- All of these foods deplete magnesium and potassium from the body.

Friendly Foods
- Plenty of fresh fruits and vegetables, especially bananas, raw cauliflower and jacket potatoes; fresh fruit juices; dried apricots and dates; seafood; all leafy greens, especially watercress, spinach, spring greens and kale. Avocado, lean steak, mackerel and beans are all good sources of magnesium and potassium.
- Eating a banana before going to bed helps to reduce cramps, as bananas are rich in potassium and magnesium.
- Snack on almonds, sesame seeds and Brazil nuts – all rich in minerals.
- Calcium-rich foods are dried skimmed milk, sesame seeds, sardines, muesli, Parmesan cheese and curry powder.
- Some breads and milks now have added calcium – check the labels, and eat wholemeal-variety brands rather than mass-produced breads.

Useful Remedies
- A liquid multi-mineral that is easy for the body to absorb and utilize, such as Ultratrace by Higher Nature. **HN**

- Black cohosh and cramp bark; 1–2mls as needed. **SHS**
- Take 200mg of magnesium citrate twice daily with food during the day and an extra 200mg at night, which is often lacking in people who suffer cramps. **BC**

Helpful Hints
- If you tend to get cramps at night, try stretching out your calves before going to bed. If you have a friend or a dog you can walk with, take a regular evening walk.
- Exercise regularly, but not to excess, and indulge yourself with a massage on a regular basis. Use geranium, ginger and cypress oils in your mix of oils.
- Reflexology helps to improve circulation and reduce cramps if undertaken on a regular basis (see *Useful Information*).

CROHN'S DISEASE   *(see also Absorption, Candida and Leaky Gut)*

Crohn's disease affects around 90,000 people in the UK. It is an inflammatory disease of the small intestine that can also affect the bowel (large intestine). Sadly, as many as 1 in every 400 children suffer this condition – this is a 50% increase in the last 10 years. In general Crohn's disease develops between the ages of 16–30, although it can occur at any age.

This condition causes ulcers and scarring to the wall of the intestines and often occurs in patches with healthy tissues in between. Symptoms are similar to those found in ulcerative colitis and tissue samples may need to be taken. It is the scarring that narrows the passages, thus disrupting nutrient absorption and normal bowel function.

Blood in the stool, weight loss, loss of appetite, nausea, severe abdominal pain or cramps after eating, especially on the lower right side of the abdomen; diarrhoea, fever, chills, weakness and anaemia are all common symptoms of this disease. It is quite often associated with other inflammatory conditions within the body that affect the joints, eyes and skin. Malabsorption of nutrients due to inflammation and/or damage of the gut is one of the biggest problems with Crohn's and up to 85% of sufferers are known to have nutrient deficiencies – therefore it's important that you should read the *Leaky Gut* section, too. There can also be a genetic link, but Crohn's has been labelled a modern disease as in 'primitive' cultures it is virtually unknown.

Over-consumption of antibiotics and eating meat and milk from herds that have been given antibiotics and hormones are all suggested as possible triggers, as is a possible autoimmune factor – in which the body's own immune system attacks part of the intestines. Children who are breast-fed are less likely to contract Crohn's. Candida is also linked to this disease, as is a leaky gut. See under *Candida* and *Leaky Gut*. Lack of fibre, parasites, stress and food intolerances have also been implicated in causing this disease.

Fistulas – tubes that form from one part of the body to another – and fissures (cracks) around the anus are a common complication. Crohn's is also linked to osteoporosis, because of poor absorption of nutrients.

Foods to Avoid
- Over-consumption of sugar is strongly linked with the development of Crohn's and some people find that avoidance of sugar slows the rate of progression.
- Tomatoes, raw fruit and nuts are often problematic for some people.
- Yeast and dairy are two food groups that many people find difficult to digest and avoidance of them has helped many sufferers.
- Avoid and reduce foods associated with inflammation – alcohol, simple sugars, refined white rice, bread, cakes and pastries and caffeine.

- Gluten-rich foods, such as wheat, rye, barley and oats, are often a problem.
- Foods high in salicylates are a problem for some sufferers, but not all. Tomatoes, aubergines, peppers, courgettes and berries (such as black- and blueberries and strawberries), radish, olives, chicory, oranges, plums, almonds, pineapple, cherries, raspberries, prunes and guava are high in salicylates. Keep a food diary.
- Aspirin contains salicylates.

Friendly Foods

- Oily fish, which is a rich source of EPA and DHA, two essential fatty acids, have been found to reduce the severity of Crohn's and the frequency of attacks via their anti-inflammatory action. Crohn's sufferer's tend to be low in EFAs. Organic-farmed salmon, mackerel, sardines, herrings and anchovies should be OK.
- It is important to eat unprocessed foods in their fresh state. Fresh organic fruits and vegetables are best.
- Protein is important for the healing and repair of the intestines. Most sufferers can tolerate meat once or twice a week; if this is a problem, lightly steamed or grilled fish and grilled chicken are often easier to digest. Quinoa and cooked tofu are good forms of protein. Eat with plenty of lightly cooked vegetables.
- If raw fruit is a problem, lightly stew or grill fruits which makes them a little easier to digest. Papaya is very healing.
- Sweet potatoes, cantaloupe melons, carrots, persimmons, pear, mango, marrow, red cabbage, green beans, lentils, lettuce, rhubarb, celery, potatoes, pomegranate, apple, nuts (except almonds) and figs should all be OK to eat.
- A couple of teaspoons of apple cider vinegar in a little warm water sipped throughout the morning helps to correct the pH level within the bowel and aid liver function.
- Drink the water that you cook any cabbage in, as it helps to heal the digestive lining. If you can't face drinking this, at least make your gravy with cabbage water.
- Try wheat- and gluten-free breads, such as Genius, which are available at supermarkets and health stores.

Useful Remedies

- Green powders help to alkalize the body and the chlorophyll is also healing to intestinal walls. Try Viridian's Organic Green Food Blend. **VN**
- As malabsorption is likely to be a problem, liquid vitamins and minerals are a better choice, as they are more easily absorbed. **BC**
- As magnesium and calcium are usually low, make sure that any multiformula contains around 300mg calcium and 400mg of magnesium.
- Quercetin is a type of flavonoid known for its anti-inflammatory action. Take 300mg, 1–3 times per day. Solgar's Quercetin Complex is available from the Nutri Centre. **NC**
- Make sure you take a high-potency B-complex tablet every day, as low levels of folic acid and B12 are often lacking in Crohn's patients.
- Glutamine and butyrate are the primary fuels for the repair of the digestive lining, helping repair and healing. Studies show that both are low in Crohn's patients. Take 4–6 x 500mg of glutamine capsules, split throughout the day, before main meals. Alternatively, you can take the glutamine powder in water half an hour or more before meals. Whey protein and hemp seed protein are also useful for the condition, as they are rich in highly absorbable proteins. **HN, NC**
- Butyric acid can also be taken separately to aid bowel healing. Take as directed. **BC**
- A high-strength carotene complex, which will convert naturally to Vitamin A in the body, vital for soft tissue healing.

- Zinc, 30mg a day, to aid tissue-healing.
- Take 2 grams of omega-3 fats daily.
- Researchers at McGill University in Montreal have linked vitamin D3 deficiency as a contributing factor to Crohn's Disease. Take 1000iu of vitamin D3 daily. Due to genetic links, children of people with Crohn's would be wise to take vitamin D3 daily to help switch on the NOD2 gene, which is often defective or deficient in Crohn's sufferers.
- Take Polyzyme Forte, a digestive enzyme that is needed to help absorption of nutrients with meals, after the first few mouthfuls. If you are having a large or rich meal you may need 2 capsules. **BC**
- Make sure you take friendly bacteria daily – acidophilus and bifidus are available at all good health stores and should be taken after meals. These really help to reduce food sensitivities.
- Organic-source aloe vera really aids healing – take one egg cupful 3 times daily before meals.
- Curcumin from turmeric has anti-inflammatory properties in the bowel. Take a concentrate capsule with main meals. **SHS**
- Omega-7 essential fats extracted from sea buckthorn help heal the mucosal gut lining. Take 2 grams daily initially and then reduce to 1 gram daily for the long term. **PN**

Helpful Hints
- You may need supplementation of the hormone DHEA – have a blood test to check for levels.
- When beginning to use digestive enzymes and other digestive supplements, it is best to do so gradually, so as not to shock the system. For example, if the directions suggest 1 three times per day, build up to this over a week.
- Evidence that food intolerances trigger Crohn's is thin on the ground, but it is widely acknowledged that they may aggravate and irritate the intestines – thus making the condition worse. It may be worth checking for intolerances and avoiding offending foods. Genova Diagnostics offer a FACT food intolerance test and can be contacted on 020 8336 7750, or check out their website at www.gdx.uk.net.

- Smoking has been linked with the development of Crohn's disease.
- Lymph drainage massage and skin brushing help to eliminate toxins from the body.
- Buy foods as fresh as possible – they will be more nutrient rich. Everything will taste better and you'll appreciate the effort in the long run.
- Crohn's disease is greatly exacerbated by stress, so any techniques known to reduce stress, such as yoga, t'ai chi, meditation, massage or hypnotherapy, will help. Spiritual healing has helped many sufferers (see *Healing*).
- Adequate rest is essential for any Crohn's sufferer, and gentle exercise, such as walking and swimming, will also help.
- To re-balance your diet and make sure you are taking the right supplements and herbs in the correct amount for your case, I strongly suggest that you consult a doctor who is also a nutritionist (see *Useful Information*).
- Avoid wearing tight clothing around the waist, as this can make you more uncomfortable.
- For further help, contact The National Association for Colitis and Crohn's Disease (NACC), 4 Beaumont House, Sutton Road, St Albans, Hertfordshire AL1 5HH. Information Line: 0845 130 2233 (weekdays 10am–1pm). Email: info@nacc.org.uk. Website: www.nacc.org.uk.
- A helpful website for children with Crohn's can be found at www.cicra.org. It includes finding penpals, how to cope at school and what to expect when you go to hospital. They can also be contacted via post – Crohn's in Childhood Research Association (CICRA), Parkgate House, 356 West Barnes Lane, Motspur Park, Surrey KT3 6NB – or call them on 020 8949 6209.

CYSTITIS

(see also Candida and Thrush)

Cystitis is far more common in women than in men and can also affect children. One-third of all women contract a urinary tract infection such as cystitis before the age of 25. It is caused by a bacterial infection in the bladder and symptoms include a frequent and urgent urge to urinate, plus a burning sensation when passing urine. With cystitis or thrush there can be a whitish/yellow discharge – but this is more common with thrush, which is a yeast overgrowth. Whatever the cause, the entire outer area can swell, which makes sitting extremely uncomfortable indeed.

If lymph nodes in the groin begin to swell (near the bikini line) or if you have pain in the loins, blood in your urine, or a fever, this denotes a kidney infection and you **must** see a doctor. A urine test can confirm which bug is responsible and usually antibiotics are then prescribed. Women who suffer candida and food intolerances regularly suffer thrush or cystitis (see also *Candida*).

These types of infections are more likely to occur in warm, moist, humid atmospheres. If you are run down, you are more prone to an attack, as your immune system is functioning under par. If you suffer thrush regularly you may be diabetic, in which case a blood test should be taken to eliminate this possibility.

Foods to Avoid
- While symptoms are acute, avoid as much as possible all foods and drinks containing sugar and yeast – especially cheeses, malt vinegar, ketchups, soy sauce, miso, pickled foods, yeast-based breads, mushrooms and alcohol.
- Sugar in **any** form including honey, maltose and so on, as all sugars will feed the yeast. For the first week also avoid all cakes, biscuits, pizza or fizzy cola-type drinks and desserts.
- Avoid junk-type burgers and fried foods, which are hard to digest and add to the toxic load.
- Also you will need to avoid high-sugar fruits, such as grapes, melons and bananas, for the first few days.
- Dried fruits are very high in sugar.
- See also this section under *Candida*.

Friendly Foods
- Eat plenty of live, low-fat yoghurt that contains the friendly bacteria, acidophilus and bifidus.
- Try cranberry juice without sugar or eat fresh or frozen cranberries – they are rich in hippuric acid, which helps prevent bacteria clinging to the bladder walls. The concentrate in capsules is in this case is more effective.
- Drink plenty of fluids but no sugary drinks.
- As these types of conditions thrive in an acid environment, eat plenty of salads and green vegetables, especially watercress, cabbage, spring greens, kale and so on, as these foods are all alkaline.
- Include apples, cherries, pineapples, papaya and pears for fruits.
- Eat more garlic and onions, which are highly anti-bacterial.
- See also this section under *Candida*.

Useful Remedies
- Cranberry Plus is a supplement made from 100% cranberry fruit solids and is sugar- and preservative-free. One 500mg capsule daily will help to fight and prevent urinary tract infections. **BC**
- Bromelain, extracted from pineapple, because it has anti-inflammatory properties. Take 500mg twice daily.

- A high-strength, natural-source carotene complex, which converts naturally to vitamin A in the body, helps support immune function when taken daily.
- To help re-alkalize your system, which will benefit your immune system and thus reduce incidence for problems such as candida, take Green pH, which is made by Metabolics (www.metabolics.com) – take one small level teaspoon daily in water, preferably taken 30 minutes before a meal or in between meals; it is a mixture of green beans, garden peas, pea leaf, dry apple cider, watercress, broccoli and nettle leaf. Available from the Wholistic Medical Centre. **WMC**
- Vitamin C and flavonoids help to fight the infection. Take up to 4 grams daily with food for the first week and then reduce to 1 gram daily. When you take large doses of vitamin C, make sure it's in an ascorbate form, which is gentle on the stomach.
- Take two acidophilis/bifidus capsules daily with food for at least six weeks. Jarro-Dophilus EPS, take one daily with food. **NC**
- Include a high-strength multi-vitamin and mineral in this programme.
- Try Higher Nature's Citricidal Grapefruit Seed Extract, which comes in liquid form, and is anti-fungal. Take a few drops in water or juice. **HN**
- Alternatively, take oregano tincture – 4 drops in half a cup of water; it has powerful anti-bacterial and anti-fungal properties. **NC**

Helpful Hints

- To make your own sodium citrate (which is what chemists sell for this problem), squeeze half a lemon into a glass, add a quarter of a glass of water, and then add a third of a teaspoon of bi-carbonate of soda. The mix will fizz; stir and drink while it is still fizzing. Do this three times daily starting before breakfast and between meals until the symptoms have gone. If you took this blend every day before breakfast it would help stop this condition re-occurring.
- Urinate as soon as possible after having sexual intercourse to stop transmission of bacteria into the bladder. If symptoms are acute, avoid intercourse for at least one week, as you can pass the bacteria from one partner to another.
- Consuming live yoghurt on a daily basis can help reduce the incidence of developing cystitis or thrush.
- Drink organic aloe vera juice containing extract of cranberry and cherries three times daily.
- Drink three to four cups of nettle tea daily. Goldenseal tea may also be helpful, as it contains berberine, an alkaloid that inhibits bacteria from adhering to the wall of the bladder.
- Drink plenty of water each day to help flush out unhealthy organisms from the bladder.
- Avoid perfumed soaps and vaginal deodorants at all times.
- Wear cotton underwear. Avoid tightly fitted jeans, especially in hot weather.
- As much as possible when you are at home, wear a skirt and no underwear to keep the vaginal area cool.
- If you have to sit all day, get up and walk around regularly.
- Get plenty of rest.
- Use a pH-balanced soap.
- Douche daily with diluted tea tree oil, crushed garlic and lavender oil or add a few drops to your bath.
- Acupuncture and homeopathic remedies such as Cantharis 30c will help reduce the burning sensation, while Apis 30c can be taken if stinging is a problem (see *Useful Information*).

D

DANDRUFF *(see Scalp Problems)*

DEEP VEIN THROMBOSIS (DVT) *(see also Jet Lag)*

DVT occurs when a blood clot forms within a deep vein, most commonly in the lower leg, the calf area, although in rarer cases it can occur in your thigh or even your arms. DVT can be mistaken for leg cramps or sore muscles, but as DVT is life threatening, urgent medical attention is needed. Symptoms are swelling in the leg affected by the clot, pain and tenderness, difficulty in placing any weight on the bad leg, skin that becomes red and feels warm to the touch. If you have any of these symptoms seek immediate medical advice, especially after a lengthy flight or if you have been bedridden for any reason. DVT can also occur after lengthy periods of stationary activity, such as sitting at a desk or in a car.

Pulmonary embolism is a serious complication of DVT, which happens when a piece of a blood clot travels via the bloodstream to the lungs. This can be fatal if immediate medical intervention is not available. Typical symptoms would be chest pain, breathlessness, possibly coughing blood or fainting. Dial 999 immediately.

It's worth noting that people who have Type A or Type AB blood are more prone to clotting disorders.

Foods to Avoid
- See this section under *Circulation*.

Friendly Foods
- Drink plenty of fluids to keep the lymph system functioning.
- Eat light meals when travelling and when in hospital – see this section under *Circulation*.

Useful remedies
- If you are worried about being cramped and contracting DVT, take some high-strength ginkgo biloba and gotu kola (500mg daily), a few days before and during your flight. These natural remedies increase circulation. The gotu kola helps increase circulation in the lower limbs, and a positive side effect is sometimes a slight loosening of the bowels!
- Bromelain from pineapples help thin the blood naturally. Take 500mg three times daily, starting 2 weeks before travel. **NB If you are on Warfarin, check with your GP before taking this supplement.**
- Natural-source, full-spectrum vitamin E thins the blood and reduces the risk of clotting on long flights. Take 400iu at least two weeks prior to travel and during the journey. **If you are taking blood-thinning drugs, check with your GP.**
- There is also a supplement called Zinopin, which contains pine bark extract (pycnogenol) and ginger. It contains the anti-clotting activity of aspirin – without the negative side effects. Ginger is also useful against travel sickness. Available from all good pharmacies or log on to www.zinopindvtsupplement.co.uk.
- Take a teaspoon of bicarbonate of soda twice daily in warm water – well away from food to re-alkalize your body fluids. This is because when the body is acid you're more likely to get

too much stickiness in the blood. Start taking this remedy a week before the flight and continue until a week after.

■ Take 2 grams of omegà-3 fish oils daily.

■ Nattokinase is an extract of Natto, which helps break down fibrin in the blood to help prevent blood clots. Take in between meals for a few days before, during and after travelling. **NC NB This should not be taken by people on Warfarin.**

Helpful Hints

■ Buy some good support stockings or socks. These are now sold at all major airports and chemists. A neck pillow can also be useful, because then you can try to relax and sleep more comfortably.

■ Keep walking around the plane as much as you can. Use the aisles to do a few squats and raise your arms up and down; stretch out as much as you can.

■ If you are in hospital or laid up in bed, then with medical supervision, start moving about, as and when you can.

■ Keep in mind that DVT can also occur after long car journeys and in people who sit too long at their desk. To keep blood flowing, and when safe to do so, press both feet firmly into the ground and flex your leg muscles. Or flex your feet up and down and round and round to get your circulation moving.

■ People more at risk for pulmonary embolism are those undergoing major surgery, women who are pregnant, and people who have had bed confinement, women taking HRT or the contraceptive pill, or those who are obese or suffer from high blood pressure.

■ Smoking more than 25 cigarettes daily can increase risk.

■ Walk and move regularly, have a good stretch.

■ Massage your lower legs from the feet upwards every hour or so – go quite deep to 'rev' up your circulation.

DEMENTIA
(see Alzheimer's Disease)

DEPRESSION
(see also Adrenal Exhaustion and Stress)

According to the NHS, one in four Britons suffers some type of mental problem, and anxiety and depression are the most common. Around 10–12% of the population struggle with depression and its effects on self-esteem, work and home life and relationships. Women tend to suffer more depression than men and growing numbers of children – around one in ten under the age of 15 – have a mental health problem including depression.

There is a world of difference between having a bad day and suffering full-blown depression. Older people tend to suffer more incidences of depression due to poor nutrition, the loss of a loved one, feelings of no longer being useful and so on. And persistent mild depression at any age lowers immunity and the ability to fight off disease.

A truly depressed person has an all-pervading feeling of sadness. Other typical symptoms include feeling worthless, inadequate or incompetent. And if you also suffer from loss of interest or pleasure in your job, family life, hobbies or sex, difficulty concentrating or remembering, insomnia, over- or under-eating, unusual irritability, a sense of humour failure, a feeling of being downhearted that just won't go away, frequent unexplained crying spells or recurrent thoughts of death or suicide, then you may be clinically depressed and you should seek help.

Depressed people often isolate themselves by withdrawing from friends and family. Not all symptoms denote clinical depression. For example, if you are feeling total apathy, like you just don't want to get up in the morning, then such symptoms can most definitely be linked to adrenal exhaustion (see *Adrenal Exhaustion*). Hormonal imbalances, low blood sugar and poor thyroid function can also trigger depressive-type symptoms (see these specific sections for extra help).

The more junk, pre-packaged, high-saturated fat, sugary-type foods and drinks you ingest, the more likely you are to feel depressed. This is because you are deficient in vital nutrients and essential fats and your body's demand is exceeding its supply. When violent and hyperactive and depressed people are given a healthier diet and take more exercise and the right supplements, their personalities usually alter completely for the better. Sugar and stimulants alter brain chemistry and alter behaviour. This has been proven time and time again, and it's now time for us to take notice and act.

Foods to Avoid
- Avoid or reduce alcohol. It can make depression worse, as it lowers levels of the feel-good hormone serotonin, as well as B-vitamins needed for energy and nerve health in the mind and body.
- If you eat too much refined sugar, your blood sugar levels keep fluctuating, which can greatly affect your mood (see *Insulin Resistance* and *Diabetes*).

- Excessive consumption of refined, processed, fatty foods and caffeine can make your depression worse, as they deplete vitamins B (needed for healthy nervous system) and C and the mineral chromium (if you do not have sufficient chromium, your blood sugar levels will become unbalanced, triggering mood swings).
- Avoid the sweetener aspartame at all costs; it can have neurological side effects and has been shown to interact negatively with antidepressants. For further information, log on to www.dorway.com.
- Which foods do you tend to crave and eat the most? I'll bet it's wheat and sugar. If this is the case for you, you should be aware that the foods you crave are usually the ones that will make your symptoms worse. It takes discipline, but for 7 days try to avoid these foods and replace them with fresh fruits, vegetables and grains like brown rice and see how much better you feel.
- Lack of iron is also linked to depression, but iron accumulates in the body and is linked to heart disease in those over 50. Your doctor can find out via a blood test if you are deficient.

Friendly Foods
- The brain is made up of around 60% fats, so eat more of the right kind of fats including oily fish such as farmed organic salmon, mackerel, anchovies and sardines, linseeds (flax seeds), hemp seeds, soya beans and wheat germ; all of these foods are all rich in omega-3 essential fats.
- Sardines are high in DMAE, a brain stimulant that helps to elevate mood. (See below: vitamin B5 encourages the body to produce more DMAE.)
- Walnuts, pecans, Brazil nuts and hazelnuts, plus sunflower and pumpkin seeds are all rich in omega-6 essential fats.
- Use unrefined nut and seed oils for salad dressings (see *Fats You Need To Eat*).
- Make sure you always eat breakfast – make porridge with half rice or almond milk and water. Sweeten it with a little honey and raisins, and add a few blueberries, banana or chopped apple for further taste. Even better, you could also sprinkle a few sunflower seeds into the porridge for EFAs.

- Increase your intake of fresh fruits, vegetables, whole grains such as brown rice, quinoa, non-wheat pastas, barley and lentils.
- To help raise serotonin levels, eat more foods containing tryptophan, such as fish, turkey, avocado, cottage cheese, organic meats, beans, lentils, cooked tofu, wheat germ and bananas.
- Foods containing the amino acids phenylalinine and tyrosine can also help to raise mood and boost motivation; these include low-fat meats, fish, eggs, wheat germ, dairy foods, oats, nuts, avocados, bananas and chocolate. This is why eating chocolate often makes you feel good. But eat dark chocolate, not milk. If you are a chocoholic, try taking 250–500mg of DLPA (DL-phenylaline) with 2mg of vitamin B6 and 500mg of vitamin C on an empty stomach before breakfast.
- Spicy foods that contain cayenne pepper produce endorphins that help raise your mood.
- Drink 6–8 glasses of water daily to help remove toxins.

Useful Remedies
If you are taking prescription drugs for clinical depression, you must check with your doctor before trying these remedies.

- First, begin taking a high-strength multi-vitamin and mineral to give you a good nutrient base plus the B-vitamins, a lack of which can trigger depression and low mood.
- Various B-vitamins play a major role in maintaining proper brain chemistry and deficiencies of B-vitamins are common in depressed people. Therefore, take a high-strength complex that contains at least 50mg of all the Bs. B2 turns your urine bright yellow – but this is normal!
- As well as the B-complex, take 250–500mg of B5 (pantothenic acid), which supports your adrenals and increases levels of DMAE in the brain, which raises mood.
- Most people over 65 are deficient in Vitamin D, a lack of which is now linked to 17 conditions. There is no doubt it raises mood. Take 800–1000iu of vitamin D3 daily.
- Take 1 gram of vitamin C daily with food.
- Omega-3 fats are vital for improving depression and have been shown in many cases to be more effective than antidepressant drugs. If you are not eating oily fish 3 times a week, then take 2 grams of omega-3 daily.
- Sprinkle one tablespoon of non-GM soya lecithin granules over cereals and fruit dishes, as lecithin is high in the brain nutrient, phosphotadyl serine.
- 5-Hydroxytryptophan (5-HTP) helps raise serotonin levels in the brain. Extracted from the griffonia plant from Africa, 5-HTP helps balance mood, aids you in falling asleep more easily, reduces aggression, reduces appetite and creates a more relaxed waking state within 45 minutes. Recommended dose: 50mg up to 300mg per day. For best results, start on a low dosage; take at bedtime along with a small carbohydrate snack, such as an oat cake. If you need to, gradually work up to 3000mg. If your mood stabilizes, gradually lower the dose until you find how much you need. Taking more than you need will not be helpful in the long run. This supplement is more effective if taken with B-vitamins and 10mg of zinc. Be patient, as it can take a few weeks for the full effects of 5-HTP to work. **HN**
- Or try Patrick Holford's Chill Food, which contains amino acids, a blend of vitamins, plant extracts and 5-HTP. Available from all good health shops or BioCare. **BC**
- In a study, DHEA hormone supplementation was tested on middle-aged and elderly patients with major depression for 4 weeks. Depression ratings and memory performance significantly improved. DHEA in other human studies significantly elevated mood in elderly people. Recommended dose: 50mg a day for men and 15–20mg per day for women – not available in the UK unless you have a prescription, but DHEA can be bought freely in health shops in the US or log on to www.lef.org.

- Ginseng is an adrenal tonic that is useful for people that are depressed, as their adrenal glands (see *Adrenal Exhuastion*) are usually functioning under par. Take two Panax Red Ginseng capsules, one with breakfast and one with lunch. Not at night. **NB Do not take the ginseng if you are on blood thinners.**
- The herb St John's wort has been proven to help milder forms of depression. In more than 25 double-blind studies of more than 1,500 people, St John's wort demonstrated its effectiveness in improving mood, lessening anxiety and reducing sleep disorders. St John's wort helps to reduce the sadness, stress and feelings of helplessness from depression. Recommended dosage: 900mg daily of 0.3 per cent hypericin concentration, 600mg with breakfast and 300mg with lunch. **NB Do not take St John's wort if you are pregnant or on the contraceptive pill and avoid intense sun exposure while using it, since this herb can make the skin more sensitive to sunlight. Do not take St John's wort with 5-HTP and drugs such as Prozac, Zoloft and Paxil.**

Helpful Hints

- Natural sunlight helps to suppress production of the hormone melatonin, which is produced by the pineal gland at night; this is why we tend to feel more depressed and sleepy during the winter months. Melatonin aids sleep and acts as an important antioxidant, but if you are depressed then you need less melatonin. Therefore, get out into daylight as much as you possibly can, especially in the mornings, and if you work in an office without full-spectrum lighting, make sure you use full-spectrum light bulbs at home and where you can at work.
- Try using Real Sunlight lamps, available at several specialist clinics in the UK. The harmful frequencies of UVA and UVB have been filtered out, making this sunlight safe. Developed in Sweden, and now used in many homes to boost immune function and relieve depression. These lamps increase levels of vitamin D3 naturally, boost immune function and reduce depression. Details via info@wholisticmedical.co.uk, or call 0207 580 7537.
- Regular exercise is vital in the fight against depression. Exercise and sunlight release endorphins, natural antidepressants, which raise your mood. Regular exercise can help you sleep better, feel better, look better, and provide you with an enhanced self-image. A German study showed a significant reduction in depression when patients walked for 30 minutes a day and other studies show that regular exercise is as effective as antidepressants and more effective against relapse than drugs.
- Studies have shown that having control over roles, such as being a parent, grandparent or provider, can add value to an elderly person's life. Many companies are at last waking up to the fact that people over 65 are more committed, take less time off sick, and are more experienced workers who tend to be more cost effective than younger people. Take charge of your life!
- Ask your doctor if you can see a counsellor – a problem shared is a problem halved; and counselling is often far more successful than taking antidepressants. Talk your innermost fears through with a friend or relative; they may not even realize you are depressed. For details of your nearest qualified counsellor, contact the British Association for Counselling, BACP House, 15 St John's Business Park, Lutterworth LE17 4HB. Tel: 01455 883300. Website: www.bacp.co.uk.
- Do volunteer work, as helping others can boost self-esteem.
- Watch videos, DVDs and films that make you laugh. Laughter produces natural mood-boosting chemicals in the body.
- Be sure to get enough quality sleep, but get up after 8 hours or so.
- Blend pure oils of bergamot, clary sage, geranium and neroli in a base of almond oil and ask a friend or relative to give you a massage. These aromatherapy oils help lift your mood.

- For further help, read *New Optimum Nutrition for the Mind* by Patrick Holford (Piatkus).
- MIND is the leading mental health charity in England and Wales and has lots of local centres throughout the UK. Find them through the MIND information line on 0845 766 0163, or check out their website at www.mind.org.uk.

DERMATITIS
(see also Eczema and Leaky Gut)

Seborrheic dermatitis is basically a type of eczema that commonly occurs on children's scalps. This is why it's often called cradle cap. In most infants it tends to clear up in the first year or so. Symptoms are thick scaly tissue on the scalp, in particular, and sometimes around the eyes and ears. The problem is linked to a deficiency in essential fatty acids and one of the B-vitamins, biotin. Eliminating allergens from the diet usually helps clear cradle cap. You can also suffer varying degrees of dermatitis in adult years – triggered by exposure to hair colourants, paints, hairsprays and all manner of chemicals in cosmetic products and household cleaners and detergents. Non-specific skin rashes can also be linked to liver toxicity (see *Liver Problems*) and food intolerances (see *Allergies* and *Leaky Gut*). Dermatitis is basically a form of eczema (see *Eczema*).

Fungi are also implicated in this problem because as children's immune systems develop, they are more susceptible to various organisms.

In adults, dermatitis is linked to food intolerances, poor immune function and liver congestion. See *Liver Problems*.

Foods to Avoid
- The most common offending foods for causing cradle cap and eczema are cow's milk and produce, wheat and eggs. As with any problem that may be influenced by food intolerances, it is important to identify the problematic foods. (See *Allergies*.)
- Avoid mass-produced, refined, white-flour-based foods and any foods and drinks that are high in sugar.
- Colourings, additives, preservatives in shampoos, toiletries, toothpastes, foods (especially sweets and drinks) are well known to trigger reactions, especially in children.

Friendly Foods
- Make your child nutrient-rich fruit blends – chop any fruit you have to hand, such as bananas, papaya, apple and pears, and place in a blender. Add a couple of teaspoons of sunflower seeds and flax seeds that have been soaked overnight in cold water (flax seeds/linseeds are rich in essential fats). Add a low-fat, live yoghurt – try goat's or sheep's yoghurt – and blend for 30–40 seconds. This makes a healthy dessert. Children can usually digest goat's and sheep's products more easily than cow's.
- Oils such as Udo's Choice, a blend of omega-3 and -6 fats, can be added to food once cooked – a teaspoon a day should be fine. I find that if you cook some sweet potatoes and mash them with a little almond or oat milk and then add the oil as they are cooling, the child cannot taste the oil. Otherwise, add to thick vegetable soups and stews before serving.
- For adults with dermatitis, eat plenty of fruits, vegetables, whole grains such as brown rice or quinoa, barley and oily fish. See this section under *Eczema*.

Useful Remedies
- Many companies make liquid multi-vitamins and minerals for children, which you can add to cold dishes to make sure your child is not malnourished. Nature's Plus makes an excellent children's range. **NP**

- Alternatively, you can add organic-source green food powders rich in vitamins, minerals and essential fats to breakfast cereals or desserts. Viridian make a 100% organic version.
- Biotin, a B vitamin that is often lacking – 6mg daily.
- As all the B-vitamins work together in the body, if you are breast-feeding or an adult with this condition, also take 1 x B-complex daily. Children would get this in their multi.
- If the child is being breast-fed, it is useful for the mother to take 10mg of biotin – which will in turn be delivered through the milk – or to eat more biotin-rich foods, such as liver and egg yolk.
- Essential fats can be applied directly to the affected areas. It should be applied twice a day for 2–4 weeks. Use either evening primrose or borage oil. You can also take 2000mg of evening primrose oil daily.
- Adults should take a high-strength multi-vitamin and mineral plus an essential-fatty-acid formula daily.
- Colostrum, which is found in breast milk, helps support the immune system and aids healing of a leaky gut – it's very helpful for babies and children suffering from eczema. Up to the age of 2, take a quarter of a teaspoon twice daily on an empty stomach. Over 2 years – half a teaspoon twice daily. Take this just for one month. **NC**

Helpful Hints

- Buy products in their most natural and unadulterated state, which are gentler on a child's delicate skin. For anyone who suffers dermatitis or skin allergies, The Green People Company makes organic lotions for skin, body and hair, sunscreens and toothpaste, and it also has an advice line on 01403 740350. Email: organic@greenpeople.co.uk or log on to www.greenpeople.co.uk.
- Note that many toothpastes, shampoos, soaps, detergents and perfumes contain a myriad of chemicals. I have met several dozen hairdressers who suffer this condition caused by all the chemicals they are in contact with daily.
- Apply a little Manuka honey cream from Living Nature or the Organic Skin Rescue Oil from the Organic Pharmacy. Or contact their pharmacist, who can suggest a specific remedy for your particular symptoms. **OP**
- Use aloe vera gel topically to help calm the itching.

DIABETES – Types 1 and 2

(see also Circulation, Insulin Resistance and Weight Problems)

Approximately 3 million people in the UK suffer diabetes. Only 15% have Type 1 – a life-long condition that requires insulin – but 85% of people have Type 2, which is triggered by our ever-escalating rates of obesity and poor diets. Most alarmingly, children as young as eight are now developing late-onset diabetes – which 20 years ago would only be seen in people over 50. This is shocking, especially when you consider that around 80% of late-onset diabetes patients will die of cardiovascular disease. Make no mistake, late-onset diabetes can shorten your life – and yet it is for the most part preventable.

Type 1 diabetes is caused by the failure of the pancreas to secrete adequate insulin. Type 2 diabetes, however, is generally characterized by adequate insulin production, but the body has become resistant to it and simply doesn't respond to the insulin as it should. Type 1 diabetes is a life-long condition, which usually starts during early childhood. Both types of diabetes involve too high a level of sugar in the blood. The hormone insulin is responsible for lowering blood sugar levels.

Symptoms of Type 1 and 2 diabetes are increased thirst, fatigue, unexplained weight loss, blurred vision, increased urination (especially at night) and regular episodes of thrush. Complications associated with diabetes include peripheral neuropathy such as numbness, tingling or throbbing in extremities, poor circulation, slow wound healing, and, in adults, impotence and eye problems. There is also a greater risk for gangrene, heart disease and blindness.

The cascade of late-onset diabetes is placing a huge burden on the NHS, costing approximately £7 billion annually to treat. This situation has been triggered by our over-consumption of refined, sugar-based carbohydrate foods such as cakes, biscuits and sugar-filled fizzy drinks. Therefore, despite high levels of insulin, glucose is not properly transported into the cells and it increases to unacceptable levels in the blood. Your body tries to get rid of excess sugar in the urine, which is why doctors test for diabetes through urine – although a blood test is more accurate.

While diabetes can have a hereditary link, your genes interact with your environment (including your diet) to either improve or worsen your health. We can inherit more from our parents than just their genes; their eating habits are often passed on, too.

If you are diagnosed as diabetic by your doctor via a fasting blood test, you will very likely be offered various courses of action. In mild cases, late-onset diabetes can be kept in check by diet alone. If severe, the diet is accompanied by oral medication or injections to either increase the production of insulin or improve your sensitivity to insulin. Over the years I have interviewed many elderly diabetics and have been appalled that they have not been offered any advice on diet – and yet most cases of late-onset diabetes can be kept in check by eating a healthier diet. It's also worth noting that if you suffer from thrush regularly, you may be diabetic.

Foods to Avoid

- See also diet in *Insulin Resistance*.
- Sugar and foods containing sugar, such as fizzy drinks, chocolate, desserts and sweets, which release their sugars too quickly into the bloodstream. According to the American Heart Association, sugary drinks alone contribute to 130,000 cases of Type 2 diabetes annually in the US – and these figures are rising fast.
- You should avoid all refined, mass-produced 'white' flour and rice-based foods, such as pizza, white rice and pastas, white breads, cakes and biscuits, which are all usually high in saturated fats and sugar.
- Honey, maltose, dextrose are still sugars and can exacerbate the problem.
- Be aware that most foods advertised as being low in fat are often high in sugar.
- Don't drink concentrated shop-bought fruit juices. Make fresh juices or dilute low-sugar juices with one part juice to two parts water.
- Reduce saturated fats from animal sources to less than 10% of your daily food intake. Cheese, chocolates, full fat dairy, red meats, pies, sausages and fried foods need to be kept to a minimum.
- Cut out red meats or only occasionally eat organic lean steak, turkey, pork, venison or chicken with fat removed.
- Too much iron and copper in the body increases the risk of diabetes and heart disease – read labels, especially on fortified cereals – and cut right down on red meat. Eat more curcumin (turmeric), which detoxifies the body of these metals.
- Reduce your use of sodium-based table salts; look for magnesium-rich sea salts and only add a little to the food on your plate. Otherwise, used powdered kelp or nori flakes as a salt

substitute. Himalayan Crystal Salt – available from good health shops – is also healthier than sodium-based salt.

Friendly Foods

- Eat more unrefined, high-fibre carbohydrates, such as wholemeal or rye bread, oat biscuits, amaranth crackers, brown rice, buckwheat, oats (especially porridge), sweet potatoes, plus low-fat proteins such as beans, pulses, lentils and barley.
- Eggs, tofu, low-fat meats, fish, hemp seeds, lentils, chick peas and all pulses help balance blood sugar.
- Fruits and vegetables are high in antioxidants and soluble fibre; eat them raw as often as you can.
- Fish oils have been shown to improve the pre-diabetic condition and insulin resistance, and help to prevent full-blown late-onset diabetes developing, therefore eat more oily fish and fresh fish. But don't fry it – poached or grilled is best.
- Eat more unrefined sunflower, pumpkin, sesame and linseeds (flax seeds) and their unrefined oils, which are rich in omega-3 and -6 essential fats.
- Blend these oils half and half with extra virgin olive oil for salad dressings.
- Vitamin E-rich foods help to lower the risk of many conditions associated with diabetes, such as circulation and eye problems. Food sources are soya beans, raw wheat germ, sprouting seeds, avocados, green vegetables, eggs, unrefined and unprocessed nuts especially almonds and hazelnuts. Look for a low-sugar muesli that is rich in nuts, oats and sprinkle raw wheat germ onto the muesli.

- Eat fresh bilberries, blueberries, blackberries, papaya, spinach, watercress, sweet potatoes, pumpkin, apricots, as these fruits help to protect the eyes.
- Use lots of cinnamon in your foods, because it has been shown to help reduce glucose levels in the blood.
- Eat more curries, as curcumin has been shown to reduce the chances of developing diabetes if you are overweight.
- Organic agave syrup and xylitol (found in fruit fibre) are natural sugars that have low glycaemic counts and therefore a minimal impact on blood sugar levels – use small amounts. Available from health stores.

Useful Remedies

- A high-strength, multi-vitamin and mineral complex taken every day provides a good baseline of nutrients.
- The mineral chromium (200mcg) is vital for helping to control and prevent late-onset diabetes. Scientists in the US found that taking 200mcg of chromium daily helped reduce the incidence of late-onset diabetes by up to 50%. Chromium also helps to reduce cravings for sweet foods. And in time, chromium should enable you to reduce your medication, which you would need to discuss with your doctor.
- Lipoic Acid and L-carnitine are two potent nutrients that help to dramatically lower blood sugar. Take 250 mg of Lipoic Acid daily and 500mg of L-carnitine twice daily.
- Vitamin C x 1gram twice daily can lower glucose response.
- Magnesium, which is needed to process insulin, is usually lacking in diabetics. Take a multi-mineral daily that contains 300–450mg of magnesium, 20mg zinc, and a trace of copper.
- Take a B-complex, as diabetic patients are usually deficient in B-vitamins, needed for energy production and nerve health.
- If you do not eat oily fish regularly, then take 2 grams of Omega 3 fish-oil daily, free from PCBs and dioxins. BioCare, Higher Nature, FSC and Seven Seas all make pure fish oil capsules. BC, HN

- The hormone DHEA (see *Menopause*) helps to lower insulin levels, and protect vital organs, particularly the kidneys, against damage due to high blood glucose. Don't take hormones unless you have been shown to need them.
- Aloe vera juice helps to lower blood-sugar levels in non-insulin dependant diabetes.
- Nettle tea helps to lower blood sugar.
- As we age we produce less Co-enzyme Q10, a vital vitamin-like nutrient that protects against heart disease. Take 100mg daily with either breakfast or lunch.
- Researchers at the University of Granada in Spain found that taking olive leaf extract helps to stimulate the production and utilization of insulin. Take 500mg twice daily.
- **NB Taking supplements can affect blood sugar levels. Diabetes must be supervized by a medical practitioner, so any supplement regimen should only be undertaken with the help of a medical doctor and/or a nutritionist.**
- Pine Bark Extract, known as pycnogenol, has been shown to help protect against diabetic retinopathy. Take 80mg daily. **PN**

Helpful Hints

- If you are overweight you greatly increase your risk for diabetes, especially after 50 (see *Weight Problems*).
- Regular exercise is vital, because it reduces the need for insulin, reduces blood cholesterol and prevents obesity. It doesn't have to be intense exercise, but try and walk for at least 30 minutes daily, as regular walking has been shown to improve insulin sensitivity and glucose management. If you have been a 'couch potato' for a long time, just start gently: walk for 15 minutes a day and then build up over a month to 30 minutes daily and within another month to 45 minutes to an hour.

- Have regular eye check-ups and see a chiropodist who can keep an eye on your feet, as both can be affected by diabetes.
- Have regular reflexology on your feet, which improves circulation (see *Useful Information*).
- For further help, contact Diabetes UK, Macleod House, 10 Parkway, London NW1 7AA. Tel: 020 7424 1000 or 0845 120 2960. Website: www.diabetes.org.uk.
- Try reading *How To Prevent and Treat Diabetes with Natural Medicine* by Dr Michael Murray. Call the Nutri Centre bookshop on 020 7323 2382, or have a look at the author's website on www.doctormurray.com.

DIARRHOEA   *(see also Crohn's Disease, Colitis and Irritable Bowel Syndrome)*

Diarrhoea can have several causes including infectious bacteria, food poisoning, food allergy or intolerance, IBS or yeast overgrowth (see also *Candida*). It may also be associated with more serious conditions, such as Crohn's disease and ulcerative colitis. If it is a chronic problem it is more likely to be associated with a food intolerance or a parasite. Severe diarrhoea, especially in babies and children, must be treated quickly, as the body can rapidly become dehydrated and the person can eventually lose consciousness. Adequate intake of fluids, particularly water, and electrolyte sachet drinks should be given hourly to prevent severe dehydration. Babies and children must see a doctor.

Foods to Avoid

- Many people who have a sensitivity to wheat and possibly gluten suffer chronic diarrhoea.
- Certain foods or drinks – for example, concentrated fruit juices or overripe fruits – can make the situation worse. It's also important to discover if you have food intolerances; to find out

which foods you may have an intolerance to, you should keep a food diary in which you make a note of when symptoms are worse.

■ Avoid sorbitol, which is used as a sweetening agent.

■ Lactose, the sugar in milk, is a common cause of chronic diarrhoea.

■ If you are a regular coffee-drinker, it's worth giving it up for a few days to see if this helps.

Friendly Foods

■ Try arrowroot, tapioca or semolina – made with rice milk – as they are less likely to make the situation worse and provide much-needed nourishment.

■ Drink barley water and keep up your fluid intake, or try ginger ale.

■ If you cook rice, drink the water it's been cooked in, once cool.

■ Although we tend to associate fibre with ensuring adequate bowel movement and frequency, it can also help to control diarrhoea as the fibre will give bulk to the stool. Try soluble fibres like oat or rice bran, linseeds (flax seeds that have been soaked overnight in cold water, then drained), psyllium husks, and plenty of water or electrolyte drinks.

■ Drinking 3–4 cups of camomile, fennel or black tea a day has been used for centuries as a gentle way of dealing with diarrhoea.

■ Eating either dried bilberries or bilberry juice can also help (but not fresh bilberries as they can actually aggravate the problem).

■ Fresh vegetable soups with a little root ginger, or a small portion of poached fish and brown rice are usually well tolerated. Move on to solids only when symptoms begin to ease, as sometimes diarrhoea is your body's digestive system telling you it needs a rest.

■ Eat plenty of low-fat, live yoghurt to replenish healthy bacteria in the bowel.

■ For acute diarrhoea, grate an apple, let it go brown and then eat it. Greenish bananas are very binding.

■ Slippery elm powder can be mashed into a paste with banana and honey. **SHS**

Useful Remedies

■ While symptoms last, take 10,000iu of vitamin A daily for one week – **but no more than 3000iu if pregnant** – as it helps protect the lining of the gut. Plus 30mg of zinc, as lack of zinc has been shown to trigger diarrhoea.

■ Thereafter, take a good-quality vitamin/mineral to help prevent malnutrition. Liquid formulas are easy to absorb. **BC**

■ The herb pau d'arco helps to kill many harmful organisms. Take 2–3ml of tincture 2 or 3 times a day, or 1 gram of capsules 2–3 times a day.

■ If you are susceptible to diarrhoea when you travel abroad, taking acidophilus for two weeks prior to your trip can help increase the number of healthy bacteria in the gut, which reduces the risk of picking up a tummy bug. You should take these for at least a week after suffering a bout of food poisoning to help repopulate your gut with healthy bacteria and eliminate any remaining bacteria. Jarro-Dophilus EPS is a good formula. **NC**

■ Floraguard by BioCare contains healthy bacteria plus garlic, oregano oil, clove oil and cinnamon and rosemary. It can be taken daily with food when you are abroad to help kill off any invading bacteria. It can be very handy for holidays, but do not take it if you are pregnant. **BC**

■ Bee propolis, grapefruit seed extract and olive leaf extract are all natural anti-bacterials.

Helpful Hints

■ Drink water from cooked brown rice or mix 15 grams of carob powder with some apple purée to make it palatable. Carob has a history of helping alleviate diarrhoea.

■ Never drink tap water unless you are sure it is safe to do so. Avoid salads and fruit washed in local tap water in places like India, Africa, the Far East and in any country you think the water may be questionable. Avoid ice cubes made from local tap water. Eat only thoroughly cooked foods. Use bottled water and fizzy drinks, but only if they have sealed tops.

- If the diarrhoea resembles water coming out of a hose, try homeopathic Podophyllum 30c every few hours for a day. Charcoal tablets are also useful for stopping diaorrhea.
- For teething children who have this problem, use homeopathic Chamomila 30c, 3 times daily.
- If you suffer persistent diarrhoea, you **must** see a doctor.

DIVERTICULAR DISEASE or DIVERTICULITIS

Diverticulitis is a disease of modern Western civilization, as it rarely occurs in people or cultures that eat a high-fibre diet. Years ago, it occurred in older people usually over 50, but these days, thanks to our over-processed diets and 24/7 lifestyles, younger people in their 20s and 30s are regularly diagnosed with this condition.

Diverticular disease occurs when the mucous membranes lining the colon form small finger-like pouches, known as diverticula, that protrude out of the intestinal wall. Thirty to forty per cent of people over the age of 60 have diverticular disease and generally these pouches do not cause problems. If, however, they become inflamed and infected, diverticulitis results. It causes extreme pain – primarily in the descending colon, which is situated on the left-hand side of the abdomen. Symptoms include pain, bleeding, diarrhoea and fever. Chronic constipation is the most common underlying cause of this condition, as a soft, bulky stool is easy to push along the colon and a hard, dry stool makes the muscles of the colon work too hard. Also, if we don't evacuate impacted faeces, then the muscular walls of the colon lose their integrity and thereby increase the risk for herniated pockets. Most sufferers tend not to drink sufficient water and ingest insufficient fibre (see also *Constipation*). Occasionally, a pouch may burst, which requires urgent medical attention.

Foods to Avoid
- Foods containing seeds such as tomatoes, grapes and strawberries, and poppy, sesame and pumpkin seeds, as the seeds can lodge in the pockets and cause inflammation and pain.
- Although fibre is necessary for a normal bowel movement, the abrasive fibres in wheat bran or high-fibre breakfast cereals, such as All Bran, can temporarily aggravate the problem.
- For many people wheat found in bread, cakes, biscuits, pizza bases, pasta and so on, can have a constipating effect – try avoiding these foods for 2 weeks to see if it helps.
- Avoid fried or spicy foods.
- Reduce saturated fats such as full-fat milk, cheese and chocolates, as these can trigger inflammation, are mucous forming and can make constipation worse.
- Avoid as much as possible white bread and pasta, white rice, cakes, biscuits, take-aways and mass-produced burger-type foods.
- Greatly reduce your intake of red meat, which takes a long time to pass through the bowel, as does cooked cheese. Pizza is one of the worst foods to eat with this condition.
- While symptoms are acute, also avoid all yeast-based foods including Marmite, Bovril, cheese, soy sauce, vinegar and so on.
- Avoid all sweeteners containing fructose, sorbitol and aspartame.
- Carageenan is a milk protein stabilizer often used in ice cream that causes problems for people with digestive/bowel problems.

- Tea, coffee, fizzy drinks and alcohol can dehydrate the bowel.

Friendly Foods

- When the bowel is inflamed, eat soothing foods such as vegetable soups with cabbage, celery, ginger, plus lightly stewed apples, apricots, prunes, papaya and porridge made with non-dairy light soya, almond or rice milk.
- Mashed pumpkin and sweet potato are rich in carotenes to help heal the gut.
- Once the inflammation is under control, introduce a little steamed or grilled fish and low-fat, organic meat such as skinless poultry.
- Gradually, increase your intake of high-fibre foods such as brown rice, gluten- and wheat-free breads and pastas, fresh vegetables, pulses, oat-based cereals and fruit (especially figs). There are many excellent organic high-fibre mueslis and cereals made from grains such as amaranth, kamut and quinoa. Remember it's important to check which foods are making your condition worse before you remove too many foods from your diet – see *Allergies*.
- Live, low-fat yoghurt containing acidophilus and bifidus helps maintain the level of bacteria in the bowel and stool, which encourages regular bowel movement.
- Drink at least 8 glasses of water daily to make sure there is adequate fluid in the bowel.
- Use extra virgin, unrefined olive or sunflower oils for your salad dressings.
- Eat more garlic and onions for their antiseptic qualities.
- Add ginger to foods and juices, which soothes and heals the gut.
- If you cook cabbage, leave the cooking water to cool and then drink. It contains cabigin, a nutrient that helps to heal the bowel.

Useful Remedies

- The anti-inflammatory essential oils found in evening primrose oil also promote healing and repair; take 1–2 grams or take 1 gram of GLA (gamma-linolenic acid) daily. **BC**
- Add half a cup of aloe vera juice to fresh vegetable juices daily to help heal the gut, soothe the mucous membranes and increase bowel movements. Aloe Pura make a good stomach formula that you can take.
- Slippery elm is gentle, soothing and nourishing to the digestive lining. Drink as a tea, chew on the bark, or take 2–3 tablets before meals. Contact Specialist Herbal Supplies, who make pure slippery elm tea, and they will be able to recommend specific herbs for your particular symptoms. **SHS**
- Good bacteria (acidophilus/bifidus) can help fight infection while it is active and help to reduce constipation. During a flare-up, take 2 capsules three times per day. To protect for the future, take 1 capsule twice a day.
- Prebiotics are plant compounds that encourage the growth of healthy bacteria in the bowel. Try Agave Digestive Immune Support. One scoop daily with breakfast really helps to keep you regular. See www.lef.org or call the Nutri Centre. **NC**
- Take a natural-source carotene complex to aid soft tissue healing. Take 60mg daily.
- Calcium fluoride tissue salts help to strengthen the intestinal walls. Take 4 daily.
- Chlorophyll found in green plants is very healing to gut lining. Take an organic green food complex, such as Viridian Green Food Blend Powder, twice daily in between meals.

Helpful Hints

- Exercise regularly – gentle walking and swimming help to work the stomach muscles and encourage bowel movements.
- Leave time to visit the loo – relax and don't rush.
- Remember to drink plenty of fluids, which helps to prevent constipation.
- Stress makes any digestive, gut or bowel problem worse. Look at your lifestyle and take time out to practise meditation, yoga or t'ai chi.

- Anxiety of any kind affects the bowel.
- An informative website can be found at www.digestive.niddk.nih.gov.
- Lots of useful fact sheets about diverticular disease can be found at www.corecharity.org.uk, or you can contact them at CORE, Freepost, LON4268, London NW1 0YT or call them on 020 7486 0341.

DIZZY SPELLS

(see Adrenal Exhaustion, Low Blood Pressure, Low Blood Sugar and Vertigo)

EARACHE   *(see also Glue Ear, Ménière's Syndrome, Tinnitus and Vertigo)*

Most earaches are caused by the build-up of fluid in the middle ear, which can lead to an infection causing pain, fever or loss of hearing. Children under the age of 5 are particularly prone to ear infections, usually triggered by a sensitivity to foods such as corn, eggs, peanuts, cow's milk and wheat. Cow's milk and milk products are without doubt the most likely culprits. Soya milk and products can also trigger mucous in many people. I have vivid memories as a child screaming with chronic earache until eventually both my eardrums burst. My poor mother had no idea that it was our diet of cow's milk, cream trifles, cheese, chocolate treats and lots of lard and dripping (solidified beef, lamb and pork fat) sandwiches that caused the problem.

I was prescribed with almost continuous antibiotics, which undoubtedly contributed to my acne, thrush and chronic fatigue during my teens. So if you have young children, try as much as possible to avoid antibiotics by changing your child's diet and giving them supplements to boost their immune function.

Cutting down on sugar also helps, as most foods containing saturated fats also contain sugar, which converts to fat within the body if not used up during exercise. Note that many yoghurts and 'low-fat' foods are high in sugar! If the earache is persistent, many doctors suggest the insertion of grommets through minor surgery, but in the majority of cases this procedure can be avoided. To make sure your child does not become malnourished, I suggest you consult a qualified nutritionist. (See *Useful Information*.)

Foods to Avoid

- Any food to which there is a sensitivity, particularly dairy produce from cows, plus wheat-based foods and eggs. Greek yoghurts are very high in fat and should be avoided.
- Generally, while symptoms are acute, avoid mucous-forming foods, such as chocolate, milks, soya (in some people), cheese and so on – but note that any foods to which you have an intolerance will trigger mucous production.
- Any sugar as it tends to weaken the immune system and leaves children more susceptible to infections. This includes fizzy drinks and desserts, which are often packed with sugar.
- Excessive amounts of fruit juice, as these are often citrus based, which sometimes adds to the problem. Remember that most canned fizzy drinks contain up to 10 teaspoons of sugar.

Never use drinks containing aspartame, as they place too much of a strain on the liver, which can further exacerbate the problem.

Friendly Foods

- Once you have identified any problem foods such as cow's or soya milk (see under *Helpful Hints*), look for alternatives, such as oat, rice or almond milk. I would not recommend soya milk and foods for any child under the age of 5 years.
- There are plenty of wheat-free pastas now available based on lentils, buckwheat, quinoa, rice, corn and vegetables.
- Wheat can be replaced by rye or rice bread, or rice, rye or amaranth crackers and oatcakes.
- Eat plenty of fruit and vegetables to keep the immune system in good shape, particularly those rich in the carotenoids, such as sweet potatoes, pumpkin, papaya, mango, apricots, carrots, watercress and spinach. Other useful foods for the immune system are cauliflower, broccoli, kale and Brussels sprouts.

Useful Remedies

- The herb echinacea. If used as a tincture, take one drop per 6kg (13lb) of body weight. Take 3–4 times a day for up to 3 weeks at any one time.
- To help fight infection and boost immunity, take 1 gram of vitamin C with food daily. Children generally find it easier if vitamin C powder is dissolved in diluted low-sugar apple juice.
- Beta Glucans, derived from yeast cells walls, are safe for children to take and improve their innate immune system functioning, which can help reduce the severity of reaction to foods. Dr Paul Clayton, who is a former scientific advisor to the Government's Committee on the Safety of Medicines, says: 'Thanks to our modern over-sanitized environment and intensive farming methods, which have removed virtually all Beta Glucans from our diet, our ability to resist infections has become compromised. You can break a capsule of the Beta Glucans 1–3,1–6 daily into cold foods – and children can safely take 250–500mg daily. Most parents report that when their children are given the Beta Glucans regularly, they suffer fewer infections.' **NC**
- Children's multi-vitamins and minerals can make sure children are not deficient in any nutrients, which can impair their immune system. Nature's Plus makes an excellent children's range. **NP**
- As antibiotics destroy healthy bacteria, encourage your children to eat low-fat live yoghurts once daily, containing the friendly bacteria acidophilus. Try them on goat's or sheep's yoghurts, which are usually better tolerated than those made from cow's milk. If they hate the taste of plain yoghurt, add any fresh fruit you have to hand and whiz in the blender for a few seconds. Make low-sugar jellies with fresh fruit juices and serve with low-fat yoghurt instead of ice cream.
- To sweeten desserts use a little agave syrup or xylitol – natural sugars that have a low glycaemic factor. Available from health shops.

Helpful Hints

- If you smoke, it is definitely worth trying to cut back or not smoking near the children, as this has been strongly linked to the development of ear infections.
- A warm hot-water bottle wrapped in a towel can be placed by the ear. Or buy a wheat bag – and warm through, then place near the ears.
- Warm an onion and place the core of the onion just inside the affected ear wrapped in muslin, or squeeze a small amount of onion water into the ear. Onion and garlic are natural decongestants.
- It is important to have an allergy test to find your worst offenders. One of the best I have found is available from the York Test Laboratories. Call 0800 458 2052 or log on to

www.yorktest.com. Alternatively, Genova Diagnostics do a FACT test that looks for inflammatory markers indicating that the body is reacting to certain substances. Call 020 8336 7750 or log on to www.gdx.uk.net.

- Another excellent method is the Bio Meridian Test for food intolerance and leaky gut, in which the practitioner measures, via electrodes, your reactions to a large list of foods and substances. For practitioners, see www.biomeridian.com or call Sheila Partridge on 0207 580 7537.
- Taking homeopathic Pulsatilla 30c or Belladonna 30c every 3–4 hours helps if the earache is in the right ear. If it is in the left ear, try Hepar Sulph 30c. If there is a sticky discharge, try Kali Bic 30c.
- Do not let a child swim under water if their ears become infected.
- Children who are given dummies are more prone to ear infections.
- Consult an allergy specialist who can test for food intolerances, which can exacerbate and trigger this problem.
- See a cranial osteopath or chiropractor to check the alignment of the head and neck, as misalignment and poor drainage can cause earache (see *Useful Information*).
- For irritations in the ears and sinuses, mucous and catarrh, use ear candles, which gently remove excess ear wax without pain. These are excellent for children as they are fun to use and not painful. Available from all good health stores, or for details, call Revital on 0800 252 875 or visit www.revital.co.uk.
- The Neil Med sinus rinse is simple to use and hugely helps to reduce sinus and ear infections. Available from all good chemists. See www.neilmed.com.

E

ECZEMA

(see also Allergies, Asthma, Leaky Gut, Irritable Bowel Syndrome and Liver Problems)

According to the NHS, around 6 million people in the UK are affected by varying types of eczema, and 1 in every 15 adults and 1 in 5 children now suffers mild to severe forms of eczema. It can be an inherited condition and is also linked to asthma and rhinitis/hayfever.

During flare-ups the skin can become very inflamed, itchy and sometimes develops into open bleeding sores. Eczema is sometimes triggered by an external irritant, such as perfumes, washing powders, shampoos, paint, house dust mites, or cat hairs; but most commonly it is linked to a food intolerance (as many as 80% of sufferers show a positive reaction to allergy-testing) or a leaky gut. Therefore, please make sure you read the *Leaky Gut* section.

It can also be associated with an under-functioning immune system.

Eczema can appear at any age, seemingly from nowhere. It tends to be aggravated by stress, exhaustion, sometimes by heat and frequently by exercise. Eczema does tend to come and go.

For most people, symptoms worsen when they are under stress, but others notice that the condition is aggravated by certain foods, especially sugar, wheat, orange juice and cow's milk, or drinking too much tea or coffee. If it starts in early childhood, the most likely culprit is cow's milk and products. Either the child has been fed formula milk or the residues are ingested via the mother's breast milk. The most common triggers for eczema in babies are dairy products, eggs, citrus and wheat. Avoidance of the offending food often resolves the problem.

It is very important to remember that by the time the eczema shows up on the skin it has worked its way through the body and you really need to address the root cause of the problem. With any skin condition it is a good idea to support the liver, which is the most important cleansing organ of the body. If the liver becomes overloaded with toxins, it tends to start dumping them into the skin – so anything you can do to keep your liver functioning more efficiently will, in the long term, help your skin.

Also, drugs such as Ibuprofen have been known to trigger an attack in some people, as this drug can contribute to a leaky gut.

Foods to Avoid
- As much as possible, avoid or greatly reduce your intake of all dairy products from cows, as well as coffee, tea, chocolate, beef, citrus fruits, eggs, wheat, alcohol, tomatoes and peanuts. This is a long list of foods, but if you have eczema and cut out all of these foods, the eczema is virtually guaranteed to improve. Start keeping a food diary, too, and note when symptoms are worse.
- Sugar greatly affects the immune system, so again try to cut down on sugary foods and drinks.
- It is important to note that even decaffeinated coffee causes problems in people who are sensitive to coffee – it's not just the caffeine. The solvent used to extract the caffeine can affect a number of skin conditions.
- As much as possible, avoid preservatives, additives, pesticides, food colourings (such as in the bright red glacé cherries on fancy cakes) and refined sugar-based, mass-produced cakes, biscuits and pies (see also *Allergies*).

Friendly Foods
- Wherever possible, go organic and eat plenty of fresh fruits and vegetables.
- Include plenty of cabbage in your diet – and drink any water the cabbage has been cooked in. It contains L-glutamine, which helps to heal a leaky gut.
- Beetroot, artichokes, celeriac, celery and radicchio are foods that cleanse the liver.
- Freshly made vegetable juices with celery, apple, cucumber, carrot, kale with a half a cup of aloe vera juice will all help re-alkalize the body and heal the gut (see *Acid–Alkaline Balance*).
- Diluted pear juice is a good alternative to orange juice.
- If you react to cow's milk, there are plenty of alternatives such as rice, oat and almond milk, all of which have a much lower incidence of reaction.
- Oily fish can be particularly beneficial, as the essential fatty acids in fish are anti-inflammatory and have been shown to improve eczema conditions. Eat more sardines, organic-farmed salmon, mackerel, anchovies and herrings.
- Sunflower seeds, sesame seeds, linseeds (flax seeds) and pumpkin seeds – and nuts with the exception of peanuts. The fatty acids and high levels of zinc and protein in these foods will help nourish the skin and speed up the healing process.
- Wheat germ and avocados are rich in vitamin E, which also aids skin healing.
- Use extra-virgin olive oil, plus unrefined walnut and sunflower oil in salad dressings.
- Use non-hydrogenated spreads such as Biona and Vitaquell in preference to mass-produced hard fats (see also *Fats You Need To Eat*).
- Orange-coloured fruit and vegetables contain beta carotene, the vegetable source of vitamin A, known to be beneficial to skin health. Try squashes, pumpkin, red grapes, sweet potatoes, mango, cantaloupe melon, peppers, carrots and apricots.

Useful Remedies
- There is now good research showing that people who take healthy bacteria (probiotics) regularly are less likely to suffer eczema, as healthy bacteria help improve digestion and reduce any immune response. Have a word with the nutritionist at BioCare or at your local health store to find out which probiotic would suit you best. **BC**
- Or take Jarro-Dophilus EPS, which is a good probiotic – one daily. **NC**
- Prebiotics are plant compounds that encourage the growth of healthy bacteria in the bowel.

Try Agave Digestive Immune Support. One scoop daily with breakfast really helps to keep you regular, which takes the burden off the liver. See www.lef.org or call the Nutri Centre on 0845 602 6744.

- Cabbage contains the amino acid L-glutamine, which greatly aids healing of the gut. Take a teaspoon twice daily in water 45 minutes before main meals. **HN**
- Colostrum, which is found in breast milk, helps support the immune system and aids healing of a leaky gut. It's very helpful for babies and children suffering from eczema. Up to the age of 2, an infant can take a quarter of a teaspoon twice daily on an empty stomach. Over 2 years – half a teaspoon twice daily. Take this just for one month. **NC**
- Evening primrose oil, take 1–4 grams a day. This has been shown to help heal eczema. It is also available on prescription.
- Also take 400iu of full-spectrum, natural-source vitamin E daily. The vitamin E will also help prevent scarring and itching.
- The mineral zinc is needed to ensure adequate absorption of fatty acids, and it's invariably deficient in eczema sufferers. It also speeds skin-healing – take 30mg twice daily for a couple of months, then reduce to 20mg per day.
- Research shows selenium levels are low in people with inflammatory conditions such as eczema. Make sure your multi-vitamin provides 200mcg, as it works well with vitamin E.
- Vitamin A is really important for skin healing. For one week only each month (for up to 6 months) take 10,000 iu of vitamin A daily to boost levels in the body. **NB If you are pregnant or planning a pregnancy, then never take more than 3000 iu of vitamin A per day.**
- Include a high-strength multi-vitamin and mineral that includes a full spectrum of B-vitamins, which help reduce stress and improve digestion and the absorption of fatty acids.
- Nettle works as a mild antihistamine, which can reduce the itching. This tincture can be applied both externally and taken internally. Ideally, do not apply to broken skin, as the small amount of alcohol would sting the skin. For young children use 1 drop per 6kg (13lb) of body weight – this will ensure you don't give them too much.
- The herb milk thistle has been shown to help regenerate and support liver function. Take 500mg twice daily with meals.
- Omega-7 fats, extracted from sea buckthorn berries, are highly effective at relieving dry skin. Made by Pharma Nord. Their advice line is 0800 591756 (freephone). **PN**
- Also take one gram of omega-3 fish oils, which are anti-inflammatory.

Helpful Hints

- Many people have found that aloe vera juice taken internally, and the gel used topically, have proved helpful for eczema.
- Allergenics cream is available from Health Imports. This cream soothes the majority of cases, and some people have said it has actually cleared their eczema up. For details, call Wellbeing on 0121 444 6585.
- To help relieve the itching, place 2 cups of any kind of bran or oatmeal in your bath and soak for 20 minutes.
- It is important to have an allergy test to find out the triggers for the eczema. Either try the York Test Laboratories. Tel: 0800 458 2052 or log on to www.yorktest.com; or Genova Diagnostics do a FACT test that looks for inflammatory markers indicating that the body is reacting to certain substances. Tel: 020 8336 7750. Website: www.gdx.uk.net
- Do something positive to help relieve the stress that may be aggravating the eczema. Try meditation, yoga, t'ai chi, or some other means of relaxation. If you can, get away and bask in some sunshine – and salt water, which usually aids eczema.

E

- If you have access to, and can afford, a reflexology treatment or aromatherapy massage, not only will the oils improve the condition but they are also incredibly relaxing. A few drops of essential oils of lavender, Roman camomile, geranium, rose and cedarwood mixed in a good base carrier oil, such as calendula, can be applied to the affected areas.
- Exercise is generally beneficial for both reducing stress and improving the condition, however, wear lightweight, cotton, loose-fitting clothing, as if you get too hot and sweaty this may aggravate the condition.
- Relief Cream, made from calendula, manuka honey, aloe vera and gotu kola, works really well on eczema and psoriasis and is great for babies. For details, log on to www.planetblueshop.com. Or try Ultra Dry Skin Cream by the Organic Pharmacy. **OP**
- Constipation, and a liver under stress from too many toxins, is also associated with eczema, as toxins cannot be broken down and removed from the body efficiently (see also *Constipation* and *Liver Problems*).
- If a sensitivity to certain foods is suspected, then avoid the offending food (see *Allergies*).
- Avoid mass-produced soaps and soap powders. Ask at your health store for pH-balanced soaps – or natural soaps that contain, say, olive oil or vitamins A and E.
- Chinese herbs have proved helpful in many cases, but you need to see a qualified Chinese herbalist and may need to have your liver function checked before and during treatment. Others report great success through homeopathy (see *Useful Information*).
- Reduce your exposure to house dust mites by using a vacuum cleaner with an allergy filter, and vacuum mattresses once a week.
- Putting duvets and pillows out in bright sunlight for a few hours a month will help to kill off the mites.
- For further help, contact the National Eczema Society, Hill House, Highgate Hill, London N19 5NA. Helpline: 0800 0891122 (Monday to Friday, 8am–8pm). Website: www.eczema.org.

ELECTRICAL POLLUTION and ELECTRICAL HEALING

In 2000 there were 31 million mobile phones in use. By 2010 around 75 million mobile phones had been connected in the UK – many for use by children – in spite of our and other governments, including France and Austria, having issued warnings that children under 12 should not use mobile phones and that masts should be situated well away from schools.

There is now a considerable body of evidence from highly accredited sources, including SAGE, the UK's Government Advisory Body and the Bioinitiative Working Group (scientists from the USA, Sweden, Denmark, Austria and China, who in 2007 released a 650-page report citing more than 2000 studies), linking electromagnetic fields from computers, mobile phones, household electrical goods, satellite receivers, transmitters, TVs, fluorescent light bulbs and dimmer switches, microwaves, and other electronic devices to childhood cancers, depression and suicide, brain tumours, dizziness and headaches, short-term memory loss, Alzheimer's, tinnitus and extreme fatigue.

Roger Coghill based in Torfaen in Wales, a bio-electromagnetics research scientist and one of the UK's leading authorities on this subject who sits on the SAGE committee advising the UK Government on how to mitigate EMF exposure, says: 'First, people need to understand that we are electrical beings in a physical shell and electricity can be used to harm or to heal us. Every cell in the human body emits its own unique range of frequencies. These frequencies are as unique to us as our DNA. When functioning properly, our cells or groups of cells, such as our liver or kidneys, emit a harmonic signal (denoting that the organ is healthy), which can clearly be seen on specialist scanners. If we become ill, cells begin emitting a disharmonic set of frequencies, which again can be detected. Every food you eat also emits a specific range of frequencies, as does every nutrient and everything on the planet – even rocks. This is how scientists measure what other planets and stars are made of, by measuring their spectral frequencies. But electrical pollution from external sources, such as WiFi equipment, which is now referred to as 'dirty electricity', is without doubt a major contributing factor to many illnesses and we need to protect ourselves.

'For instance, a study in Sweden has suggested that a person has a five-times increased risk of brain cancer if they start using a mobile phone in their teens. Israel has banned the placement of cellular antennae on residences, and we now believe that up to 3% of the population are clinically hypersensitive.

'In 1981, a study by a British Doctor, Dr Stephen Perry, was published which clearly demonstrated that significantly more suicides occurred at locations of high magnetic field strength.

'There is now a critical mass of evidence to show that excessive use of mobile phones, and the EMFs that come off various sources, can trigger a variety of cancers, impair immune functioning and contribute to Alzheimer's Disease, heart disease and other health disorders.'

Coghill continues: 'The hands-free kits are also linked with health problems and if you use these phones for more than ten minutes at a time you are at a much greater long-term risk of brain tumours. We are living in a sea of artificial frequencies and because animals, especially whales, dolphins, insects and birds, are more sensitive to these man-made emissions, their sensory abilities are being greatly affected – which is why so many whales are beaching themselves. Humans are also becoming more electro-sensitive, and there are even societies that help people who are either affected by, or whose fields affect, electrical equipment.

'Also if you have subterranean flowing water under your home or office, this often compounds health problems, as the water can create an inharmonious electromagnetic field. Hundreds of years ago, builders would watch carefully where sheep settled at night and would not build in places where sheep refused to sleep. Studies show rats also avoid areas of high electromagnetic fields. Every time you turn on a light switch or any electrical equipment, your brain's rhythms change immediately. Spending too much time under fluorescent lighting or in front of a computer screen can suppress the brain chemical melatonin, which can have negative effects as diverse as sleep disturbance, depression and infertility.'

Foods to Avoid
- Junk foods have a dull energy field frequency that will eventually trigger negative symptoms if you eat junk foods to excess. But it is important to note that all foods emit their own frequency: if you eat certain foods, whether considered healthy or not, that emit a frequency that is incompatible with your own frequency range, this too can trigger symptoms in sensitive individuals.

Friendly Foods
- Foods in as near a natural state as possible. For example, if you look at the energy field of a raw cabbage it has a really bright energy field – but once cooked, the energy field is greatly reduced. See *General Health Hints*.

Useful Remedies

- One of the best ways to help protect yourself is by taking the hormone melatonin. EMF pollution reduces your pineal glands' ability to synthesize melatonin – which is why exposure affects sleep patterns. Radiation creates free radicals in the body, and highly potent antioxidants, such as melatonin, help protect you from electrical pollution – as melatonin passes the blood brain barrier into the bloodstream. Coghill has developed a supplement called Asphalia, which contains natural melatonin extracted from certain grasses to maintain melatonin levels. Roger has permission from the MHRA (Medical Healthcare Regulatory Authority) to sell this supplement in the UK. For more details or to find your nearest supplier, log on to www.asphalia.co.uk or call 01495 752122.

Helpful Hints

- The Bicom Resonance machine developed in Germany picks up the electromagnetic frequencies emanating from the body, which an experienced practitioner can interpret and then determine which frequencies should be amplified back into the patient's energy field, to enable the body to heal itself. Cells carry a memory of certain diseases that you thought long ago had left your body. For example, when I was tested with the Bicom my cells showed a positive reading for the memory of glandular fever, which I suffered during my teens. To counteract this the therapist inverted the frequency of the Epstein Barr virus (from a tiny phial containing Epstein Barr) back into my body to neutralize any remaining memory. The Bicom is good for helping people eliminate allergies, chronic fatigue, endometriosis, treating intestinal parasites and eczema. For more details contact Peter Smith at the Hale Clinic in London. Tel: 020 7631 0156.
- Another excellent method similar to the Bicom is Bio Meridian Testing. Via electrodes placed on acupuncture meridian points, the practitioner can measure electric currents being emitted by various organs and musculoskeletal systems, which gives the therapist accurate feedback as to the health of various systems. This method can also determine which supplements and/ or drugs agree with your unique physiology and determine what foods and substances to which you have sensitivities. For practitioners, see www.biomeridian.com or call Sheila Partridge on 020 7580 7537. Sheila works with Dr Shamin Daya at the Wholistic Medical Centre in Harley Street, London, and is one of the most experienced practitioners of the Bio Meridian practices I have ever encountered.
- Electro-crystal healing, invented by bio-physicist Harry Oldfield, works on similar principles. First, patients' energy fields are scanned via a specialist scanner, which enables therapists to view negative frequency emissions and thus determine which areas in the body are under-functioning. An experienced practitioner then pulses calming or stimulating frequencies through crystals suspended in saline solution to encourage healing of areas affected. I have interviewed dozens of people crippled with arthritis and other conditions who have been greatly helped by this type of therapy. Harry has trained hundreds of therapists worldwide. For details of your nearest therapist, log on to www.electrocrystal.com.
- The basic rule is that moving electric fields – for example, mobile phones or power lines – are harmful, while static magnetic fields, such as the earth on which we all evolved, are beneficial to health.
- Avoid using a mobile phone inside a car, building, or any enclosed space, because the phone is forced to increase its output power, which can affect your health more quickly. Never use a mobile phone for more than 5–7 minutes at a time.
- Never charge your mobile phone by your bedside.
- If you are pregnant, do not sleep with an electric blanket on and keep mobile phone use to a minimum.

- When you attach a phone ear piece directly into your ear, Roger says that you risk pulsing radio waves straight into the brain; you need to look for sets that have ferrite components, which block radiation from travelling up the wire.
- Keep electrical appliances in the bedroom to a minimum. Turn off all mains switches in the bedroom at night. If you live near an electrical power station, put large copper jugs or ornaments in the windows. Avoid placing 'touch lamps' with thyristor dimmers anywhere near your bed. Also turn off computers and TVs at the mains at night. Leaving TVs and other equipment on 'standby' wastes huge amounts of energy and still creates an electrical field.
- Turn off your Wifi router box at night.
- Avoid sleeping with an electric blanket on; instead, warm the bed thoroughly before you get into bed and then switch it off for the night. However, if you are over 60 and have poor circulation and have been specifically told to sleep with it on, for goodness sake don't get too cold!
- Studies show that microwave ovens alter the chemistry of food. Irradiating (x-raying) food could, in the long run, prove very dangerous. If any foods like strawberries are still healthy looking after being in your fridge for a few days, then they have most likely been irradiated.
- DECT (digital enhanced cordless telecommunications) cordless phones give out some of the worst EMF signals that arc across the room. So change to a low-radiation cordless phone. Contact Orchid on www.lowradiation.co.uk or call 020 8398 9925.
- Avoid having too many CT scans and X-rays unless they are deemed essential. One CT scan is equivalent to 400 X-rays.
- The Coghill Research Laboratories can supply an ELF Meter to tell you the field strengths in your home. For details, call 01495 752122. Or read Roger's book, *Something in the Air*. To order or for more information, log on to www.cogreslab.co.uk.
- Have your home dowsed by an expert if you are worried about suffering from overexposure to electricity. Contact The British Society of Dowsers. Tel: 01684 576969. Website: www.britishdowsers.org.
- For further news on pollution issues, visit www.pollutionissues.co.uk.

EMPHYSEMA   *(see also Bronchitis)*

A group of conditions including emphysema and chronic bronchitis are termed as chronic obstructive pulmonary disease (COPD).

Bronchitis means 'inflammation of the bronchi'; the inflammation increases mucous production in the airways and a sufferer will produce more phlegm as they cough.

Emphysema is a serious disease when the air sacs or alveoli (the place where carbon dioxide is exchanged for oxygen, which is the main job of the lungs) lose their elasticity and the airways narrow. This means that your lungs are not efficient at getting oxygen into the body, so you need to breathe harder, which triggers shortness of breath.

Any chronic lung condition that causes narrowing of the airways, such as asthma or bronchitis, may contribute to emphysema, but 80% of cases are triggered by smoking.

As this condition can take years to develop, and usually manifests in mid life or later, official Government figures in the UK state that as many as 3.5 million people are at various stages of developing COPD.

Other potential triggers for COPD are exposure to coal dust, toxic moulds, cotton, flour, wood or grain dusts, welding fumes and minerals such as cadmium and vanadium. Pollution from industry and our roads definitely plays a part in chronic lung disease.

It's a sad fact that many patients lose up to 70% of their functional lung tissue before they realize that they have a chronic disease – therefore the earlier a diagnosis can be made, the less damage is done.

Low levels of protective antioxidants (such as vitamin C, E and so on) and high levels of oxidative stress, caused by damaging free radicals (from burnt food, pollution, chemicals and so on) alongside exposure to toxins will only exacerbate onset of this condition.

Symptoms might begin as a chronic cough or bouts of bronchitis, phlegm or shortness of breath – especially in winter. As the condition progresses the patient will suffer from shortness of breath more regularly, until it happens daily.

Other symptoms include skipped breaths, wheezing, insomnia, fatigue, swelling of feet, ankles or legs, irritability and unexplained weight loss. Emphysema patients have an increased risk of contracting pneumonia, so keeping the immune system strong is essential. See *Immune Function*. Heart disease is another risk factor, as the heart has to work extra hard to make up for the lungs. The more you can avoid developing infections, the better.

Foods to Avoid

- Avoid foods that contain hydrogenated/trans-fats and oils found in many pre-packaged and processed foods, as these can trigger inflammation. They also compete with the healthy fats that help keep the alveoli in the lungs supple so that they can do their job more easily. See *Fats You Need To Eat*.
- Any foods to which you have an intolerance – the most common being wheat and any dairy food/milk from cows.
- If you find that you are making too much phlegm, this is almost always linked to eating high-fat foods, including full-fat cheese, chocolate, cow's or soya milk, white bread, croissants and bananas.
- Fried and barbecued foods, as they have high levels of damaging free radicals.
- Generally, cut down your intake of red meat and if you choose to eat meat make it organic and always cut off the fat first.
- Eggs are hard to digest for some people and it's well worth being tested to see if they are a problem. See Genova and York Test details under *Allergies*.
- Sugary foods and drinks suppress immune function, which leaves you more susceptible to infections. Also, most foods high in sugar are also high in animal fats. And keep in mind that many low-fat foods are high in sugar which, unless burnt during exercise, will be converted to fat within the body.

Friendly Foods

- People who eat fruit and vegetables on a regular basis seem less likely to develop emphysema, so focus on foods rich in natural sources of carotenes, which help to protect mucous membranes in the lungs. Eat more apricots, mangoes, green vegetables, pumpkin, parsley, red peppers, spinach, sweet potatoes, watercress and cantaloupe melon.
- Vine-ripened tomatoes are rich in the carotene lycopene, which helps support the lungs. Cook in a little olive oil to help release the lycopene. Guava and pink grapefruit also contain a fair amount of lycopene.
- Go for organic whenever possible, as fruits, such as apples, which are great for lung health, can otherwise be covered in up to eighteen pesticides.
- Quercetins – flavonoids found in apples, pears, cherries, grapes, onion, kale, broccoli, garlic, green tea and red wine – help protect the lungs from the harmful effect of pollutants and cigarette smoke. Eat more fresh pineapple.

- Use organic rice or almond milk as non-dairy alternatives. Some people find low-fat goat's or sheep's milk better.
- Choose low-fat dishes including cottage cheese and replace butter with spreads such as Biona, Vitaquel, Olivio. Or try organic raw walnut, hemp seed or almond butter. From Higher Nature (**HN**) or call Sun & Seed on 020 7267 7799.
- Use olive oil for salad dressings and eat plenty of brown rice, lentils, barley, oat-based dishes, wheat-free breakfast cereals (Nature's Path make a great range). There are also plenty of wheat-free pastas available such as lentil, rice, corn and potato pasta and flour.
- Liver, kidney, butter, and skimmed milk contain retinol, the animal form of vitamin A, which is good for tissue-healing. Don't go mad on the butter – and make it organic.
- Eat more garlic and onions, as these help to fend off infection and clear the lungs.
- Fenugreek or liquorice tea can help to soothe the lungs.
- See *General Health Hints*.

Useful Remedies

- People with lung conditions tend to be low in Vitamin A. If you are not pregnant or aiming to become pregnant, then take 25,000iu of vitamin A daily for one month and then reduce to taking 2 natural source carotene complex daily. **SVHC, VN**
- N-acetyl cysteine (NAC): take 500mg 1–2 times a day. This amino acid is one of the best-researched nutrients for emphysema, as it helps break up mucous and has been shown to reduce the frequency and duration of attacks of COPD when taken twice daily over a period of at least 6 months. NAC also helps the body to produce the powerful antioxidant glutathione in the liver.
- Vitamin C: take 1–2 grams daily with food in an ascorbate form to help clear mucous and improve respiratory ailments. It works well with NAC (above).
- L-carnitine: take 2 grams daily, if breathing is made worse by exercise.
- Microcell Nutri Guard Plus contains high-potency lycopene, selenium, zinc, alpha-lipoic acid and vitamins A, C and E, which all help to support lung tissue. **BC**
- Include a high-potency multi-vitamin and mineral in your regimen.
- Bromelain, extracted from pineapples, is great for helping to break up mucous and is anti-inflammatory. Take 500mg twice daily.
- Co-enzyme Q10 is a powerful antioxidant that helps restore energy to damaged lung cells. Take 100mg, twice daily with food, but do not take it at night, as CoQ10 also increases general energy levels.
- Magnesium helps to relax bronchial muscles for easier breathing. Take 200mg three times a day. See www.positivehealthshop.com.
- The amino acid taurine is able to help to improve breathlessness. Take 1000mg twice a day before meals.
- Lipoic acid is a very important antioxidant for lungs: take 200mg daily.

Helpful Hints

- Don't smoke, and if you do smoke – give it up. Avoid smoke-filled rooms and sources of second-hand cigarette smoke.
- Regular exercise before the onset of COPD can help increase lung capacity and strengthen the heart.
- To help break up any thick mucous that may collect in the lungs, drink plenty of fluid.
- Avoid air pollutants such as dust, aerosol sprays, herbicides, pesticides, fumes from fuel and exhausts, smoke from bonfires and barbecues, and dust stirred up by house-cleaning.
- Use an Ultrabreathe – a small, inexpensive device that helps to exercise the lungs. For details, visit their website at www.ultrabreathe.com.

- Gentle exercise can help relieve the symptoms of this condition by building lung capacity and cleansing the lungs of stale air. Start slowly and build up gradually. Choose walking, swimming or cycling.
- Reflexology has proved to be successful with some sufferers. Yoga can also be beneficial, since this therapy will teach you relaxation techniques and how to breathe properly (see *Useful Information*).
- Aromatherapy has also been of benefit to some sufferers. Fill a basin with boiling water and add three drops of eucalyptus essential oil. Put your head over the basin with a towel over and inhale the steam.
- Be careful about visiting high altitudes, as this makes it harder to breathe.
- An ionizer in the home may be useful for lowering levels of dust in the house.
- Sing when you can, as this helps increase lung capacity. Take deep breaths regularly. You can increase the efficiency of your lungs a thousandfold by increasing your air intake by 5% on each breath.
- Environmentally friendly cleaning products are kinder to your lungs, as they don't contain harsh chemicals that can be breathed in. Try Ecover products – available from health stores and supermarkets.
- www.lef.org – a US research site (The Life Extension Foundation) – offers a wealth of information for people with emphysema.

ENDOMETRIOSIS   *(see also Thyroid underactive)*

Around 2 million women in the UK suffer from this problem, which most commonly occurs between the ages of 25 and 45. Endometriosis is a condition where tissue that normally lines the womb grows outside the womb. The endometrial tissue can be found in places such as the ovaries, fallopian tubes or pelvis, in the cervix, colon, appendix and vagina. In more severe cases, adhesions of endometrial tissue are found on the bladder, kidneys, lungs or even in the nasal lining. Some doctors believe that endometriosis is an autoimmune disease, as higher rates of rheumatoid arthritis, MS, and lupus are found in women suffering this condition.

The chemical dioxin (from vinyl, plastics and produced during incineration and forest fires) and numerous other toxic chemicals found in our air and water have also been linked to this condition. This is because dioxins can interfere with the metabolism of B-vitamins, needed for optimum liver function, which in turn is needed to break down excess oestrogen. Also excess pollutants mimic oestrogen in the body, triggering hormonal imbalances.

Most nutritional practitioners also believe there is a strong link between endometriosis and candida overgrowth (see *Candida*), because when it is treated symptoms are greatly alleviated. Many of the women suffering this condition find that symptoms are definitely worse when they are stressed or really tired.

The current theory is that, during menstruation, womb tissue flows not only down to the vagina but also up through the fallopian tubes, eventually sticking to other structures. The displaced tissue acts in the same way it would if it had stayed in the womb, and has a monthly bleed. In mild cases the blood is reabsorbed, but in more severe cases cysts can form and irritate the pelvis. It can be very painful, particularly during ovulation, menstruation and sexual intercourse. Pain can also be triggered by a bowel movement or emptying the bladder. Internal examinations are necessary to diagnose the condition, but sometimes these can aggravate the condition. Nevertheless, they are necessary to rule out anything more serious. Endometriosis is one of the more common causes of infertility.

Foods to Avoid

- Avoid alcohol and saturated animal fats found in red meat and dairy produce as these can elevate oestrogen levels and place a greater workload on the liver, which in turn can increase the pain and inflammation.
- Sugar and sugary foods trigger inflammation in the body, so sweets, puddings, cakes, sugary fizzy drinks, and pastries are best avoided or greatly reduced.
- Caffeine reduces the body's ability to cope with pain and blocks absorption of some minerals.
- If you suspect candida – symptoms include bloating, constipation and/or diarrhoea, thrush, food cravings and chronic fatigue – then avoid sugar, refined carbohydrates, cheese, mushrooms, concentrated fruit juice and yeasted breads for a couple of weeks to see if this helps (see *Candida*).
- As with so many other conditions, if there is a food intolerance it will almost certainly aggravate the problem. Avoid wheat and dairy produce from cows for at least one cycle. Keep a food diary and note when symptoms are worse.
- Peel all fruit and vegetables, if they are not organic, as this is where the pesticides and herbicides that disrupt hormones are more concentrated.
- Reduce your intake of wheat and wheat bran in the diet as they contain phytic acid, which binds to essential minerals such as zinc and magnesium that are needed for hormone balance and muscle relaxation.

Friendly Foods

- Eat more foods known to eliminate excess hormones from the body, such as broccoli, cauliflower, cabbage and Brussels sprouts. They are rich in I3C (indole-3-carbinol), which aids detoxification of excess hormones out of the body. Or take one Triple Action Cruciferous Vegetable Extract capsule daily, by Life Extension (www.lef.org or call the Nutri Centre on 0845 602 6744).
- Fermented soya-based foods, such as tempeh, miso, natto and tofu, have an ability to help control excessive oestrogen levels, as do beans, lentils, chickpeas, cauliflower, Brussels sprouts and broccoli.
- Add sunflower, pumpkin, sesame and ready cracked linseeds (or, if whole seeds are used, soaked overnight in cold water and drain) to your breakfast cereal, as they provide essential fatty acids and zinc that are vital for soft tissue healing. Nuts, with the exception of peanuts, are a good source of fatty acids and zinc.
- Eat more oily fish – farmed, organic salmon, trout, mackerel, sardines, pilchards and anchovies – along with nuts and seeds for their anti-inflammatory properties.
- Pineapple is rich in bromelain, which has a potent anti-inflammatory affect. It should be eaten before main meals.
- Ginger and turmeric (curcumin) are also anti-inflammatory, and ginger is very soothing within the gut.
- Eat foods high in natural carotenes – spinach, carrots, apricots, pumpkin, watercress, papaya, parsley, mangoes, cantaloupe melons and sweet potatoes.
- Dark fruits including blueberries, prunes, cherries and blackberries are high in bioflavonoids, which ease inflammation.
- Natural wheat germ and avocados are rich in vitamin E, which is known to help reduce scar tissue associated with endometriosis.
- Eat more magnesium-rich foods – cashew nuts, almonds, broccoli, bananas and prunes – as these will help to reduce cramping.
- Brown rice, millet and oats contain lots of fibre, which binds to excess oestrogen so that it can be removed from the body.

E

- Dandelion coffee helps to support the liver so that it can remove excess hormones more easily.
- Add fresh coriander and sea vegetables such as nori (available from www.clearspring.co.uk) and kombu to your diet, as they help remove toxic metals from the body.

Useful Remedies

- Gamma-linolenic acid (GLA) is the omega-6 essential fatty acid found in evening primrose and borage seed oil. Taking GLA really helps reduce inflammation. Take 500mg twice daily (available from BioCare) or 3 grams of evening primrose oil daily. **BC**
- Omega-3 fish oils (DHA and EPA) are vital for controlling the inflammation associated with endometriosis. Take three grams daily.
- Full-spectrum, natural-source vitamin E helps protect cell membranes. Take 400iu daily.
- Take one soya/isoflavone supplement daily if you do not eat fermented soya foods or chick peas daily. Take 50–100mg daily. **HN**
- Include a high-strength multi-vitamin and mineral in your regimen that is suitable for your age.
- Pycnogenol – pine bark extract – helps reduce inflammation, bleeding, pain and the forming of endometrial tissue. Take 120mg daily.
- Vitamin C is vital as an antioxidant needed when excess oestrogen is a problem. Take 2 grams daily in divided doses with food.
- Beta-carotene, which converts naturally to vitamin A in the body, is important as it helps protect against the harmful effects of dioxins found in our air, water and foods. Take 20,000iu daily.
- Most sufferers are lacking in the mineral magnesium. Take 200–600mg daily.
- If your multi-vitamin has a daily total of 30mg, this is fine. If not, you need 30mg of zinc daily, as most sufferers are deficient, and zinc, which ensures proper absorption of fatty acids and aids hormone balance.
- A strong B-complex will help absorption of fatty acids and support liver enzymes in the breakdown of excess oestrogen. If you have a high-strength multi-vitamin, the Bs should already be included.
- Take 500mg of the amino acid L-methionine, which helps detoxify oestrogen from the liver. Take 1–3 capsules daily, 30 minutes before food.

Helpful Hints

- Almost all cases benefit from using natural progesterone cream. For an information pack, contact the Natural Progesterone Information Service, PO Box 24, Buxton SK17 9FB. Tel: 07000 784849. Also see details of natural progesterone bio-identical hormones plus suppliers under *Menopause*. **NB Do not self-medicate with hormones – have a blood or saliva test and find out if you need them. Do not take progesterone if you might be pregnant or are breast feeding.**
- Anthony Porter, a reflexologist since 1972, went to China and the Far East to teach reflexology during the 80s and found that their methods combined with his own gave even better results. He has taught his advanced techniques to thousands of reflexologists internationally and says: 'With Advanced Reflexology Techniques (ART) we can not only balance various parts of the body (which is what happens with normal reflexology), but we can also feel more subtle changes within the 7000 nerve-endings or reflex areas of the feet, and after working on them this has a profound therapeutic affect. Medical research with a leading gynaecologist has shown huge success with easing the pain and distress in these types of conditions.' To find an ART therapist in your area, log on to www.artreflex.com.
- Naturopathy and Chinese medicine have proven beneficial to many sufferers. If you decide to try Chinese herbs, make sure your doctor keeps an eye on your liver function, too. (See *Useful Information*.)

- Epsom salts added to a hot bath relaxes and soothes; add a drop of lavender oil to relax.
- Avoid heating foods in plastic containers and heating foods that are covered in cling film – once heated, these plastics can leach chemicals that act like oestrogens, which are 'builders' in the body.
- As much as possible, remove chemicals from your home, which can have a hormone-disrupting action, and use biodegradable products whenever possible. Use Ecover products, available in most supermarkets and health food stores.
- Use a hot water bottle or alternatively a heat pad, available from www.conformuk.com, or call 0870 762 4841, to help relax cramping muscles.
- Massage your abdomen with gentle strokes, using lavender and neroli essential oils, as they both have a calming and anti-spasmodic effect and will help cramping.
- Acupressure: you may be able to alleviate cramping by applying pressure to Spleen 6, located on the inside of the leg 5–7.5cm (3–4in) above the centre of the ankle bone.
- Always use pure cotton towels that are guaranteed free from dioxin. Beware of tampons, as they can exacerbate symptoms.
- Light exercise will help to raise levels of endorphins, which make you feel good and help pain relief. In winter, double the benefit by walking in daylight as this can also lift your spirits.
- To reduce tension, drink soothing herbal teas made with herbs such as hops and valerian.
- Read *Women's Encyclopedia of Natural Medicine*, by Dr Tori Hudson (McGraw Hill).
- Contact the Natural Health Advisory Service, Mon–Fri 9am–5.30pm. Tel: 01273 609699 or log on to www.naturalhealthas.com.
- Further help is available from The National Endometriosis Society, 50 Westminster Palace Gardens, Artillery Row, London SW1P 1RL; or call their help line on 0808 808 2227, which is open every day, 365 days a year. Website: www.endo.org.uk.

E

EXHAUSTION *(see also Adrenal Exhaustion, ME and Stress)*

Being 'Tired All The Time' or 'Tired and Toxic' have become modern-day mantras. If you are a Type A person, who lives life in the fast lane, eats in a hurry, and if you suffer bloating/and or constipation, or food cravings, especially for carbohydrates such as bread, cakes and pasta, first read the *Adrenal Exhaustion* section – as adrenal problems are now at epidemic levels.

As well as adrenal stress, being tired much of the time can also be linked to toxicity in the body (see *Liver Problems*), long-term stress (see *Stress*), and/or being overweight (see *Weight Problems*). It is also heavily linked to food sensitivities, most especially to wheat and cow's milk. However, the list of possible causes is fairly extensive, and you may also need to have your thyroid checked as chronic exhaustion is also linked to an underactive thyroid.

One of the most common causes of constant tiredness may simply be lack of sleep. And the quality of sleep is very important. When you are under pressure you have more difficulty getting to sleep, and then you have to get up for work feeling almost as tired as you did the night before. There is no right or wrong amount of sleep, we are all unique; Margaret Thatcher could manage on 4 hours, but I need 8. Everyone knows how much sleep they need to be fully functioning the next day, but the average is 7–8 hours. See *Insomnia*.

Obviously, there are varying levels of exhaustion, but if you find you are suffering bouts of palpitations during the day, chronic headaches, have an urgency to keep going to the loo or experience a red flushing in your upper chest and throat area, this is most likely your adrenal glands telling you that your body is exhausted. And if you start crying without cause and begin to suffer a total sense of humour failure, you urgently need to listen and take note of the signals – or worse is to come. Your immune system is lowered and you are more likely to pick up anything that's going. Rest is your best option at this point. Know when to walk away. It's not worth dying for – literally.

Foods to Avoid
- Unfortunately, stimulants such as coffee, tea, alcohol and sugar give a short-term energy boost, but this soon wears off, leaving you craving more sugary, refined foods. Therefore, greatly reduce your intake of colas and fizzy drinks, chocolates, biscuits, cakes, snacks, croissants and mass-produced refined foods. Not only do these foods leave us feeling tired, but they also deplete important nutrients such as magnesium, chromium and the B-vitamins, and we become even more exhausted.
- Don't eat heavy protein meals late at night as they take a long time to digest.

Friendly Foods
- Eat more high-energy foods such as alfalfa or aduki bean sprouts, wheat grass and fresh fruits and vegetables.
- Include more wholegrains such as brown rice, oat-based cereals and millet, which are packed with B-vitamins and so help support your nerves.
- Try The Village Bakery, or Genius gluten-free breads, which are delicious, but generally avoid wheat-based foods which can trigger an energy dip in many people.
- Try almond or oat milk in preference to cow's milk.
- Eat breakfast every day. Good-quality protein will keep you feeling fuller for longer and reduce cravings, and increase energy. Eggs, fish, lean meats, hemp seed protein powder, and peanut, almond or walnut butter would all be fine.
- Magnesium and calcium are known as nature's tranquillizers, so eat more green vegetables such as kale, cabbage and broccoli, as well as almonds, Brazil nuts, sesame seeds, pineapple, papaya, Parmesan cheese, fish, dried apricots, pilchards and skimmed milk. Chocolate is also high in calcium, but the benefits are offset by the caffeine content. Just eat it in moderation; and make it dark and organic.
- At night, eat wholewheat pastas, and jacket potatoes (especially sweet potatoes), pumpkin and oats, which are more calming. Make thick vegetable soups, too, which are easier on digestion.
- Turkey, bananas, oats and avocado are high in tryptophan, which aids natural sleep.
- Generally, try to control your blood sugar levels – eating small meals regularly instead of bingeing on junk foods is important to help to reduce the constant exhaustion. See *Low Blood Sugar*.
- Drink herbal teas throughout the day, which are free from caffeine, and choose a calming blend such as liquorice, yerba mate or camomile. Green tea is rich in L-theanine, known to induce feelings of calm.
- As your digestive system is bound to be stressed, eat a low-fat, live yoghurt with meals.

Useful Remedies
- Take a high-strength B-complex to help calm your nerves and aid digestion, plus 500mg of pantothenic acid (B5), which helps support adrenal function. If you wake regularly between 3 and 5am, this can be linked to adrenal exhaustion; also, if you find you need to urinate regularly but don't have a bladder infection, this can also denote that your adrenals are on limits. See *Adrenal Exhaustion*.
- As the digestive system begins malfunctioning when we are really tired, take a digestive enzyme or betaine hydrochloride (stomach acid) with meals to improve the absorption of nutrients. Do not take the betaine if you have active stomach ulcers; instead, take a digestive enzyme capsule (without HCl) with main meals.

- Co-enzyme Q10 is a supplement well proven to improve energy levels. The body produces CoQ10 naturally, but as we age or when stressed we produce less. And as most people no longer eat organ meats, rich in Co-enzyme Q10, it is best taken as a supplement of 100mg daily with breakfast.
- Calcium and magnesium are often depleted. Take 300mg of calcium with 200mg of magnesium an hour before going to bed. Stress and exhaustion make the body more acid, and these minerals help to re-alkalize your system; they have become known as nature's tranquillizers. **SVHC**
- Siberian ginseng is useful as a general tonic that helps to support adrenal function. There are plenty of liquid formulas and this can be taken for a month. Holos Health makes an advanced stress formula containing Siberian ginseng, ashawagandha and gotu kola, which help regulate cortisol levels. Website: www.holoshealth.com.
- L-carnitine – an amino acid helps to improve energy levels; take 1 gram a day before meals for a month.
- Take L-Theanine and Lemon Balm formula before retiring. They really do help. See www.lef.org.

Helpful Hints

- If you are at rock bottom, a few vitamin pills and a couple of nights' sleep will help, but will definitely not provide the long-term solution. You have to try to address the root cause of your exhaustion.
- Generally try to take at least 1 day a week for yourself and make dates in your diary for exercise or time simply to call your own.
- Breathe deeply into your tummy every hour. Get up, walk around, have a stretch.
- If your exhaustion is linked to personal problems, ask your doctor to refer you to a counsellor. Talking problems through gives you a better perspective. See also *Depression*.
- Never take work to bed and always finish work at least one hour before going to bed – otherwise your mind simply keeps churning your thoughts over and over.
- Gentle exercise like yoga, t'ai chi, qigong, or walking at leisure in nature helps to make you feel more positive and re-build energy levels.
- Find a practitioner who can really sort out your diet, such as a nutritionist or naturopath, and make a determined effort to improve your food intake (see *Useful Information*).
- If at all practical, treat yourself to three days at a health spa to rejuvenate and rest.

E

EYE PROBLEMS

(see also Cataracts, Conjunctivitis, Glaucoma and Macular Degeneration)

Eye problems are highly varied ranging from simply being tired, to suffering blurred vision, redness, dark circles and so on. I have covered several of the more common problems – but please, if any eye problems become chronic, you must see either an optician or your doctor. Your eyes can become bloodshot if you cough too much, sneeze a lot, and if you have high blood pressure.

Generally, if the whites of your eyes look yellowish, it means that your liver is somewhat toxic and you need to take steps to clean up your diet. If you suffer 'floaters' in your vision, this can denote poor liver function, and possibly candida, a yeast/fungal overgrowth. But if there are large numbers of floaters and you also have a curtain-like darkness coming across your eyes from the outside in, this can indicate a detached retina and you **must** seek urgent medical attention.

Blepharitis

If red eyes are accompanied by a burning sensation, excessive tearing, itching, sensitivity to light, swollen eyelids, blurred vision, frothy tears, dry eyes or crusting of the eyelashes on awakening, then blepharitis (inflammation of the eyelid caused by an infection) should be considered. Visit an eye-care specialist to check this out (see also *Red-rimmed Eyes*).

Foods to Avoid
- Avoid saturated fats found in red meat and dairy foods, and sugar, as these foods create inflammation in the body, and can block the essential lubricating fats found in oily fish, nuts and seeds from doing their job.

Friendly Foods
- Eat plenty of dark-purple fruits like bilberries, blueberries, blackberries and cherries, as they are rich in bioflavonoids, which protect and strengthen the eyes and help reduce the risk of eye damage from other diseases.
- Eat more green vegetables, especially raw spinach, cabbage, kale and watercress, plus sweet potatoes, pumpkin, papaya, cantaloupe melons and carrots, which are all rich in carotenes that nourish the eyes.
- Eat more oily fish – salmon, trout, mackerel, tuna, sardines, pilchards and anchovies – along with nuts and seeds. These are rich in essential fats, which help to lubricate the eyes from the inside out.
- Immune-boosting foods rich in vitamin C and zinc are essential, as these will help the body to fight off any infection. Eat more red and yellow peppers, kiwi fruit, green leafy vegetables, whole grains, nuts and seeds.
- Green and white teas supply catechins, which reduce oxidative stress in the eyes. Drink them black without milk

Useful remedies
- Higher Nature's Visual Eyes contains a good combination of vitamins and antioxidants. These antioxidants are believed to help protect the retina from free radical damage. **HN**
- If the blepharitis is severe, an eye-care professional may prescribe antibiotics. Healthy bacteria found in the gut need to be taken alongside the antibiotics. Take 1 BioCare bio-acidophillus as far away from the antibiotics as possible. See *Antibiotics*. **BC**
- Bromelain, extracted from pineapples, really helps reduce the inflammation. Take 500mg twice daily while symptoms are acute.

Helpful Hints
- Castor oil has been used traditionally as an anti-inflammatory remedy for treatment of blepharitis. Eyelid inflammation may initially increase after starting treatment, but with repeated use over a week, the inflammation should be reduced. Refresh Endura contains castor oil and is available from most health stores. Use 1–2 drops a few times a day.
- Gently massage the eyelids through a clean, warm, steamy flannel (change each time) for 5 minutes, 2–4 times daily. Wipe all debris off the lids with cotton wool soaked in warm, salty water.
- Note that many eye drops are on based on urine (urea). Therefore, if you can stand it, use fresh urine – which is a sterile liquid – and dab it around the eyes.

Dark circles under the eyes

(see also Adrenal Exhaustion, Allergies, Hayfever and Thyroid)

The obvious culprit for dark circles is lack of sleep, and if you are chronically short of sleep, then the adrenal glands become exhausted, which will make your eyes even darker. Panda-like 'black' eyes are also a common symptom of thyroid problems – see *Thyroid*. Dark circles can be triggered by sensitivities either to products (creams, hair sprays and so on) that you are using, or by foods to which you have an intolerance. And if you suffer from hay fever, then rubbing your itchy eyes can make dark circles worse.

If you have truly 'black', panda-like eyes, ask your doctor to check for an underactive thyroid or low iron levels. Food intolerances are one of the most common causes of dark circles and wheat is usually the main culprit. In a few cases it can also be hereditary (see below). Pregnancy and menstruation can cause skin under the eyes to become more pale, which allows underlying veins to show through, thus making the circles look darker, as can certain medications used to dilate blood vessels, which cause circles under the eyes to darken. Too much ultraviolet light – from the sun or sunbeds – and smoking can also make dark circles worse, as can water retention caused by kidney problems (in Chinese medicine the eyes relate to the liver) or PMT (see *Pre-menstrual Tension*). If you have a tendency for dark circles under your eyes, as you grow older, they are likely to become more noticeable and permanent. Excess folds of skin under the eyes will also make dark circles more pronounced. Therefore, it makes sense to first make sure you are getting enough sleep, and if you are, but still suffer dark circles, try eliminating wheat for seven days. You will be amazed at the difference.

Also, it's important to realize that as we age, some people develop what is known as periobital volume loss. Consultant ophthalmic surgeon Mr Raman Malhotra, based at Gatwick Park Hospital in the UK, says: 'This is a combination of loss of bone volume and soft tissue volume, including fat and thickness of skin under the eyes, which can give rise to the appearance of under-eye dark circles partly due to the concavity that occurs as a result of hollowing. In addition, darkness occurs due to the visibility of the underlying orbicularis eyelid muscle underneath thinner skin.'

My mother suffered with this dark hollowing under the eyes and so have I. For years I always looked 'tired all the time' until I discovered that Mr Malhotra has developed a method of injecting fillers such as Restylane directly into the hollow, dark, under-eye circles. His injections have completely (unless I'm really exhausted) eradicated this hollow look. This treatment, which is done in central London, is well worth looking into. Details can be found on www.ramanmalhotra.com or call 01883 712888.

Foods to Avoid
- Cut down on alcohol and salt and drink plenty of water to flush toxins from the body.
- Processed foods, packet sauces and ketchup-style foods often contain huge amounts of hidden salt, so are best avoided.
- If you are sleeping well but still have circles after 3 or 4 good nights' sleep, then eliminate wheat for a week and see if this helps. If there is no change, then also try eliminating cow's milk. These are the most common triggers.

Friendly Foods
- Drink plenty of water to eliminate toxins and generally eat a clean diet, avoiding too much refined food and sugar. See *General Health Hints*.
- Green leafy vegetables, seaweeds, kelp, lentils and peas are all rich in vitamin K, which has been shown to help reduce bruising and under-eye circles.

- Natural-source carotenes, especially lutein, plus vitamin C, are great eye nutrients – eat more strawberries, kiwi fruit, red, yellow and green peppers, squashes, sweet potatoes, pumpkin, papaya, oily fish, spinach, watercress, mangoes and green leafy vegetables.

Useful Remedies

- If you are totally exhausted, see Useful Remedies under *Adrenal Exhaustion*.
- Eyecare contains bilberry extract, antioxidants (vitamins A, E and C, plus selenium), potassium, grapeseed extract, ginkgo biloba, lycopene and chromium. **BC**; otherwise all companies mentioned on pages 15–16 make good eye complex formulas.

Helpful Hints

- Do not drag or rub the delicate skin under the eyes when using cleansers and make-up.
- Use skin-care products made especially for the eyes, as regular moisturizers can be too heavy and lead to puffy, dark circles.
- Beware of using concealers, as many are too heavy for this delicate area and actually make the problem worse. However, one of best I have found is Jane Iredale's mineral make-up. Available at good pharmacies and the Organic Pharmacy. **OP**

Detached retina

This is when a separation occurs between the retina and the wall of the eye at the back of the eye – much like wallpaper peeling off a wall. This can occur if there is a trauma to the eye (such as being hit by a squash ball), in diabetics, and sometimes during cataract surgery.

  If you suddenly begin to experience large numbers of floaters in your vision, and if you also have a curtain-like darkness coming across your eyes from the outside in, this can indicate that the retina has indeed become detached or developed small holes, in which case you **must** seek urgent medical attention. Otherwise, you risk blindness in that eye.

Follow diet as above.

Dry eyes   *(see also Sjogren's Syndrome)*

Dry eyes can be triggered by being in a dry environment for lengthy periods, such as on an aircraft or working at a computer all day, and contact lens users often complain of dry eyes. Chronic dry eyes is also a classic symptom of Sjogren's Syndrome – see under this heading.

  There are two types of dry eyes. The first and less common is known as aqueous or tear deficiency (linked to Sjogren's), whilst the second type, which is more common, is known as evaporative dry eye. Evaporative dry eye occurs as a result of meibomian gland dysfunction. The meibomian glands are oil glands along the eyelid margin that produce oil as a component of tears to prevent evaporation. Treatment includes regular use of artificial tears (available at all chemists) and regular warm compresses help to maintain good meibomian gland function and healthy oil turnover.

  A hormone imbalance can play a significant role in dry eye related to meibomian gland dysfunction and in particular, androgen deficiency, which can occur post-menopause but also in the perimenopausal period. Certain types of hormone replacement therapy can be androgen suppressing and can therefore exacerbate dry eyes. If a patient is found to be androgen deficient, then switching to a more androgen-friendly hormone replacement therapy may be of some help. See *Hormones associated with the menopause* under *Menopause*.

  For foods to avoid and eat more of, see *Blepharitis*.

Useful Remedies
- Essential fats are vital for healthy eyes – take 2 grams of omega-3 fish oils daily.
- Flax seed oil has been shown to be of benefit for people with meibomian gland dysfunction. Take 500mg daily. **BC**
- Omega 7 found in sea buckthorn is particularly useful for reducing dry eyes. Take 2 grams daily for one month then reduce to 1 gram daily. **PN**
- Natural-source beta-carotene is also crucial for healthy eyes. Take 7–10mg daily. **SVHC, VN**
- Take a good quality multi-vitamin with 15–30mg of zinc.
- Natural-source, full-spectrum vitamin E helps nourish and protect the eyes. Take 400–500iu daily.
- Hyaluronic acid (HA) is a naturally occurring protein in the body. HA is what makes young skin look plump and supple. It also helps to keep your eyes moist from the inside out. But it can also be taken internally in a liquid formula. Take 1ml daily in water on an empty stomach; it takes time to work but it does help. It will also help your skin and joints to remain supple. For more details, ask at your health store or call Modern Herbals on 01274 889047. Website: www.modernherbals.com.

Itchy eyes   *(see also Conjunctivitis and Hayfever)*

Itching of the eyes can be due to an infection such as conjunctivitis, allergies or hayfever, or exposure to a smoky or polluted atmosphere. As I can attest, dry eyes can also be due to over-exposure to computer screens. Eyes also become irritated on long-haul flights and when they are tired. If you suffer dry, itching eyes after a long flight, then use Natural Tears Eye Drops regularly and take more essential fats, which help nourish your eyes from the inside out. (See *Fats You Need To Eat.*)

E

If the problem is linked to your PC, then take regular breaks, get out in the sunshine and get some rest. Dry, itching eyes are also a classic symptom of Sjogren's Syndrome, an autoimmune condition – see under that section.

Foods to Avoid
- Avoid dehydrating beverages such as caffeine and alcohol. Just like every other part of the body, the eyes need plenty of fluid intake to keep them in good shape – drink more water.
- Processed flour dries out the body – therefore reduce your intake of flour-based foods.
- Avoid saturated fats, found in red meat and full-fat dairy foods, as these create inflammation in the body, and can block the essential lubricating fats found in oily fish, nuts and seeds from doing their job.

Friendly Foods
- Eat plenty of dark-purple fruits like bilberries, blueberries, blackberries and cherries, as the bioflavonoids in these fruits not only protect and strengthen the eyes but also help reduce the risk of eye damage from other diseases.
- Eat more green vegetables, sweet potatoes, pumpkin and carrots, which are all rich in the carotenes that nourish the eyes.
- Eat more oily fish, which are rich in essential fats that help prevent the eyes from drying out.
- Eat more unsalted nuts (not peanuts) and seeds, which are high in zinc and selenium.

Useful Remedies
- Vitamin A, 25,000iu a day for 1 month. **NB You can only take 3000iu of vitamin A per day if you are pregnant or planning a pregnancy.** After the month then take around 10–15mg of natural-source carotenes daily. These convert naturally to vitamin A in the body. Carotenes are safe even in higher doses and fine to be taken in pregnancy. **SVIIC, VN**

- Zinc, 30mg a day, is essential for enhancing vitamin-A absorption.
- A strong B-complex: B-vitamins – in particular B2 – are necessary to aid the prevention of dry eyes.
- Take a high-strength multi-vitamin, mineral and EFA formula. No need to take the extra zinc or B if you are taking a high-strength multi.

Helpful Hints
- Eyebright, raspberry and pau d'arco can be made into an infusion, strained and, when cooled, applied to each eye using an eye bath. Make sure you sterilize the eye baths before using them. The infusion has anti-inflammatory, astringent, antiseptic and anti-catarrhal properties. **SHS**
- I often find that if I sleep in an air-conditioned room this can make my eyes very sore; similarly in rooms that are too hot. In winter, keep a small bowl of water near radiators to keep the air in the rooms moist.
- The homeopathic version of eyebright, euphrasia, can be used for bathing the eyes and is very soothing. Use Euphrasia Mother Tincture about 4 times a day using a disposable eye bath. Most good health stores should stock this.
- Heel Homeopathics makes disposable remedies in single phials. Order Oculoheel through your local pharmacy or any homeopathic pharmacy. **OP**
- Another way to relieve itchy eyes is to brew a pot of camomile tea and lay the tea bags, when they've cooled, on the eyelid. Ideally, leave on the eye for about 15 minutes.
- Don't use anyone else's face cloth or towel just in case the problem is infectious. If your eyes are inflamed, Chloride Compound is useful to reduce redness around the eyes. **BLK**
- Traynore Pinhole Glasses help to take the strain off the eyes and help your eyes to focus properly. Sold at all good health stores, or visit the Body and Mind Shop online store at www.bodyandmindshop.com, or call 01237 478818.
- If you suspect allergies are the problem, keep your home free from pet dander and house dust, and stay inside when a lot of pollen is in the air. Air ionizers can help to keep the air clean. Find one at www.healthproductsforlife.com (see also *Allergies*).

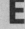

Macular degeneration   *(see under Macular Degeneration)*

Optic neuritis

This is an inflammation of the optic nerve, which carries information from the seeing part of the eye, the retina, towards the brain. It can cause partial or complete loss of vision, which comes on over a few hours or days and may be accompanied by pain in the eye. Optic neuritis can be one of the symptoms of multiple sclerosis, but it can also be triggered by sinus problems, severe high blood pressure, post-viral and post-meningitis infections or more serious problems – so always check out symptoms with your doctor.

Foods to Avoid
- Foods that would aggravate inflammation, including red meat and dairy foods (butter, cheese, cream and milk).
- Try to avoid alcohol and caffeine, which can interfere with blood circulation to the eyes.
- Cut down on sugar in any form, as sugar triggers inflammation in the body. All the usual suspects, I'm afraid: cakes, biscuits, sweets, puddings and fizzy drinks.

Friendly Foods
- Pineapple is a rich source of bromelain, an anti-inflammatory enzyme, which is really good for the eyes.
- Oily fish is rich in essential fats, which are anti-inflammatory. Eat more mackerel, sardines, anchovies, organic salmon, pilchards and herrings.
- Spices such as ginger, turmeric and cayenne are all great at reducing inflammation as well as improving circulation to the eye.
- Bilberries, blueberries and blackberries, and all blue and orange fruits, will help to nourish the eyes.
- Resveratrol is an anti-inflammatory compound that helps to relieve pain associated with inflammation. You can find it in red grapes – enjoy a glass of red grape juice daily, or an occasional glass of red wine (preferably organic).
- Sugar-free blueberry, plum, cherry or damson jams are fine.

Useful Remedies
- Bromelain, 500mg twice daily, can reduce the inflammation and improve circulation.
- The herb ginkgo biloba helps to strengthen the capillaries in the eye and improve the circulation; take 120–240mg of standardized extract a day.
- Vitamin A – take 10,000–25,000 units a day, for one month **NB Take only 3000iu if you are pregnant or planning a pregnancy.** After a month take a natural source carotene daily, which is safe at any dose. Take 10mg daily. **SVNC, VN**

Puffy eyes

Puffiness and bags under the eyes can denote kidney problems and a build-up of toxins within the body. The condition also signifies that the sodium and potassium levels within the body are out of balance. In this case, take 100mg of potassium daily for a week or so, and reduce your intake of sodium-based salts. Puffiness can also be associated with food intolerances and conditions such as hayfever (see *Hayfever*). Drink more water to flush the kidneys, and for at least three days, avoid wheat and dairy products and note if your eyes go down. Puffy eyes can also indicate an underactive thyroid, so if the problem continues after making these changes, have a check-up with your doctor.

Foods to Avoid
- If the area underneath the eyes is both puffy and dark, it is very likely that you have food intolerances, so it is important to identify these. The most common intolerances are dairy produce from cows, and wheat, citrus fruits, eggs and nuts. Salt is a major trigger, and definitely exacerbates any water retention and increases swelling in all parts of the body.
- Mass-produced breakfast cereals often contain more salt than the average bag of crisps.
- Dairy products from cows, cheese and cottage cheese are high in sodium.
- Most pre-packaged, refined foods will have additional salt, and a lot of foods that are naturally sweet have salt added partly as a preservative, but also to help take the edge off the sweeteners.
- Look out for hidden sources of salt/sodium found in high quantities in ketchups, pickles and relishes, olives, and frankfurters from such things as sodium benzoate E211 – a preservative – and monosodium glutamate (MSG), also known as E621
- Cut down on all foods and drinks containing caffeine and alcohol, which further dehydrate the body.
- Reduce your intake of heavy red meat to reduce the burden on the kidneys.

Friendly Foods
- Water is really important, drink 6–8 glasses a day.
- Eat lots of fruit and green vegetables – especially celery and dark green leafy vegetables, dried fruits, nuts, sunflower seeds, and seafood. These are all rich in potassium, which can improve the balance of minerals in the body, particularly if your salt intake is high.
- Eat more artichokes, beetroot, celeriac, celery and fennel.
- If you are not a big fan of fruit and vegetables, at least try drinking a couple of glasses of non-concentrate fruit juice or freshly made vegetable juice daily as they are rich in potassium. Avoid orange juice, which is a common trigger for puffy eyes.

Useful Remedies
- Dandelion tea or tincture taken with every meal; total 5ml daily.
- Take a digestive enzyme with all main meals.
- A good multi-vitamin and mineral suitable for your age and gender
- Vitamin C: take 1 gram daily as potassium or magnesium ascorbate to encourage lymph drainage. **BC**
- Celery seed extract; take 500mg twice daily to aid drainage. **BC**

Helpful Hints
- One of the most effective ways of getting rid of puffy eyes (as well as the enclosed hints) is to have regular acupuncture – which can help tone up the kidney meridians, which in turn should reduce the swelling. Facial acupuncture is great for reducing eye problems. (See *Useful Information*.)

- Manual lymph drainage (MLD) can also aid this condition (see *Useful Information*).
- Dry skin brushing will help to break up toxins stored under the skin, so that the body can eliminate them. Combine the skin brushing with an Epsom salt bath to really help flush out toxins. Use 1 cup per 27kg (60lb) of body weight and add to a warm bath. Soak for 15 to 20 minutes and rub your skin all over with a flannel. Don't rinse off before getting out of the bath; just dry off and retire for the evening. Keep some drinking water handy by the tub as a warm bath can make you thirsty.
- Make an infusion with camomile tea bags and, when cool, apply to the eyes.
- Take the homeopathic remedies Apis 6c and Kali Carb 6c, which are excellent for reducing puffy eyes.
- Lymph drainage done mechanically through massage, reflexology or even bouncing up and down on a rebounder can be quite helpful.
- If you suspect a food intolerance, get this checked out through York Laboratories. They offer a home test kit called The Food Intolerance Test for £9.99. This checks for the most common culprits, and gives you the option of going on to a more thorough test should you have a positive result. Contact them at www.yorktest.com or call 0800 0746185.
- The puffy eyes may be related to an underactive thyroid, so it is worth checking with your GP and getting a thyroid test.

Red-rimmed eyes

Consistently red-rimmed eyes can be a sign of malnutrition or lack of B-vitamins, and can also be a sign of malabsorption of nutrients within the gut from your diet (see also *Absorption* and *Leaky Gut*). It can also be associated with hay fever or hangovers – and if symptoms also include a burning sensation, excessive tearing, itching, sensitivity to light, swollen eyelids, blurred vision, frothy tears, dry eyes, or crusting of the eyelashes on awakening, then blepharitis (inflammation of the eye lid) should be considered. Visit an eye-care specialist to rule this out. Red-rimmed eyes can also, of course, simply denote extreme tiredness; make sure that you get some rest.

Foods to Avoid
- Refined carbohydrates, such as biscuits, cakes, white bread, pizza and pasta, which all deplete the B-vitamins you need for good eye health.
- Avoid caffeine in foods and drinks, as these tend to over-stimulate the system and deplete B-vitamins still further.

Friendly Foods
- See *Friendly Foods* under *Itchy Eyes*.

Useful Remedies
- A high-strength B-complex.
- Dandelion and burdock tincture, 1–3ml a day. If the red-rimmed eyes are due to a build-up of toxins, these herbs can help eliminate them from the body, as well as improving liver function and digestion. **OP**
- Always include a high-strength, multi-vitamin and mineral and essential fats formula in your daily regimen.

Helpful Hints
- Bathe the eyes in cooled camomile tea bags, which are very soothing, or apply cooled slices of cucumber.
- Soak some pads in witch hazel and rose water and lay them on the eyes for 10 minutes. Use a soothing eye balm made from cucumber extract.
- If the condition is linked to blepharitis, then massage the lids through a clean, warm, steamy flannel (change each time) for 60 seconds, and wipe all debris off the lids with cotton wool soaked in warm salty water. If the blepharitis is severe, an eye-care professional may also prescribe antibiotics or steroid eye drops, which need to be followed by a course of healthy bacteria; take BioCare Bio-acidophillus Forte for a month. **BC**

General hints for eye problems

- If the whites of your eyes are dull or yellowish in colour, this indicates that your liver is struggling. Eat more green vegetables, fruits and whole grains, try dandelion coffee, and take the herb milk thistle to help cleanse the liver. Eat fewer saturated fats, and less sugar, alcohol and coffee. See also *Liver Problems*.
- Trayner Pinhole Glasses help strengthen weak eye muscles. Available from the Body and Mind Shop Ltd at www.bodyandmindshop.com, or call 01237 478818.
- Dr Hauschka's Eye Solace is an organic and environmentally friendly solution that you can just add to cotton wool pads, lie back and enjoy. It contains eyebright, anthyllis and camomile extracts, which soothe and refresh sore, reddened, overtired eyes. Available from many good beauty salons and online at www.drhauschka.co.uk.
- For people like me who spend a lot of time reading and working in front of a computer screen, take breaks as often as you can. While sitting at your desk, look into the distance to stretch your eye muscles, and get out in the fresh air and natural sunlight as often as possible.
- Get plenty of sleep.

E

FATIGUE

(see Adrenal Exhaustion, Exhaustion, ME and Stress)

FATS YOU NEED TO EAT

For more than 16 years I have been telling people about the health benefits of essential fats – as have many other health writers, doctors, scientists and nutritionists – and at long last the message is finally filtering through. It needs to.

After all, your brain is almost 60% fat, but it needs more of the right type of fats to function effectively. Essential fats (EFAs) are essential to life, hence their name, and, as we cannot manufacture them in our bodies, we must take them in from external sources through our diet. Most people consume approximately 42% of their calories from fat, but unfortunately it's usually the wrong type of fat.

Dr Udo Erasmus, a Canadian-based bio-chemist and world-renowned authority on fats and oils, says: 'A huge proportion of degenerative health conditions are triggered not only by eating excessive animal fats, but also by over-consumption of mass-produced fats and oils. The majority of vegetable oils found in supermarkets have been refined, bleached and deodorized and then used for frying, which introduces huge amounts of ageing free radicals into the body.' To compound the negative health affects, a commercial practice called hydrogenation, in which liquid oils are turned into spreadable fats called trans-fatty acids, found in some margarines, mass-produced cakes, biscuits, cereal bars, flapjacks, chocolates, crisps and so on, are also unhealthy fats.

Some stores, such as Marks and Spencer's, have taken the positive step of banning trans- and hydrogenated fats from their ready meals. Let's hope more follow.

Erasmus adds to this list sweet and starchy foods – desserts, high-sugar fizzy drinks, filled pastries, chocolates and so on – which tend to be high not only in sugar, but also in saturated fats. If it is not utilized during exercise, sugar converts to fat in the body and sits on your hips, thighs and stomach. But before sugar turns into fat, it triggers cross-linking in the skin, which means you develop wrinkles faster; bacteria thrive on sugar, which will impair your immune system; and sugar increases inflammation in the body, and inflammation can trigger practically every disease from arthritis to Alzheimer's, cancers to Parkinson's.

Having said this, some children, especially young girls, are becoming obsessed with eliminating all fat from their diets – this is dangerous. If the body becomes too low in fat, then chronic depression and a host of skin disorders, such as eczema, can result. Children (and adults) need fats for vital functions, such as the manufacture of hormones and energy. That said, I would not encourage really overweight children, who do little or no exercise, to eat lots of junk fatty foods; but I would never recommend that normal-weight children give up all fats. We all enjoy treats, but we do need to stop living on them. The body also needs essential fats to encourage weight loss, as EFAs help to burn stored fat.

There are two main types of EFAs, omega-3 (alpha-linolenic acid) and omega-6, which comes in two forms, linoleic acid and gamma-linolenic acid (GLA). There is more about GLA under *Useful Supplements*.

The best source of omega-3 is oily fish, which contains EPA and DHA (easily utilized types of omega-3 fats). Eating lots of oily fish is why Eskimos rarely suffered heart disease – until they began eating a Western diet. Linseeds (flax seeds), walnuts, hemp seeds and pumpkin seeds also contain omega-3 fats, which the body then converts into the useful EPA and DHA forms; in fish oil this has already been done by nature. There are a few people who cannot easily convert the essential fats in seeds and nuts into EPA and DHA, which is known as atopic tendency, and common characteristics of this condition are asthma, eczema and hay fever.

Therefore if you suffer these conditions, take fish oils as your first line of defence. Omega-3 fats help to transfer oxygen around the body, relax blood vessels, and are vital for hormone production, healthy eyes, gut function, weight loss, reducing inflammation, speeding wound-healing, and so on. Unfortunately, because most people eat 80% less oily fish now than we did in the 1940s, and 60% of people are deficient in omega-3 EFAs.

The second type of EFAs, omega-6, is found in evening primrose, starflower, blackcurrant, walnut and sesame oils. Walnuts, Brazil nuts, pecans, almonds, and sunflower, pumpkin and sesame seeds are also rich in omega-6 EFAs. These fats help to lower blood pressure, thin the blood, and help insulin to work, which keeps blood sugar levels in balance and helps reduce the cravings for sweet foods.

Most people ingest plenty of omega-6s from nuts and non-hydrogenated vegetable oils and margarines, but normally from poor-quality sources, such as bread, biscuits, cakes and so on, which are usually made with vegetable oils.

To absorb **any** essential fatty acids, the minerals zinc and magnesium, plus vitamins B3 and B6 are necessary, and are often depleted by our over-consumption of omega-6s.

'Undoubtedly,' says nutritionist and my co-author Gareth Zeal, 'we need to take far more omega-3, plus these co-factors daily and to address our modern dietary deficiencies we need to consume twice as much omega 3 as 6.'

Another beneficial fat, omega-9, is found in unrefined extra-virgin olive oil, a monoun-saturated fat, which is far more stable for cooking (but never heat until it spits and produces smoke). A lesser-known EFA is omega-7, also known as palmitoleic acid. This polyunsaturated fatty acid is found in the sea buckthorn berry. It is useful for dry skin and dry eyes, and for mouth and vaginal dryness. (For more help with omega-7, call Pharma Nord on 0800 591756.)

Polyunsaturated fats (also found in seeds, nuts and their oils) are healthy in their cold, unrefined form, and they are rich in omega-6 EFAs. So if you use sunflower, walnut, sesame seed or grape seed oils in their unrefined forms in salad dressings, they are healthy. However, once the polyunsaturated oils that you find in most biscuits, flapjacks, margarines, and mass-produced vegetable oils are heated, they become unhealthy.

Many people cook (mostly frying) with oils and margarines labelled 'polyunsaturated', believing them to be healthier – but it is not so. If the oils that you buy are mass-produced, all the processes I mentioned earlier will have long ago destroyed the majority of any health benefits. Butter is actually better for cooking at low temperatures, as it does not turn rancid like the essential fats. Coconut oil has similar properties. Butter contains vitamin A and butyric acid, which has anti-cancer properties, and a little butter, preferably organic, is OK, if you have sufficient EFAs in the body.

All essential fats need to be kept cool and never heated, as the heat destroys their delicate make-up; this includes all oil-based supplements, which should be kept in the fridge.

Typical symptoms of insufficient EFAs are dry skin and eyes, cracked lips, water retention, increased thirst, physical and mental exhaustion, mood swings, inflammatory conditions such as eczema and arthritis, frequent infections, hay fever, allergies, mental health problems including depression, poor memory and learning difficulties and cardiovascular disease. Most

F

of these conditions we tend to accept as we age, but if you take sufficient EFAs then you should avoid such symptoms for many more years.

Foods to Avoid

- Reduce your intake of full-fat milk, cheeses, chocolates, crisps and refined mass-produced cakes and biscuits, which are usually high in hydrogenated or trans-fats, and are not good for your health.
- Avoid as much as possible all refined vegetable oils, typically found in margarines, biscuits and cakes, and, of course, mass-produced vegetable oils.
- If you like red meat, just eat lean organic meat once a week. Hugely reduce or eliminate meat pies, sausages and so on, and if you do eat meat choose a lean cut. With chicken, turkey, duck, venison, buffalo, quail, or other game, cut off the skin. If you eat bacon, make it only a rare treat, then grill it and cut off the fat.
- Eliminate or greatly reduce the amount of fried foods you eat.
- Remember that sugar, if not used up during exercise, converts to fat inside the body and many foods advertised as being low in fat are usually packed with sugar!

Friendly Foods

- Look for non-hydrogenated spreads such as Vitaquell, Biona and Olivio or try organic raw walnut, almond, hemp or pumpkin seed butters. Higher Nature or Sun and Seed make these; call 020 7267 7799 for stockists.

- You can also buy coconut oil/butter to use as a spread – but make sure it's raw, organic and non-hydrogenated. Reported to lower LDL cholesterol.
- If you need to shallow fry, use a little organic olive oil or raw, organic coconut oil/butter. Although butter is a saturated fat, it does not turn rancid like vegetable oils when heated. I also use a little butter for baking cakes. For biscuits and flapjacks, I use extra-virgin olive oil.
- Nutritionist Gareth Zeal recommends blending extra-virgin olive oil with butter to use as a healthier alternative to hydrogenated/ trans-fat-based margarines, also for spreads and making cakes and biscuits.
- If you like stir-fries, use a little olive, canola, coconut or ground nut (peanut) oil. Heat through (but not until 'spitting or smoking', which means the oil has become carcinogenic), then add vegetables and so on and stir for a minute. Then add a little water and 'steam fry' for a couple more minutes. This helps to reduce the amount of free radicals that are produced when you fry food.
- Oily fish, such as mackerel, organic salmon, trout, sardines, anchovies and herrings, are all rich in omega-3 fats.
- Soya and kidney beans also contain some omega-3 fats, but try to use only GM-free and organic soya beans.
- Walnuts, pecans and almonds are all rich in omega-6 fats.
- If you use linseeds (flax seeds) to increase your omega-3 intake, buy them ready cracked (available from most supermarkets). Keep cracked linseeds in the fridge. Or, grind them first. Use a coffee grinder, which breaks them up in seconds, or simply crush them with a pestle and mortar. Otherwise, soak whole linseeds overnight in cold water and drain before eating.
- Seeds, such as sunflower and pumpkin, which are high in omega-6, can be eaten as a snack or sprinkled on soups or salads, and added to meals.
- Hemp seed is readily available and is a good blend of omega-3 and -6 fatty acids. You can also buy excellent organic-source hemp seed protein powders.
- Eat more (but not to excess) monounsaturated fats, such as those found in avocados and olive oil.

- Eat more raw wheat germ and rice bran, rich in vitamin E, which helps you to also absorb the EFAs more effectively.
- Buy good-quality, unrefined and preferably organic sunflower, walnut and sesame oils and mix them half and half with olive oil to make delicious salad dressings, or drizzle them over cooked foods (once they are on your plate). Keep them in the fridge to protect the EFAs.
- Once a week I pop a tablespoon each of sunflower, pumpkin, sesame seeds, hazelnuts, hemp seeds, walnuts, almonds, and Brazil nuts into a food mixer and pulse for a few seconds. I then place them in a glass jar in the fridge and use them over breakfast cereals, yoghurts, desserts, fruit salads and so on. This is a great way to get more EFAs.

Useful Remedies

- If you are not vegetarian, then take 1–3 grams of fish oil capsules daily. Many people no longer take fish oils, as they worry about the concentrations of toxins, such as PCBs and dioxins, but Higher Nature, BioCare, Pharma Nord, Seven Seas One-a-Day fish oils are all guaranteed to be free from toxins. **HN, BC, PN, FSC** Eskimo 3 stable fish oil capsules are one of the best and are distributed by PPC Galway Ltd, 27–28 Mulvoy Business Park, Sean Mulvoy Road, Galway, Ireland. Tel: 00353 91 753222, or email info@ppcgalway.ie
- Gamma-linolenic acid (GLA), is an omega-6 EFA, which is found in evening primrose oil, blackcurrant oil and borage oil. It has anti-inflammatory properties and helps increase your metabolic rate, and reduces symptoms of PMT. Most supplement companies sell GLA and you can take around 250mg daily. **BC**
- If you want pure linseed (flax seed) oil try Omega Nutrition from Higher Nature. **HN**
- Udo's Choice Oil is made from organic flax, sunflower and sesame seeds, plus rice and oat germ oils, in the perfect ratio for good health. Dr Udo Erasmus says we need approximately 1 tablespoon for every 23kg (50lb) of body weight, and we need more EFAs in winter than in summer. It is available as an oil, which either can be blended with other oils for salad dressings, or a little can be drizzled over cooked dishes. It is also available in capsules. These oils are highly unstable, should never be heated, and need to be kept in the fridge. Udo's Choice is available from health stores worldwide, or to find your nearest stockist in the UK, contact Savant Distribution Limited, Quarry House, Clayton Wood Close, Leeds LS16 6QE, or call 08450 606070. Website: www.savant-health.com or e-mail: info@savant-health.com
- Another good blend of omega-3 and -6 oils is called 'IQ', available at chemists and health stores.
- When supplementing with fatty acids, either in capsule or liquid form, it is very important to take a natural-source, full-spectrum vitamin E, at least 100iu a day
- For anyone who has had their gall bladder removed, suffers from Crohn's disease or colitis, or has a sensitive gut or irritable bowel and cannot tolerate too much oil (as the liver has to metabolize all fats and oils), use DriCelle Omega Plex essential fatty acid powder by BioCare. The EFAs have been micro-encapsulated into water-soluble fibre and then freeze-dried, using no oxygen or heat. This powdered formula is therefore stable, which increases absorption dramatically. It bypasses the liver and is 100% absorbed in the intestines. **BC**
- Read Dr Udo Erasmus's book, *The Fats That Heal and Fats That Kill* (Alive Books). He has also written *Choosing the Right Fats*, which contains recipes that show you how to integrate healing oils and fats into your daily meals naturally. To order call 0845 060 6070, or log on to www.savant-health.com

F

FIBROIDS

A fibroid is a benign tumour made up of muscle and fibrous tissue that grows in the muscular wall of the womb. Fibroids often produce no symptoms at all, but they are known to cause heavy menstrual bleeding and may contribute to infertility. The growth of fibroids seems to be related to a hormone imbalance, especially an excess of the hormone oestrogen. If you are on the combined pill or HRT, both of which contain oestrogen, you may wish to discuss coming off these drugs with your GP in order to prevent further growth. If you suffer heavy periods over several months, please have this checked out. With any condition that is linked to hormones, you really need to detoxify and support the liver – see *Liver Problems*. Basically, fibroids are another symptom of the body holding onto excess toxins.

Foods to Avoid
- Any foods that can trigger elevated oestrogen levels or will recycle oestrogen into its more aggressive form. These include alcohol, animal fats, such as red meats, or any fat on any meats including chicken, cheese, milk other than fully skimmed, cream, ice cream, butter and chocolates.
- Most importantly, don't heat ready-made meals in plastic containers as the plastic residues leach into the food, which again has an oestrogen affect. Never heat cling film if it's next to food.
- Avoid as much as possible non-organic foods that are often high in pesticides and herbicides, which migrate to fatty tissue and increase oestrogen activity in the body.
- Avoid refined soya milks and products.

Friendly Foods
- Chick-peas, broccoli, cabbage, Brussels sprouts and cauliflower are all beneficial foods, as they encourage excretion of excess hormones.
- Fermented soya-based foods, such as tempeh, miso and natto, have a regulating effect on oestrogen levels and are protective against aggressive oestrogens.
- Linseeds (flax seeds) contain lignan, which also helps to balance hormones naturally. I soak a tablespoon of Linusit Gold linseeds in a cup of cold water overnight and then use in fruit breakfast blends, in porridge or over cereals.
- Don't overcook your vegetables. Make fresh vegetable juices every day and drink immediately after juicing.
- Eat plenty of foods containing natural carotenes such as cantaloupe melons, apricots, sweet potatoes, parsley, carrots, spring greens, watercress, pumpkin and spinach. Eat more almonds, cod liver oil, avocados, wheat germ and hazelnuts, which are all rich in vitamin E.
- Eat more oily fish rich in omega-3 fats.
- Use plenty of rosemary and pineapple, which are anti-inflammatory.

Useful Remedies
- Soya isoflavones: take 50–100mg, for regulation of hormone levels, and wild yam to help curb excessive bleeding, 1–3ml of tincture or 1–3 grams of tablets.
- Triple Action Cruciferous Vegetable Extract by The Life Extension contains broccoli, watercress and rosemary, which include I3C, a compound known to neutralize harmful oestrogens. www.lef.or or call the Nutri Centre on 0845 602 6744. Take one capsule daily.
- You need plenty of essential fats, which play a vital role in hormone production. Take 2–3 grams of omega-3 fish oils daily.
- A high-strength multi-vitamin and mineral for women. **BC, HN, NC, SVHC or VN.**
- Some women stop ovulating at some point between their 35th and 40th birthdays and

therefore no longer make progesterone, but continue to make oestrogen. Talk to your GP about using natural bio-identical progesterone cream, which can help reverse fibroids. This cream is freely available to buy outside the UK, and you can order it for your own use via Pharm West. Tel. UK and Ireland: 00 353 46 943 7317.

■ Within the UK, natural progesterone needs a prescription. For a list of doctors who work with natural progesterone, send a large SAE with £1 in stamps to NPIS, P.O. Box 24, Buxton SK17 9FB. Call them on 07000 784849 www.npis.info/contactus.htm Otherwise, log on to www.lef.org, The Life Extension Foundation in America, who also supply bio-identical hormones. **Never self-medicate with hormones unless you have had a blood or saliva test showing that you need them.** Dr Shamin Daya at 57 Harley Street also prescribes bio-identical hormones if they are required. Call 0207 580 7537.

■ Silica and calcium fluoride tissue salts can help to break down the fibroids. Take 4 of each daily.

Helpful Hints

■ Once you go through menopause, the fibroids should shrink naturally.

FIBROMYALGIA *(see also Candida, Irritable Bowel Syndrome and Leaky Gut)*

The word 'fibromyalgia' is derived from the Latin *fibra*, meaning 'fibre', and the Greek word *mys*, meaning 'muscle'. This syndrome generally affects more women than men and is characterized by aching and stiffness in the large muscle groups – especially in the neck, shoulders and pelvis. There may be pain in the chest and ribcage, stiffness in the morning, nausea and/or a low-grade fever. Anxiety, depression and sleep problems are also common. Some sufferers experience an irritable bowel and bladder, even when no bladder infection is present. In virtually every case this condition can be greatly alleviated or cured by dietary changes, as fibromyalgia is very much linked to the yeast fungal overgrowth candida and a leaky gut. See both these sections.

Many people confuse polymyalgia with fibromyalgia, but polymyalgia rheumatica (PMR) is an autoimmune condition linked to rheumatoid arthritis, involving inflammation of the muscles, whereas fibromyalgia is associated with low pain tolerance in the muscles and connective tissue. If you are diagnosed with PMR, see also *Rheumatoid Arthritis* and *Sjogren's Syndrome*.

People who suffer chronic fatigue, such as ME, also tend to suffer fibromyalgia. High homocysteine levels (a toxic by-product from digesting proteins) may also be linked to these types of conditions – for more information on homocysteine, see *High Blood Pressure*.

Doctors have also noted that several other conditions, such as thyroid problems, lupus and rheumatoid arthritis, can trigger fibromyalgia-type symptoms. Blood tests could confirm if any of these conditions are an underlying cause for the fibromyalgia.

Foods to Avoid

■ Any food to which you have an intolerance will make this problem worse. Without doubt, it's usually the foods you tend to eat and crave the most – the most common being wheat, sugar, cow's milk, soya, corn, citrus fruits or tomatoes.

■ Avoid caffeine and alcohol, which are stimulants. These affect hormones in the body linked to pain receptors. Caffeine drinks include cola-type drinks, chocolate, coffee and so on. Alcohol also acts like a depressant.

■ Greatly reduce your intake of sugar, which can trigger inflammation and low blood sugar.

■ Read labels and avoid hydrogenated and trans-fats – found in mass-produced meat pies, salami, sausages, margarines, cakes and biscuits. See *General Health Hints* and *Fats You Need To Eat*.

■ See this section under *Candida* and *Leaky Gut*.

F

Friendly Foods

- Eat more cold-water fish, such as herrings, mackerel, and organically farmed salmon and trout, as they are high in omega-3 essential fats, which reduce inflammation. If you are sensitive to fish, then include flax and hemp seeds in your diet.
- Eat more whole foods (preferably organic) including fruits and vegetables, especially squash, carrots, pumpkin, papaya, watermelon, watercress, cantaloupe melon, mango, sweet potatoes, cabbage and kale.
- Grains can be a problem and flour really dries out the body. Avoid white flour and wheat, which can irritate the gut. Try millet, buckwheat, quinoa and amaranth grains – in breads, biscuits, pastas and crackers from any good health store, and in numerous supermarkets.
- Eat more brown rice.
- Eat fresh pineapple before main meals, as it has anti-inflammatory properties and aids digestion.
- Eat more cabbage and drink cooled water in which you boil cabbage as it contains L-glutamine, an amino acid that really heals your gut.
- Take aloe vera daily. Aloe Pura make a great Stomach Formula.
- Use more turmeric in curries, as it is highly anti-inflammatory.
- Drink nettle leaf tea.
- As dehydration is often a problem, drink more water.
- See *General Health Hints* and the dietary advice given in *Rheumatoid Arthritis*. It is worth pointing out that, although Fibromyalgia is not strictly an inflammatory condition, it would be helpful to avoid foods that cause inflammation (as above) and eat the anti-inflammatory foods suggested. This will help reduce the overall burden on the pain receptors.

Useful Remedies

- Beta Glucans 1-3, 1-6, derived from yeast cell walls, are proven to strengthen the body's innate immune system (the immune system you were born with). People and children who take beta glucans suffer fewer food intolerances; take 250–500 mg daily. If you make ALL the dietary changes and eliminate foods that you have a sensitivity to, your immune system will improve naturally and you will not need the beta glucans! Beta Glucans are a type of yeast that can kill pathogenic yeasts such as candida.
- Take a multi-vitamin/mineral for your age and gender with plenty of B-group vitamins.
- B-vitamins – especially B6, B12 and folic acid – are needed to support the nerves and they help lower a high homocysteine level. Therefore, if you don't take a multi, make sure you take a B-complex daily.
- Minerals such as magnesium help to relax the muscles – so does calcium. You can buy these minerals in a duo formula; you need 600mg of magnesium and 400mg of calcium. Of the two, magnesium is the most important – if you buy this in capsule form, ask for magnesium citrate and take your last 200mg before bed. To help absorb the calcium, take 1000iu of vitamin D3 daily. **BH, SVHC**
- Omega-3 is usually deficient in this condition – take 2–3 grams daily.
- MSM – a type of organic sulphur – really helps to reduce pain and inflammation, and is good for reducing muscle spasms. Take 2 grams daily spread throughout the day.
- The amino acid L-theanine, extracted from green tea, acts like a natural tranquillizer. You can take 100mg three times daily to help calm the brain and reduce anxiety.
- If you suffer from insomnia, the hormone melatonin may be useful – see *Insomnia*.
- Take a digestive enzyme with all main meals.
- Taking liquid hyaluronic acid (a natural component of skin, joints and tendons) daily in water helps to keep joints more supple and reduces pain. Take one sachet in a full glass of water before breakfast. For details call Modern Herbals on 01274 889047 or visit www.modernherbals.com.

- Healthy bacteria – known as probiotics – often help, as sufferers from both these conditions tend to also suffer from a leaky gut (see *Leaky Gut*).
- Capsaicin cream (the active ingredient in chilli peppers), applied topically to painful areas, is effective in reducing pain in these conditions. Apply three or four times over the day; it may take two weeks before the effects are felt. Don't use on broken skin or if pregnant or breastfeeding.

Helpful Hints

- It is important to have an allergy test to find your worst food offenders. Try the York Test Laboratories. Tel: 0800 458 2052 or log on to www.yorktest.com; or Genova Diagnostics do a FACT test, which looks for inflammatory markers indicating that the body is reacting to certain substances. Tel: 020 8336 7750. Website: www.gdx.uk.net.
- Another excellent method to test for food intolerance and leaky gut is the Bio Meridian Test. The practitioner measures your reactions, via electrodes, to a huge list of foods and substances. For practitioners, see www.biomeridian.com or call Sheila Partridge on 0207 580 7537.
- People who don't get sufficient sleep tend to suffer more muscle pain; therefore, get more sleep. Sleep is very important for these conditions.
- Moderate exercise, such as swimming, walking, cycling and so on, will help.
- Have a regular massage using therapeutic grade oils – such as diluted oil of wintergreen – which is anti-inflammatory.
- Regular acupuncture is wonderful for reducing pain and stiffness with this condition.
- Soak in warm baths with Epsom salts or sea salt to help relax the muscles.

F

FLATULENCE   *(see also Candida, Constipation and Irritable Bowel Syndrome)*

Flatulence, wind and bloating is, to say the least, very unsociable and sometimes extremely uncomfortable. It can be due to partly digested foods being fermented in the gut and/or to an imbalance of the organisms that reside in the bowel. The yeast fungal overgrowth *Candida* is often the root cause, as unhealthy bacteria thrive on less healthy foods, particularly sugar, but also the bi-products of partial digestion.

It is very important that you chew your food properly, as the digestive process begins in the mouth. Almost 60% of carbohydrate digestion is done in the mouth if foods are properly chewed. The majority of protein digestion is done in the stomach, so it is crucial that we have adequate levels of stomach acids and enzymes to break down the foods. Various factors can weaken our ability to digest foods properly: smoking is notorious, but alcohol, sugary foods, high-fat foods, caffeinated beverages, and prolonged stress can all progressively weaken the digestion. Another important factor is food intolerances, most especially to cow's milk, wheat and, in my case, chocolate, which causes me to bloat!

Foods to Avoid

- Beans such as cannellini, kidney, black-eyed and so on, plus lentils, artichokes, broccoli, Brussels sprouts, fizzy drinks and beer are all famous for causing wind. In some people, taking a digestive enzyme with these foods does help.
- Some people also have problems with cabbage and onions.
- Also avoid any food to which you have an intolerance, the most common being dairy products from cows.
- Cheese, especially melted cheese is incredibly hard to digest. Avoid pizzas!
- Try to note any foods that make you feel bloated or cause a lot of wind and see if there is a common denominator.

- If you have eaten a large meal, don't eat large amounts of fruit directly after the meal, as the fruit will ferment in the gut as it becomes stuck behind the other food, and fruit likes a fast passage through the gut. Eat fruit before or in between meals. Generally, avoid large meals that place a huge strain on your gut and liver.
- I often begin a meal with a few chunks of fresh pineapple or papaya, which aid digestion.

Friendly Foods
- Certain foods help to improve digestion, noticeably fennel, celeriac, radicchio, young green celery, and watercress. They all help to stimulate gastric juices.
- Try wheat-free breads, such as Genius and Village Bakery, or use amaranth crackers or oat cakes.
- Rice, corn, lentil and lentil pastas are now freely available.
- Drinking peppermint, fennel or camomile teas, or a combination of them, after meals can often make digestion easier and make you feel more comfortable. Fennel seems to be the most effective.
- Add a strip of dried kombu seaweed when cooking any bean dishes; this helps to predigest the enzymes that cause the wind and bloating.
- Include more fresh root ginger in your cooking, which aids digestion.
- Eat more low-fat, live yoghurts.
- Try low-fat goat's milk, or almond or oat milk instead of cow's milk.

Useful Remedies
- With breakfast take one scoop of Agave Digestive Immune support powder, extracted from the agave plant, as it contains inulins that help you to naturally produce more healthy bacteria. Very useful for helping to keep you regular. www.lef.org or call the Nutri Centre.
- Otherwise, Bioforce make Molkosan Vitality, a prebiotic drink made with concentrated whey, maize starch and green tea, which has been shown to help improve bowel transit times. For stockists, call 01294 277344 or log on to www.avogel.co.uk
- Betaine hydrochloride; taking 1 capsule with meals helps improve digestion, which tends to weaken as we get older. If you have active stomach ulcers, do not take this remedy – take a digestive enzyme that does not contain hydrochloric acid.
- Acidophilus and bifidus; 1–2 capsules, taken at the end of a meal helps replace healthy gut flora, which in turn helps manufacture gastric enzymes and keeps candida under control, if this is the root cause of the problem.
- Take peppermint oil capsules before meals. But generally once you remove the foods, such as wheat, that trigger these types of problems, your digestion works altogether more efficiently.

Helpful Hints
- Try to eat smaller meals, which place less strain on the digestive tract and liver. This really helps.
- Stress can trigger bloating and flatulence.
- Eat far fewer grain-based foods.
- Many people have benefited from following the principle of food combining, separating carbohydrates and proteins.
- Chronic flatulence can also be a symptom of food intolerance, irritable bowel syndrome, candida, or gut infections. If you are concerned, see a qualified nutritionist (see *Useful Information*).

FLU
(see Colds and Flu)

FLUID RETENTION
(see Water Retention)

FLUORIDE

(see also Bleeding Gums and Thyroid)

No essential function for fluoride has been proven in humans. Fluoride compounds generally have a toxicity between that of lead and arsenic. Calcium fluoride occurs naturally in most UK drinking waters at a fluoride concentration of 100–200 parts per billion (ppb). However, artificial fluoride, such as fluorosilicic acid – a waste product from phosphate fertilizer plants – is one of the more toxic fluoride compounds. It is added to drinking water by water companies to a concentration of 1,000 ppb (1 part per million) at the request of health authorities – not to make water safe to drink, but to medicate those who drink it. To put these levels into context, lead and arsenic in drinking water are limited to 25 and 10 ppb, respectively.

Five and half million people in the UK receive fluoridated water, mainly in the West Midlands and the North East of England. The number drinking artificially fluoridated water worldwide is 300 million.

Regardless of fluoride intake, mother's milk is very low in fluoride, at 4–10 ppb. This means a baby fed formula feed reconstituted with fluoridated water will ingest up to 250 times more fluoride than a breast-fed baby. In late 2006, the American Dental Association issued advice to dentists on how to address parental concerns. Their advice was that formula feed should be reconstituted with water that has no or a low level of fluoride. This advice was not issued by health authorities directly to parents in any country that fluoridates.

The problem today is that we get fluoride from so many sources – certain foods, toothpastes, mouthwashes, medicines (Prozac is fluoxetine), anaesthetics, pesticides and polluted air. Volcanic dust also contains fluoride. Half of the fluoride ingested is retained in our bodies. Dental fluorosis (mottled teeth), a manifestation of systemic toxicity, is common in areas where the water is fluoridated. The accumulation of fluoride in bone and soft tissue causes many health problems, including irritable bowel, bone deformities, arthritic pain and hypothyroidism. The NHS carries out no tests to link these problems to fluoride.

In 2006, a team of Harvard University scientists led by Dr Elise Bassin published a study that reported a five-fold increased risk of teenaged boys exposed to fluoridated water between the ages 6 and 8 developing osteosarcoma.

In his analysis of the 2000–2003 National Diet and Nutrition Survey, Dr Peter Mansfield, a York Review Advisory Panel member, found that a quarter of the UK population exceeds the safe intake defined by the Committee on Medical Aspects and Food Policy. In fluoridated areas, this rises to two-thirds!

Since 1997 the FDA in the US has required a poison label on all toothpastes containing fluoride, but in Britain there is currently no such requirement. In 1999, the US Centers for Disease Control and Prevention conceded that the predominant 'benefit' of fluoride is topical. This means for the 'benefit' perceived by the promoters of fluoride, we do not need to swallow it! In areas with added fluoride, many doctors have noticed an increase in thyroid problems – see *Thyroid*. This is because fluoride is a halide (a group of chemicals that competes with iodide receptor sites in the body) and can therefore interfere with proper hormone production.

Foods to Avoid

- Read labels carefully and note that tea, salmon and sardines are rich in fluorides. As much as possible, avoid non-organic foods that have more than likely been sprayed with pesticides containing fluoride. If you live in a fluoridated area, as much as possible drink bottled, distilled or reverse osmosis de-ionized water. Visit www.pureh2o.co.uk.

Friendly Foods
- Organic foods that are free from harmful pesticides and herbicides. Drink plenty of fluoride-free water in between meals.
- See *General Health Hints*.

Helpful Hints
- If you drink fluoridated tap water, do not use fluoridated toothpastes or mouthwashes.
- To avoid fillings, greatly limit your child's intake of sugary foods and drinks.
- Buy fluoride-free toothpastes, such as Aloe Dent, containing aloe vera, co-enzyme Q10, tea tree oil, silica and so on, which all promote healthy gums and teeth. For your nearest stockist, visit www.williamransom.com Otherwise, ask at your local health store as there are several good natural brands available including The Green People Company, Kingfisher, Waleda, Tom's and Sarakan.
- Young children tend to swallow toothpaste – therefore, make sure it is fluoride free.
- Consider having a fluoride-removing water filter fitted at home. The Fresh Water Filter Company Ltd offers a broad range of water filters. Call them on 08451 770896, or visit their website at www.freshwaterfilter.com
- The Doctors' Laboratory will test for levels of fluoride in the body. You do need a referral from a health professional, such as a doctor or nutritionist. The Laboratory can be contacted at 60 Whitfield Street, London W1T 4EU. Tel: 020 7307 7373. Website: www.tdlplc.co.uk
- Read *The Fluoride Deception* by Christopher Bryson (Seven Stories Press) and *Fluoridation: Drinking Ourselves to Death* by Barry Groves (Newleaf).
- Support The National Pure Water Association, which has fought fluoridation in the UK for 50 years. Website: www.npwa.org.uk

FOOD POISONING (see also Diarrhoea, Irritable Bowel Syndrome and Vomiting)

Each year an estimated 5.5 million people in the UK – that's one in every ten people – suffer from some kind of food poisoning. And this figure is on the low side, as many mild cases go unreported. Approximately 500 people die annually from food poisoning, which is mainly caused by various bacteria found in food, mainly meats, reheated foods and shellfish, home-made ice creams and jams, but can also be caused by viruses, parasites and toxins in foods such as those in many wild field mushrooms.

The most common and widely known bacteria are salmonella, campylobacter, E-coli, listeria, staphylococcus, shigella and botulism. The more bacteria present on a food, the more likely you are to become ill.

These bacteria are hard to detect, as they don't usually affect the taste, appearance or smell of food. Having said this, if foods such as fish, shellfish or meat smell extra strong or 'high', then to be safe, don't eat them.

Food poisoning is more likely to affect people with lowered resistance to disease, such as the elderly or sick, babies, young children, and pregnant women. Symptoms of food poisoning are nausea, vomiting, diarrhoea, abdominal pain, headache, and low-grade fever.

The most serious types of food poisoning are due to bacteria, which can cause poisoning in two different ways. Some bacteria infect the intestines, causing inflammation and problems with the normal absorption of nutrients and water, which triggers diarrhoea. Other bacteria produce toxins on the food that are poisonous to the human digestive system. When eaten, these chemicals trigger nausea and vomiting, kidney problems and, in extreme cases, death. Bacteria multiply very fast, especially in warm, moist conditions. The presence or absence of oxygen, salt, sugar and the acidity of the surroundings are also important factors. In the right conditions, one bacterium can multiply to more than 4 million in just 8 hours.

Bacteria generally like temperatures between 5°C (41°F) and 63°C (145°F), where they can multiply easily. They are killed at temperatures of 70°C (158°F). Most bacteria multiply very slowly at temperatures below 5°C (41°F) and some bacteria die at very low temperatures. Unfortunately, many can survive these low temperatures and can start to multiply again if warm conditions return. This is why proper handling and storage of food, plus sensible hygiene precautions, are of utmost importance in preventing food poisoning.

Foods to Avoid

- Beware of eating wild mushrooms unless you are absolutely certain of which types you aim to eat. Only gather mushrooms that you can positively identify; however, I personally would **never** eat a wild mushroom that had not been identified or picked by an expert, as some varieties are deadly (such as Death Cap and Destroying Angel).
- To help prevent an attack, avoid food that has been reheated more than once, especially rice dishes.
- Avoid eating any foods that have been left standing in warm conditions such as at garden fêtes and buffets – and which you know have been there a while.
- Food that is not piping hot – especially chicken or any meat dishes.
- Food that has come into contact with raw meat or poultry.
- If you are in any country that has poor-quality drinking water, take the following precautions:
- Drink only bottled water, and avoid salads at all costs, as the salad has likely been washed in local water. The worst case of food poisoning I ever had was in India, because I thought, 'Oh, raw food is fine.' Big mistake! Hot food that has been well cooked is preferable.
- Similarly, if you are offered bottles of water or other drinks that are not properly sealed, say no thanks.
- It may sound ridiculous, but if cutlery has been washed in local streams in, say, India, you would be wise to take your own cutlery.
- Peel fruit.
- Beware of ice cubes unless made with bottled water.
- Do not eat any of the following under-cooked or rare: poultry, burgers, sausages, chicken nuggets and kebabs. Also avoid uncooked fish, which can be lethal.
- Short episodes of vomiting and small amounts of diarrhoea lasting less than 24 hours can usually be cared for at home. When a bout of food poisoning is under way, it is best to rest and starve yourself of solid food for 24 hours, as this will also starve the bacteria. But if you are not holding down any fluids, you **must** seek medical help, as dehydration can kill you. This is especially true for young children and babies.

Friendly Foods

- During an attack, drink plenty of boiled or bottled water, or sip ginger ale to avoid dehydration.
- Try and sip an electrolyte drink, such as Emergen-C available in sachets from any chemists, regularly. Dissolve the contents of the sachet in water.
- After 24 hours of avoiding all foods, and when you are successfully tolerating fluids, start eating small amounts of brown rice, soups, and dry toast or crackers and see how you go. Don't try to eat anything heavy for the first couple of days – be kind to your system.
- Try making porridge or semolina with almond or oat milks. Don't use cow's milk.
- Mashed pumpkin, sweet potato and a little grilled fish should be fine.
- Hemp seed protein powders mixed with a banana and a small amount of aloe vera juice and

rice milk should be well tolerated and give you some much-needed nutrients.

Useful Remedies

- One or two drops of liquid grapefruit-seed extract can be added to water and sipped throughout the day, as it has strong anti-bacterial action. **HN** or contact www.positivehealthshop.com
- Whenever you have had an episode of food poisoning, probiotics – healthy bacteria found in the bowel – are really essential. They help re-populate the bowel and help protect against further growth of the offending bugs. If you are susceptible to diarrhoea when you travel abroad, taking acidophilus for two weeks prior to your trip can help increase the number of healthy bacteria in the gut, which reduces the risk of picking up a tummy bug. Jarro-Dophilus EPS is a good broad-spectrum formula. **NC**
- Floraguard by BioCare contains healthy bacteria plus garlic, oregano oil, clove oil and cinnamon and rosemary. It can be taken daily with food when you are abroad to help kill off any invading bacteria. It can be very handy for holidays, but do not take it if you are pregnant. **BC**
- Homeopathic Arsen Alb is good for reducing stomach cramps, Nux Vomica helps reduce feelings of nausea and Mag Phos is also great for cramps.
- Once symptoms have begun to settle and nausea and vomiting have ceased, you can try the following: goldenseal is a useful herb once initial symptoms have subsided. It helps to increase appetite and reduce nausea and vomiting. It also has strong properties for fighting off bad bacteria and it has a soothing effect on the mucous membranes in the gut. Solgar's Goldenseal Root Complex provides 500mg. Available from all health stores. Initially, take one a day with food and then increase to one, three times day for two weeks.
- Charcoal capsules or tablets may help in the case of diarrhoea. The charcoal will help bind on to the toxins that will be produced from the bug and will be excreted through the bowel. These are available at most health food stores and some chemists.

Helpful Hints

- Most cases of food poisoning clear up on their own after a few days, but you should visit a doctor if the symptoms of food poisoning last for more than 2 or 3 days. Also, if there is a fever and the diarrhoea is very watery, or there is blood, pus or mucous mixed in with the stools, please seek medical help.
- Signs of dehydration are intense thirst, dry lips and tongue, increased heart rate and weakness.
- Bacteria thrive on dirty, damp cloths. So it's very important to wash kitchen cloths, tea towels and sponges regularly. Choose the hottest wash that your washing machine permits to make sure all bacteria are killed.
- Bacteria love to travel and will hitch a ride on anything they can – hands, chopping boards, knives or tongs – and find their way onto foods such as bread or salad. Make sure you thoroughly wash hands and utensils in warm soapy water after touching raw meat and poultry, going to the toilet, touching the bin, and touching pets.
- Don't forget to dry your hands thoroughly, because if they are wet they will spread bacteria more easily.
- Cook meats thoroughly – especially poultry. If you are serving poultry cold, make sure it's kept really cool; and if re-heating, make sure it's hot right through. Chickens need to be roasted at 200°C (400°F), or gas mark 6, for 20 minutes per 450g (1lb), plus an extra 20 minutes.
- Citricidal – grapefruit-seed extract – has wonderful anti-bacterial and anti-parasitic actions and has been proven in laboratory tests to be 10 times more effective as a disinfectant than chlorine. Available from health stores.

- If you have cooked food that you aren't going to eat straight away, cool it as quickly as possible (ideally within 1–2 hours) and then store it in the fridge. Do not cool it down in the fridge, as this can raise the overall temperature in the fridge, which will enable bacteria on food already stored in the fridge to grow.
- Don't store leftovers for longer than 2 days.
- Never use cracked raw eggs, although well cooked eggs are fine for anyone recovering from food poisoning.
- Don't put raw chicken or meat next to cooked food on the grill or barbecue.
- Don't add sauce or marinade to cooked food if it has been used to baste raw chicken or meat.
- Store raw chicken and meat on the bottom shelf of the fridge, where it can't touch or drip onto other foods.
- Use separate tongs and utensils for raw chicken and meat and for cooked chicken and meat.
- Keep raw meat and ready-to-eat food separate in the fridge and also in the kitchen area. This is especially important regarding raw meat and ready-to-eat foods, such as salad, fruit and bread. As these foods won't be cooked before you eat them, any bacteria that get onto them won't be killed.

FOOT PROBLEMS

All too many of us spend far too long on our feet. A typical person walks 116,500km (about 71,000 miles) during their lifetime. Our often-neglected feet contain 26 bones, 56 ligaments and 38 muscles, so there is an awful lot that can go wrong with them. Wearing shoes that are too high can trigger back problems, and if your shoes are too tight they will restrict circulation, triggering problems such as blisters, corns and chilblains. One of the best ways to keep your feet pain free is to visit a chiropodist regularly.

Cold feet

Cold feet usually relate to poor circulation (see *Circulation*), but can also be associated with low thyroid function (see *Thyroid*). If your feet are chronically cold, even when the weather is warm, ask your doctor to check you for an under-active thyroid or for Raynaud's disease (see *Raynaud's Disease*).

Regular exercise, massage with essential oil of black pepper (mixed with a base oil), acupuncture, and reflexology will all help alleviate cold feet. Wearing bed socks helps – and keeping a magnet in your shoes encourages better circulation to the feet. For all foods and supplements, see *Circulation* and *Raynaud's Disease*. One very useful herb for cold feet is gotu kola, as it increases circulation in the lower limbs. You can also include more fresh root ginger in your diet, or take ginger capsules as they bring more warmth to the body.

Cracked heels   *(see also Thyroid)*

Also referred to as fissures, for most people cracked heels just look unsightly, but for others they can become quite painful. Cracked heels are mainly due to excessive callus build-up as well as very dry thin skin on the outside of the heels. But they can also be due to a thyroid problem, lack of essential fats, prolonged standing, inactive sweat glands, obesity, wearing flip-flops or open-backed shoes, flat feet (see *Fallen Arches*, below), use of excessively hot water, walking abnormally, eczema and psoriasis. Cold weather greatly dehydrates the whole body and therefore this problem is more likely to occur during the winter months.

Foods to Avoid
- Avoid alcohol and caffeine found in coffee, tea, power drinks and some painkillers, as these dehydrate the body.
- Reduce saturated fats found in red meat and dairy – trim all fat from the meat, and grill rather than fry your food. These 'bad' fats prevent the good fats from doing their job (see also *Fats You Need To Eat*).
- Grains in the form of flour of any type will dehydrate the body if eaten to excess.

Friendly Foods
- Aim to drink plenty of water per day to help rehydrate your body and skin.
- Zinc-rich foods, such as brown rice, lentils, and pumpkin, sunflower and sesame seeds, plus almonds, are rich in minerals and essential fats that nourish your skin from the inside out.
- Use more organic olive, walnut, sesame and avocado oils in salad dressings or drizzle over cooked foods. Eat avocado twice weekly.
- Generally, eat more oily fish, organic salmon, trout, anchovies, mackerel and sardines, as they are high in essential fats.
- Magnesium-rich foods are dark green leafy vegetables, cashew nuts, broccoli, bananas and prunes; selenium-rich foods are Brazil nuts, oats, and brown rice.

Useful Remedies
- A good all-round multi-vitamin for your age and gender.
- Break open a vitamin E capsule and apply to the affected area.
- There are dozens of nutrient-dense creams made for the feet such as Heel from Germany that will help keep the area nourished. Ask at your pharmacy or health shop or call The Organic Pharmacy on 020 7351 2232.
- Take 3 grams of omega-3 essential fats daily if your skin is dry.

Helpful Hints
- Avoid thick creams on fissures, which can sit on the skin and make the problem worse – use a trans-dermal moisturizer that contains Emu Oil, which soaks into the hard skin on the feet more easily. For details, call Margaret Dabbs Chiropody on 020 7487 5510 or log on to www.margaretdabbs.co.uk
- Find a really good cream for extra-dry skin. Apply twice daily, especially before going to bed, and then put on old cotton socks so that the cream can really soak into the dry areas.
- Soak your feet daily in warm soapy water for 15 minutes, then use a good pumice stone or foot scrub on the thick skin on your heels, thickly apply a moisturizing cream, sit back and let it soak in. Avoid open-backed or thin-soled shoes and buy shoes with a good shock-absorbing sole. Never try to cut back the hard skin yourself with a razor blade or a pair of scissors – see a chiropodist. Ask in any large Boots the Chemists, or call the Institute of Chiropodists and Podiatrists on 01704 546141 to find a qualified chiropodist in your area. Website: www.locp.org.uk

Fallen arches

Most people when standing have a gap between the inner side of the foot and the ground they are standing on – this is called the arch. Fallen arches – also known as flat feet – happen when there is a flat arch and the foot rolls over, so there is little or no gap. Symptoms depend on the severity of the condition, but corns, hard skin under the sole of the foot, and a tender arch area are common and shoes will tend to wear out quickly. In severe cases calf, knee, hip or back pain can be experienced. Fallen arches may be hereditary, but in most cases are caused by abnormal walking where the joints in the foot roll in too much. Fallen arches can also cause plantar faciitis, a painful condition where the tight band of connective tissue in the arch of the foot becomes highly inflamed. A ruptured tendon can also lead to a flat foot, as can cerebral palsy, spina bifida and muscular dystrophy.

Helpful Hints
- Find a good local health clinic that deals with sports injuries. If they have an in-house chiropodist or podiatrist, you can be fitted for individual orthotics – inserts made specifically for your feet, which give your foot all the support it needs. Otherwise, large chemists and foot specialists, such as Scholl, offer a variety of orthotic inserts especially to support the arches. One of the best inserts I have found is Orthaheel, which is available worldwide. Log on to www.orthaheel.com.
- To find a qualified chiropodist in your area, ask in any large pharmacy or chemist, or contact the Institute of Chiropodists and Podiatrists at www.locp.org.uk, or call them on 01704 546141.
- MBT shoes (Masai Barefoot Technology) are state-of-the-art shoes that support the feet really well. These shoes greatly alleviate many structural problems, including back, knee and joint pain. Have a look at www.swissmasai.com

Hot, burning feet

F

Poor circulation is often the cause of this problem (see *Circulation*). It is also common in people suffering from diabetes who frequently have problems with nerves within the feet, which can be linked to a deficiency in B vitamins. Alcoholics often suffer this problem as they are greatly deficient in B vitamins. Other than diabetes, circulation can be affected by eating too many of the wrong type of fats, which tend to clog up the system. Dehydration can compound the problem, as it makes it harder for fluid and nutrients to move around the body. Improving circulation to the feet can often relieve symptoms.

There may also be a link with trapped nerves in the lower spine, therefore it may be a good idea to consult a chiropractor.

Foods to Avoid
- Avoid saturated animal fats found in red meat and full-fat dairy produce, plus hydrogenated and trans-fats rich in processed foods – especially burger-type foods, and cakes and pastries. See *Fats You Need To Eat*.
- Reduce or avoid alcohol, as this is dehydrating.

Friendly Foods
- The essential fats found in oily fish, such as mackerel, sardines, organic-farmed salmon and anchovies, plus nuts and seeds.
- Blueberries and cherries. These contain bioflavonoids that help to keep the walls of blood vessels strong so that they can carry fluid and nutrients around the body more easily and efficiently.

Useful Remedies
Take a high-potency B-complex daily – aiming for 50mg of the majority of B-vitamins.
- Higher Nature's Essential Oil Balance contains the correct ratio of the essential oils. Take 3 capsules daily, or buy the oil and drizzle it over cooked vegetables, or rice dishes, or use it for salad dressings.

- Otherwise take 2–3 grams of omega-3 fish oils daily.
- The herb gotu kola is very useful for increasing circulation to the feet. Try 1–3 grams daily with food for a month and see if this helps.

Helpful Hints

- Acupuncture and reflexology are also very useful for alleviating this condition (see *Useful Information*).
- Exercise is great for stimulating the circulation. Take a regular 30-minute walk each day. Any exercise that gently pounds the bottom of the feet will help to improve circulation. Try dancing, skipping or rebounding.

Numb and tingling feet

It is very important if you have this problem for more than a few days that you see your GP to find out if there is anything more serious going on, as numb or tingling feet can be due to peripheral neuropathy, which can denote late-onset diabetes. A blood test is all that's needed to clarify if this is the case. A lack of calcium may also cause this problem. Try taking 1000mg of calcium daily for a couple of weeks. Epidurals are also associated with this problem.

If you have numb and tingling feet, take the supplements suggested under *Circulation*, and get plenty of exercise, such as walking, skipping or rebounding, which really helps bring more blood to the feet.

Consult a chiropractor, who can check for trapped nerves and any spinal misalignments that may be triggering this problem. See *Useful Information*.

Try reflexology and acupuncture to further improve circulation.

Smelly feet   *(see also Athlete's Foot, Body Odour and Candida)*

Smelly feet also known as bromihydrosis, can be highly embarrassing for you and those around you – and in most cases are easily preventable. Initially, wash your feet a couple of times a day with warm water with a little added tea tree oil, and then use natural talcum powder to help keep them drier. Several companies, such as Crystal, make foot sprays that help kill bacteria on the feet (available from good health stores www.thecrystal.com). Always wear 100% cotton socks and leather shoes, as synthetic fibres lead to increased sweating and it is the bacteria in the sweat that create the unpleasant smell. Change your shoes often – alternating pairs daily would help, as this gives your shoes a chance to breathe. Also, avoid wearing closed shoes without socks. Going without shoes whenever possible is also a good idea, as the fresh air will help reduce sweating. Some people find that if they put their shoes in a freezer overnight it helps to kill off the bacteria responsible for the odour. Eat more coriander, which helps destroy 'smelly' bacteria in the body.

Swollen feet and ankles   *(see also Water Retention)*

As we age, the ratio of water found inside and outside our cells changes and we find it harder to properly absorb water into the cells. This extra fluid triggers oedema (collection of water in the body's tissues), which with gravity heads south toward our feet. This problem is common in middle-aged and older ladies, and can also happen during pregnancy. Again, this is mainly linked to circulation and the body's ability to remove excess fluid (see *Circulation*). Any injury of the feet, ankles or legs can also contribute to swelling in this area.

Foods to Avoid

- Avoid all foods high in salt and sodium, such as preserved meats and fish, crisps, processed foods, packet sauces and ketchup-style foods, which often contain huge amounts of hidden salt. Salt exacerbates any water retention and increases swelling in all parts of the body if you suffer fluid retention.
- Check the salt content of breakfast cereals and cereal bars – look for low salt/sodium alternatives such as Himalyan Crystal Sea Salt or use nori flakes.
- Look out for hidden sources of salt/sodium. It is found in high quantities in ketchups, pickles and relishes and olives, and in sodium benzoate E211 – a preservative – and monosodium glutamate (MSG), also known as E621. Cut out adding salt to your food and cooking or use nori or kelp flakes for their natural salts.
- Avoid burger-type meals that are high in salt and fat; also avoid sausages and mass-produced pies, cakes and biscuits.
- Avoid caffeine in any form (watch out for it hidden in energy drinks and some painkillers), plus tea and alcohol, as these will dehydrate the body.
- Cut back on saturated fats found in red meat and dairy produce. These clog up the lymphatic system, which is responsible for removing excess fluid. See *Fats You Need To Eat*.
- See also *General Health Hints*.

Friendly Foods

- Eat foods rich in potassium, such as green vegetables, fresh fruit, dried fruits, unsalted nuts (not peanuts), fresh fish, bananas, potatoes, and unsalted sunflower and pumpkin seeds.
- Eat more oily fish and use unrefined walnut, olive, hemp and sunflower oils for your salad dressings.
- Try a little magnesium-rich Solo Salt – easily available and found in the majority of supermarkets and all good health food stores.
- Otherwise use nori or kelp flakes.

F

Useful Remedies

- Celery seed extract acts like a diuretic. Take 2 capsules twice daily until symptoms ease. **BC**
- Also take 1 gram of vitamin C as potassium ascorbate to improve lymph drainage. This should help to remove excess fluid. **BC**
- Silica and sulphur compound for three months will help to improve tissue tone. **BLK**
- On days when your ankles are very swollen, take 15 drops of dandelion tincture 3 times a day before meals. Dandelion leaves are a potassium-rich diuretic, which also help to cleanse the liver. A. Vogel makes a good one. Tel: 0800 085 0820. www.avogel.co.uk
- As a lack of B vitamins is linked to this problem, take a B-complex daily and look for one that contains 50mg of B6. Otherwise, take a good-quality multi-vitamin and mineral that contains a full spectrum of B vitamins.

Helpful Hints

- Reflexology and acupuncture are usually highly effective for helping to alleviate this condition. See *Useful Information*.
- Sit with your feet at hip level for at least 15 minutes every day, moving your feet back and forth to improve circulation.
- Rebounding (mini-trampolining), gentle jogging and skipping are especially good for boosting lymphatic drainage. Deep-tissue lymphatic drainage can help if the problem is one of a stagnant lymph system.
- Dry skin brushing helps remove excess fluid. Buy a natural (not synthetic), long-handled brush, which shouldn't scratch the skin. Begin by brushing the soles of the feet as the 7,000 nerve endings there affect the whole body; next, brush the ankles, calves and thighs; then

brush across your stomach and buttocks; and lastly brush your hands and up your arms. Always brush in the direction of the heart. Follow this with a warm bath or shower and complete the process with a cool rinse to really invigorate circulation. I find this a great way to wake up every morning and it really helps my skin to stay soft and in good condition.

■ Call at a homeopathic pharmacy, which can suggest a remedy to suit your particular symptoms. Or call the Organic Pharmacy. **OP**

■ If the symptoms persist after following the advice given here for more than six weeks, ask your GP for a thorough check-up, as occasionally swollen feet and ankles may be a sign of heart, liver or kidney problems.

FROZEN SHOULDER

This condition is often characterized by pain and limited movement in one and very rarely both shoulders. It is triggered by inflammation of the muscles, ligaments or tendons around the shoulders. Exercise can be very painful, especially if you try and lift your arm higher than the shoulder joint; however, gentle exercise that encourages blood flow and does not overstrain the joint or tendons is often helpful. Frozen shoulder is common between the ages of 40 and 60, and affects between 2 and 5% of the population.

Foods to Avoid

■ Avoid any foods and drinks containing caffeine, which greatly reduces our body's ability to make pain-killing endorphins.

■ Animal fats from meats, butter, cheese and milk will tend to increase inflammation in the body, as they are acid-forming – see *Acid–Alkaline Balance*.

■ Sugar and alcohol greatly increase inflammation in the body.

Friendly Foods

■ Oily fish contain anti-inflammatory essential fatty acids – especially organic-farmed salmon, mackerel, sardines, pilchards, trout, black cod or red snapper.

■ Cherries are high in bioflavonoids, which are mildly anti-inflammatory. Eat more pineapple for its bromelain content, which is also anti-inflammatory.

■ Ginger, turmeric, and cayenne pepper are all spices that, used liberally, can help decrease pain.

Useful Remedies

■ Ginger, curcumin and boswellia; take up to 4 tablets a day, which should help reduce the inflammation. **HN**

■ Magnesium helps to relax the muscles; while symptoms are acute, take 1000mg per day.

■ Taking liquid hyaluronic acid (a natural component of skin) daily in water helps to lubricate joints. Take one sachet daily before breakfast in a full glass of water. For details call Modern Herbals on 01274 889047. Website: www.modernherbals.com

■ Glucosamine with MSM (a type of sulphur) is very useful for easing the discomfort and gradually healing the joint. Take 2 grams of glucosamine and 1 gram of MSM. Health Perception make a duo formula. **NB This supplement is usually derived from crab shells, so if you have an intolerance to shellfish take the vegetarian version.**

■ Bromelain is highly anti-inflammatory – take 500mg twice daily, as this will also help improve elasticity in tissues.

Helpful Hints

■ Creams made with cayenne pepper can bring rapid pain relief. **NC**

■ Glucosamine gels with capsicum and MSM can also be applied daily.

- Bags of cherry stones or wheat can be either heated or frozen and then applied to the affected area for 10 minutes at a time to ease pain and inflammation.
- Traditionally, frozen shoulder is treated with regular physiotherapy. Find a local sports injury clinic, as they have experts who deal with these types of conditions on a daily basis. Alternatives are chiropractic and osteopathy, which are available on the NHS in some areas.
- Use your local swimming pool, as gentle movement in warm water loosens the shoulder.
- Acupuncture is highly effective for reducing the acute pain associated with frozen shoulder, and aromatherapy massage with essential oils of eucalyptus, ginger and juniper is helpful (see *Useful Information*).

GALL-BLADDER PROBLEMS

(see also Gall Stones and Liver Problems)

Gall-bladder and gall-stone problems are far more common in women than men and many people end up having surgery that could be prevented by making dietary changes. The gall bladder is a small pear-shaped organ (sac), which sits underneath, and is connected to, the liver. The gall bladder's main function is to store bile that is made in the liver. Water is removed from the bile, thereby concentrating it to be stored in the gall bladder. The gall bladder passes bile into the small bowel, where the bile helps to break down fat during digestion. If the liver is overloaded, this prevents efficient gall bladder function. The gall bladder can be affected by gall stones, inflammation and infection. Each of the problems may produce pain on the right side encasing the centre of the abdomen. In some cases the pain can be so severe that the patient feels nauseous and faint. Food intolerances definitely play a part in gall-bladder problems and you can avoid the need for surgery once the diet is balanced.

Foods to Avoid
- Anyone who has a tendency to gall bladder problems usually eats too much fatty foods, plus eggs and cheese, which can cause problems in some people, especially melted cheese which is very hard to digest.
- High-fat and fried foods put an extra load on the gall bladder and its ability to digest fats.
- Alcohol, coffee and chocolate place an extra strain on the liver, which can make the problem worse. Many people who have gall-bladder problems are overweight and tend to love creamy, naughty foods. Cut these out, and generally eat less, otherwise you end up having your gall bladder removed and then your body finds it difficult to metabolize fats and you will put on even more weight.
- See also *General Health Hints* and the dietary advice in *Liver Problems*.

Friendly Foods
- People who eat more beans and lentils are less likely to end up with gall-bladder or liver problems.
- Foods such as celeriac, artichokes, beetroot and celery are all good for liver and gall-bladder function.

- Try making fresh vegetable juices daily with celery, artichoke, parsley, raw beetroot, apples, carrots, and any green vegetables you have in your fridge. Add this to half a cup of organic aloe vera and drink daily to help detoxify your liver and gall bladder.
- Use unrefined extra-virgin olive, walnut or linseed (flax seed) oil in small amounts in salad dressings, all of which help to diminish the risk of developing problems.
- Drink plenty of fluids.

Useful Remedies
- Milk thistle and dandelion are very effective for maintaining a healthy gall bladder. Milk thistle encourages better liver detoxification and dandelion stimulates bile flow.
- Sprinkle 1 tablespoon of lecithin granules over breakfast cereals, fruit whips or yoghurts, which helps to emulsify the LDL cholesterol within the body.
- Swedish Bitters is a bitter tonic that aids the liver by enhancing the flow of bile. Put a few drops in a little water before main meals.
- Sodiphos contains sodium sulphate and sodium phosphate, which helps the flow of bile; take 3 tablets daily. **BLK**
- See also *Useful Remedies* under *Gall Stones*.

Helpful Hints
- Generally, to avoid gall-bladder problems you need to control your LDL cholesterol levels and levels of stress. See also *Cholesterol* and *Stress*.

G GALL STONES

Although up to 25% of the population have gall stones, only 15–20% eventually develop symptoms. Gall stones are four times more common in women, especially after 40. The classic description for a gall stone patient is 'fair, female, fat and forty!'

Many women end up having their gall bladder removed, yet changes in diet could prevent this major surgery in most cases. After surgery it's harder for the body to metabolize any fats, so prevention is definitely preferable.

People who tend to eat high saturated-fat and sugary diets without sufficient fibre, or those who are obese, constantly dieting but rapidly gain weight, or suffer Crohn's disease, are at a higher risk. Multiple pregnancies, the contraceptive pill and HRT are other factors, as is a high stress level. The gall bladder can become congested with substances such as cholesterol, which causes stagnation. Most gall stones consist of a sediment made up primarily of cholesterol, bilirubin and bile salts, and occur in individuals with excess cholesterol in the bloodstream or as a result of stagnation of bile flow in the gall bladder.

Small gall stones often produce no symptoms, but if they become large enough to obstruct the bile duct they can cause jaundice, inflammation, intense pain and vomiting. Symptoms tend to be much worse after high-fat meals or after foods to which the individual has a sensitivity, such as eggs. Constipation can be linked to the risk of gall stones, so it is very important that adequate fibre is eaten to reduce the likelihood of constipation and thus re-absorption of toxins.

Foods to Avoid
- To avoid gall-bladder attacks and gall stones, you really do have to stick to a low-fat diet by greatly reducing your intake of animal fats from any source.
- Low-fibre foods, such as white bread, cakes, biscuits, ice cream, most puddings, and pre-packaged meals should be avoided as much as possible.

- Foods such as eggs, pork, onions, pickles, spicy foods, peanuts and citrus fruits are likely triggers.
- Regular coffee-drinkers (that's real coffee, not decaffeinated) have a much lower risk of developing gall stones, but if you have a sensitivity to coffee then you do need to avoid it.

Friendly Foods

- Drink plenty of water/ fluids to prevent the bile from becoming too concentrated – around 6–8 glasses daily.
- Small amounts of lean cuts of lamb (without the fat), plus brown rice, and peas, pears and broccoli are usually no problem.
- Keep a food diary and eliminate any foods to which you have a reaction within an hour of eating them.
- Include more beetroot, artichoke, chicory, radicchio (Italian chicory), dried beans (aduki, kidney, pinto, haricot and so on), linseeds (flax seeds soaked overnight in cold water, drained and eaten with any cereals), and oat or rice bran – all of which are high-fibre foods – to reduce constipation.
- Sprinkle a tablespoonful of lecithin granules over a low-sugar, oat-based muesli or cereal, as soya lecithin helps to break down the fat in foods.
- Eat more porridge.
- Use wholemeal bread, and pasta made from corn, lentil, rice and potato flour.
- Include fresh fish, a little chicken without the skin, plenty of salads and fresh fruit in your diet.
- Replace full-fat milks with skimmed and try more herbal teas. Use organic rice, almond or oat milks.
- Use organic extra-virgin olive, sunflower and walnut oils for salad dressings – these are all rich in essential fats, which help to dissolve stones.
- Freshly made carrot, beetroot and cucumber juices help support better gall-bladder function.

G

Useful Remedies

- Milk thistle and dandelion in combination as tablets or capsules, or dandelion formula. Take 1 or 2 tablets with every meal, or 10–20 drops of tincture with every meal.
- As people suffering from gall stones process large amounts of toxins, they are frequently deficient in B vitamins, which are crucial for enzyme production and helping the liver function. Therefore, take a multi-vitamin that contains 50mg of each of the B-group vitamins.
- People with gall stones tend to be deficient in vitamins C and E. Take 2 grams of C daily with food, which is needed for the conversion of cholesterol to bile acids. Take 200–400iu of full-spectrum natural-source vitamin E.
- Take betaine hydrochloride (stomach acid) – 1 capsule with meals – as many people with gall stones have food intolerances and digestive problems. Many practitioners find that gall-stone sufferers are deficient in stomach acid. **Don't take this remedy if you have active stomach ulcers – instead take a digestive enzyme that is free from hydrochloric acid.**
- New Era silica and calcium fluoride tissue salts can help to break down and expel the stones. Take four of each daily.
- Please remember to use non-GM lecithin granules daily – they are very important to help prevent this condition.
- L-methionine is an amino acid that greatly aids detoxification of the liver. Take 500mg twice daily an hour before breakfast and supper. **PN**

Helpful Hints

- As multiple food sensitivities are linked to gall-bladder problems, it is well worth your while to consult a qualified nutritionist or naturopath who can sort out your diet. The initial few weeks may be hard, but there are plenty of foods you can eat. See *Useful Information*.

- It is important to have an allergy test to find your worst food offenders. Try the York Test Laboratories. Tel: 0800 458 2052 or log on to www.yorktest.com; or Genova Diagnostics do a FACT test, which looks for inflammatory markers indicating that the body is reacting to certain substances. Tel: 020 8336 7750. Website: www.gdx.uk.net
- Another excellent method is known as the Bio Meridian Test for food intolerance and leaky gut, in which the practitioner measures via electrodes your reactions to a huge list of foods and substances. For practitioners see www.biomeridian.com or call Sheila Partridge on 0207 580 7537.

GENERAL HEALTH HINTS

- Make time for breakfast, which is the most important meal of the day. You are literally breaking a fast and to keep your blood sugar on an even keel you need to eat, or you will end up craving sugary snacks by mid-morning.
- Oat, quinoa, kamut, amaranth and low-sugar-based cereals or sugar-free muesli make an ideal breakfast for most people. Gluten is now a problem for many people – try more gluten-free foods. Low-gluten breads are easier to digest, therefore you can try sprouted wheat bread, spelt or 100% rye breads. Eat cereals and porridge with skimmed milk (unless you are intolerant to animal-based milks) or try organic oat, rice, almond, sheep's or low fat goat's milk.

- Quality protein really helps to wake up your brain, which is why eggs (not fried), grilled fish or lean meat also make great breakfasts. Buy organic or free-range eggs. Otherwise, wholemeal/stone-ground bread, toasted, with a non-hydrogenated spread, such as Vitaquell, Biona, Olivio or organic raw walnut, hemp seed, coconut or almond butter, and a little honey or low-sugar jam, is fine. If you cannot face breakfast, at least take with you an apple or a couple of bananas and a low-fat, live yoghurt to eat later.
- Otherwise, make a protein shake the night before and swallow on your way to work. (See recipe, below.)
- Eat as great a variety of foods as possible, preferably locally grown and organic, which contain higher levels of nutrients than foods flown thousands of miles. Buy fruit and vegetables that are grown locally and allowed to ripen naturally. Unripe fruits and vegetables do not contain as many nutrients from the soil as those that have been allowed to ripen naturally on the vine. The price of organic foods is coming down and I believe that 100% organic food will help reduce many cancers and greatly alleviate the toxic load on the planet and its inhabitants. Many pesticides, especially the organophosphates (OPs), seep right through the vegetables and fruit and cannot be washed off. They are now linked with many cancers and lowered sperm counts.
- As much as possible, use organic products on your skin and hair – we ingest several kilos of chemicals annually through our skin alone. Also try to eliminate chemical-based cleaners and so on from your home.
- In winter, eat heart-warming cooked foods and in summer choose lighter meals with plenty of raw foods and fresh fruit. In winter, I make fruit compotes or I lightly grill fruits – which are more warming and easier on the digestion – especially with added freshly grated root ginger to aid circulation.
- Very few people make the effort to drink sufficient clean water, which is vital for good health. Every day we lose around 3 litres (6¼pt) of water; 1.5 litres (3pt) are excreted in urine; 750ml (24 fl oz) through the skin (and more during exercise); 400ml (13 fl oz) from simply breathing

and 150ml (5 fl oz) from faeces. We ingest just under a litre (1¾pt) from food and generate about half a litre (about ¾pt) by burning fats and carbohydrates, so we need to drink about one and half litres (about 2½pt), around 6 large glasses of water every day simply to cover our losses. Under normal circumstances, don't drink more than 2 litres (3½pt) daily as this can overburden the kidneys. As in all things, find a balance. Dr Sebagh, a plastic surgeon in London, says that 80% of his patients are dehydrated and their skin could greatly improve if they would just drink more water. Even the smallest degree of water loss can impair physical and mental function. Also the body siphons what it needs from the colon, and faeces can become hard and dry, thus contributing to constipation and increased toxicity in the body. Throughout the book we have re-iterated the need simply to drink more water – it's a quick and easy way to stay healthier.

- Cut down on coffee, alcohol and caffeinated soft drinks, which dehydrate the body. For every caffeinated or alcoholic drink, you need 250ml (8 fl oz) of water.
- The additives, artificial sweeteners (especially aspartame) and sugar in soft drinks and foods can trigger hyperactivity and mood swings. Sugar depletes the body of vital minerals, such as chromium. Forget low-calorie drinks, they place a strain on your liver, which slows weight loss. If you find yourself craving sweet foods, take 150mcg of chromium daily. After a few days it will kick in and you will notice that you crave sugar less. A fair amount of self-discipline is also needed.
- Organic agave syrup (a plant extract), xylitol and stevia can be used as sugar substitutes, as they have a low glycaemic Index. Available at all good health stores.
- Remember it's often the foods and drinks you crave the most that are causing most of your health problems.
- Drink more herbal teas, especially organic green and white teas.
- Try to eat at least five pieces of fresh, whole fruit and five portions of vegetables daily. Aim to have one salad a day in summer that includes some fresh, steamed or raw vegetables. Otherwise, lightly roast the vegetables, and allow to cool, then serve in the salad. The darker green the leaves, the more nourishing they are. Three portions of cabbage a week can reduce the incidence of colon cancer by as much as 60%.
- Steam or lightly stir-fry vegetables when possible, as boiling destroys vitamins.
- Keep food simple – say no to rich foods with rich sauces and to fried, barbecued and burnt foods, which are carcinogenic. See also *Cancer*.
- Avoid pre-packaged, take-away and tinned foods whenever possible, as they often contain plenty of fat, salt, sugar and additives. Also a great majority of these foods are packed in aluminium containers, and aluminium is linked to Alzheimer's and senile dementia.
- Do not add sodium-based salt to your food, as it can aggravate water retention and cause blood pressure to rise. Our typical diet contains 9 grams of salt a day and it has been estimated that if we could reduce salt consumption to 3 grams per person per day it would save 70,000 deaths in the UK each year. There are plenty of magnesium- and potassium-based sea salts readily available from supermarkets and health stores. Try Himalayan Crystal Salt, or try nori or kelp flakes (from seaweed) as a healthy salt substitute. Available from all health stores.
- Do not become fanatical about fad diets. Everything in moderation and keep a balance of foods at all times for good nutrition. I bake cakes with butter or I use organic olive or coconut oil, which do not become rancid like hard margarines when cooked. You can also try organic walnut, hemp seed or coconut butters from Higher Nature or Sun and Seed, available at health stores. Use a little organic agave syrup, honey, xylitol or fresh fruit instead of sugar; or soak some dried fruits in warm water, drain, chop and add to the cake mix.

G

- Use extra-virgin, cold-pressed olive or coconut oil in cooking and try walnut, avocado, organic sunflower or sesame oils for salad dressings. These oils have many health benefits, from lowering cholesterol to keeping your skin looking younger.
- Eat your meals sitting down – or at least standing still. Chew your food thoroughly; if you bolt down your food your body will tell you. Aid digestion by eating fruit between meals and not as a dessert. Fruit can ferment when eaten after a large meal, causing wind and bloating.
- Cow's milk is often a problem for many people. Skimmed milk is higher in sugar (lactose) and some people are intolerant to this. Try organic oat, quinoa, coconut (one of the better tasting is Karawww.karadairyfree.com), almond (try Ecomil) or organic rice milks, which are non-dairy. Also try sheep's or goat's products and eat plenty of live, low-fat yoghurt, which contains beneficial gut bacteria and is a rich source of calcium.
- Throughout the book we have regularly re-iterated how animal dairy produce – especially cow's milk – often has a negative effect on many conditions. Cow's milk is difficult for many people to absorb, which can trigger bloating. It is also acid forming after digestion. However, low-fat bio yoghurts, which are also low in refined sugars, are somewhat easier to digest as they are fermented. This is why we sometimes recommend avoiding cow's milk, while also advocating that small amounts of yoghurt may be OK. Sheep's and goat's milk yoghurts are even easier to absorb. We are all unique and you need to listen to your body and act accordingly.
- Avoid any foods and oils that contain hydrogenated or trans-fats – these are the bad guys.
- Wheat-based cereals, especially wheat bran, trigger bowel problems for many people. Use oat or quinoa-based cereals, or oat, soya and rice bran or wheat germ instead. Try lentil, rice, corn, spinach and potato-based flours and pastas, now available at health stores.
- Try to avoid red meat, which can putrefy in the gut and may contain antibiotic, hormone and chemical residues. If you adore meat: gentlemen, please don't eat more than 100g (3½oz) at one meal and ladies keep it to 50–75g (1¾–2½oz). Go for organic whenever you can to avoid the extra chemicals that non-organic meat contains. Other great proteins are fish, free-range eggs, low-fat cheese, chicken, turkey, tempeh, beans and lentils.
- Avoid smoking and smoky atmospheres.
- Make time to relax. When we are stressed the body starts pumping the hormones adrenaline and cortisol, ready for the fight-or-flight response. Eventually this can cause us to blow a fuse. It can be a gastric fuse, leading to ulcers, or a heart fuse causing heart attacks, and so on. The body and mind are one. If you are stressed, something has got to give in the end – which is why adrenal exhaustion has now reached epidemic proportions. Vitamins, minerals and diet alone will not keep you healthy. Stress is a major factor in many of today's health problems. Remember that you are special: give yourself the odd treat and make space in your diary for yourself.
- Get plenty of fresh air and learn to breathe deeply; this aids relaxation. Deep breathing also helps to alkalize the body. Stress makes it too acid.
- Sunlight is great for your health and without it you can become very ill indeed. Moderate sunbathing is fine with sunscreens; just stay out of the midday sun. As a general rule, never let your skin go red.
- Learn to have a good laugh regularly and don't be afraid to laugh at yourself – lighten up.
- Take regular, sensible exercise, which is one of the best favours you can do for your health. Try brisk walking, cycling, light jogging, swimming, skipping, aerobics and/or aqua aerobics, as these exercises have the most health-related benefits. You will be amazed at the difference regular exercise can make to your overall wellbeing. If you do nothing else, try to walk for 30 minutes daily, preferably away from main roads.

- Gradual lifestyle changes are of much greater benefits than 2–4 day fad diets.
- Over time, your taste buds will come to love healthier foods.
- Eat when you are hungry and don't let your blood sugar drop too much as this is when you start filling up on sugary snacks. I tend to eat breakfast, lunch and supper – and if I don't snack in between, I definitely feel better. Other people find it easier to have small meals at more regular intervals. Listen to your body. Large meals place a strain on the liver and digestive system. Losing weight is easier if you practise this way of eating, which also keeps blood sugar on an even keel, thus preventing mood swings.
- **Breakfast Smoothie Recipe** Get into blending and juicing. This is a fantastic way to ingest large amounts of nutrients quickly. Buy yourself a blender and learn to love smoothies. For breakfast daily, I place all the following items in a blender: 1 tablespoon of organic sunflower seeds, 1 tablespoon of non-GM lecithin granules, 1 tablespoon of linseeds (flax seeds that have been soaked overnight in cold water and drained), 1 scoop of organic hemp seed green powder protein mix (or a good whey, pea, rice or soya protein-based powder), half a cup of organic blueberries, a chopped apple (minus the pips but with the skin) and a banana – you could use any fruit you particularly like, especially papaya, pomegranate or pineapple. To this I add a tablespoon of aloe vera juice and a cup or so of organic rice milk and then I blend the lot for 30 seconds. Your smoothie makes a wonderful meal replacement. If it's thick, use more milk to make it into a drink, or eat it with a spoon. It's neat fibre, vitamins, minerals and essential fats.
- For added benefits, you can also add a teaspoon of any organic-source green powder, such as Green Magic Powder – which contains Hawaiian spirulina, chlorella, lecithin, barley and wheat grass, kamut, pectin apple fibre, kelp and wheat sprouts, CoQ10, royal jelly, artichoke powder and lactobacillus acidophilus – as a great all-round way to ingest good nutrients, healthy bacteria, keep the body more alkaline and help keep you regular. Details on www.itsgreenmagic.com or call Helen Cruikshank on 08453 279688.
- With a juicer, make yourself fresh raw vegetable juices, again adding any extras such as the aloe, fresh root ginger, a few drops of any herbal tinctures you like, especially dandelion and burdock, to cleanse the liver, and drink immediately after juicing, while the beneficial enzymes are still active.

G

GLANDULAR FEVER

(see also Adrenal Exhaustion, Candida, Immune Function and ME)

Glandular fever is caused by the Epstein Barr virus. It is most common in younger people, between the ages of 15 and 25, when the immune system is developing, hence the nickname of the 'kissing virus'. Symptoms include a severe sore throat, fever, swollen glands in the neck, and a feeling of overwhelming exhaustion. Initially it can appear similar to a bad dose of flu, but after a few days it becomes obvious that it is not flu and symptoms can continue for several months. The liver can be affected and some sufferers develop a mild hepatitis caused by the virus. (See also *Hepatitis* and *Liver Problems*.)

Antibiotics are inappropriate, because it is a viral infection and certain strengths of antibiotics can actually make this illness much worse. Bed rest and good nutrition are essential to help prevent a relapse, but unfortunately the illness often coincides with stressful academic studies, making life rather difficult. It is one of those diseases where you can appear to make a recovery and then a month later experience a relapse. For some individuals this can lead to chronic fatigue syndrome or ME. The more you rest when the problem is first diagnosed, the more likely you are to make a complete recovery. The yeast fungal overgrowth candida often occurs with glandular fever (see *Candida*), because the immune system is compromised from lymphatic congestion.

Adrenal exhaustion may result from glandular fever – see this section.

Foods to Avoid
- Sugar is the most important food to avoid, as it lowers immune function and adds to adrenal exhaustion. Colas and fizzy drinks often contain up to 10 teaspoons of sugar, and sugar in any form will greatly deplete immune function.
- Avoid all pre-packaged, ready-made meals, which are usually low in nutrients and high in additives, fats and sugar. Stores such as Marks and Spencer and Waitrose have greatly reduced sugar, salt and additives in food, and most stores now sell organic soups and other products.
- Try to eliminate hamburgers and sugary snacks.
- White bread, croissants, Danish pastries, cakes, chocolate snacks, crisps, pork and sausage pies, and all these instant-type foods should be avoided for a few weeks.
- If you know you have a problem with certain foods, the most common being gluten from wheat and dairy from cow's milk, then eliminate them for two weeks.
- Stimulants such as caffeine and alcohol can overload the body, giving brief bursts of energy, but actually reducing it in the long-term. See *Insulin Resistance*.
- See general Health Hints.

Friendly Foods

- Try to eat plenty of fresh fruit and vegetables that are rich in magnesium and natural-source carotenes, such as spring greens, cabbage, artichokes, kale, sweet potatoes, pumpkin, watercress, papaya, pineapple, dried apricots, parsley, broccoli, spinach, and all orange fruits.
- If you have a juicer, try a mixture of carrots, raw beetroot, apple and small amounts of garlic and onion. Garlic and onions are highly anti viral.
- Cook with garlic and onions.
- Make rich soups and stews with added fresh ginger.
- Plenty of good-quality, high-protein foods, such as fresh fish, chicken, tempeh, beans and lentils, plus free-range eggs, which all help to support the immune system. If you are really low, then add hemp seed or whey protein powders to breakfast cereals and smoothies (a good smoothie recipe is included under *General Health Hints*).
- Eat more wholemeal/stone ground breads and pastas, and jacket potatoes, brown rice, quinoa or amaranth. Make porridge with organic rice, almond or low-fat goat's or sheep's milk and look for low-sugar cereals.
- Eat more low-fat, live yoghurts to help replenish healthy bacteria in the gut.
- Drink plenty of fluids.
- Coriander and parsley are packed with nutrients.
- Drink liquorice tea to help support your adrenal glands, which are usually exhausted.

Useful Remedies
- Beta Glucans 1–3, 1–6, derived from yeast cell walls, are proven to strengthen the body's innate immune system (the immune system you were born with), making it more resistant to pathogens from food and air. Helps fight viruses. Take 250–500mg daily. Also safe for young children.
- Vitamin C is anti-viral and anti-bacterial. While symptoms are acute, take 5–6 grams daily in divided doses with food. Use an ascorbate or esther form and after a couple of weeks reduce this to 1 gram daily for several months. If this causes loose bowels, reduce the dose to just below bowel tolerance. **BC**

- Take a high-strength, multi-mineral and vitamin, as when we're fighting an infection we are often depleted in minerals especially calcium, magnesium and zinc.
- As vitamin A is vital for immune function and for fighting viruses, take 30–60mg of natural-source carotenes daily while symptoms are acute, as they naturally convert to Vitamin A in the body. When you start to improve, reduce to 15mg daily. **PN**
- Herbs such as echinacea, olive leaf extract, golden seal, astragalus, wild indigo, goldenseal and Siberian ginseng are all anti-viral. Take 3 grams daily of either the single herbs or a combination formula. Astragalus and golden seal also support liver function, which is often impaired in glandular fever. See *Liver Problems*.
- Co-enzyme Q10 is a vitamin-like substance that the body produces naturally to produce energy. Take 100mg twice daily until you improve, then take 100mg with breakfast daily.
- Propolis has been shown to be highly anti-viral; try taking 1–3 grams daily for the duration of your illness. **NB Avoid this remedy if you are severely allergic to bee stings.**
- If for any reason you end up taking antibiotics, then take some probiotic capsules for a month. **BC**
- Fructo-Oligosaccharides (FOS) is a powder that can be used as a sweetener, and acts as a prebiotic, which helps the body to make more healthy bacteria in the gut, which in turn boosts immune function. **BC**

Helpful Hints
- A gradual return to normal life is necessary because over-activity too soon can cause a relapse.
- Gentle exercise is really important to get you moving again.
- Homeopathic Ailanthus Glandulosa 6c, or Gelsemium 6c, 3 times daily for 10 days should help reduce symptoms dramatically.
- Check for possible iron deficiency with your doctor and take iron if necessary (see under *Anaemia*).
- You should also ask your doctor to check for parasites (see under Irritable Bowel Syndrome). If, after two months, your energy and appetite have not returned, contact a qualified nutritionist (see *Useful Information*).

GLAUCOMA   *(See also Eye Problems and Macular Degeneration)*

Glaucoma is a group of eye diseases that cause vision loss through damage to the optic nerve. In the UK around three people in every 100 over 40 years of age have this condition. Experiencing high pressure inside the eyes, without actually having glaucoma, is common and affects one in 10 people over 40. Diabetics are twice as likely to develop glaucoma, which is the leading cause of blindness worldwide. Afro and Caribbean people also tend to suffer more glaucoma, as do people with high blood pressure or a family history of glaucoma. If a family member suffers from glaucoma, it's important that you see an optician annually after the age of 35 to check your eye pressure. Glaucoma can also occur if the eye is injured in any way or suffers repeated inflammations, such as iritis.

The most common type is chronic (open angle) glaucoma, which develops slowly. Acute (closed angle) glaucoma happens when the pressure in your eyes rises very quickly. This occurs when the drainage angle between the cornea and the iris narrows suddenly, which stops the fluid from leaving the eye. When this happens, intraocular pressure (IOP) increases, which can be very painful and needs urgent medical attention; otherwise your sight can be lost in 2 to 5 days.

Symptoms of glaucoma differ depending upon the type of glaucoma diagnosed. In the majority of cases, typical symptoms would be progressive loss of side vision, followed by reductions in central vision plus watering eyes, headaches, an inability to adjust the eye to darkened rooms, difficulty focusing on close work and a frequent need to change eyeglass prescriptions. You may also experience nausea, vomiting, pain, blurred vision and the whites of your eyes may be inflamed. If you have any of these symptoms, consult an optician or go to your local hospital immediately so that the pressure in your eyes can be tested and immediate action taken.

Foods To Avoid
- Reduce or eliminate caffeine and cola-type drinks, which can contribute to a rise in blood pressure.
- Avoid the artificial sweetener aspartame and greatly cut down on your sugar intake from foods and drinks, as it depletes magnesium which is often low in glaucoma sufferers.
- Avoid all mass-produced vegetable oils, including canola oil and especially margarines. Eliminate deep-fat fried foods from your diet.
- Avoid monosodium glutamate (MSG), which is a potential optic nerve toxin.
- Limit your alcohol consumption. Alcohol interferes with liver functions, and reduces levels of protective glutathione, an amino acid.
- See also *Diet* section under *Eye Problems*.

Friendly Foods
- Crucial foods to supports your eyes are flavenoids found in dark purple fruits – red grapes, blueberries, prunes, blackcurrants, blackberries and cherries.
- Natural-source carotenes, found in watercress, pumpkin, sweet potatoes, papaya, apricots, cantaloupe melons, are all great foods to nourish the eyes, which require large amounts of carotenes.
- Eat more flax (linseeds) and oily fish, such as organic salmon, anchovies, trout, mackerel, sardines and pilchards, as omega-3 fats are necessary for healthy eyes.
- Eat more avocados and wheat germ, rich in vitamin E.
- See also *Diet* section under *Eye Problems*.

Useful Remedies
- Vitamin C is vital, as it helps to stabilize intraocular pressure (IOP) and plays an important role in the prevention and treatment of glaucoma. Take 2–4 grams daily with food in divided doses. You can take Vitamin C to bowel tolerance as a way to lower IOP. Once your bowel movements start to become loose, cut back your dose.
- The mineral magnesium has been shown to improve blood supply and visual field, as it relaxes constricted blood vessels. Take 200–800mg per day with food.
- The mineral chromium not only helps to balance blood sugar, but also helps the eyes to focus and low levels of vitamin C and chromium are associated with IOP. Take 200mcg daily.
- Essential fats, especially fish oils, are vital for healthy eyes. Take 2 grams of omega-3 fish oils daily.
- Pycnogenol – pine bark extract – supports healthy collagen. Take 80mg twice daily for one month and then 80mg daily.

Helpful Hints
- Glaucoma is linked to stress, which thickens the blood and constricts circulation. Avoid emotional upsets and upheavals. External pressure increases internal ocular pressure (see under *Stress*).
- Make sure you get sufficient sleep.

- According to research from Florida University, contact lenses infused with vitamin E help to keep the prescription eye drops in the eyes for longer periods, making them more effective. Speak to your specialist about this.
- Climates with great temperature variances are thought to be detrimental. Temperate-even climates and temperatures appear better tolerated by the glaucoma patient.
- Don't smoke, as smoking constricts blood vessels, reducing the blood supply to the eye.
- Avoid prolonged eye stresses, such as long movies, excessive TV viewing, or excessive reading and staring at computer screens for hours on end. Take regular breaks, preferably outside.
- For more help and to find details of where to have laser surgery, log on to the Glaucoma Research Foundation website at www.glaucoma.com

GLUE EAR
(see also Earache)

The Eustachian tube is a pathway that allows the equalisation of air pressure between the middle ear and the back of the throat, through which bacteria can enter the middle ear. Ear infections are one of the most common childhood ailments. They are also likely to re-occur over a relatively short space of time. These infections can be very painful. It is understandable that parents would want to give the child immediate relief, the normal treatment being either antibiotics or the insertion of a grommet in the ear drum. Neither of these treatments is particularly effective. In fact, almost 90% of children with glue ear have food intolerances (see *Allergies*). Identifying which foods are a problem is important, and the most common culprits tend to be wheat and dairy produce from cows. But don't eliminate a whole group of foods and leave the child malnourished. Children who are breast-fed are less likely to develop ear infections. One other odd thing that seems to increase the risk of inner-ear infections is the use of dummies when children are very young.

Nutritionist Gareth Zeal has seen many children with glue ear who also suffer ADHD (Attention Deficit Hyperactivity Disorder) – see under *Hyperactivity*.

Foods to Avoid
- Sugar is top of the list as it weakens the immune system, leaving children more prone to infections. Other than sugar it is very important that the food intolerances or allergies are identified as these are likely to be the primary cause. Typically they would include dairy produce from cows, eggs, wheat and citrus fruits such as oranges, grapefruit, lemons and limes; but it could be any one of a number of other food groups.
- Keep your child off mucous-forming food, such as full-fat cheeses, pizzas, Greek yoghurts, white breads and cakes, full-fat milks from any source, soya milk and foods, chocolates and so on. Mucous will also be formed as a reaction to any foods to which the child has a sensitivity.
- Remember that many canned drinks and mass-produced desserts and jams can contain up to 10 teaspoonfuls of sugar, and artificial sweeteners are often a problem for people with allergies.
- Try to avoid preservatives and additives in foods and toiletries such as toothpastes.

Friendly Foods
- Fresh fruit and vegetables are rich in vitamin C, which will boost the immune system.
- Garlic helps to fight infections – but note that garlic is a common allergen, so keep a food diary and note reactions.
- Chewing gum made with xylitol seems beneficial, as children who chew xylitol-sweetened chewing gum have a much lower rate of inner ear infections. You can also buy xylitol as a

sweetener. **HN.**

- Introduce your child to foods lower in saturated fats, but highly nutritious, such as brown rice, barley, lentils and pulses, and try rice, amaranth or oat cakes.
- There are numerous health cookery books giving great recipes for cookies, biscuits and cakes that are low in fat and sugar.
- There are plenty of low-fat, live fruit yoghurts freely available that replenish healthy bacteria in the gut, which helps fight infection.
- Use rice, almond or oat milk and bake cakes with barley, buckwheat, rice, potato or spelt flours.
- Use non-hydrogenated spreads such as Vitaquell, Olivio or Biona.

Useful Remedies

- Colostrum, which is found in breast milk, helps support the immune system and aids healing of a leaky gut, also normally associated with glue ear. It's also very helpful for babies and children suffering from eczema. Up to the age of 2 give a quarter of a teaspoon twice daily on an empty stomach. Over 2 years give half a teaspoon twice daily. Give this just for one month. **NC**
- Echinacea either as tincture or tablets. An alcohol-free tincture is often easier for children, as it can be added to fruit juice or yoghurt. If the child is very small, use 1 drop per 6kg (3lb) of body weight. It can be used several times a day while symptoms last. For more help call the Organic Pharmacy. **OP**

- Vitamin C – for children give 250–500mg daily. For adults 1–2 grams daily. Again, as a lot of children don't like tablets, vitamin C is often available as a powder, some of them fairly pleasant-tasting, or you can find ones that can be added to fruit juice and the flavour of the fruit juice is what the child will taste. Alternatively, use a vitamin crusher. Available from Lemon Burst: www.lemonburst.co.uk
- Zinc lozenges and zinc supplements can be given to a child. Give 1–2 lozenges a day while the child has an infection. Zinc boosts the immune function and helps to fight the infection. 25mg daily for adults and 10–15mg daily for a child over 8.
- A child's chewable multi-vitamin and mineral. For details call Nature's Plus. **NP**
- The celloid potassium chloride helps to unblock the Eustachian tube – take or give100mg daily. **BLK**; or you can buy Ionic Potassium Chloride by Metabolics from the Nutri Centre. **NC**

Helpful Hints

- It is important to have an allergy test to find your worst food offenders. Try the York Test Laboratories. Tel: 0800 458 2052 or log on to www.yorktest.com; or Genova Diagnostics do a FACT test which looks for inflammatory markers indicating that the body is reacting to certain substances. Tel: 020 8336 7750. Website: www.gdx.uk.net
- A humidifier placed in the main living room or the child's bedroom has been found to reduce the risk of inner-ear infections.
- Many nutritional doctors advocate that your child should not be subjected to vaccinations until the cycle of ear infections is cleared, as vaccines place a strain on the child's immune system.
- Try Dr Christopher's B & B ear Formula as ear drops. Call 0845 345 3727.
- Gently warm through a few drops of olive oil (to no more than body temperature) which can be placed in the ear overnight and kept in place with a little cotton wool. This can help to soften the wax and therefore make it easier to remove.
- Cranial osteopathy helps as it encourages lymph drainage. See *Useful Information*.
- Do not let the child be exposed to cigarette smoke – it increases the incidence of glue ear by 80%.

GOUT

(see also Acid–Alkaline Balance and Arthritis)

In the 18th century you were considered fortunate to develop gout, as it was believed this prevented you from contracting fatal diseases. It was seen as a rich person's disease because only those who could afford large amounts of meat, cheese and wine were likely to suffer. Gout is a form of joint inflammation, which is caused by high levels of uric acid in the blood creating crystal deposits in the joints. It is very common in the big toe, but can also affect other joints and the kidneys. The vast majority of gout sufferers are men, but more and more women are beginning to suffer gout, which is totally avoidable. An attack can be triggered by ingesting overly rich food and drinks; typically this would include shellfish, cheeses such as Stilton, port, red meat and red wine. Most people who suffer gout tend to drink a lot anyway – especially champagne. Occasionally, an accident or trauma to the body can also precipitate an attack.

Foods to Avoid

- Generally, eat a lot less meat, plus reduce beer and cheese, which are the main triggers in gout.
- Any foods that are high in purines, found in high-protein foods, such as offal and oily fish (including anchovies, herrings, cod and mackerel), plus chicken, caffeine, shellfish (including crab, lobster, scallops and mussels), roe, kidney beans, lima beans, navy beans, yeast-based drinks, such as Marmite and Bovril, oatmeal porridge and lentils. Once the attack has subsided, you can eat small amounts of these foods.
- Avoid full-fat cheeses, especially Stilton and Brie.
- Most forms of arthritis usually benefit from taking cod liver oil or eating oily fish; with gout, however, these foods would almost certainly make it worse.

Friendly Foods

- Cherries and pineapple should be eaten on a daily basis, cherries in particular. They are one of the easiest ways of keeping gout under control and of preventing it, as they increase excretion of uric acid from the body. You can also try pure, low-sugar cherry concentrate and dilute in water.
- Also include blueberries, blackberries and bilberries in your diet. Many people report that by boiling a few cubes of green papaya with fresh green tea and sipping as needed helps eliminate uric acid from the body.
- Prunes, although acid forming, help mobilize uric acid out of the body. Eat daily or try prune juice.
- Eat plenty of fruit and vegetables, especially celery, quinoa, millet, brown rice, and pastas made from corn, rice, amaranth, potato or buckwheat flours.
- Free-range or organic eggs, cooked soya tofu and lamb should not cause any problems.
- Make a healthy drink containing a small box of blueberries, some pineapple, frozen or fresh pipped cherries, a pear, an apple and a banana. Add a teaspoon of any good organic green food powder (which will help alkalize your system), and a tiny piece of fresh root ginger. Put in a blender with half a cup of rice or almond milk, whiz for one minute and drink immediately.
- Drink at least 6–8 glasses of water every day, to encourage excretion of the uric acid.

Useful Remedies

- Vitamin C: 1–2 grams a day taken with food will gradually help lower uric acid levels.
- Bromelain: take 500mg twice a day; this is a very powerful anti-inflammatory.
- Ginger, curcumin and boswellia: take 4 capsules, or more, a day. These herbs in combination provide relief from any type of inflammation discomfort. Pukka and Higher Nature make these formulas. P, HN

G

- Cat's claw, 400mg 3 times a day for 3 months or more. This herb can gradually help lower uric acid levels, as well as improving bowel function. It can also help protect your gut lining against the negative side effects of anti-inflammatory painkillers – known as NSAIDs. **HN**
- Omega-3 fats found in flax (linseeds), hemp seeds, and extracted from oily fish, will help dampen the inflammation. Although we say to avoid eating oily fish, once you have the pure fish oil, the proteins that cause the problem have been removed. Take 2–3 grams daily with food.

Helpful Hints
- Lose weight, as this is quite often part of the problem. Remember that gout is pretty much self-inflicted and almost entirely brought on by a rich diet. Be prepared to make some changes.
- Nettle tea will also aid with excretion of uric acid.
- Massage the painful joint with essential oil of Roman camomile, juniper, wintergreen and ginger to help reduce the pain and inflammation.
- Homeopathic Ledum 30c twice daily for 2–3 days will reduce symptoms.
- Do not take aspirin if you are taking anti-gout drugs.

GUMS
(see Bleeding Gums)

HAEMORRHOIDS
(see Constipation and Piles)

HAIR LOSS
(see also Absorption, Circulation and Stress)

The average person loses between 70 and 100 hairs a day, and as we age our hair becomes finer and/or thinner. Most of us tend to associate balding and thinning hair with men, and yet many women experience thinning hair, too. In fact many trichologists, who 10 years ago tended to see more men than women experiencing hair loss problems, are now seeing just as many women suffering hair loss – even Asian and Caribbean women, who traditionally have beautiful, thick hair. Our Western lifestyle seems to be a major factor.

There are a number of causes for hair loss, such as hormonal changes at menopause or after childbirth – but for the majority of women with hair problems, stress is probably the most likely culprit. Stress robs us of major nutrients that are essential for healthy hair growth. When a person is very stressed the scalp becomes tight, which restricts circulation; and the hair follicles becomes malnourished resulting in further hair loss. Adrenal exhaustion, an underactive thyroid, and certain prescription drugs are also factors in hair loss.

Naturopath Stephen Langley says: 'In Chinese medicine the lung *chi* governs the shine or lustre of the hair and the thickness and strength is governed by the kidney *chi*. Roughly translated, this means that the shine and lustre is dulled by our reduced capability to oxygenate our blood cells fully. We can all see evidence of dull-looking hair when we are tired and don't exercise enough, or through anxiety, which causes us to shallow-breathe. Smoking will have the same effect.

'The kidney *chi* is depleted through poor nutrient supply that helps make up our essence or primary energy reserves. This happens also when we are run down or our adrenal glands become exhausted through burning the candle at both ends. Our requirements for nutrients under these circumstances will be much greater. We literally feed off our own body, and nutrients will be taken from less important areas (such as the scalp) to supply more important tissues, such as the organs. And if tissues are too acid, which they are when we are stressed, then minerals needed for healthy hair, such as iron, magnesium and zinc, are taken from the hair follicles to buffer this acidity.' See *Acid–Alkaline Balance*.

Mainly then, the health of your hair depends upon the circulation to the root of the hair and the amount of nutrients present in the blood. Hair is composed of a protein-like substance called keratin, and requires a healthy balanced diet for proper nourishment. Many drugs are claimed to increase hair growth, but some have negative side effects, which include an inability for men to maintain an erection. So before trying any of these drugs, always discuss any implications with your doctor or trichologist.

Another important factor is the male hormone testosterone, which is also found in women. Although this hormone is responsible for making men hairy during puberty, it also has a large role to play in hair loss in later life, in both men and women. Some women have too much testosterone, which shows up in excess facial hair and can trigger male-type thinning. In this case, taking the herbs *Vitex agnus castus* or saw palmetto helps to reduce testosterone levels.

Hereditary factors are also important. The more hair loss there is/was in your father, uncles and grandfathers, the more likely you are to lose your own hair. However, dietary supplements and regular daily firm-scalp massage can help slow down hair loss. Hair loss in much younger people is also becoming extremely common, showing that stress is definitely a trigger. Stress and a toxic bowel prevent production of some of the B-vitamins that are necessary for maintaining hair colour and healthy hair.

Hair loss in women is common after childbirth and the menopause, and a lack of protein can trigger thinning hair or even cause it to fall out. Hair loss is also linked to heavy metal toxicity. I have seen several cases of alopecia in young women due to stress, which triggered a leaky gut; when they started taking a digestive enzyme with an easily absorbed multi-nutrient with meals, the hair grew back.

It is thought that men lose hair on the tops of their heads rather than the backs and sides because the blood flow to the top of the scalp is reduced in comparison to the sides.

Hair grows faster in summer and a single hair can live for several years. On average human hair grows between 12 and 15cm (5 and 6in) a year.

Foods to Avoid
- Although protein is needed for healthy hair, too much protein such as red meat and cheese without sufficient fruit and vegetables leaves the body very acid, which depletes reserves of important alkaline minerals necessary for healthy hair.
- Reduce caffeine from any source. Caffeine increases stress (as it triggers adrenaline and cortisol to be released) and weakens the adrenal glands.
- Avoid sugar and refined carbohydrates, such as pastries, cakes, desserts, pies and so on, all of which deplete nutrients needed for hair growth.
- Reduce the amount of sodium-based salt in your diet.

Friendly Foods
- Quality protein is the most important food for your hair. Eat organic lean meats, chicken and game, including venison, in moderation, plus fish and eggs (particularly egg white).

- Whey, milk, yoghurt and cheese are also rich in protein. But don't eat too much cheese, as it's very acid forming – like all dairy foods.
- If you cannot tolerate whey protein from cows, then use organic hemp seed protein powders; for a healthy smoothie recipe, see under *General Health Hints*.
- Vegetarian-based proteins are found in seeds, nuts, vegetables, wholegrains such as brown rice and quinoa, plus legumes, such as peas, lentils, soya beans, tofu, tempeh, lentils and peanuts.
- Eat more iron-rich foods, such as egg yolks, green leafy vegetables (for example, spinach, curly kale and watercress), wholegrain breads and cereals, meat (especially organic liver) and fish.
- Try adding seaweeds such as kombu, arame and wakame to meals. You use them as you would a green vegetable and they are a rich source of minerals needed for healthy hair.
- Essential fats are vital for healthy hair and a healthy scalp; therefore eat more oily fish, plus walnuts, pumpkin seeds, sunflower seeds or linseeds (flax seeds soaked in cold water overnight, drained and then eaten) and their unrefined oils, mixed half and half with olive oil. Use them for salad dressings and drizzle on cooked foods. Essential fats help you to avoid a dry, scaly scalp, and they nourish the hair follicles. See *Fats You Need To Eat*.
- Coriander, chlorophyll (and selenium) detoxify heavy metals from the body and are full of nutrients, especially B-vitamins. Most organic green food powders contain plenty of chlorophyll. A good version is Green Magic Powder, containing Hawaiian spirulina, chlorella, lecithin, barley and wheat grass juice, kamut, pectin apple fibre, kelp, wheat sprouts, CoQ10, artichoke powder and healthy bacteria – for details log on to www.itsgreenmagic.com or call Helen Cruikshank on 07798 873266.

- Muesli, cereals and oats are all high in B-vitamins.
- Eat one avocado a week to help your hair shine.
- Good sources of copper needed for healthy hair are Brazil nuts, almonds, walnuts, hazelnuts, along with lecithin granules sprinkled over your morning cereal.

Useful Remedies

- Take a good-quality multi-vitamin/mineral daily; most of the companies listed at the beginning of the book supply specific hair-nutrient formulas. You will need at least 15–30mg of zinc and 1–2mg of copper in your multi-, as lack of copper is linked to greying hair.
- A Finnish company called Viviscal make good multi hair products – call 01923 852790 for stockists or details.
- Romanda Healthcare makes an excellent formula that contains all the nutrients needed for healthy hair, plus a growth serum and shampoo (see *Helpful Hints*, opposite, for contact details).
- Naturopath Stephen Langley has formulated a blood cleanser, called Essential Detox Combination, that has been shown to help restore hair loss due to stress and mineral depletion. The quality of your scalp depends on the quality of the blood supplying the roots. As we age, the quality of our blood is reduced because of the accumulation of toxins. Once the blood is able to carry more oxygen and nutrients, hair can improve. Take 1 teaspoon in a glass of water 3 times daily, preferably before meals. www.holoshealth.com
- The B-group vitamins are vital if you want to keep your hair, and many people who take a full spectrum of B-vitamins report that their grey hairs disappear. B5, PABA, biotin and folic acid are the anti-greying nutrients and you would need 1000mcg of biotin daily. Check the content of your multi before taking extra Bs.
- Vitamin B6 x 50mg per day is helpful for women taking the contraceptive pill, which can affect hair loss. **You do not need this if your multi contains 50mg of B6.**
- Find out if you are low in iron, in which case take a liquid, easily absorbable formula such as

Spatone. Available from health shops worldwide. Don't take iron unless you need it. If you cook in iron pots, you will absorb some of the iron in your food. **NB Never leave iron supplements near children.**

- CT241, plus Colleginase, which contain vitamin C, rutin, hesperidin, cellulose, silica, and vitamins A and D to strengthen hair and nails. **BC**
- Herbs that help balance hormones naturally if your hair is thinning because of the menopause include dong quai, black cohosh, sage and soya isoflavones. All the companies mentioned at the front of the book sell these supplements.
- Thinning hair in men, caused by excess dihydrotestosterone, can be balanced by taking saw palmetto (500mg daily, under supervision – it may need to be higher) and zinc (30mg daily).

Helpful Hints

- Take regular exercise, which will stimulate your heart and circulation, thus increasing oxygen flow, reducing stress, and promoting scalp and hair health.
- There is a myth saying that the more you brush your hair, the thicker and healthier it will grow – it's not true. Too much brushing pulls hair out, breaks it and scratches the scalp.
- Don't over dry your hair as this makes it more brittle.
- 'Women who lose a lot of hair after giving birth should stop panicking,' says London- and New York-based trichologist Philip Kingsley. 'During pregnancy oestrogen levels are higher and this hormone prolongs the natural life span of a hair. The average person loses 70–100 hairs a day, but during pregnancy hair falls out less, because of the oestrogen. Then 4–6 weeks later the woman gives birth and hormones return to normal levels – and all the normal shedding that should have happened during the previous months occurs all at once. As long as these women eat a healthy diet and take the right supplements, the hair should soon get back to normal.'

- Philip Kingsley has formulated various hormone drops for men and women that nourish the follicle and help prevent hair loss. They don't make hair re-grow if the hair loss is permanent, but they help you to keep the hair that you have. For details in the UK call 020 7629 4004. In New York call 001 212 753 9600. Website: www.philipkingsley.co.uk. For more help on hair, read Philip Kingsley's book *The Hair Bible* (Aurum Press).
- Some doctors have noticed that smokers tend to lose their hair faster than non-smokers.
- Shampoo your hair regularly; this helps to re-moisturize the hair.
- Jojoba oil mixed with a little essential oil of rosemary and massaged into the scalp removes dead skin cells and increases circulation. Be firm, you need the skin on your scalp to move so that blood can circulate more freely. Do this before going to bed and leave the oils on overnight.
- Some yogis say that by doing head and shoulder stands they have kept their hair because the circulation to their heads is greatly increased. If, like me, you are not into head stands, simply lie on the floor and put your calves up on a chair or a bed. This not only helps gives your leg veins a rest, it encourages more blood to the head.
- Chlorine from swimming pools damages your hair and is also linked to asthma and heart disease.
- To find your nearest qualified trichologist, call 08456 044657 or visit the Institute of Trichologists website at www.trichologists.org.uk
- Try Romanda lotion and shampoos, along with Romanda hair formula powder supplements. Call Jan Adams on the Romanda Advice Line on 0208 346 0784, or e-mail jan_romanda@hotmail.com or log on to www.romanda-healthcare.co.uk. Jan is very helpful and formed the company after suffering hair loss. She also helps people with hair loss after chemotherapy, plus alopecia and patchy hair loss.

- Numerous salons offer hair transplants, which are becoming more sophisticated. Professor Nick Lowe, a dermatologist, offers the latest technique called Micro Grafting, which gives a more natural-looking hairline, rather than hundreds of 'puncture marks'. The surgery is expensive, but the results are amazing. For details in the UK, call the Cranley Clinic on 020 7499 3223.
- Philip Kingsley recommends Dr Patricia Cahuzac in Paris. He says her transplant work is the best he has ever seen anywhere. Dr Cahuzac often sees patients for their initial consultation in London – but she works in Paris. Her address is 16 Rue Clément-Marot, Paris 75008, France. Tel: 00 33 15 65 20 101.
- The Hair Clinic at John Bell and Croydon in London also offers a Micro Grafting service at 50–54 Wigmore Street, London. Tel: 020 7224 4640.

HALITOSIS (bad breath) *(see also Liver Problems)*

Bad breath is often caused by poor dental hygiene and/or poor digestion, gut functioning and a sluggish bowel. A build-up of plaque, infected gums, abscesses, and insufficient brushing and flossing are mostly to blame. Make sure you see a qualified dental hygienist at least twice a year. Use fluoride-free floss and mouthwash daily, change your toothbrush regularly, and clean your teeth at least twice a day – but not immediately after eating fruit.

Foods such as meat take a long time to digest and can putrefy in the bowel. One of the simple things you can do is to chew properly, as this enhances carbohydrate digestion and makes it easier for the rest of the digestive process. Try not to eat too much food at one sitting, which overloads the stomach and bowel.

One of the Atkins Diets, which suggests a high-protein, low-carbohydrate way of eating, was notorious for triggering constipation and bad breath. Some people find their digestion improves if they avoid eating proteins and carbohydrates together in one meal. For example, if you are eating a meal of chicken or fish (protein), accompany it with vegetables only and not with starches. Conversely, if you are eating a rice or pasta dinner, eat it with vegetables only and not with protein.

Long-term bad breath can also indicate problems with the liver or kidneys, or diabetes, in which case you must consult a doctor. If the bowel is severely congested with impacted matter, the body re-absorbs the toxins into the blood and hence the lungs, and toxins are then breathed out. See under *Constipation*.

Foods to Avoid
- Avoid too much caffeine, sugar and low-fibre, high-fat foods, which all weaken the digestion and cause sluggish bowel movements. This includes white breads, cakes, biscuits and pastas.
- Smoking not only causes bad breath directly, it can also cause it indirectly as it weakens digestion.
- Cut down on the amount of milk and dairy produce from cows, which is mucous forming and slows bowel function.

Friendly Foods
- Leafy green vegetables, such as pak choy, spring greens, kale, watercress and cabbage are rich in chlorophyll. Chlorophyll is useful in helping to clear the bowel, thus helping to improve the smell of the breath.
- Eat more artichokes, celeriac, radicchio (Italian chicory) and chicory – see dietary advice in *Liver Problems*.

- Eat plenty of fresh whole fruits. Pineapple or papaya, eaten either before or after a meal, are useful, as the enzymes in these fruits can help break down the proteins, ensuring proper digestion.
- A 'bio' or live yoghurt containing acidophilus and bifidus, either for breakfast or as a dessert, improves the quality of the bacteria in the bowel, enhancing digestion and making bad breath less likely.
- Add more coriander and fresh mint to foods, and eat fennel or caraway seeds, which help kill the bacteria that cause bad breath.
- Drink fenugreek tea and also green tea, which help to kill bacteria in the mouth.
- Aloe Pura make an excellent Stomach Formula Aloe Juice; drink a capful before main meals to further aid digestion.
- Fructo-Oligosaccharides (FOS) – a powder – can be used as a sweetener, and acts as a prebiotic that helps the body to make more healthy bacteria in the gut, which in turn can help reduce bad breath. Take 5–20 grams daily sprinkled onto cereals or smoothies. **BC**
- Drink plenty of water.

Useful Remedies

- Sprinkle 1–3 dessertspoons of linseeds (flax seeds that have been soaked overnight in cold water and drained) into porridge or mix in a smoothie. You will find a good recipe under *General Health Hints*. Otherwise, use ready-cracked linseeds, such as Linwood's, which do not need soaking.
- Also use organic sunflower seeds over salads, breakfast cereals and so on to encourage toxins to move more quickly through the bowel.
- Betaine hydrochloride (stomach acid): 1 capsule taken with main meals improves protein digestion and ensures that foods are completely digested and don't arrive at the bowel causing fermentation. **Not to be taken if you have active stomach ulcers, in which case take a digestive enzyme free from hydrochloric acid. BC**
- Acidophilus and bifidus capsules with FOS (fructo-Oligosaccharides), which increase healthy bacteria. One to two capsules taken at the end of the meal can increase healthy bacteria in the bowel and enhance digestion. **BC**
- Take 5–6 drops of chlorophyll daily to help eliminate bad breath
- Most organic green food powders contain plenty of chlorophyll.
- Try Green Magic Powder, containing Hawaiian spirulina, chlorella, lecithin, barley and wheat grass juice, kamut, pectin apple fibre, kelp, wheat sprouts, CoQ10, artichoke powder and healthy bacteria – for details log on to www.itsgreenmagic.com or call Helen Cruikshank on 07798 873266.
- Try Lepicol capsules or powder (also includes beneficial bacteria) – take daily. Available from health stores and some pharmacies.
- Make a mouthwash of one capful of hydrogen peroxide mixed with four capfuls of water – swill around the mouth, hold for one minute and then spit out. This helps to oxygenate the gums and kill off bacteria.

Helpful Hints

- Make up your own healthy mouthwash using a few drops of essential oils of tea tree, peppermint, thyme and lemon. Mix with warm water and use regularly after meals and before bed. I make up mine with boiled water, which I allow to cool, and then I keep the blend in a dark bottle in my bathroom and it lasts for ages.
- Exercise regularly as this ensures healthy bowel function.
- If the bad breath is severe, with your doctor's permission, have a colonic irrigation, which gently washes out the bowel helping to reduce toxicity (see *Useful Information*).

- Contact the Fresh Breath Centre, 2 Devonshire Place, London W1G 6HJ; or call 020 7935 1666. Website: www.freshbreath.co.uk
- Ask at your chemist for a tongue scraper; use regularly to help clear bacteria off your tongue
- For immediate breath freshening, use a drop of pure peppermint oil on the tongue.

HANGOVERS
(see Alcohol)

HAYFEVER
(see also Allergies, Allergic Rhinitis and Liver Problems)

Dr Jean Monro, an allergy specialist at the Breakspear Hospital in Hertfordshire, says: 'Before the industrial revolution, conditions such as hayfever did not exist. But since then we have done a great job of polluting our atmosphere and thus our bodies, which is why hayfever is actually more common in city-dwellers than in people who live in the country. We now know that an accumulation of a variety of pollutants, such as paint sprays or pesticides (there are hundreds of others), acts as the initial trigger; these chemicals became the sensitizers – and in most cases the membranes within the nose and throat begin to react by becoming inflamed. Then the body treats the next thing that comes along, such as grass pollens, as a threatening foreign invader, which increases any inflammation and induces allergic-type symptoms. But it's important to realize that it's the chemicals that sensitize the body in the first place. Chemicals can have a local effect, such as on the skin, and then this effect is communicated to the rest of the body by neural (nerve) pathways and a sensitivity is born.'

This is important news to anyone suffering from hayfever, as Dr Monro and her colleagues have developed vaccines that can help to neutralize any reaction to substances found to trigger a response. For more details, see under *Allergies*.

Meanwhile, symptoms vary from sore, puffy, itchy, watering eyes to continual sneezing and a runny or congested nose. Hayfever is sometimes confused with a condition called allergic or perennial rhinitis, as the symptoms are similar to those of hayfever but occur all year round. Common causes of allergic rhinitis include dust, food allergies and atmospheric pollution. Many people with hayfever and allergic rhinitis are also likely to have a sensitivity to certain foods, the most common being wheat and potentially dairy produce from any source, but some sufferers have problems with anything from eggs to bananas. As this has been linked to digestive problems for some people, see also *Leaky Gut*.

Foods to Avoid
- Greatly reduce your exposure to any foods with additives and/or preservatives, and that have been sprayed with pesticides and herbicides – eat organic. Keep in mind that non-organic apples, for example, can be sprayed up to 18 times before being sold.
- Any foods to which you have an intolerance; typically these would include wheat, dairy products, eggs, and citrus fruits – especially oranges.
- Dairy foods are mucous forming and without doubt can exacerbate the problem. While symptoms are acute, avoid milk in any form for at least one week, plus cheeses, chocolate and foods high in saturated fats, such as croissants, Danish pastries, meat pies and white-flour-based cakes and biscuits.
- Many foods high in sugar, such as puddings and sweets, are also high in dairy and fats. Too much sugar will greatly lower immune function.
- Reduce salt, caffeine and alcohol.

Friendly Foods
- Ingesting sufficient fluids is important, as researchers have found that people who are dehydrated tend to suffer more hayfever-type symptoms.
- Garlic and onions are high in the flavonoid quercetin, which can help reduce the severity of allergic reactions.
- Nettle tea helps to ease the symptoms of allergic rhinitis.
- Dairy-free alternatives to cow's milk are organic rice, almond, oat and pea milk. You can also try low-fat coconut milk; look for Kara Dairy Free – it's one of the better tasting non-dairy milks (www.karadairyfree.com). If animal-source dairy produce is a problem, try these milks in small amounts and note if they trigger a reaction.
- Have a freshly squeezed vegetable juice, especially beetroot, artichoke, a little garlic, ginger, apple and carrot, which boosts the immune system and helps eliminate toxins.
- Bioflavonoids are important protectors of mucous membranes, so eat plenty of blueberries, blackberries, plums, red grapes, strawberries and cherries.
- Include plenty of fresh vegetables, brown rice and whole grains in your diet.

Useful Remedies
- Quercetin, 400mg, 3 times a day, is a natural antihistamine, which helps reduce puffy eyes and reduces irritation in the nose.
- While symptoms are acute, take up to 2–3 grams of vitamin C daily in an ascorbate form with food, which again acts like a mild antihistamine.
- Beta Glucans 1–3, 1–6, derived from yeast cell walls, are proven to strengthen the body's innate immune system (the one you were born with), making it more resistant to airborne pathogens. It also helps reduce incidence of food intolerances. Can also be taken by children. Take 250–500 mg daily. **PN**. To see good research on beta glucans, see Dr Paul Clayton's site on www.healthdefence.com

- Butterbur, a plant, taken in capsule form can help treat hay fever. Take 500mg twice daily.
- Nettle tablets or tincture 3 times a day has proven to be effective for allergic rhinitis.
- Onion and horseradish concentrate, as all of these herbs can ease congestion and reduce the symptoms of hayfever. Take 1–2ml as needed. Herbs Hands & Healing supply this on 0845 345 3727.
- Histazyme contains calcium, vitamin C, the amino acid lysine, zinc, vitamin B6, silica, bromelain, vitamin A and manganese, which all help if you suffer seasonal disorders. Take 1 capsule twice daily. **This formula is not to be taken if you are pregnant. BC**
- If nothing else, take a high-strength multi-vitamin and mineral that contains plenty of the B-group vitamins.
- Take probiotics daily – these healthy bacteria help to boost immune function and heal the gut wall, thus reducing the toxins that enter the bloodstream. **BC**
- Alka Life is a green herbal food supplement rich in bee pollen. Sprinkle daily over breakfast cereal for at least one month prior to the hayfever season to help reduce the severity or onset of an attack. Available from health stores, or for your nearest stockists contact Best Care Products on 01342 410303, or log on to www.bestcare-UK.com **NB. Do not use if you are highly allergic to bee stings.**

Helpful Hints
- It's well worth checking for food intolerances – see details of the York or Genova Tests under the *Helpful Hints* in *Allergies*.
- Begin subscribing to *Allergy* magazine; details under *Allergies*.
- Ask your GP to refer you to the Breakspear Medical Group, which specializes in the treatment of allergies and environmental illness. The NHS will pay if your GP agrees.

Otherwise, you can call them direct and pay privately. Telephone 01442 261333 or log on to www.breakspearmedical.com.

■ Buy a pot of honey from your local area, preferably with the honeycomb still in it, and take a dessertspoonful daily for about a month before the onset of the hayfever season. The pollen in the honey may protect you from developing full-blown hayfever.

■ Homeopathy has been successful in treating hayfever with remedies such as allium cepa, euphrasia or 'mixed pollens'. Ask for details at your local homeopathic pharmacy or see *Useful Information* to find a qualified practitioner in your area. The Organic Pharmacy makes a combination mixture in a tablet, which makes this easier. **OP**

■ Place a few drops of essential oil of basil and melissa on a handkerchief to help clear the sinuses. Massage these oils into the chest and throat once mixed with a base carrier oil, such as almond or jojoba.

■ Treat yourself to a good-quality ionizer and place it near your bed to help reduce any allergens in the air around you.

HEAD LICE
(see Scalp Problems)

HEALING AND HEALERS
(see also Electrical Pollution)

There is now such a huge body of validated independent scientific evidence that hands-on healing and prayer have in many cases positive physical affects that the efficacy of healing itself is no longer in doubt. Some hospitals and doctor's surgeries offer healing on the NHS and there are hundreds of Reiki healers working in alternative treatment centres globally. Some people still believe that healing cannot work unless one has a specific religious belief or strong faith that the healing will work. Yet there are hundreds of documented cases where young babies, plants, children and animals have responded positively to healing. To understand how healing works, it is imperative first to comprehend that we are all electrical beings in a physical shell. If you take a photograph using Kirlian cameras, you can clearly see the energy or auric field surrounding a person, animal, plant, vegetable; in fact any object, even a stone will have an auric field. Roger Coghill, a bioelectromagnetics research scientist based in Wales, says: 'An individual's energy field or aura is as unique to them as their DNA. When we become ill, our field's characteristics change; this was proven by the American neurologist Albert Abrams in 1916.'

After my near-death experience in 1998, which is documented in my book *Divine Intervention* (Cico Books), I truly began to comprehend how healing works. Professor Gary Schwartz at the University of Arizona conducted experiments during 2002 in which a well-known healer, Rosalyn Bruyere, taught 26 doctors and nurses how to give hands-on healing. After the training it was found that the nurses and doctors were able to absorb more gamma cosmic rays (which are the highest frequencies we can measure) – and then their bodies acted like transformers, literally 'turning down' the cosmic ray frequencies into subtle x-ray frequencies, which they then focused and pulsed into patients' energy fields. There are also machines that mimic this process. Biophysicist Harry Oldfield spent 20 years developing a PIP scanner, which can 'read' the energies being emitted from our bodies. During his early research at some of the UK's leading teaching hospitals, Harry began to notice that when he compared patients' energy emissions before and after treatments such as chemotherapy, the treatments triggered energy distortions, which eventually manifested as negative symptoms.

Over the following 20 years he became an expert at correctly interpreting these energy distortions – and eventually concluded that if these distortions could be treated with correcting harmonic frequencies, this could normalize the person's energy field, which would encourage the body to heal itself. Years later, he designed electro-crystal healing for this purpose.

When we become sick, cells begin emitting disharmonic frequencies, which can clearly be seen in our energy field on his specialist scanners. Harry has found that every illness shows up in our energy field before appearing in the physical body. To counteract various medical conditions, he simply pulses the correct tonal frequency back into the patient to encourage the body to heal itself. This is what healers have been doing intuitively for thousands of years. Harry has trained hundreds of therapists in the UK and globally; for more information on your nearest therapist, Harry Oldfield's PIP scanners and his electro-crystal therapy, visit www.electrocrystal.com

New frequency-based vaccines for allergies work on similar principals – see *Allergies*. This is how dolphins heal. They have been on the planet for 30 million years longer than humans and their brains are highly developed. They can 'scan' someone, much the same as a good healer can, and they then pulse harmonic, healing frequencies back into the patient, which over time can encourage the body to heal itself. And when Harry has scanned healers while they are working, he says the transfer of energy can be clearly seen on his equipment. I have seen film of this myself. Also Harry has said that sometimes the healing energy emanates from inside the healers – usually from within their heart or solar plexus energy centres – while at other times they can clearly see energy from outside the healer being absorbed into the healer and then out through their hands.

However, both Oldfield and Schwartz and other scientists, such as those based at the Institute for Noetic Science in America, make it clear that, in the majority of cases, without a clear intention from the healer, little or no energy transfers take place. Also they say that it's vital that the healer should be in a positive frame of mind and not be sick themselves when they offer healing to a patient.

Of course, some healers are better than others – just as there are better pianists, computer experts, or surgeons. Recalling that we all emit our own unique range of frequencies, you need to find a healer who is on a compatible range of frequencies to your own, then you generally receive a more beneficial effect. You will soon know after 3 or 4 sessions whether their healing is making any difference, and if you are no better, simply find another healer. It is also possible to facilitate a transfer of healing energies over distances – and the science as to how this is possible is detailed in my book, *Countdown to Coherence* (Watkins Publishing).

Remember, energy can neither be created nor destroyed – it can only change into other forms of energy. Your thoughts are energy – they go somewhere – and when the intention is done with the whole heart and is for the receiver's greater good, your prayers will reach their destination. And the more people who pray at the same time with the same intention, the more powerful the prayer becomes. According to well-known healers such as Seka Nikolic, it is imperative that we transmit only positive thoughts and visualize the person as looking 100% well in our mind's eye or imagination. I have also detailed more information on healing and the science of miracles, plus the science behind how spontaneous healing occurs, in my book *The Evidence For The Sixth Sense* (Cico Books).

Helpful Hints

■ The human mind is far more powerful than most people can even begin to imagine; therefore if you also truly believe the healing will work, this really helps. Remember, there is a huge difference between wanting something to work and believing 100% that it will.

- I find healing a great additional therapy when used in conjunction with eating the right diet and so on. It literally recharges your internal batteries, which gives your body more energy to heal itself. Most healers find that the great majority of their patients are looking for a single magic bullet to heal their ills. But if they continue eating junk foods (or foods to which they have an intolerance), take no exercise and so on, obviously it's like trying to put out a fire while you remain standing in the flames.
- Then again, I have witnessed many miracles. Cancers have disappeared, crippled people have walked again. How can this happen? I firmly believe this is a combination of the power of the sick person's mind believing they are well and the ability of the healer to transmit a strong healing signal. Also, spiritual masters can without doubt effect healing miracles without the person's knowledge. But I also know that if a person believes 100% with their mind and heart that they are truly healed, in that instant they are.
- Read *The Biology of Belief* by cell biologist Bruce H. Lipton Ph.D., which documents dozens of validated case studies in healing and the mind.
- To find out more about Reiki, log on to www.reikiassociation.org.uk For non-membership enquiries call 07704 270727.
- Although there are hundreds of good healers in the UK alone, there are two I would mention. The first is Seka Nikolic, who practices in London. Contact her via 0207 443 5544. Her books are well worth a read or log on to her website www.sekanikolic.com. The second healer is Kelvin Heard, who specializes in chronic fatigue or ME. He is based in France, but treats people in the UK once a month. Email him at kelvinheardhealer@kelvinheardhealer.org.
- To find your nearest registered, insured healer call The Healing Trust on 01604 603247. They have a worldwide network of healers. Visit their website on www.thehealingtrust.org.uk
- The Nutri Centre bookshop on 020 7323 2382 can also help you with any number of books on healing.

HEARTBURN
(see Acid Stomach, Indigestion and Low Stomach Acid)

HEART DISEASE
(see also Angina, Atherosclerosis, Cholesterol, Circulation and High Blood Pressure)

Heart disease and diseases of the circulatory system account for the death of one in every four men and one in every six women. Around 300,000 people in the UK suffer a heart attack each year and the faster you can receive medical attention, the more likely you are to survive. Eighty percent of people who suffer a heart attack now receive potentially life-saving drugs within 30 minutes of their arrival at hospital.

The majority of younger people who die with heart disease are male. Once women go through the menopause, their risk of dying from heart disease increases threefold (see *Menopause*). And symptoms of a heart attack can vary somewhat between men and women.

Your heart is an amazing organ – a simple pump that can beat around 70 times a minute non-stop for 100 or more years, pumping more than 10 million litres (2.6 million gallons) of blood around your 100,000km (62,000 miles) of blood vessels every year. While it works, we tend to take it for granted – and yet if more people could think of their heart health from their 30s onwards, heart and arterial disease would not be the number one killer in the Western world.

For some people, there is a genetic predisposition towards developing heart disease – but if you eat healthily and change any negative and unhealthy lifestyle patterns practised by your parents and grandparents, then in most cases you can stack the cards in your favour and add decades to your life. The heart, like any other muscle, needs its own blood supply and receives this via three main vessels called the coronary arteries. Over time, one or more of the arteries can become blocked and if an artery becomes completely blocked, some of the heart muscle may die during a heart attack.

Typically, symptoms of a heart attack include a severe pressing band of pain across the chest that can spread up the neck and into the jaw or across the shoulders and down into the left arm. This is often termed a 'myocardial infarction' (MI), which means death of the heart muscle due to an interrupted blood supply. The muscle may simply stop beating or, more commonly, it goes into an irregular pattern, which no longer works like a pump. Sweating, breathlessness and a feeling of nausea can accompany a heart attack, which needs **urgent** medical attention.

A heart attack can be fatal, unless someone can apply immediate cardio-pulmonary resuscitation (CPR is something everyone should learn and one day you may save a life with this simple skill). Luckily, many people survive their first heart attack. Specialists may recommend drugs and/or by-pass surgery or other operative procedures, but it's important to consider that none of these medical or surgical treatments attempts to solve the underlying cause of the problem, only the result of the problem.

While some heart attacks appear to strike out of the blue, there are usually warning signs telling us that something wrong. Some women (and men) report feeling as though they have indigestion, but in women the pain seems to be centred more in the middle of the chest rather than towards the left side and discomfort or pain is felt between the shoulder blades. Some people report having spasms that travel up their spine and that the jaw pain on both sides can be severe, while others report a sense of 'impending doom'. **Please take notice.**

And just because you don't have a high cholesterol level, don't think, 'It cannot be a heart attack', as myocardial infarction can be triggered by long-term stress and inflammation in the body. **Call an ambulance.** Do not think, 'I'll see how I feel in the morning'... Better to have a false alarm than to die!

Another common warning of heart problems is angina – a constrictive pain in the chest that is provoked by exertion. It's the body's signal that the blood supply to the heart is inadequate, owing to narrowed arteries or spasms in the coronary arteries. If you experience angina, it's time to act. You can still turn it around and live another 40 years or more. Some people have gone on to run a marathon after their first heart attack. If you suffer angina or have had a heart attack, then you need to radically change your diet, increase exercise (gently) and reduce stress.

Other known risk factors for heart disease include smoking, excessive alcohol consumption, high blood pressure, high homocysteine levels (see *High Blood Pressure*), high LDL cholesterol levels, being overweight, diabetes, taking insufficient exercise, eating a high-fat, -salt and -sugar diet, insufficient intake of fresh fruit and vegetables, excessive stress and inflammation. Stress thickens the blood, which in the long term can kill you, and a Type-A personality, who becomes angry easily, is more prone to heart disease.

There are also links with heart disease via inflammatory conditions caused by the parasite chlamydia pneumonia, and poor root canal treatment is also linked to heart disease. Mercury is also linked to heart disease, as are unbalanced hormone levels – including thyroid hormones, progesterone and testosterone. Also statins, now used by 7 million people in the UK to control their high cholesterol levels, place a strain on all muscles including the heart muscle, as they block production of a vitamin-like substance, CoQ10, which is produced naturally in the liver. This is needed for a healthy heart – but as we age, production of this vital heart-protecting substance slows and statins exacerbate the problem further.

Foods to Avoid

- Cut down on saturated fats found in meats, butter, cheese, cream and hard margarines. Keep in mind that many low-fat foods are high in sugar, which will convert to fat in the body if it is not burned off during exercise.
- Reduce the amount of concentrated shop-bought fruit juices, fizzy drinks, desserts, cakes and pastries you eat.
- Reduce dairy foods, especially milk. Research published in *The Lancet* in 1999 showed how changes in a country's milk-consumption pattern, either up or down, accurately predicted changes in coronary deaths 4 to 7 years later.
- Especially avoid any foods and mass-produced oils containing hydrogenated or trans-fats, which are found in most mass-produced biscuits, pies, cakes and so on.
- Don't eat too much fried food, as frying damages fats and turns them into dangerous fats that heart surgeons find in your arteries.
- Cut down on sodium-based table salts. Use a low-salt alternative or a little magnesium or potassium-rich sea salt, available from all good health stores and most supermarkets. Try nori flakes or kelp flakes, which are rich in minerals and do not cause the damage that sodium-based salts do.

- Greatly reduce your intake of mass-produced burgers, pies, sausages, pastries, cakes and desserts.
- Avoid excessive alcohol consumption; even though a moderate intake – that is, 1 glass a day – is slightly protective. Large amounts of alcohol over time is a known risk factor for heart disease. Red wine, such as Pinot Noir, seems to confer the most health benefits, as it's high in polyphenols, bioflavonoids that help protect the arteries. Aim for around no more than 6 units a week on average. See *Alcohol*.

Friendly Foods

- Pomegranate has been proven in several trials to disrupt formation of plaque, and has also shown some benefit in reducing blood pressure. I eat at least a tablespoon daily. Otherwise, drink the juice daily. Trials in America found that when patients drank the juice daily for a year, atherosclerosis was reduced by as much as 25%. The most potent form to take includes pomegranate whole fruit, flower and seed extracts. See www.lef.org for details.
- Oily fish are rich in omega-3 essential fats: farmed organic salmon, black cod, sardines, pilchards, red snapper, mackerel, trout and herrings are good sources, as are linseeds (flax seeds). Try to eat oily fish two or three times a week.
- Generally, eat more fish of any kind in preference to meats.
- Unrefined, unsalted seeds, such as pumpkin, linseed (flax seed), sesame and sunflower, and their unrefined oils, are also a good source of essential fats. Use unrefined organic linseed oil for salad dressings, as people who consume more linseed oil, which contains omega-3 essential fats, have a lower risk of developing heart disease.
- Lean meats such as venison, boar, buffalo, rabbit, chicken (preferably breast meat with skin removed) and turkey are fine in moderation.
- Avocado oil contains monounsaturated fats and is great for salad dressings, as is walnut oil. Make them organic and always keep cool. Never cook with these oils.
- Eat plenty of fruits and vegetables that are high in carotenes and antioxidants – such as carrots, asparagus, French beans, broccoli, Brussels sprouts, watercress, pumpkin, papaya,

cabbage, spinach, sweet potatoes, spring greens, apricots, mangoes and tomatoes – which help lower your risk of heart disease.

- Include brown rice and pastas, porridge oats, beans, wholemeal/ stone-ground bread and other grains, such as quinoa, amaranth and barley in your diet.
- Eat more garlic and onions, which help thin the blood naturally.
- Fibre, derived from fruits and vegetables, is very protective and additional fibre from linseeds (flax seeds), oat or rice bran or psyllium husks all help lower the risk.
- Eating pistachios, walnuts, pecan nuts and macadamia nuts on a regular basis have been shown to help lower LDL cholesterol.
- Wheat germ and soya beans are rich in natural vitamin E, which has been shown to reduce the risk of heart disease. This is particularly true for people who have stickier blood such as Type A or AB blood.
- Use non-hydrogenated spreads such as Biona, Vitaquell or Olivio. There is nothing wrong with a little butter, as long as you are eating sufficient omega-3 essential fats. Otherwise, try organic raw walnut, hemp seed or almond butters, available from health stores.
- A vegetarian diet, using a lot of beans, vegetables, grains and pulses, dramatically lowers your risk of developing heart disease.
- Sprinkle 1 dessertspoon of soya lecithin granules over breakfast cereals and desserts, which really helps to break down the 'bad' LDL fats and, as a bonus, nourishes your brain. **SVHC**
- Olive oil raises HDL (the good cholesterol) levels, lowers bad LDL cholesterol, and contains antioxidants that protect the LDL from damage.
- Drink more fluids.

Useful Remedies

- One of the most important nutrients for your heart is Co-enzyme Q10, which is a vitamin-like substance that your body manufactures naturally in the liver. As we age, we make less, and if we take statins, they block production of CoQ10. Therefore, to protect your heart and maintain good energy levels, take 100mg daily with either breakfast or lunch. If you have had a heart attack, you would need 200mg daily in divided doses.
- Take a multi-nutrient formula to support your heart. Most companies featured at the beginning of the book will happily help you. Otherwise try Solgar's Cardiovascular Support.
- There are several formulas that contain pure cocoa, concentrated pomegranate, and either blueberry extract or superoxide dismutase, an enzyme known to defend the body against oxidative stress. The Life Extension Foundation make a good one called Endothelial Defence. Details are on www.lef.org The Life Extension Foundation products from America are mostly available via the Nutri Centre in the UK. Take as directed
- Otherwise take a pomegranate concentrate formula. **NC**.
- Take a garlic capsule such as Allimax daily, which helps thin the blood naturally.
- After the age of 50, unless you have a medical condition that requires iron, do not take extra iron supplements as excessive iron in the body is linked to heart disease. This applies more to men than women.
- Vitamin C and the amino acid lysine can help to reverse arterial blockages. You need approximately 3 grams of each per day. Take the vitamin C with meals and the lysine 30 minutes before meals. **HN**
- Take a high-strength B complex or take Homocysteine Formula by Metabolics – one three times daily. For stockists call 01380 812799. (You may not need this if you are on a high-strength multi that contains a full spectrum of B vitamins; it depends how high your homocysteine level is.)
- Include a good-quality multi-vitamin and mineral for your age and gender that contains at

least 400iu of natural-source vitamin E, 150mcg of selenium, 30mg of zinc, 100mcg of chromium and 400mg of magnesium. Almost all the vitamin companies listed on pages 15–16 supply such formulae.

■ Try the herbs hawthorn (100–500mg of standardized extract) and ginkgo biloba (60–120mg of standardized extract) daily, either as tea, tincture or capsules. Both are known to improve circulation. Specialist Herbal Suppliers make a formula containing hawthorn, motherwort, lime blossom and dandelion to help balance the heart and circulation. Start with 5 drops a day and then increase gradually. **SHS NB Always tell your doctor if you decide to take hawthorn, which can lower blood pressure.**

■ Several studies have demonstrated that lack of vitamin K2 *accelerates* arterial calcification, whereas taking K2 daily (approx 100mcg) can help keep excess calcium in the bones and out of your arteries. **NB Vitamin K should not be taken by people on Warfarin without a doctor's advice.**

■ Carnitine is an amino acid that helps remove fat deposited in the arteries. Take 500mg three times daily, 30 minutes or so before food.

■ Low vitamin D levels are also linked to heart disease. Research from the University of Colorado has demonstrated a link between low vitamin D levels and an increased risk of heart disease, even in younger people. As low Vitamin D levels are associated with numerous problems, from cancers and high blood pressure to osteoporosis and depression, most nutritional physicians now state that everyone should take 1000iu daily and make the effort to expose their skin to sensible amounts of sunshine.

■ Take 2 grams of omega-3 fish oils daily.

Helpful Hints

■ People who are generally happy, positive and enthusiastic are less likely to develop heart disease than their unhappy counterparts.

■ Make sure you get a good night's sleep, as research has shown that women who are chronically short of sleep are more at risk of heart problems.

■ If you are overweight, lose weight (see *Weight Problems*).

■ Gentlemen, unless you are very tall, a good rule is to not let your waist exceed 99cm (39in); for ladies, the figure is 90cm (35in) if you want to avoid heart problems.

■ Learn to test your heart health. What's your resting pulse? For 1 minute place your first two fingers on the vein crossing the bony protuberance on the thumb side of your inner wrist and check your pulse. While your blood pressure tells you about the health of your arteries, your pulse is a measure of your heart health. If your heart is strong and able to pump blood easily around the body, it will pump slowly and rhythmically, around 60–70 beats per minute. If it's weak, and therefore can't pump as much blood as it should with each beat, it will have to beat more often to keep your cells properly oxygenated, so your pulse will be higher. This is why your pulse goes up when you exercise – your cells need more oxygen, so the heart pumps more rapidly. In time, this strengthens the heart and it will be able to pump more blood with each beat, so your resting pulse will slow down. A raised pulse is now considered a 'normal' result of ageing, although there is no reason you can't have a pulse of 70 when you're over 70.

■ Under medical guidance, try chelation, an intravenous therapy that has saved thousands of people from undergoing major heart surgery. It helps to clear clogged arteries, and this reduces the likelihood of strokes and heart disease. For more details contact the Arterial Disease Clinic, who have several clinics in the UK, on 01942 886644, or call Dr Wendy Denning on 020 7224 2423.

■ Reduce stress in your life, because stress is now proven to increase coronary arterial disease (see *Stress*).

- There is now an easy test to discover your plasma homocysteine levels. Made by York Laboratories and backed by the British Cardiac Patients Association, it's a simple pinprick method that can be done by post. For details call York Labs on 0800 458 2052 or log on to www.yorktest.com.
- Get some exercise. If you have a heart condition, then with your doctor's permission start walking for 30 minutes every day and gradually build up to an hour a day. Join a gym and go regularly. If you don't have access to a gym, walking, swimming, jogging or cycling along quiet roads or nature trails are good alternatives. A little exercise every day is far more effective than a lot of exercise once a week. Even though exercise raises your heart rate while you're doing it, the overall effect is to strengthen the heart and slow your resting heart rate. Research has shown that even moderate exercise after having a heart attack is one very effective way of preventing a second one. If you have had any heart problems, undertake an exercise programme only under professional supervision.
- Stop smoking and avoid places where you will be exposed to second-hand smoke. The chemicals in cigarette smoke damage your arteries, oxidize the cholesterol that forms plaque in your arteries, and increase the likelihood of clotting.
- Reduce your exposure to toxic metals such as lead, cadmium and mercury. Eat more coriander, which helps to eliminate toxic metals from the body – as does chelation (see above).
- People who are angry and argumentative suffer more heart problems. Millions of people are dying because they don't get things off their chest. Learn to deal with anger and internal emotions. See a counsellor – your life may depend on it.
- Contact the British Heart Foundation, 14 Fitzhardinge Street, London W1H 4DH, or call the Heart Help Line on 03003 303311. Website: www.bhf.org.uk.
- Read Patrick Holford's *Say No to Heart Disease* (Piatkus), which is an excellent book explaining the causes of arterial damage and what you can do to prevent or correct high blood pressure and heart disease.
- Another good book is *Put Your Heart in Your Mouth* by Dr Natasha Cambell-McBride (Medinform Publishing).
- See *High Blood Pressure* for more on protecting your whole cardiovascular system.

HEPATITIS A, B & C   *(see also Liver Problems)*

Hepatitis A (Hep A)

Hepatitis A is the most common of the seven known types of hepatitis and is caused by a virus that triggers inflammation of the liver. It is 100 times more infectious than HIV. The Hep A virus is found in the faeces of someone who is infected, and can easily be passed from one person to another with poor personal hygiene if even a fraction of faeces residue gets into another person's mouth. Hep A is common in countries where sanitation and proper sewage is poor. You can become infected by eating or drinking contaminated water. It can also be passed on sexually – and washing the genital area and using condoms can help prevent transmission.

Symptoms may include flu-like symptoms, nausea, vomiting or diarrhoea, loss of appetite, weight loss, yellowing of the skin and of the whites of the eyes and abdominal pain. Symptoms are not always present when a person is infected, but the virus is still active and can still be passed on. If you suspect that you have hepatitis it is important that you visit your doctor or local sexual health clinic, where a simple blood test can confirm the presence of hepatitis.

If you are run down before the onset of the virus, you may feel fatigued for some months afterwards. There is no standard medical treatment for Hep A, but once the virus is cleared from the body you are immune from repeated attacks for life. Hep A immunization offers effective protection against the virus and is worth considering, especially if you are going to travel abroad out of Europe, or are living with someone who is infected.

Foods to Avoid
- Water if you are at all unsure of its purity – such as in India and the Far East.
- When you go abroad, avoid eating salads that have been washed in local water. See *Food Poisoning*.
- Raw or partially cooked shellfish.
- **All** alcohol, as this adds to liver damage.
- Foods full of saturated animal fats, red meat and dairy (cheese, cream, butter and milk), as these put an additional burden on the liver, as do deep-fried foods such as crisps, samosas, fried breakfasts and chips. Avoid curries, too.
- Simple carbohydrates, such as white rice, pasta, bread, cakes and pastries, give the liver extra work to do, so keep them to a minimum.
- Caffeine, from tea, coffee, cola-type energy drinks and some painkillers, adds to the overall load of the liver, so they are best avoided.
- Try not to consume excess amounts of preserved meats, such as pizza meats, jerky, salami, provolone, sausages, hot dogs or hamburger meats, as these are often high in unfriendly bacteria, which the liver has to clear from the body.
- Toxicity is linked to aspartame, so avoid artificial sweeteners; look out for aspartame hidden in hundreds of foods, drinks and chewing gums.
- A high-potassium diet, low in sodium, is known to have a positive effect on the liver. Avoid salt and salty foods, such as chips, sauces, ready-made processed foods and savoury snacks, to reduce salt intake, and increase intake of fresh fruits and vegetables to increase intake of potassium.

Friendly Foods
- Eat more organic food as non-organic food often contains antibiotic, steroid, hormone and pesticide residues, all of which place a strain on the liver.
- Include salads in your diet – made with fresh raw vegetables, such as tomatoes, shallots, sliced red onion, cucumbers, broccoli, lettuce, endives, radicchio, celery, red radish, avocado, shredded cabbage, carrots and beets, grated horseradish, ginger and so on. You can use a dressing of cold-pressed oil, apple cider vinegar, and/or lemon and lime juice. Try to have a salad 4 to 5 times a week, or ideally every day.
- Drink several cups of antioxidant-rich green tea daily. Green and white teas are also rich in polyphenols, which have strong anti-viral properties.
- Make yourself raw vegetable and fruit juices regularly. Ideally, you should do this every day; however, even if you make raw juices only two to three times a week, you will see tremendous benefits. A basic juice to improve liver function can be made with equal parts of apple, carrot and/or beetroot, and cabbage of different colours – one week use a purple–red cabbage and the next week, a green cabbage.
- Linseed (flaxseed) oil is essential for improving liver function. It is beneficial for damaged liver cells, whilst reducing inflammation. Use instead of butter on baked potatoes and for salad dressings.
- Sprinkle a tablespoon of non-GM lecithin granules over cereals, fruit salads, porridge and so on. It helps the liver metabolize fats and lowers LDL cholesterol. It also nourishes the brain. **SVHC**

- Wholegrain foods such as brown rice, millet, brown pasta and rye contain a lot of B-vitamins, which are needed for the liver to work effectively.
- Sulphur-rich foods, including, onions, garlic and leeks, enhance liver function, so try to eat a little of one of these daily.
- Globe artichoke, celeriac, kale and beetroot are all great liver foods.

Useful Remedies

- Linseed oil is a good source of omega-3 and -6, essential fats for repairing damaged liver cell membranes and reducing inflammation. This helps cell walls become more resistant to infection. Use with olive oil in salad dressings or take BioCare's easily absorbable Linseed Oil 1000; 1 capsule, three times per day with meals.
- Otherwise, take 1–3 grams of pure omega-3 fish oils daily.
- Liquorice is known for its anti-viral and immune-enhancing action, as well as being beneficial to the liver. Take 1–2 grams of powdered whole root once a day, or 250mg of solid root extract once per day. Available from www.positivehealthshop.com. If you are taking liquorice for long periods, increase the amount of fresh fruit and vegetables you are eating to address your potassium balance, which can be upset by liquorice.
- Milk thistle extract is highly protective for the liver as it boosts levels of glutathione, a very important amino acid for liver function, which is often low in hepatitis patients. In all cases of hepatitis, take 500mg three times daily.
- Methionine is an amino acid that hugely supports liver function. Take 500mg, three times per day, 30 minutes before meals.
- Take selenium, 200–500mcg per day, as selenium is strongly anti-viral. Do not take more than 500mcg daily for more than a month, then reduce to 200mcg.
- A high-strength vitamin B complex to improve clearance of toxins from the liver.
- Vitamin C has strong anti-viral properties. Take to bowel tolerance levels; 5–10 grams per day. BioCare's magnesium ascorbate powder can be added to a bottle of water and drunk throughout the day.
- Lipoic acid, a major antioxidant, helps protect oxidative damage in the liver. Take 200mg daily.

Helpful Hints

- Avoid chemical cleaning products in the home as the liver has the job of breaking these down. Instead opt for natural products. Look out for the Ecover range available in most supermarkets.
- Travellers to areas such as Asia, Africa, India, Haiti, Eastern Europe and Central and South America are at high risk. While travelling, drink only boiled or bottled water, avoid eating all raw fish and shellfish, and use disinfectant soaps for the hands. (For more help see under *Food Poisoning*.)
- If you have Hep A get plenty of rest and above all practise good hygiene.
- Cigarettes weaken your immune system, compromising its ability to fight the virus; do your best to give it up (see *Smoking*).

Hepatitis B (Hep B)

The Hepatitis B virus (HBV) is very common worldwide and more than 350 million people are infected. The virus can survive on dry surfaces for up to 7 days, making it one of the most communicable diseases and the 9th most common cause of death worldwide. Ninety percent of sufferers recover but 10% are chronically infected – meaning they could develop liver damage, which can be fatal. This virus can be spread via blood or other bodily fluids. The most common routes of infection are via unprotected penetrative sex – especially if blood is produced – or by sharing contaminated needles during drug use. Hep B is also contracted by blood transfusions and non-sterile needles, which may be used in hospitals in certain developing countries (all blood used in the UK is tested for Hepatitis B). Non-sterilized equipment used for tattooing, acupuncture or body-piercing is also a risk. It can also be passed from an infected mother to the unborn child, usually during delivery. It cannot be spread via sneezing, coughing or coming into contact with faeces of an infected person. Symptoms are the same as those of Hep A (see above) and may need hospital treatment. As vaccination is 95% effective, it's worth considering if you are travelling abroad or living with an infected person.

Foods to Avoid
- See dietary advice for *Hepatitis A*.

Friendly foods
- See dietary advice for *Hepatitis A*.

Useful Remedies
- (see also *Useful Remedies* for *Hepatitis A*)
- Selenium reduces Hepatitis B infection by 77%, as well as helping to prevent liver cancer – a secondary complication common in chronic Hepatitis B sufferers. Take 200–500mcg daily. Do not take more than 500mcg daily for more than one month, then reduce to 200mcg daily.

Helpful Hints
- (see also *Helpful Hints* for *Hepatitis C*)
- If planning to travel outside Europe to developing countries, it is possible to get a small first-aid kit that contains sterile needles to prevent infection. The kit is available from the Hospital for Tropical Diseases in London, or ask at pharmacies.

Hepatitis C (Hep C)

Hepatitis C is a cancer-causing, infectious, blood-borne virus that often goes undiagnosed. As many as 250,000 to 465,000 people may be infected in the UK alone.

It can take from 15–150 days or more to develop, and around 8 out of 10 people are unaware that they have it. Unlike Hepatitis A and B there is no vaccine for Hepatitis C. Infection occurs from blood transfusions, needle-sharing (including acupuncture, piercing and tattooing), the sharing of notes used to snort cocaine, working in a medical environment, and sexual contact – especially if a woman is having her period or genital sores are present and bleeding. Hep C is usually passed from the male to the female if internal tissue is damaged. On very rare occasions it can be passed from an infected mother to her baby, mainly during delivery. If you have ever received a blood transfusion in a country where blood is not tested for the Hepatitis C virus (many developing countries), or if you received a transfusion in the UK before 1991 (all blood for transfusion in the UK is now tested), or if you have received medical or dental treatment abroad where equipment may not have been sterilized properly, you may want to have a blood test. As with all types of hepatitis, symptoms may not occur but the virus can still be passed on. Evidence suggests that about 20% of individuals who have Hepatitis C appear to clear the virus from the blood, whilst about 80% will remain infected and can pass on the virus to others. If a person continues to be infected over a number of years, he or she may develop chronic hepatitis, liver cirrhosis or liver cancer. Hepatitis C virus is not spread by sneezing, hugging, coughing, food or water, sharing eating utensils or drinking glasses, or casual contact.

A simple blood test can detect Hep C.

Foods to Avoid
- (see *Hepatitis A*)

Friendly Foods
- (see also *Hepatitis A*)
- Drink plenty of water: try to drink 8 full glasses a day. If you vomit a lot, you should drink more clear liquids.
- Include salads in your diet. Make them with fresh, raw vegetables, such as tomatoes, shallots, sliced red onion, cucumbers, broccoli, lettuce, endives, radicchio, celery, red radish, avocado, shredded cabbage, carrots and beets and grated horseradish, ginger and so on. You can use a dressing of cold-pressed oil, apple cider vinegar, and/or lemon and lime juice. Try to have a salad 4 or 5 times a week, or ideally every day.

Useful Remedies
- (see also *Hepatitis A*)
- Keep iron levels to a minimum and do not supplement with iron. Approximately 30% of Hep C sufferers have high iron levels due to the massive amounts of oxidative stress in their livers. Ask your doctor to investigate this possibility. Alpha-lipoic acid, a potent antioxidant, reduces oxidative stress by raising levels of glutathione in the liver. Take 200mg twice daily.
- Take 4 green tea extract capsules daily with food, which will help to block iron absorption. **NC**

Helpful Hints
- (see also *Hepatitis A*)
- Blood spills should be wiped up with bleach and all cuts and wounds covered with adhesive dressings. Bloodstained tissues, sanitary napkins and so on must be disposed of safely.
- Tell your healthcare provider and dentist that you have the virus to avoid infecting them.
- Do not share toothbrushes, razors, nail files, clippers or scissors, or any object that may come into contact with your blood.
- Do not share food that has been in your mouth and do not pre-chew food for babies.
- Tell sexual partners you have the virus, advise them to see their doctor and in the meantime use a condom.
- For more help call the NHS Hepatitis C helpline on 0800 451 451, open from 7am–11pm, 7 days a week.
- An informative Hepatitis C website can be found at www.hepatitis-central.com
- To find details about your local STD clinic, go to www.nhs.uk/livewell/sexualhealth

H

HERPES
(see also Cold Sores)

There are two types of herpes simplex virus: Type 1 causes cold sores, Type 2 is sexually transmitted and is the most common. It can cause extreme pain and swelling of the genital area and is sometimes accompanied by fever. You never eradicate the virus once you have it, but you can keep attacks under control by using supplements and eating a healthier diet.

There can be a stigma associated with herpes, suggesting that the person must be promiscuous, but nothing could be further from the truth! It is very common and millions of people in the Western world suffer from it. The virus needs only a depressed immune system to take hold and can spread most easily through sexual contact.

Lack of sleep, poor nutrition, too much alcohol and cigarettes, as well as allergies to certain foods will all encourage the virus to multiply. In addition, sunburn, over-exercising or excessive sexual activity can also lead to a recurrence.

Those with sensitive nervous systems, and who are prone to anxiety or depression, are more vulnerable to recurrence. The virus will lie dormant and resides in a nerve centre or ganglia. When activated, the virus moves down the nerve and can show up anywhere in the genital area (depending on which nerves are involved), as well as the buttocks, back or legs. Vegetarians may be more prone to attacks because they do not eat enough foods rich in the amino acid lysine, which helps starve the virus.

Foods to Avoid

- Avoid alcohol, especially fortified wines such as sherry and port as well as wine and beer.
- Caffeine, and smoking should also be curtailed.
- During an attack, avoid all foods high in arginine, which feed the virus. This includes chocolate, nuts (especially peanuts, almonds, cashews and walnuts), seeds (especially sunflower and sesame), coconut and grains, such as wheat and oats.
- Avoid all foods high in sugar and pre-packaged 'junk' fast–foods as they will all greatly deplete your immune function, as will alcohol.

Friendly Foods

- High lysine foods, including fish (especially halibut), milk, eggs, chicken, turkey, lamb and potatoes. Lysine suppresses arginine, which tends to feed the virus, so remove or cut out foods high in arginine.
- Vegetarians can eat more corn and soya-based foods, which also contain good amounts of lysine.
- Make sure the diet is rich in all fruits, vegetables, eggs, brown rice and breads.
- Eat more garlic and onions as they are highly anti-viral.

Useful Remedies

- Vitamin C: take 1 gram as a preventative, and between 2 and 3 grams daily with meals during an attack.
- The amino acid lysine inhibits replication of the virus. If you suffer attacks regularly, take 500–1000mg daily as a preventative measure, and up to 3 grams daily, spread throughout the day and taken 30 minutes before food, while suffering an attack.
- Beta Glucans 1–3, 1–6, derived from yeast cell walls, are proven to strengthen the body's innate immune system (the immune system you were born with), and nutritionist Gareth Zeal says, 'Within 2 days of taking beta glucans, which are highly anti-viral, most patients say that genital pain is hugely reduced.' Can also be taken by children with cold sores. Take 250–500mg daily. **PN**
- Propolis cream is highly anti-viral. Use daily on affected areas.
- Olive leaf extract acts like a natural antibiotic and boosts immune function. Take 2–3 capsules daily.
- Take a daily multi-vitamin and mineral that contains around 30mg of zinc.
- Lemon balm (*Melissa officinalis*) helps to stop the spread of the virus and speeds the healing process. Take 20–40 drops daily in water. You can also dilute the drops and gently bathe the affected areas. **OP**

Helpful Hints

- Avoidance of sexual intercourse when you have an attack of Type 2 is very important, as the virus is extremely contagious. If you must have sex then use a condom, but you may well find it is too painful and need to wait until the sores have either healed or completely disappeared.
- Avoid oral sex when you have an attack of Type 1 or 2. Remember that oral sex is one way of transferring a cold sore and turning it into genital herpes.
- For further help contact the Herpes Viruses Association helpline on 0845 123 2305. Website: www.herpes.org.uk

HIATUS HERNIA

(see also Acid–Alkaline Balance, Indigestion and Low Stomach Acid)

The gullet or oesophagus takes food from the mouth to the stomach and passes through a sheet of muscle called the diaphragm. A hiatus hernia occurs when a part of the stomach pushes up through the diaphragm and allows acid to escape into the gullet, causing heartburn, reflux of food, and indigestion, especially when lying down. It can also cause a fair amount of chest pain, which obviously needs looking at quickly by a doctor. Most hiatus hernias can easily be seen on an X-ray. Being overweight is a common factor for hiatus hernia. Believe it or not, too much exercise – especially jogging or weight lifting to excess – can on occasion trigger this problem.

Sometimes, people think that they have excess stomach acid because they are experiencing acid reflux, but low stomach acid is far more likely to be the problem – see *Low Stomach Acid*. But if you suffer indigestion-type pain after eating over several weeks and find that you wake in the night with heartburn, then please see a doctor.

Foods to Avoid

- Generally, avoid large meals, especially ones containing red meat, fried foods such as chips, and creamy-type sauces, which can trigger an acid reflux attack. Melted cheese is especially hard to digest, so keep away from pizzas.
- Alcohol, strong tea, coffee, fizzy drinks, sugar, chocolate, dairy products and all high-fat foods can cause an 'acid' rebound reaction, as they are all acid-forming foods within the body.

- Chew food thoroughly and don't drink too much fluid with food.
- If symptoms are acute, avoid eating for a short time, or, at most, eat only lightly cooked small meals regularly.
- Avoid artificial sweeteners, such as aspartame, and artificial additives, which can aggravate symptoms.
- Avoid chewing gum, as the body produces stomach acid thinking that food is on its way. This depletes levels of stomach acid (needed for digestion) when you finally eat a meal.
- Eating pasta with a glass of wine can be a lethal combination for people with this condition.

Friendly Foods

- Aloe Pura make a Stomach Formula juice containing aloe, slippery elm and peppermint, which really helps soothe symptoms. Take one capful in a little water 20 minutes before food. If stomach acid has damaged the back of your throat, the aloe will also help soothe this problem.
- Slippery elm and liquorice both soothe the oesophagus, as well as providing a gentle fibre, which can reduce discomfort. Ask at your health shop for de-glycyrrhized liquorice, and chew 20 minutes before each main meal. Liquorice works as well as many drugs, without the negative side effects.
- Try decaffeinated beverages, and drink more herbal teas such as camomile, liquorice and peppermint.
- Try dandelion root coffee.
- Food combining has proved very useful to people who have this condition. The basic rule is to avoid eating proteins, such as meat or fish, with potatoes, pasta, rice or bread. And when eating potatoes, pasta, rice or bread, do not eat proteins, but eat vegetables and salads.
- Generally, eat a low-fat diet, but see *Fats You Need To Eat* and *General Health Hints* to ensure that you get all the essential nutrients you need.

- Steam, boil, poach, stir-fry, roast or grill your food.
- Eat more wheat germ, soya beans, alfalfa and dark green vegetables (especially cabbage, watercress and kale – these are rich in glutamine, which heals the gut), plus a little avocado rich in vitamin E to aid soft tissue healing.
- Sprinkle lecithin granules over a low-sugar breakfast cereal daily, which helps to emulsify fats.
- Eat more garlic and fresh root ginger.

Useful Remedies

- Slippery elm: 2 tablets taken at the end of each meal can help reduce discomfort.
- L-glutamine, found in cabbage, helps to heal any ulceration in the gut. Take 1–2 grams daily before food for 6 weeks. **HN**
- Take a good-quality multi-vitamin and mineral for your age and gender.
- Calcium fluoride tissue salts: 4 a day to help strengthen the diaphragm.
- Healthy bacteria, known as probiotics, are essential for healthy digestion and gut function. Jarro-Dophilus EPS is a good formula. Take 1 daily with meals for a couple of months. **NC**
- prebiotics are certain foods that encourage healthy bacteria in the gut to multiply. These are good to use, as levels in hiatus hernia patients are likely to be low. They are also a great way to stay 'regular' and thus avoid any discomfort from straining on the loo. I have found a great one based on the agave plant, called Agave Digestive Immune Support, which I take every morning in my breakfast whiz. Or just dissolve one scoop of this powder in water. Really helps keep you regular! See www.lef.org or call The Nutri Centre.

Helpful Hints

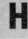

- Eat smaller meals, which are easier on the digestion. Avoid large, rich meals at any time.
- Try to relax as much as possible and avoid lying down immediately after eating.
- Do not smoke near meal times. Smoking and alcohol relax muscles, thus allowing food from the stomach to return more easily up to the oesophagus.
- Go for a gentle walk after meals, but do not get involved in heavy exercise.
- Many people report relief from symptoms after seeing a chiropractor. See *Useful Information*.

HIGH BLOOD PRESSURE

(see also Atherosclerosis, Circulation, Stress and Stroke)

High blood pressure makes you more susceptible to heart disease, strokes and kidney disease. Blood pressure of 150/100 or more is classified as high. A normal reading is 120/80, but 140/90 or less is deemed as raised, but acceptable. There is no reason why you shouldn't have a blood pressure of 120/80 when you're 80 if you take good care of your arteries.

While your pulse is a measure of your heart health, your blood pressure tells you about the health of your arteries. High blood pressure, also known as hypertension, is often considered a 'normal' part of ageing, but the fact that something is common doesn't mean it's normal. It's important to remember that high blood pressure is a symptom of a problem, not the problem itself. The problem is that your arteries are too constricted, or 'furred up', to properly relax when your heart pumps the blood through. And narrower arteries make you age faster, because the oxygen supply to your tissues is reduced, so the heart works harder, which raises your blood pressure even more, exposing arterial walls to damage. This triggers further hardening or furring up, and the problem gets worse still.

Think of your arteries as being like a complex system of garden hoses, coming off a single pump – your heart. Every time your heart beats, it's sending oxygen and nutrient-rich blood around your body via your arteries to nourish each of your trillions of cells. These gushes of blood, forced through the arteries with every heartbeat, exert pressure on the walls of your arteries, and this pressure can damage the delicate cells lining your arteries. To reduce the pressure and ensure smooth blood flow, rather than blood flow in spurts, the arterial walls are flexible, and are surrounded by smooth muscle that is able to expand and contract in response to the pressure being exerted on the arterial walls by the pumped blood. Over time, many people's arteries become gradually harder and narrower, a process called arteriosclerosis; if the arteries are furred up, the condition is called atherosclerosis.

Arteriosclerosis is a major recognized cause of dementia in the elderly (see *Alzheimer's Disease* and *Atherosclerosis*). The kidneys, liver and other organs suffer reduced blood flow, too, and so cannot perform effectively in detoxifying the body. Lumps of thickened matter (called 'plaques') build up in the artery wall and reduce the diameter of the vessels that the blood flows through. We now know why this occurs, and it all starts with damage to the arterial wall. This can occur due to abrasion (from high blood pressure), viral or bacterial infection, high homocysteine levels (a toxic amino acid formed as a by-product of the metabolism of proteins), or free radical damage. Once the damage is done, the body tries to repair the area, causing scar tissue, and this is made worse by high levels of low-density lipoprotein (LDL – 'bad cholesterol') that can pass into the walls of the artery where it is oxidized by free radicals into dangerous rancid forms. This in turn is gobbled up by macrophages (part of your immune system), which become engorged 'foam cells'. The whole area attracts more and more oxidized cholesterol, more immune responses, more inflammation, and inevitably the arteries grow stiffer and narrower.

Homocysteine, now thought to be one of the key agents involved in damaging the arterial walls, is a harmful compound produced in the body that's normally recycled or broken down by vitamins B6, B12 and folic acid – nutrients often deficient in overly refined foods.

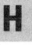

Another key cause of raised blood pressure is a lack of the mineral magnesium. Magnesium is needed for muscles to relax after they've contracted (muscle cramps or eye ticks are a symptom of magnesium deficiency), and research has shown that arteries are considerably narrower in those who are deficient in magnesium. In some countries, paramedics inject magnesium directly into the heart of heart-attack victims to relax the muscle and the blocked arteries supplying it. Many heart attacks and strokes are now thought to be due to arterial spasms blocking blood supply to the heart or brain, rather than a clot.

Stress and excessive exercise are known to deplete magnesium, which may be deficient if you don't eat enough dark green leafy vegetables, whole grains and seeds. This may explain why fit, apparently healthy people sometimes die suddenly of a heart attack or stroke.

A dangerous side effect of arteriosclerosis is an increased tendency toward and greater dangers from blood clotting. This is especially true for those with A or AB blood types. Turbulence in the blood caused by rough areas in the normally very smooth arterial walls can increase clotting. Also the plaques can break off and travel along the artery until they get stuck in a narrower blood vessel; this is commonly known as 'thrombosis'. If these clots reach an area sufficiently narrowed by arterial plaques, they can block the vessel completely and starve the tissues 'down stream' of blood, oxygen and nutrients. If this happens in the vessels supplying the heart or brain, a heart attack or stroke can occur.

Eighty-five percent of all cases of high blood pressure can be treated without drugs, if the person is willing to change their lifestyle and diet. For example, in societies where salt is virtually absent, hypertension is equally absent. Too much caffeine, alcohol and smoking, when combined with high blood pressure, greatly increases your chances of suffering heart disease or stroke. Stress is a **major** factor in high blood pressure, because adrenaline is released into the bloodstream, which increases your heart rate, breathing and blood pressure, but also constricts arteries.

Foods to Avoid

- Reducing or eliminating wheat grains, corn starch and sugars can really help reduce blood pressure. This includes white bread, pasta, biscuits, pre-made pies and so on.
- Avoid all highly refined hydrogenated oils and fats found in mass- produced cooking oils, margarines, biscuits, pastries and cakes.
- One-third to a half of people with high blood pressure benefit from lowering salt intake. Keep the sodium level in your diet low: sodium causes more water to be retained by the kidneys, and more water means more blood volume, and therefore higher blood pressure, so eliminate sodium-based table salts. There are plenty of magnesium- and potassium-based salts, such as Solo Salt, and Himalayan Crystal Salt available from health shops. Use sparingly on the food that's on your plate.
- Reduce stimulants. Blood pressure has been shown to drop as much as 20 points when all caffeine is eliminated, because caffeine ultimately causes arteries to constrict. Some decaffeinated drinks contain formaldehyde, so look for decaffeinated drinks and coffee that has been decaffeinated using the more natural water method.
- Sugar is also a problem, as sugar converts into fat in the body if not used up during exercise. Be aware that many low-fat foods are high in sugar. Always check the labels.
- If you have eliminated all of the above and still have a tendency towards high blood pressure, it might be worth consulting a nutritionist who can check for food intolerances, particularly if you are a migraine sufferer. See *Useful Information*.

Friendly Foods

- Eat more pomegranate, which helps arteries not to become clogged in the first place. Also eat plenty of blueberries, blackberries, strawberries and raspberries, which all help to balance blood pressure.
- Eat green vegetables, fresh fruit, unprocessed and unsalted nuts, fresh fish, whole grains such as brown rice, breads and pastas, to increase your intake of the B-vitamins B6, B12 and folic acid, which are involved in breaking down homocysteine.
- Butterbeans, currants, dried figs, apricots, almonds, black treacle and sunflower seeds are all rich in minerals such as magnesium and potassium.
- Use nori flakes or kelp flakes, which are rich in minerals, as a salt substitute; they are great over fish and stir fries. Available from health stores.
- Another useful salt is Organic Herb Seasoning Salt by Bioforce. It is made from organic sea salt, dried celery, leeks, cress, parsley, kelp, garlic and basil, and sold globally in health stores and supermarkets. Website: www.bioforce.co.uk.
- Try Solo instead of table salt, which is potassium- and not sodium-based. Potassium can help lower blood pressure because it balances sodium.
- Two bananas or four sticks of celery a day (rich in potassium) have been shown to help lower blood pressure over time.
- If you are not a fan of eating fresh fruit and vegetables, at least drink a couple of glasses of freshly made fruit or vegetable juice. You will miss out on the fibre, but still get much of the nutrient content.
- Try switching to a more vegetarian-based diet, as the more fruit, vegetables, beans and lentils you eat, the greater your potassium intake and, generally speaking, the lower your sodium intake. And vegetarians tend to have much lower blood pressure.
- Chick-peas and soya beans contain isoflavones, which can help reduce LDL.

- Eat more garlic, onions, broccoli (which are antioxidant, anti-viral and anti-bacterial) and celery (which is diuretic).
- Use unrefined organic virgin olive, walnut, pumpkin, linseed (flax seed) or sunflower oil for your salad dressings, and eat oily fish 3 times a week (see *Fats You Need To Eat*).
- As high levels of toxic metals, such as lead, can contribute to high blood pressure, buy a good-quality water filter. The fibre in apples (pectin), plus coriander and seaweed, which are high in chlorophyll all help to detoxify metals from the body.
- Natural-source vitamin E helps to thin blood naturally, therefore eat more soya beans, wheat germ, alfalfa sprouts, dark green vegetables, hazelnuts, almonds and avocados. This is especially important for those with type A or AB blood.
- Add more cayenne paper to your food, or take 1 capsule 3 times daily, to help balance your blood pressure. Check with your doctor if you are taking drugs such as Warfarin.
- See also *Friendly Foods* in *Constipation*, as constipation can aggravate blood pressure.
- Lycopene, found in tomatoes and watermelon, has been found to slow accumulation of arterial plaque.
- Try hibiscus tea, which has been shown to lower blood pressure.

Useful Remedies
- If you are taking blood-pressure medication, tell your doctor about any supplements you are taking, as in time your prescription drugs may be able to be reduced, and these supplements help to lower blood pressure naturally and you don't want your blood pressure to go too low.
- Take 500–1000mg of magnesium with 400mg of calcium daily. Both of these minerals have been shown to lower blood pressure.
- Taking Pycnogenol – pine bark extract – regularly has been shown to help patients lower their medication. Take 125mg daily. **PN**
- The spice turmeric contains curcumin, which has highly anti-inflammatory properties, and as atherosclerosis is basically inflammation of the arteries, taking this spice daily in a concentrated form with meals can greatly reduce plaque forming. Take around 1 gram daily in divided doses with food. **NC** or log on to www.lef.org
- Essential fats thin the blood, and reduce inflammation in your arterial walls. Take 2 grams of fish oil daily or 2 grams of linseed (flax seed) oil, both of which contain omega-3 fats (see *Fats You Need To Eat*).
- Take garlic; 900mg a day. When used long term, garlic can help gently lower blood pressure and thin the blood.
- Hawthorn, either as tincture or as tablets, is a gentle way of bringing blood pressure back down to normal. 1–3ml of tincture or 1–2 grams of the tablets. **NB You must tell your doctor if you want to try hawthorn as he/she may be able to reduce your medication.**
- Take 100iu of natural-source, full-spectrum vitamin E and gradually increase to 500iu a day. Vitamin E thins the blood, protecting from clotting, and prevents LDL cholesterol from oxidizing.
- Include a high-strength multi-vitamin/mineral in your programme, as the B-vitamins help to support your nerves, controlling muscle contraction and improving your tolerance to stress.
- If your homocysteine level is high, take an extra 10–50mg of vitamin B6, 400–1000mcg of folic acid plus 10mg of B12. To find your plasma homocysteine levels, use a simple pinprick method that can be done by post. Made by York Laboratories and backed by The British Cardiac Patients Association. Call 0800 458 2052, or log on to www.yorktest.com.

Helpful Hints
- High blood pressure can occur during pregnancy, in which case seek medical attention.
- Cigarettes, plus the chemicals in cigarette smoke, damage your arteries and make the blood more likely to clot, raising your risk of developing heart disease.

- Reduce stress, which in the long term can kill you. Try to find a method of relaxation that you enjoy, whether it's meditation, t'ai chi, yoga, exercising, walking or swimming. See under *Stress* and *Adrenal Exhaustion*.
- Have a regular aromatherapy massage, using relaxing essential oils such as rosewood, ylang ylang, clary sage, lavender and marjoram.
- Get a pet. Researchers from the State University of New York have shown how having a pet can protect against the effects of stress better than drugs designed to lower blood pressure.
- Exercise is vital for reducing blood pressure. With your doctor's permission, start walking briskly for 30 minutes daily. People who are overweight and don't get much exercise are much more likely to suffer high blood pressure.
- Breathe deeply regularly – this helps to re-alkalize the body and helps you stay calm.
- Toxic metals in the body are also linked to high blood pressure. If you have tried all the dietary guidelines without impact, have your metal levels checked.
- Have a nutrition consultant conduct a hair mineral analysis. This test costs around £40–£50 and determines your level of calcium, magnesium and other important minerals and identifies any raised heavy metals in your system. For further information call Sarah Stelling of ARL (UK) on 0131 229 1077, or write to ARL (UK), Edinburgh Centre of Nutrition and Therapy, 11 Home Street, Edinburgh EH3 9JR. www.ecnt.co.uk

- Have your doctor obtain an ordinary cardiac risk blood profile. This will check your total cholesterol, HDL (good cholesterol), LDL (bad cholesterol), and triglycerides. There is no doubt that raised triglycerides put you in the high-risk category, although this does not mean that triglycerides are necessarily to blame. If you're prescribed cholesterol-lowering drugs, get a second opinion (see *Cholesterol*).
- Have your homocysteine level checked: it is not tested routinely and you will need to ask for the test. It should be below 8; above 10 is poor; above 12 is definitely not great. Homocysteine levels rise with age and can be controlled by supplementing B6, B12 and folic acid. If yours is high, you need higher levels of these vitamins than you can get in your diet alone. There is an easy test to discover your plasma homocysteine levels (see above).
- Many men who suffer arteriosclerosis have low levels of testosterone – therefore, gentlemen over 45 should ask their GP to test their hormone levels.
- Patrick Holford's *Say No to Heart Disease* (Piatkus) is an excellent book explaining the causes of arterial damage and what you can do to prevent or correct high blood pressure. He has also written *The H Factor*, which gives all details of homocysteine. Website: www.patrickholford.com

HIRSUTISM   *(see Body Hair, Excessive)*

HYPERACTIVITY   *(see also Allergies)*

Hyperactivity is also often referred to as Attention Deficit Disorder (ADD), or Attention Deficit Hyperactivity Disorder (ADHD), and they are all closely related. These conditions occur predominantly in children, but sometimes symptoms can continue into adulthood. There is no hard-and-fast definition of this disorder and consequently children who are merely rebellious, find it difficult to pay attention for great lengths of time, or find it difficult to learn generally may tend to be labelled as having ADD. And children that also constantly fidget and are always on the go may well be diagnosed as having ADHD. Typical symptoms include an inability to concentrate or sit still for any length of time, or rapid and severe mood swings, and these children often need very little sleep. Children that are affected often find themselves in trouble and are shunted from school to school. They can become delinquent teenagers and often end up using drugs and alcohol.

Nutritionist Gareth Zeal says: 'In clinical practice, it's been noted that children with eye problems such as short-sightedness, astigmatisms or a 'lazy eye' are more likely to be genuine ADHD cases. We encourage all pregnant women to take 3–5 grams of omega-3 fish oils during pregnancy, as they are crucial for healthy brain and eye development'

All of these conditions are associated with an excessive intake of artificial sweeteners, colourings and preservatives that are found in prescription medicines and thousands of foods and drinks. Sensitivities to various foods also play an enormous role in hyperactive children and adults. Other substances, such as bubble bath, air fresheners, spray deodorants, perfumes and toothpastes can also trigger these types of behavioural problems. Far too many children still eat huge amounts of junk foods that are devoid of vitamins, minerals and essential fats. Junk foods deplete nutrients from the body, and without any doubt, tests have shown that these children are malnourished, and the lack of proper nutrients can have a devastating effect not only on their bodies, but most importantly on their brains. Also, exposure to neurotoxins, such as lead from water pipes and car fumes, plus cadmium from cigarettes, can make the problem even worse, as can overexposure to these chemicals during pregnancy.

The normal drug therapy is Ritalin, from the amphetamine family, which initiates changes in brain structure and function that remain long after any therapeutic effects have dissipated. Ritalin may also increase the incidence of depression, addiction to other substances such as cocaine and smoking in later life. Understandably, many parents don't feel comfortable giving this drug to their child; however, others feel it is their only weapon in making the child controllable or easier to teach.

There is a growing body of negative evidence against this drug, and nutritionists, such as UK-based Patrick Holford, have shown time and again that if artificial additives and foods to which the child is sensitive are removed from the diet, and proper nutrition is practised, these children improve in leaps and bounds. In prisons in the US and the UK, it has also been shown that when violent prisoners are given a healthier diet, plus the right vitamins, minerals and essentials fats, they become calmer and 'kinder' people.

Foods to Avoid
- It is very important to discover which foods/and or substances that are triggering the hyperactivity. See under *Helpful Hints* for York and Genova Tests.
- Any foods containing large numbers of additives, particularly the strong colourings such as tartrazine. Many sweets are bright and rainbow-coloured and should be totally avoided.
- Greatly reduce or eliminate cola-type drinks, and any foods or drinks containing the artificial sweetener aspartame. Look out for hidden sources such as chewing gum.
- Generally cut down on foods containing sugar, such as cakes, biscuits, chocolates, and snack bars. One specialist once told me that giving sugar to hyperactive children was 'like putting rocket fuel in a Mini'. The odd treat is OK, but try to buy organic, low-sugar snack bars that have been sweetened with apple juice or honey. Most of the mass-produced refined foods (white bread, pasta and rice; packaged ready-meals and so on) should go. As an occasional treat, allow the child to eat a small amount of organic chocolate. Sugar depletes the mineral magnesium needed to stay calm, and B vitamins, which support the nerves and brain function. Sugar also depletes essential fats that are crucial for healthy brain functioning.
- Citrus fruits and juices are often a problem.

- If your child has a favourite food, be it cheese, eggs, wheat-based foods, cow's milk or orange juice, try cutting these out for 1–2 weeks and see if behaviour improves. It is usually the foods they eat and crave the most that are triggering many of their symptoms.
- Buy a book that gives you all the E numbers and note which foods have the highest amounts and avoid them like the plague.

Friendly Foods
- As much as possible feed your child organic foods, free from pesticides and herbicides.
- Try buying corn, lentil, rice and spinach-based pastas.
- Introduce more wholefoods and grains, such as brown rice, millet, oats, quinoa, lentils and vegetables into your child's diet.
- Nature's Path/ and Gillian McKeith make healthier breakfast cereals that are sweetened with apple juice. Any health shop sells ranges of wheat-free and/or low-sugar organic cereals, mueslis and snack bars these days. Chop an apple or banana into the cereal for added fibre and nutrients.
- Use sunflower and pumpkin seeds or linseeds (flax seeds), plus nuts such as pecans or hazelnuts, as they are high in essential fats, and in minerals like zinc, which is also vital for healthy brain-functioning.
- Add pumpkin seeds to a salad – they are delicious and rich in magnesium and zinc.
- Try organic rice, oat, hemp, almond or goat's milk or yoghurt, which are less likely to cause a problem.

- Use diluted sugar-free pear, apple or even grape juice, which are less likely than the citrus fruits to cause a problem.
- Encourage the child to drink water in preference to fizzy drinks and try to encourage a taste for fresh fruit rather than sugary sweets.
- Add low-sugar fruit yoghurts to colourful fruit for tasty desserts. I make jellies with a base of low-sugar cranberry or freshly squeezed orange (or mango) juice, camomile tea, or fresh grapes and chop fresh fruit into the jelly liquid and allow to set – a wonderful low-sugar treat.
- Give your child a serving of quality protein, such as chicken, fresh fish, eggs, tempeh, lentils and beans, nuts and seeds, with each meal of the day.
- Essential fats found in oily fish are really important in controlling this type of behaviour. (See *Fats You Need To Eat*.)
- Ensure plenty of iron-rich foods are included in the diet, as a lack of iron can decrease attentiveness and narrow attention span. Good choices are cooked tofu, lean meats, beans and pulses, spinach, eggs (unless your child has an intolerance to eggs), cabbage, prunes, dates and apricots and pumpkin seeds. Eat them along with some strawberries or papaya, which are rich in vitamin C, to enhance absorption.
- Use unrefined, cold-pressed, preferably organic olive, sunflower, hemp, walnut or sesame oils for salad dressings, or drizzle over cooked foods. Cook only with the olive oil or use Higher Nature's coconut oil instead. **HN**
- Make flapjacks using oats, raisins, sunflower and pumpkin seeds, chopped organic apricots or dates with olive or sunflower oil, then add organic agave syrup (which has a lower glycaemic index than refined sugar). Or use a little melted butter. Bake weekly and keep in an air-tight container.

Useful Remedies
- Magnesium is known as nature's tranquillizer and many children are low in this vital mineral; give 400mg daily. Dr Bernard Rimland, the director of the Autism Research Institute, has found that combining vitamin B6 and magnesium was up to 10 times more effective than Ritalin. 50mg of B6 can be taken in a high-strength B-complex.

- Essential fatty acids are vital. Eskimo make a flavoured omega-3 and Barlenes make a lemon version for children. **NC**
- Give your child a good-quality chewable multi-vitamin and mineral that is free from artificial additives. Solgar's chewable Kanga Vites are flavoured with natural fruit (avoid if citrus is a problem for your child). Nature's Plus also makes a great children's range of nutrients. **SVHC, NP**

Helpful Hints
- Try to avoid smoking and drinking during pregnancy, as both of these have been linked with an increased likelihood of the child becoming hyperactive.
- If the child has allergies or food intolerances, explain to the child how they affect their behaviour and tell everyone in the school or relatives, who might be giving the child food or drinks, which they think are perfectly harmless.
- For some children natural compounds found in food, called salicylates, can cause a problem (see *Autism* for more details).
- Homoeopathy has a great track record of dealing with ADD and hyperactivity so, if you can, get your child along to a good homoeopath. Be prepared to be patient, as it may not be an overnight success. See *Useful Information*, or call the Organic Pharmacy. **OP**
- It's really important to avoid exposure to air fresheners **of all types**, spray deodorants, potpourri, and perfumed fabric conditioners, washing powders and liquids. Try Ecover products, which contain far fewer chemicals, available in all major supermarkets and health stores.
- As children with ADHD are 7 times more likely to have food intolerances than other children, get these checked out. Genova Diagnostics have an in-depth food intolerance test, and you can also request that they add on food additives to the test. Contact them on 020 8336 7750, or check out their website at www.gdx.uk.net

- Otherwise contact York Laboratories, who can test for a large range of intolerances via a simple test kit that can be taken at home. For details call York Labs on 0800 458 2052, or log on to: www.yorktest.com
- Links have been found between hyperactivity and high levels of heavy metals, namely mercury, lead, copper and aluminium. Many vaccines still contain mercury. See under *Fluoride*. Get these checked out with a simple non-invasive, hair mineral analysis test. To order, call Analytical Research Laboratories on 0131 229 1077.
- Read Patrick Holford's book, *New Optimum Nutrition for the Mind* (Piatkus)
- ADD and ADHD are complex conditions, and as it is important that children do not become deficient in any nutrients, enlist the help of a qualified nutritionist. Contact the British Association for Nutritional Therapy by checking out their website at www.bant.org.uk, or calling 08706 061284 to find a nutritionist in your area.
- A great site sharing stories from children affected by ADD and ADHD can be found at www.adders.org
- For more help contact the Hyperactive Children's Support Group via www.hacsg.org.uk, or call 01243 539966.

HYPOGLYCAEMIA *(see Low Blood Sugar)*

I

IBS
(see Irritable Bowel Syndrome)

IMMUNE FUNCTION   *(see also Adrenal Exhaustion, MRSA and Stress)*

With new strains of bacteria and viruses mutating with alarming speed, the challenge for our immune systems has never been greater. Our immune system is made up of a network of cells, organs and fluids that help defend us against the millions of bacteria, viruses and fungi that bombard us in our daily lives. And one of the most important things you can do to stay healthy, throughout your life, is to keep your immune system in good shape. For example, when I was younger and did not realize how diet and lifestyle affected my ability to fight off illnesses, when I was under pressure, not getting sufficient sleep, and eating the wrong foods, I was always ill. At times when I felt ghastly, I would turn to a sugary snack to keep me going and I could literally feel my immune system going 'over the edge'. Stress alone can suppress immune function by up to 60% (see also *Adrenal Exhaustion* and *Stress*).

These days I recognize my limits, I know when to stop and get more sleep. I eat a cleaner diet and try as much as possible to keep my stress levels within limits. You need to listen to your body and take notice! Often the first signs of an immune system under threat are a chronic sore throat, regular colds or niggling infections. If this is the case with you, it's time to take action.

Meanwhile, most people don't think of their skin as being part of the immune system, but it forms a physical barrier against attack, and the immune system is in charge of cell regeneration within your skin. The more efficient your immune system, the fresher your skin will look.

Then comes your stomach acid, which also helps to destroy harmful organisms, but as we age and get stressed, stomach acid levels fall and more bacteria can get through (see *Low Stomach Acid*).

Within a child's bone marrow there are 'stem cells' which, as we grow, develop into various types of immune cells, some of which mature in the thymus gland, where they become known as T-cells. The spleen also contains immune cells that manufacture antibodies; and the lymphatic system, often called the master drain, is also a major player in immune function. The lymphatic system removes toxins and microbes from the body's tissue and, along with bone marrow, manufactures lymphocytes (a specific kind of white blood cell that comes in 3 types – B-cells, T-cells and natural killer cells – which keep your immune system in good shape). Lymph nodes are found all over the body, but the ones most people are aware of are situated in the neck, groin and arm pits. During an infection, the lymph glands can swell as they produce more white blood cells; this is very common in throat conditions, for example. If the lymphatic system becomes congested, the fluid thickens and becomes more gel-like, which inhibits proper drainage and detoxification and puts more pressure on the liver and kidneys. This is why a fully functioning lymphatic system helps you to fight off invading bacteria and viruses. The liver and thymus gland also play a huge role in immune function (see *Liver Problems*).

Unfortunately, as we age our immune system becomes less effective at protecting us and more viruses and bacteria get through our defences. Conversely, our immune system can also overreact, which produces chronic inflammation when we eat certain foods, or are exposed to pollen, pollutants and so on. The immune system may even begin attacking the body's own tissue, called an 'autoimmune response', in conditions such as lupus and rheumatoid arthritis.

High cholesterol levels are also linked to a lowered immune response, because cells containing high levels of cholesterol can disrupt our cells' ability to communicate with each other, which is vital for proper immune responses (see *Cholesterol*).

Lowered immune function is also linked to chronic fatigue, allergies, parasite infections, and some forms of heart disease. Many women also have low iron levels, which can reduce immune function – so have a blood test to check iron levels if you think this may be a problem. Prostaglandins, which are hormone-like substances, become more out of balance as we age. This has the effect of suppressing the immune system and affecting important processes, such as body temperature and metabolism. Essential fatty acids, such as EPA (from fish oil) and GLA (from evening primrose, blackcurrant, and borage oils) help to restore the proper prostaglandin ratios, thereby supporting the immune system (see *Fats You Need To Eat*).

Foods to Avoid
- As a person with a sweet tooth, I'm sorry to say that refined sugar greatly compromises your immune system. If you are run-down and then you eat one, say, mass produced sugary breakfast bar, it can literally send your immune system into free-fall – and the next thing you know, you have a cold, or develop cold sores or whatever. So if you know that you are under stress, stay away from products high in refined sugars and allow your immune system time to regroup. Use a little organic agave syrup or organic brown rice syrup as healthier alternatives to refined sugar, and generally cut down on pies, biscuits, sweets and shop-bought sugary snacks and drinks.
- Reduce your intake of caffeine and alcohol, which place an additional burden on the immune system.
- Avoid any foods containing lots of preservatives, additives and especially the artificial sweetener aspartame, which places an extra burden on your liver.
- Avoid all smoked foods and cheeses.
- Reduce your intake of saturated fats found in red meat and full-fat dairy produce including milks, cheese, Greek yoghurts, and chocolates, as well as hydrogenated and trans-fats (see *Fats You Need To Eat*).

Friendly Foods
- When the body is under attack it requires more protein, so eat fresh fish, organic tofu (cooked), fresh chicken, turkey and lean organic meats. Lentils, beans and pulses are also excellent sources of low-fat, healthy protein.
- Eat organic as much as possible. Make sure your diet is high in all fresh fruits and vegetables, which are packed with nutrients.
- Eat more fresh fish, broccoli, cabbage, cauliflower, parsley, green beans, apples, green salads, pumpkin, buckwheat, watercress, papaya, mango, quinoa, soya beans and millet.
- Eat sprouts, such as alfalfa and brown rice, and algae, such as spirulina and chlorella. Otherwise use Green Magic Powder – containing Hawaiian spirulina, chlorella, lecithin, barley and wheat grass, kamut, pectin apple fibre, kelp and wheat sprouts, CoQ10, royal jelly, artichoke powder and lactobacillus acidophilus, this is a great all round way to ingest good

nutrients, healthy bacteria, keep the body more alkaline and help keep you regular. Details on www.itsgreenmagic.com or call Helen Cruikshank on 07798 873266. Add a teaspoon of this powder to a breakfast smoothie to boost immune function – see recipe under *General Health Hints*.

- Eat more purple, red and orange foods: blueberries, bilberries and blackberries are particularly high in immune-boosting nutrients, as are sweet potatoes, apricots, pumpkin, papaya and red peppers.
- Nuts and seeds are packed with essential fats, and minerals, such as zinc and selenium (see *Fats You Need To Eat*).
- See also *General Health Hints*.
- Eat more freshly made soups – many supermarkets and take-away shops now sell freshly made organic soups. They are easy on the digestive system and full of nutrients. Add barley, brown rice, lentils and more cabbage to soups.
- Alternatives to refined sugars are organic agave syrup or xylitol (found in fruit fibres), which have a low glycaemic index and thus a minimal impact on blood sugar levels. Higher Nature make Zylo Sweet. Otherwise, try Valdivia, a totally unrefined sugar, rich in minerals. To order, call 0207 580 7537.

Useful Remedies
- Take a good-quality, high-strength multi-vitamin and mineral, as well as an antioxidant formula, daily.
- Organic -ource Hemp Seed Protein Powder (available from all good health shops), or Vianesse Protein Powder, which is free from lactose, but contains plenty of easy to absorb protein – to order, call The Wholistic Medical Centre on 020 7580 7537.
- Add organic-source green food powders to your breakfast cereals, smoothies, or vegetable juices, and drink daily. They are packed with nutrition that helps to keep your immune system in good shape. See details of Green Magic Powder, above, or try Viridian's 100% Organic Green Food Blend Powder.
- Drink more pau d'arco herbal tea, which can boost immune function.
- Echinacea and astragalus in a combination formula can be taken in capsules or fluid extract to really help boost immune function, if taken daily for 3 months. Astragalus has been shown to increase white blood cell counts. Try Ultimate Echinacea Complex by Holos Health, which is available from www.holoshealth.com or the Nutri Centre. **NC**
- Drink more alkaline waters as the immune system is weakened when the body becomes too acid – see *Acid–Alkaline Balance*. Water Filter Man supply alkalizing filters for your home. Their number is 0844 8733148, or log on to www.waterfilterman.co.uk.
- Colostrum is the pre-milk fluid produced by all mothers after giving birth. It arrives before breast milk and contains 37 natural immune-boosting factors and 8 growth factors, which support the immune system and regeneration of all types of cells. Recent studies have shown it to be extremely beneficial, not only for the newborn, but for people of all ages. Dose: 2000–4000mg per day. Try Kirkman's Colostrum for one month. This supplement is great for young children as it boosts immune function and reduces the likelihood of suffering food intolerances. **NC**
- Astragalus is a traditional Chinese herb used to strengthen the immune system. At least one clinical trial in the US has shown astragalus to boost T-cell levels to close to normal in some cancer patients, suggesting the possibility of a synergistic effect of astragalus with chemotherapy. Dose: 250mg twice a day.
- Sunlight and vitamin D are absolutely crucial to good immune health. Go out in sensible amounts of sunshine and take 1000iu of vitamin D3 daily.

- Beta Glucans 1–3, 1–6, derived from yeast cell walls, are proven to strengthen the body's innate immune system (the immune system you are born with), making it more resistant to pathogens from food and air. Take 250–500mg daily. It can also be taken by children and reduces the likelihood of food intolerances triggered by a weakened immune system. Dr Paul Clayton based in the UK and US is a medical pharmacologist. His website research on Beta Glucans is well worth a look – find him at www.healthdefence.com. Glucosan, developed by Dr Clayton, is available from Vitalize Health products on 0870 042 8423 or via www.vitalizeshop.co.uk.

Helpful Hints

- One of the simplest ways to boost immune function is to get more sleep and relax more. Take a day off to call your own; book a holiday; walk out in the countryside breathing the fresher air – and see how that alone lifts your spirits.
- Laugh a lot: watch films that make you laugh; make friends with people who make you laugh. Laughter and having some fun strengthen immune function.
- Stress alone can suppress immune function by up to 60%. Stress triggers the release of the hormone cortisol, which is thought to shrink the thymus gland (which is where T-cells mature and is situated in your upper chest area, just below the hollow in your neck). Therefore, keep your stress levels in check (see also *Adrenal Exhaustion* and *Stress*).
- Learn to say no and not feel guilty.
- Greatly reduce your exposure to external pollutants, such as cigarette smoke, car fumes, chemical-based sprays and heavy metals.
- If possible take regular holidays in the sunshine, which helps to boost your immune system.
- Think positively – people who are cheerful and who look on the bright side have stronger immune systems.
- Take regular exercise but not to excess. Don't over-exercise if you are truly exhausted.
- To help decongest your lymphatic system, apply therapeutic grade essential oils along the spine, under the arm, and in the neck, breast and groin areas – anywhere that is congested. Try a blend of 3 drops of cypress, 1 of orange and 2 of grapefruit.
- See *General Health Hints* for more help.

IMPOTENCE
(see also Libido Problems)

There are many reasons why a man may lose either his desire for sex or his ability to get and maintain an erection. Both problems are often linked to long-term stress and, by dealing effectively with stress, sexual desire and function can, in many cases, be restored. The related problem of 'brewer's droop' is mainly due to excessive alcohol consumption, which can interfere quite severely with the ability to maintain an erection. Stress, and an imbalance of male hormones such as testosterone, DHEA plus Cortisol, are also linked to this condition. Dr Shamin Daya, says 'When men's (and women's) energy levels are compromised, then libido is almost always also affected. Statins and many prescription drugs, including beta blockers, will also affect libido.'

Smoking has been linked with reduced ability to maintain an erection; this is because smoking constricts blood flow, which is essential for erectile function. Anyone with erectile problems would do well to consider a cholesterol-lowering diet.

Foods to Avoid
(see *Circulation* and *Libido Problems*)

Friendly Foods
(see *Circulation* and *Libido Problems*)

Useful Remedies
- The herb ginkgo biloba when taken regularly improves circulation.
- Take 2 grams of the amino acid L-arginine daily (unless you are suffering an attack of cold sores, as arginine will make them worse), as this amino acid has been shown to improve impotence. Or try Arginmax by Arginmax – containing L-arginine, ginseng, gingko, vitamins, antioxidants and minerals to help support sexual function. **NC**
- Stress reduces B-vitamins in the body – therefore, also include a good-quality multi-vitamin and mineral for men that includes a full range of B-vitamins.
- Muira Puama, a South-American herb, is considered nature's most potent viagra. A daily dose of 1 gram of a standardized extract has been shown to be effective as it raises testosterone levels. In one study of 100 men with impotence problems, 66% had increased frequency of intercourse, while 70% reported intensification of libido. The stability of the erection was restored in 55% of the patients, and 66% reported a reduction in fatigue. The herb is suitable for both men and women. Rio Trading make a good one. **NC**
- Pycnogenol – pine bark extract – increases nitrous oxide production, which relaxes blood vessels thereby increasing blood flow to the sexual organs. 100mg daily. **PN**

Helpful Hints
- Have your hormone levels checked by a qualified doctor, as testosterone patches are known to help increase libido in both sexes. Once hormones are balanced, sex drive often returns (see *Menopause*).
- Testosterone creams that are applied directly to the genital areas are also available. These have been shown to increase libido and erectile function in most patients. For more help, contact Dr Malcolm Carruthers at the Andropause Centre in Harley Street, London on 020 7636 8283, or visit www.centreformenshealth.co.uk.
- Measures to alleviate stress are often very effective. Take regular exercise and learn to laugh more. This releases natural endorphins, which lower stress levels and help you feel more positive. Learn to breathe more deeply.
- People who use a large amount of marijuana or take steroids may also find their erectile function diminished.
- By constantly worrying about your lack of sex drive, you often make the situation worse. Studies show that a lack of vitamins C, E, A and B, plus the minerals zinc and selenium, can cause a low sperm count and lack of sex drive. Anyone taking regular antidepressants or sleeping pills may be lacking in these nutrients.
- If the condition continues, or you are worried about infertility as well as impotency, see a doctor who is also a nutritionist (see *Useful Information*).
- Acupuncture can help with impotence by unblocking energy channels within the body to help increase blood flow.
- To help get you in the mood, try watching a sexy movie – this works for most people.

INCONTINENCE *(see also Cystitis, Leaky Gut and Prostate Problems)*

Incontinence can lead to urine leaking out when the bladder is put under pressure when you laugh, cough, sneeze or exert yourself. It can also occur when you have eaten to excess and the bloated bowel exerts pressure on the bladder. This type of problem is referred to as stress incontinence and is usually associated with a weakness in the muscle in the pelvic floor.

Exercise can help keep the pelvic floor strong, and childbirth tends to weaken it, hence it is a good idea to do plenty of pelvic exercises after giving birth. I suffered this problem during my twenties after giving birth to my daughter. It became so embarrassing that in my early thirties I found a gynaecologist who specialized in bladder repair and had surgery. It has really made a huge difference and I can now exercise without the embarrassment. Non-chronic but acute urinary incontinence is usually caused by an infection (see also *Candida* and *Cystitis*).

Also if you suffer a leaky gut, you may also be prone to a leaky bladder. See *Leaky Gut*.

Foods to Avoid
- Any food to which you have an allergy or intolerance can aggravate incontinence. The worst offenders are usually wheat and cow's milk.
- Avoid fluoridated water, toothpastes and mouthwashes. I have received many letters from people who say that when fluoride is eliminated, the problem stops. It also seems to help with children who wet the bed.
- The biggest culprits are usually yeast, wheat, dairy, alcohol and sugar.
- Don't overeat – when your bowel becomes full, pressure is exerted on the bladder.
- See also *Stress*, as when your adrenals are on limits, you often need to urinate far more often.

Friendly Foods
- Add a little cayenne pepper to your foods. It may initially aggravate the problem, but in the long term usually helps.
- See *General Health Hints* and *Friendly Foods* under *Leaky Gut*.

Useful Remedies
- A high-strength, multi-vitamin and mineral for women.
- 500mg of calcium with 250mg of magnesium to help muscle control. After 6 weeks you should see benefits.
- The mineral silica – take 75mg daily.
- The herb horsetail, which contains silica, is very useful for strengthening the bladder. You can take 5ml daily.
- Cantharis is a homeopathic remedy for frequent urination associated with any burning. Causticum and equisetum arvense (horsetail) help to reduce symptoms when there is a weakness in the bladder.
- Cranberry Plus by BioCare contains cranberry concentrate, vitamin C, and acidophilus, and helps to fight any infection (such as cystitis). **BC**

Helpful Hints
- Check with your doctor, who will be able to tell you if you have an infection that is causing this problem.
- Women can try using a set of vaginal cones containing weights to help strengthen the muscles. For information on the Aquaflex system, call the information line on 0161 925 3180. Website: www.mobilis-rolyan.com.
- Also there is a progressive resistance exerciser called the Pelvic Toner. Website: www.pelvictoner.co.uk. Tel: 0117 968 1414. This has proven really useful in improving muscle tone, which can help cure or greatly relieve this problem.

- An osteopath or chiropractor can check the alignment of bones in the pubic area. This can help because if the bones are out of balance, urine flow in both men and women is sometimes affected.
- Acupuncture has proven helpful to some people. See *Useful Information*.
- Contact The Bladder and Bowel Foundation helpline on 0845 345 0165. Website: www.bladderandbowelfoundation.org.

INDIGESTION *(see also Flatulence, Hiatus Hernia and Low Stomach Acid)*

Indigestion covers a variety of symptoms from cramping in the stomach, to heartburn, wind, belching, and even pain in the bowel. It is usually a sign that the digestive system is having difficulty coping with food, and this is frequently due to a lack of stomach acid and digestive enzymes in the small intestine. The problem can be made worse if you eat too quickly and don't chew food thoroughly. Overeating, drinking to excess, eating poor food combinations, or eating when stressed all exacerbate indigestion.

Many people who suffer chronic indigestion have the bacterium *Helicobacter pylori* – ask your doctor about a blood, breath or stool test. Well worth investigating this possibility. If you test positive you would need to remove, gluten, cow's milk and soya milk from your diet.

Severe indigestion-type symptoms in the centre of the chest may indicate a heart problem. If you are distressed in any way – call a doctor. Better to be safe than sorry!

Foods to Avoid
- Red meat and fatty cuts of meat are hard to digest. Cheese, especially melted cheese, is really hard for the body to digest. Keep cheese to a minimum.
- Chocolate can be hard for some people to digest, and any foods that you are not digesting properly, can trigger indigestion and bloating.
- Generally, try to reduce your intake of sugar and sugary foods, such as cakes, biscuits and rich puddings.
- Coffee, tea, chocolates, caffeine in any form, alcohol, peppers, citrus fruits, onions, and sometimes garlic, can be difficult to digest.
- Salt hinders digestion and assimilation of proteins, so cut down on sodium-based salts.
- Don't drink too much liquid with meals as this dilutes the stomach acid, which you need to digest your meal.
- Avoid fruit immediately after a large meal, unless it's a small chunk of pineapple or papaya.
- Avoid as much as possible rich, creamy foods and heavy desserts such as Christmas pudding.
- Avoid antacids that neutralize stomach acid, which is the very substance you need to digest your meals.
- Many people with indigestion have problems digesting wheat. Try Ryvita, low-salt crisp breads, rice cakes, or amaranth crackers, available from health shops. Especially avoid warm croissant-type treats, as freshly cooked 'dough' is really hard on your digestion. I know they are delicious, so if you are desperate, just one a week!

Friendly Foods
- Drink some ginger or dandelion root tea with or before meals to stimulate digestion.
- Small meals made from whole foods and small quantities of meat or fish are much easier on the digestion.
- Try eating small amounts of pineapple or papaya before a meal. They contain enzymes that can enhance digestion.

- Add more fresh root ginger to foods, as it is very calming.
- If you like beans and pulses, but they give you wind, soak them overnight first and/or cook them with a strip of kombu seaweed, which helps to pre-digest the beans.
- Eat more live, low-fat yoghurts.

Useful Remedies
- Take betaine hydrochloride (HCl; stomach acid); 1 capsule with main meals. If you have active stomach ulcers, or the HCl causes a burning sensation, take a digestive enzyme that is free from HCl.
- Chew 1–2 tablets of deglychyrrized liquorice before a meal. This soothes any symptoms of heartburn or indigestion.
- Acidophilus and bifidus are healthy bacteria, which encourage better digestion and elimination. Take 1–2 capsules at the end of a meal.
- Sip peppermint tea after meals.
- Bitters stimulate stomach-acid production and therefore improve digestion; Dr Theiss Swedish Bitters and A Vogel Centaurium tincture work very well (taken before meals).
- If symptoms are at the bowel level, try a good colon-cleanser, such as psyllium husks. Lepicol powder or capsules contain both psyllium husks and probiotics.
- Aloe vera is a very good digestive-system healer. Taken twice a day between meals. Try Aloe Gold Natural from Higher Nature. **HN** Aloe Pura also make an excellent Stomach Formula Aloe Drink.

Helpful Hints
- Digestive enzyme production is greatly inhibited when you are stressed, therefore your ability to digest and absorb foods is severely impaired. Don't eat when you are stressed, especially avoid glutens in breads and cereals, plus cheese and rich foods.
- Sit down and eat food in a relaxed setting.
- Go for a walk after eating, which really aids digestion.
- Eat fruit between meals, but avoid fruits you know can cause the problem, such as oranges and grapefruit.
- If symptoms are acute, avoid eating for a short time, or at most eat only lightly cooked, small meals regularly.
- Sometimes when people suffer indigestion, it is because they are unable to digest some information or something going on in their lives. If this is the case it would be worth seeing a homoeopath, who may be able to resolve the underlying issues. See also *Stress*. Meanwhile, the homeopathic remedy Nux Vomica 30c helps reduce the symptoms of indigestion.
- Consult a nutritionist who will help re-balance your system (see *Useful Information*).

INFERTILITY *(see also Adrenal Exhaustion, Polycystic Ovarian Syndrome and Stress)*

Sperm counts have dropped dramatically in the last fifty years and around 25% of couples planning to have a baby will have problems conceiving. In four out of every ten cases the problems are on the male side, with 30% of men being sub-fertile and 2% totally infertile. If the male sperm count is low, this can sometimes be a result of an infection such as mumps.

A low sperm count can be due to a poor diet, nutrient deficiencies and/or environmental toxins, such as lead, mercury and cadmium. Food additives, smoking, alcohol, food intolerances, urinary tract infections, plus stress, can all affect fertility. Common organisms such as *Mycoplasma hominis*, *Ureaplasma*, *Toxoplasma* and *Chlamydia* can infect the urinary tracts of men and women. They don't always cause infertility, but there seems to be a higher number of these organisms in the secretions of couples who have unexplained fertility problems. Smoking and alcohol can also reduce sperm count. Many scientists now openly state that sperm counts in the Western world are dropping because of overuse of herbicides and pesticides, which have an oestrogen-boosting effect within the body that counteracts male testosterone.

Female infertility may be due to blockages in the fallopian tubes, which can be triggered by an infection such as thrush or cystitis, or by chlamydia and other sexually transmitted diseases. Whatever the cause, diagnosis requires a medical examination.

Sometimes, there is a problem with ovulation, usually due to a hormone imbalance. Other conditions, such as endometriosis, polycystic ovarian syndrome (see that section), low thyroid function, a diet deficient in nutrients especially zinc, magnesium, vitamin D, and/or environmental toxins are also common causes of infertility in women.

Candida, a yeast fungal overgrowth, is also linked to infertility. When women are under a lot of stress the body releases adrenaline, eventually exhausting the endocrine system and affecting hormone levels, which can prevent conception – see *Adrenal Exhaustion*.

Foods to Avoid

- Coffee, chocolate and cola, which all contain caffeine, have been shown to affect impotence and reduce the chance of conception.
- Sugary snacks, puddings and confectionery provide empty calories and in turn upset hormone balance. Keep to an absolute minimum; see below for healthy, fertility-boosting snacks.
- Alcohol alone can reduce your chances of fertility, and the more you both drink, the more your chances of conceiving are reduced. It affects zinc levels, reduces sperm count, causes malformation of sperm, and impairs sperm motility in men, while preventing implantation in women. The effect is worse when combined with caffeine.
- Avoid foods high in saturated fats, junk foods, pre-packaged meals, sugar and salt, which deplete the body of the nutrients needed for conception.
- Avoid dairy produce from cows, which can lead to malabsorption of essential nutrients if you have an intolerance; see *Allergies*.
- Wheat is high in phytates, chemicals that block absorption of some minerals. Avoid foods containing wheat as much as possible. This includes bread, cakes, spelt-based foods, biscuits, pasta and pizza bases.
- Refined soya products including soya milk may well have a negative effect on fertility.
- Avoid food additives, preservatives and artificial flavourings and sweeteners. Individually, tartrazine is known to lower zinc levels and other additives lower magnesium. The London Food Commission found that of 426 chemicals listed, 35 were found to individually cause reproductive problems ranging from impotency to birth defects. No one knows the real effect on fertility or the foetus of a chemical cocktail.
- Non-organic food is high in pesticides and other hazardous substances, which have a hormone-disrupting effect. Offspring in cattle exposed to high levels of pesticides are known to be born with higher levels of malformation.
- For a woman, when the tissues are more alkaline, this helps with conception, because the body functions more efficiently when the pH is alkaline. For full information, see *Acid–Alkaline Balance*.

Friendly Foods

- Good-quality protein is needed for hormone health and sperm synthesis. Choose from lean organic poultry and meat, eggs, fish and vegetable sources, such as seeds, nuts and beans.
- Fibre found in wholegrains – brown rice, millet, quinoa, barley and oats – helps to reduce excess oestrogen levels and eliminate hormone residues.

- Make sperm stronger by eating more brown rice, lentils, beans, organic nuts and seeds – all rich in fertility-boosting zinc. Enzymes on the sperms' heads need zinc in order to push through the egg to fertilize it. Zinc has a huge impact on women's fertility, too.
- Eat oily fish, such as mackerel, organic-farmed salmon, trout, sardines, pilchards or herrings, at least once a week as they are rich in omega-3 essential fats needed for hormone health.
- Add some sunflower seeds, pumpkin seeds and linseeds (flax seeds) to any low-sugar breakfast cereal, as they are high in minerals and essential fats.
- A lack of selenium in the diet has been shown to reduce egg production in females and leads to reduced testicular growth and problems with sperm maturation in men. Eat more brown rice, seafood, oats, barley and garlic.
- Nuts, barley, rye, oats and brown rice are also rich in the mineral manganese, a lack of which leads to defective ovulation and testicular degeneration, as well as affecting libido in men.
- Fresh fruit and vegetables are rich in vitamin C, which helps sperm motility. Choose from papaya, mango, strawberries, broccoli, sweet potatoes, pumpkin, watercress, cabbage, red and yellow peppers, peas, blackcurrants and oranges.
- Carry a small bag of mixed seeds around for fertility-boosting snacks. These are full of the minerals zinc, manganese, chromium and essential fats.
- Use organic olive, sunflower, walnut and linseed (flax seed) oils for your salad dressings.
- If you have any iron deficiency, eat more lean meats, especially calves' liver, turkey and chicken, plus eggs and dried apricots.
- Leafy green vegetables, cereals, honey, beans and nuts are all good sources of magnesium, which may also be deficient. Having an alkaline diet is important for conception – see *Acid–Alkaline Balance*.
- Try caffeine-free alternatives, such as dandelion tea or dandelion root coffee, as these can have beneficial effects on the liver and consequently enhance hormone production.

Useful Remedies
- The most important supplements are folic acid (which can prevent spina bifida), vitamins B12 and B6, zinc, selenium, essential fats, vitamins C and E, and natural-source carotenes.
- In order to produce testosterone at optimal levels, any multivitamin for men needs to contain at least 30mg of zinc, 200mcg of selenium and 250mg of magnesium.
- Nourish has researched and developed a natural treatment plan for couples to help them take control of their reproductive health. The recommended four-month course comes in convenient monthly packs and contains nutrients and other ingredients that are vital both for conception and for your baby's healthy development. Call 01534 857197 or visit www.nourish-fertility.com.
- A multi-vitamin and mineral – many companies now make special formulas for women who are trying to conceive. The Pregnancy Pack is available from Health Plus on 01323 872277. Website: www.healthplus.co.uk.
- Metabolics makes a Pre-natal Formula balanced with nutrients needed for any woman wanting to become pregnant. For details call the Wholistic Medical Centre on 020 7580 7537. Men should also take a multi formula. Details on same number. **WMC**
- Both partners should take a B-complex plus 3000iu of vitamin A, which are needed for egg and sperm production. Once pregnant the vitamin A can be reduced to 3000iu daily. **NB If you are taking a pre-natal multi, then you should not need extra vitamin A or B.**
- Full-spectrum, natural-source vitamin E, 200iu a day, has been shown to help reduce both male and female infertility by helping to balance hormone levels and enabling egg and sperm to fuse. This should be included in most multis for men and women.
- Both partners should take 1–3 grams of vitamin C daily with meals.

- Essential fats are crucial for healthy hormone functioning in both partners. Take a 1-gram omega-3 capsule daily. See under *Fats You Need To Eat* for further details.
- The celloid mineral complex potassium chloride; 150mg can help clear the fallopian tubes. Or try the tissue salt Kali Mur by New Era. **NC**
- L-arginine and carnitine are two amino acids that are needed for sperm production and to prevent sperm becoming too 'sticky', which can interfere with conception. You could take 1.5–3 grams of each daily. Avoid arginine if you have herpes (cold sores) or shingles.
- Dr Marilyn Glenville also recommends the herb agnus castus, which has been shown to help restore hormone balance in women. It also helps to regulate periods and increases the ratio of progesterone to oestrogen. **NB Not to be used by anyone using drugs treatments or IVF to conceive.**

Helpful Hints

- Anyone wishing to become pregnant should have a full health MOT to make sure that hormone and nutrient levels are all in balance. Also conditions such as blocked fallopian tubes, PCOS, endometriosis, thyroid imbalances, diabetes and so on can then be ruled out.
- For more help read, *Natural Solutions to Infertility* by Dr Marilyn Glenville (Piatkus), one of the leading alternative doctors in this field. For more information on Dr Glenville's work, log on to www.marilynglenville.com. Her site includes an online personalized assessment and action plans to suit.
- Another good book for women struggling with their health and fertility issues is *Women's Encyclopedia of Natural Medicine* by Professor of Gynecology Tori Hudson. Order from the Nutri Centre Bookshop on 020 7323 2382.
- Anthony Porter, a reflexologist since 1972, who went to China and other parts of the Far East to teach reflexology during the 1980s, found that their methods, combined with his own, gave even better results. He has taught his advanced techniques to thousands of reflexologists internationally and says: 'With ART we can not only balance various parts of the body (which is what happens with normal reflexology), but we can also feel more subtle changes within the 7,000 nerve-endings or reflex areas of the feet, and after working on them, this has a profound therapeutic effect.' Medical research with a leading gynaecologist has shown huge success using ART to help women conceive. To find an ART therapist in your area, log on to www.artreflex.com.
- Eat organic and get more nutrients, as hormone and antibiotic residues are known to affect fertility in both men and women.
- Your weight can affect your fertility; check out your body mass index (BMI) – a measure of your weight in relation to your height. A BMI of 20–25 is ideal. Below 20 is underweight and above 25 is overweight.
- Hypnotherapy has been proven to be an effective aid when dealing with infertility. Studies show that it can also increase conception rates for couples undergoing IVF treatment. See *Useful Information*.
- Regular acupuncture has proven very successful for many couples – see *Useful Information*.
- Cigarette smoke is high in the toxin cadmium. This toxin competes against zinc, which is vital for fertility. This is one of the reasons why smokers are less likely to conceive. Stop smoking – and avoid alcohol.
- Ask to be screened for any urinary infections and sexually transmitted diseases, many of which lay dormant and are often symptom free. 69% of couples screened have an infection.
- Much of the water in the UK is contaminated with high levels of fluoride, aluminium, copper and cadmium, which compete with essential minerals in the body. Pesticide residue and traces of the contraceptive pill (which can have hormone-disrupting qualities) are excreted via urine,

which eventually finds its way into the water system, and can also affect fertility. The Fresh Water Filter Company Ltd offers a broad range of water filters. Call them on 0845 177 0896, or visit their website at www.freshwaterfilter.com.

- Limit the amount of chemicals in your home and garden, such as wood preservatives, perfumes, insect sprays and so on. Use eco-friendly products.
- Avoid too much exposure to mobile phones, computers and electrical equipment.
- If either partner is taking prescription drugs or regular over-the-counter remedies, check for their known side effects.
- Deal with stress, as stress in either partner can lower the chances of conception. I have received letters from many couples who, when they gave up trying so hard to conceive, bought a pet or adopted a child, found that a baby was on its way!
- See supplements to help reduce stress response under *Adrenal Exhaustion*.
- Sitting for long periods raises the temperature in the testicles, which may reduce male fertility. If you are deskbound, for example, or a long-distance driver, wear loose-fitting underwear and trousers, and get plenty of exercise.
- Contact Foresight, who specialize in giving couples information about how to plan for a healthy pregnancy and increase fertility naturally. The service includes nutritional status analysis, although this is usually done in consultation with a recognized Foresight practitioner. Foresight can be contacted by writing to 178 Hawthorn Road, Bognor Regis, West Sussex PO21 2UY. Tel: 01243 868001. Website: www.foresight-preconception.org.uk.

INSECT BITES (and repellents)

Apart from the obvious discomfort that they cause, insect bites can occasionally transmit serious disease and cause severe allergic reactions, such as anaphylactic shock. If you know that you or a family member has a particular sensitivity to stings and bites, it is important to discuss this with your GP to make sure you take the appropriate medication away with you. You may also find the Allergy section very useful. For people who suffer anaphylactic shock, you need to carry adrenaline injections with you at all times. For anyone travelling to tropical countries, where malarial mosquitoes exist, take precautions seriously. In Africa a child dies every 30 seconds from malaria. In the Caribbean both my husband and myself have suffered dengue fever from mosquito bites, and I would never want to feel that ill again. The key, as always, lies in prevention. If you are unfortunate enough to be attacked by a swarm of bees, immediately close your eyes and mouth and wait for help. If you happen to be near water and can swim, then jump in.

Foods to Avoid
- Sugar makes your blood taste sweeter, especially to mosquitoes. If you are visiting the tropics, greatly reduce refined sugar for at least a week before you travel. Otherwise, use small amounts of organic agave syrup or xylitol (found in plant fibres) as sweeteners, as they have a lower glycaemic index.

Friendly Foods
- Garlic eaten on a regular basis may well make you smell less appetizing to stinging insects. Or take a one-a-day garlic tablet, such as Allimax.
- Malaria-carrying mosquitoes are attracted to the smell of human feet. Limburger cheese or other strong cheeses smell just like your feet, so by putting a bit of the cheese in your room at least 2.5m (5ft) away from you, the mosquitoes are distracted.

Useful Remedies

- Thiamine (B1), 300mg and 50mg of zinc per day. When these are excreted in our sweat, they give off an odour that repels insects. As all the B-vitamins work together, take a B-complex as well.
- Brewer's yeast, either as tablets or powder, is a rich source of vitamin B1, which changes the smell of your sweat, making you less attractive to insects. Take 6–8 tablets daily for a week prior to travel and during your stay. If you have candida, then don't take this supplement.
- Some people have found that taking feverfew, the herb that contains pyrethrum (an effective insecticide), really helps. Also, the herb catnip repels mosquitoes.
- Use Bug Ban by Herbcraft – spray liberally over the body as often as is needed.
- Quantum Buzz Away is deet-free and made from a combination of essential oils, such as cedarwood, eucalyptus, lemongrass and peppermint.
- Try a calendula, arnica and echinacea spray for the bites – to reduce the inflammation and itching. OP

Helpful Hints

- Use lemongrass or citronella candles at dusk to repel insects.
- Try an essential oil preparation for repelling insects. Mix 10 drops of lavender oil, 10 drops of orange oil, 5 drops of eucalyptus, 5 drops of citronella and 10 drops of neem oil into a base of 50ml apricot or almond oil. Apply sparingly on exposed areas of skin, especially ankles and wrists. Most good health food stores will carry these oils. If you do not have the time to do all this, the Organic Pharmacy make an insect repellent spray containing most of these oils. OP
- Try Alfresco body lotion, containing melissa, geranium, lavender and other essential oils, which has been proven to help repel insects. For details, call 020 8348 6704 or visit www.alfresco.uk.com.
- Avoid wearing any perfumed toiletries at night, and use cotton night clothes that cover the arms and wrists.
- Use a mosquito net. In Africa, trials on children showed incidence of malaria was cut by 80% when nets were used at night. These are easy to buy at travel shops.
- Ainsworth Homeopathic Pharmacy can supply a general travel kit, which includes items for bites, traveller's tummy, sunstroke and so on. They can also provide individual homeopathic remedies for tropical diseases such as malaria, and Caladium, which changes the smell of your sweat making you less attractive to insects. Tel: 020 7935 5330 or log on to www.ainsworths.com.

INSOMNIA *(see also Adrenal Exhaustion and Stress)*

If there is truly one subject I could fill a book on, it's this one. I have suffered from chronic insomnia for almost 30 years and I really do know what it's like not to be able to get to sleep because your mind is racing, and then when you do drop off to be wide awake again at 3 or 4am. Thanks mainly to our modern way of life – open-all-hours, stress and anxiety – one in every four people experiences irregular sleep problems. In order to go to sleep, you need to switch your brain from its normal busy or beta-brainwave state to a more relaxed alpha state. The best way to achieve this is by regular meditation, self-hypnosis, or relaxation tapes. No one functions well when they are short of sleep, as it not only compromises your immune system but can severely affect your day-to-day performance. Studies have shown that, when it comes to driving, lack of sleep can have almost as drastic an effect as drinking alcohol. Lack of sleep has also been shown to increase inflammation in the body.

Many people, including myself, when absolutely desperate, resort to prescription sleeping pills. The problem can then become chronic and addictive. This is why it's best to use sleeping pills only on the occasional night – as a preventative to stop the body and brain becoming overtired, which often makes it even harder to get to sleep. In the long term, prescription sleeping pills can affect your memory and upset delicate brain chemistry. It's worth noting that if you tend to wake regularly between 3 and 5am you are likely to be suffering adrenal exhaustion (see *Adrenal Exhaustion*); or if you wake between 1 and 3am, then it's likely that your liver is struggling, in which case you need to cut down on fats, coffee and alcohol, and eat lightly for a few days (see also *Liver Problems*).

People who suffer muscle twitching or restless legs also tend to suffer sleep deprivation. See *Restless Legs*. There can be many explanations for not getting enough sleep, such as noise or bladder problems, but if you can get to the root cause of the problem and deal with it, this often helps to let go of the fear of not sleeping.

Foods to Avoid

- Avoid eating large meals late at night, as this promotes a high insulin release which could, later in the night, lead to low blood sugar. When this happens, adrenaline is released into the blood stream to compensate for the low blood sugar – which usually wakes us up and leaves us unable to go back to sleep.
- Don't go to bed hungry, either, as this will affect your ability to get off to sleep. See below.
- Caffeine is one of the most important substances to avoid after around 5pm. Having said that, I have friends who can drink espresso and sleep like a log. I'm not one of them; if I drink filter coffee after 4pm I can be awake until the early hours. Remember that caffeine is not just found in tea and coffee, it's also in cola, chocolate, caffeine energy-type drinks, cocoa and some over-the-counter cold remedies.
- If you drink a fair amount of alcohol you tend to feel sleepy, but unfortunately because of the way it is metabolized in the body, you might sleep for 2–3 hours and then wake up again and find it very difficult to get back to sleep.
- Food intolerances can make the problem considerably worse. In one study cow's milk appeared to be the problem but it can be any food to which you have a sensitivity. Keep a food diary. See *Allergies*.
- Avoid red meat and too much protein in the evenings, which tend to wake up the brain. Eat protein for breakfast and/or lunch.
- Avoid cheese at night – it contains amino acids that can keep you awake and is very hard on your digestion.

Friendly Foods

- Try to eat the last meal of the day before 8pm and, if possible, make it a carbohydrate-based one, such as small amounts of pasta, potatoes or brown rice. These starchy foods can have a soporific effect. Eating carbohydrate-rich foods before sleep also encourages the body to produce the brain chemical serotonin, which can reduce anxiety and improve the quality of sleep.
- Serotonin is made from a constituent of protein called tryptophan, so include more foods such as fish, turkey, chicken, cottage cheese, beans, avocados, persimmon (Sharon fruit), bananas and wheat germ in your diet.
- Sprinkle wheat germ over a healthy breakfast cereal; Nature's Path and Alara (www.alara.co.uk) make healthy cereals from amaranth, quinoa and kamut that are sweetened with a little apple juice.
- Eat more lettuce at night – it contains the natural sedative lactucarium, which encourages deeper sleep. You can also heat crisp lettuce in stir fries and so on – it's delicious.

- Some people find that eating a banana or an oat cake half an hour before they go to sleep helps them sleep longer, as bananas and oats are a good source of tryptophan, which is calming.
- Many people have porridge for breakfast, but often having it as a supper or late-evening snack made with organic rice milk and a chopped banana encourages sound sleep. If I wake at night or cannot get off to sleep, I often have a small bowl of gluten-free porridge, with a chopped banana, a few sunflower seeds and raisins, made with a little organic rice milk and water, which helps me to get to sleep almost immediately. Otherwise, use any low-sugar cereal and only eat small amounts.
- If you are a regular tea or coffee drinker, gradually switch over to the decaffeinated varieties. Don't do this too quickly, as caffeine withdrawal headaches can be quite unpleasant.
- Drink camomile tea (or any night-time formulas) before going to bed.
- If you suffer low blood sugar problems, eat a banana with a Ryvita, oat or amaranth-based biscuit, or a cracker spread with something like humous just before going to bed. See also under *Low Blood Sugar* and *Adrenal Exhaustion*.

Useful Remedies
- Calcium and magnesium are nature's tranquillizers; take a two-in-one formula with your evening meal that includes 600mg of calcium and 300–400mg of magnesium. **SVHC**
- If, like me, you are a Type A person, always on the go with a 'busy' mind and you find that you often cannot 'switch' off at night, try the supplement Cortisol Manager. It's a blend of ashwagandha, L-theanine (from green tea), magnolia bark extract and phosphatidlyserine. This blend can be used in the day if you find yourself becoming very stressed and are producing cortisol and adrenaline – it really helps to calm you. Taking this supplement just before bed helps you to wind down. Made by Integrative Therapeutics Inc in the States – see www.integrativeinc.com. **NB If you are suffering total adrenal exhaustion then you are unlikely to be producing sufficient cortisol, and so would not need this blend. To check adrenal function, you can have a simple saliva test. See** *Adrenal Exhaustion*.
- Otherwise, the Life Extension make an L-theanine and lemon balm blend. The amino acid theanine is found in green tea, and it produces calming effects within the brain but does not make you drowsy or groggy. It helps you to relax by increasing alpha-brainwave activity. It also increases levels of dopamine, a brain chemical that improves mood. Try 100mg twice daily. See www.lef.org or contact the Nutri Centre on 0845 6026744. **NB Drinking green tea during the day is a great boost to your health, but it also contains caffeine, so avoid drinking the tea at night. Otherwise, buy a decaffeinated version.**
- Take a B-complex every morning to support your nerves and keep you calmer.
- Published research in 2010 demonstrated that pure jasmine oil enhances production of GABA, a neurotransmitter in the brain that induces relaxation and reduces anxiety. Jasmine oil has been found to be as effective as sedatives and sleeping pills. Dab a tiny amount on your wrists at night.
- Melatonin is a hormone secreted by the pineal gland in the brain, which regulates our sleep–wake cycle. It is produced at night and is nature's way of preparing the body for sleep. Melatonin is one of the most efficient antioxidants known and helps protect DNA. As we age, production of melatonin declines, which means we sleep less and sometimes have more problems getting to sleep. If you choose to take melatonin supplements, try taking only 0.5mg a night, and see how you go. It has been used successfully for years for jet lag and is freely available in health shops outside the UK, but within the UK you need a prescription. It can be ordered for your own use by calling Pharm West on 001 310 301 4015. Website: www.pharmwest.com.

- However, bio-electromagnetic research scientist Roger Coghill says: 'If you take melatonin supplements that you can buy online and in the States, most synthetic tablets contain thousands of times the natural dose that your pineal gland normally produces at night.' Therefore, Roger suggests a supplement called Asphalia, containing natural melatonin extracted from certain grasses, which mimics the normal dose made by your pineal gland to induce sleep at night, rather than the larger doses that are found in mass-produced tablets. Roger has permission from the MHRA (Medical Healthcare Regulatory Authority) to sell this food supplement in the UK. For more details or to find your nearest supplier, log on to www.asphalia.co.uk or call 01495 752122. Take 1 to 2 capsules 30 minutes before bed.
- The Life Extension Foundation in the US make a Natural Sleep Melatonin formula, which also contains co-factors such as calcium and B-vitamins. Find them on www.lef.org.
- Try a homeopathic mix of oats, passiflora, valerian and coffee (*Coffea*) – put one pill under the tongue just before bed and again if you wake in the night. **OP**, or ask their pharmacist to make up a remedy that matches your constitution and symptoms.

Helpful Hints
- Aim to be in bed by 10.30pm at the latest.
- Turn off electrical switches near the bed – see *Electrical Pollution*.
- One of the most important factors in sleep management is to get up at the same or a similar time every morning, regardless of when you go to bed.
- To help your body make more melatonin naturally, get out in the sunshine during the day, and then at night sleep in a fully darkened room – the darker the better.
- Noise is a problem for many people; I use ear plugs, which are at times a godsend.
- If you tend to be near or work with electrical equipment every day, particularly computers, then in the summer months try walking barefoot on grass for 5 minutes in the evening; this helps disperse any electromagnetic radiation that you build up during the day. Then warm your feet before going to bed. In winter, wear bed socks if your feet tend to be cold.
- Try reading a novel before switching out the lights – this takes your mind away from the day's activities and helps you to wind down. If you can't get off to sleep, don't panic. Get up and do something relaxing, like reading a few more pages of a novel, until you start to relax and let go; then go back to bed. Don't try to go to sleep, allow yourself to fall asleep naturally. Eat the breakfast cereal I suggest on the previous page – it works every time for me. You can also try taking another Cortisol Manager – see above.
- Exercising on a regular basis can often improve sleep patterns, but don't exercise too late in the day as the endorphins released by the brain can be quite stimulating.
- Find a way to reduce stress levels, as stressed individuals definitely have poorer sleep patterns.
- Meditation is particularly useful, as it helps you to clear the mind and get rid of all those extraneous thoughts. People who meditate on a regular basis enjoy better-quality sleep.
- Smoking can also be a factor in insomnia so if you want another reason for giving up, poor sleep patterns might be the last push you need.
- Massage your chest with a mixture of essential oils of lavender, clary sage, marjoram and basil, or add them to a relaxing bath. Or, buy a burner and let the aroma fill your room.
- Potter's Nodoff Mixture is a traditional herbal remedy to promote natural sleep. Available from all good health stores. For your nearest stockist, contact Potter's (Herbal Supplies) Ltd. Tel: 01942 219960. Website: www.pottersherbal.co.uk.
- Don't read any work papers close to bedtime – it stimulates your mind.
- Turn the bedside clock to the wall, so you will not panic about the time.
- Advanced reflexology, homeopathy, acupuncture, and hypnotherapy have all proved useful in restoring natural sleep patterns (see *Useful Information*).

- Inner Talk also make some very good tapes – for details, call 01628 898366 or visit www.innertalk.co.uk.
- Persistent insomnia can also be exacerbated by food intolerances, in which case it would be wise to consult a doctor who is also a qualified nutritionist (see *Useful Information*).
- Invest in a really comfortable mattress – simply being cosy, and not too warm and not too cold really helps. In winter buy a sheepskin mattress cover and in summer use cotton sheets.
- Read *Alternative Medicine Magazine's Definitive Guide to Sleep Disorders* by Herbert Ross and Keri Brenner (Celestial Arts).

INSULIN RESISTANCE

(see also Adrenal Exhaustion, Candida, Diabetes, Leaky Gut Syndrome, Low Blood Sugar)

Thanks to our over-consumption of refined sugary foods, stress and eating in a hurry, blood sugar problems are truly reaching epidemic proportions. If any blood sugar imbalance is not addressed, over time it can develop further into insulin resistance, which is also known as metabolic syndrome or, Syndrome X, and finally into full-blown diabetes.

Insulin is a hormone secreted by cells in the pancreas. Its major function is to lower blood sugar levels and promote the storage of sugars as fats. Its release is stimulated by the consumption of any type of carbohydrate from fruits and grains, to starchy vegetables like potatoes and cakes. It also slows the breakdown of any stored fats.

Of all the hormones associated with ageing, insulin is the king player and Dr Shamin Daya from the Wholistic Medical Centre in Harley Street, London says: 'High insulin levels trigger inflammation, hormone imbalance and deterioration of virtually every body system. This problem is closely associated with adrenal function – mainly adrenal exhaustion.' See under *Adrenal Exhaustion*.

According to US diabetes expert, Dr Ron Rosedale MD, almost everyone eating a typical Western diet is overproducing insulin. Bread, rice, potatoes, pasta and so on are digested into simple sugars, such as glucose, when they enter the gut. Eating large amounts of carbohydrates, such as cakes and biscuits, can result in a 'sugar rush'. Basically, insulin makes cells more receptive to glucose, so they can either metabolize it, or store it for future use as glycogen or fat. This takes glucose out of your blood and into your cells, lowering your blood sugar levels.

'However,' adds Dr Daya, 'when this process has been abused for many decades, it's liable to break down. Eventually, the body ceases to respond to glucose as it should and despite ever-increasing levels of insulin, glucose in the blood begins to rise. The cells can no longer utilize it properly. Insulin receptors on the surface of cells seem to have switched off and stopped listening to the signal from insulin, hence the term for this condition. Insulin resistance is dangerous. Apart from the obvious risk of progression into Syndrome X and eventually diabetes, high insulin levels result in excess sympathetic nervous system activity, which means the individual is prone to fatigue. What's more, because insulin is usually only released when there's an excess of blood sugar, conversion of fat back to sugar for use as fuel is blocked by the hormone, so weight loss becomes increasingly difficult. Insulin resistance is also an important factor in polycystic ovarian syndrome.' A real giveaway symptom of insulin resistance is weight gain around the waist and midriff – as in apple shape against pear shape.

Foods to Avoid

- White flour, white sugar, corn syrup, white potato and other refined starch-rich foods will increase blood-sugar problems. Bread, cakes, biscuits, pasta, pastries and other confectionery items, French fries, food-thickeners, coffee whiteners, white rice, and skimmed milk (milk with the fat reduced has proportionately more sugar).

■ Avoid refined sugar and foods containing sugar, such as fizzy drinks, chocolate, sweets and many processed foods (check labels), plus reduce your intake of honey, dried fruit and juices, as they are all rich in fast-releasing sugars. Try diluting fruit juices. A healthier alternative to refined sugars are organic agave syrup or xylitol, which have a low glycaemic index. **HN**

■ Artificial sweeteners may seem like a good solution, although they do nothing to reduce your sweet tooth and because they place a strain on the liver, can add to weight gain and other health problems.

■ Caffeine found in coffee, tea and cola drinks is a powerful stimulant. A cup of coffee contains around 100mg of caffeine, cola 50mg, tea 60mg, green tea 25mg, a slice of chocolate cake 25mg, and 25g (1oz) dark chocolate 30mg. Stimulants encourage sugar to be released into the blood stream.

■ Replace chocolate with fresh fruit. Replace coffee and tea with coffee alternatives available in all health shops. Try green or white teas, peppermint or fruit teas.

■ Alcohol is such a refined carbohydrate that much of it is converted to fat in the body. We are not suggesting you eliminate it altogether, but just be aware that it is fattening.

■ Note that many foods advertised as being low in fat are often high in sugar, which if not used up during exercise will turn to fat in the body and reside on your hips!

Friendly Foods

■ Eat more lentils and beans. Dr Jeffrey Bland and fellow researchers at the Functional Medicine Research Centre in Gig Harbour, Washington, have found that legumes create a very low insulin response and that increased intake of lentils, chick peas, beans and peas is desirable in the management of blood-sugar problems.

■ In general, vegetables have a beneficial effect on blood sugar and insulin, but certain vegetables appear to be even better at maintaining blood sugar and insulin levels, including members of the brassica family (cabbage, cauliflower, broccoli), plus sweet potato and other green leafy vegetables.

■ Soya products – especially fermented soya products, such as tempeh – help balance blood-sugar levels. Soya helps improve glucose transport, as well as containing soluble fibre that slows the absorption of glucose from the gut.

■ See also the dietary guidelines under *Diabetes*.

■ Make time for breakfast: this 'kick starts' your metabolism for the rest of the day and is crucial for better energy balance. 'In 11 years of advising people on how to improve their energy levels,' says nutritionist Shane Heaton, 'I've never met anyone who skips breakfast and has good energy levels for the rest of the day.' He recommends a piece of fruit followed by muesli or porridge with added pumpkin, sunflower or amaranth seeds. Oats, rich in B-vitamins and fibre, are ideal, providing good, slow-burn energy, although the most important thing is to choose breakfast foods you enjoy. By eating breakfast your energy will improve throughout the day. Any cravings for stimulants will decline, you'll sleep better, and you'll wake feeling more refreshed in the morning.

■ Protein helps wake up the brain and keeps you feeling full for longer. Eggs, tofu, quinoa, lean meats (preferably organic), fresh fish are all great proteins. Otherwise, make yourself a delicious breakfast smoothie (recipe under *General Health Hints*) that includes hemp seed protein powder.

■ Eat more foods in their natural state. Include complex carbohydrates and wholefoods, which contain higher levels of nutrients and fibre, such as brown rice, basmati rice, quinoa, buckwheat, amaranth, stone-ground or rye bread, porridge oats, fruits and vegetables. These foods also tend to have a low glycaemic index.

- Choose more foods with a low glycaemic index. This is a guide as to how much and how quickly sugar is released from certain foods, compared with straight glucose, which is set at 100. Some foods are fast, others are slow. For example, white bread scores 70, while rye bread is just 41. Bananas are 62, while apples are 39. You don't have to choose only low glycaemic index foods all the time, but where possible, choose alternatives with lower scores, and when you do eat high glycaemic index foods, mix them with protein or low glycaemic index foods to slow the sugar release. Read *The Low GL Diet Bible* by Patrick Holford (Piatkus) – a godsend for anyone with this problem. His website is at www.patrickholford.com.
- Drink more fluids, as dehydration is a key cause of fatigue and can make you crave fast-energy foods that contribute to blood sugar imbalance.
- If you are desperate for sugar, use small amounts of xylitol (ZyloSweet, **HN**) or organic agave syrup as sweeteners.

Useful Remedies
- A high-strength, multi-vitamin and mineral complex that provides a good range of antioxidants, chromium, and plenty of B-vitamins.
- The mineral chromium is the main constituent of 'glucose tolerance factor', a substance that helps with the delivery of sugar to cells. It's used widely by nutritional therapists to help balance blood sugar and reduce cravings. Take 100–200mcg twice daily with meals. American research has shown that when people who tend to eat a high-carbohydrate diet are given 200mcg of chromium daily, this one step helps reduce the incidence of diabetes by 50%. Most multis contain around 150mcg.
- Fish oil supplementation has been found not only to improve insulin sensitivity in diabetic animals, but also to help prevent diabetes-induced nerve damage. Take 2 grams daily of omega-3 oils.
- Antioxidant nutrients have also been found to improve insulin sensitivity. Take a good-quality antioxidant formula containing 100–400mg of natural-source, full-spectrum vitamin E and 50–100mg of alpha-lipoic acid, both known to improve insulin response. **HN**
- Ultrameal Plus 360 by Nutri is a specially fortified, vegetarian, powdered beverage mix, designed for the nutritional support of glucose metabolism and insulin regulation. **NC**
- Vitamin C is involved with energy production, so if your energy levels are low and your stress levels are high, take 1000mg of vitamin C twice daily with food.
- If stress is a real problem in your life, consider trying the herbs rhodiola or Siberian ginseng. They're both adaptogenic herbs, so help you adapt to stress and can really help improve your tolerance to stress of all kinds. Take 200–300mg of a standardized extract of either herb daily with meals. See also *Adrenal Exhaustion* for more adrenal support.
- Metagenics make a formula called Insinase – a formula of acacia and hops, which has a unique ability to help reverse insulin resistance. Take one tablet 3 times a day. **NC**.

Helpful Hints
- As well as eating sensibly, another way to improve glucose control and insulin sensitivity is through regular aerobic activity. This doesn't have to be intense exercise and can be as moderate as a regular walking programme. Even 20 minutes daily will help.
- Moderate alcohol consumption is OK.
- Reduce stress. Stress is a major hindrance to stabilizing blood sugar levels, because the fight-or-flight mechanism when you produce cortisol and adrenalin floods your blood with sugar ready for action. If we constantly suffer from low blood sugar, we can sometimes learn subconsciously to use stress as a way to keep us going. We might stay in a stressful job, make situations more stressful than they need to be, seek out stressful situations, take too much on, do things at the last minute, be late everywhere we go, and so on. Blood sugar imbalance

itself is a major stress on the body and at the same time lowers your stress tolerance, so by improving your blood sugar balance, your tolerance to other stresses in your life should improve. Try yoga, t'ai chi, meditation, massage, or having 'down time' every week, and learning to relax (for more help, see *Stress*).

- Stop smoking – cigarettes are a stimulant, which many people use to keep themselves going. If you find smoking relaxing, you are very likely addicted. The feeling of relaxation is most probably the alleviation of withdrawal symptoms (commonly anxiety, stress, tension, nervousness and so on). Those who stop smoking and gain weight usually do so because they replace the cigarettes with other stimulants instead, such as sugar or sugar-containing foods and drinks.

- The worst thing you can do if your energy levels are poor is go long hours without eating. So eat small, frequent meals throughout the day – every 2–3 hours or so – and avoid skipping meals. People who miss meals often experience hypoglycaemic (low blood sugar) symptoms. Healthy snacks throughout the day can include fruit, nuts, seeds, rice or oat cakes with humous or other spreads, raw vegetables (such as carrots), rye crackers with lentil pâté and so on.

INTERMITTENT CLAUDICATION

(see also Angina, Atherosclerosis, Circulation and Heart Disease)

This condition is characterized by a pain in the legs, usually in the calves, when walking. It is caused by blockages in the arteries supplying blood to the legs and is due to the hardening of the arteries in the lower body. To deal successfully with intermittent claudication, you need to resolve the hardening of the arteries. Diets and natural therapies that help to reduce the build-up of deposits on the arteries are the most important treatment for this condition. See *Atherosclerosis*.

Dr Shamin Daya says: 'Statins, drugs used to lower LDL cholesterol levels, can contribute to this problem, and also food intolerances, particularly gluten, wheat, lack of exercise and dehydration. Smokers are more likely to develop these types of circulation problems.'

Foods to Avoid
- Greatly reduce your intake of animal fats and saturated fats, including margarines and highly refined mass-produced cooking oils. Avoid red meat, chicken skin, too much butter, full-fat milk and most mass-produced pies, sausages, cakes and so on.
- All fried foods should be avoided.
- Cut down alcohol to only 2 units a day.
- See under *Atherosclerosis*.

Friendly Foods
- Oily fish is rich in the omega-3 fats that help to thin the blood naturally.
- Use garlic and onions liberally as they help to lower LDL cholesterol levels.
- Adopt a diet rich in soluble and insoluble fibres from fruits and vegetables, nuts and seeds, linseeds, oat or rice bran and psyllium husks.
- Eggs are fine as long as they are boiled, poached or scrambled and not fried.
- Use plenty of fresh root ginger in cooking, in teas or with fruits to aid circulation.
- Look for non-hydrogenated spreads in the supermarket such as Biona, Vitaquell and Olivio. Use olive oil instead of butter.
- Higher Nature also make hemp, pumpkin seed, walnut and coconut oil butters. HN

- Drink at least 6–8 glasses of water daily.
- Eat more coriander, which helps detoxify heavy metals from the body, as does chlorella.
- See *Friendly Foods* in *Atherosclerosis* and *Circulation*.

Useful Remedies

- Take natural-source, full-spectrum vitamin E, 400iu a day, which has been shown to improve walking distance and decrease the discomfort of intermittent claudication. It needs to be taken for a minimum of six months to be effective. **NB Check with your GP if you are on blood-thinning drugs, as vitamin E will thin your blood naturally and reduce the risk of heart disease**.
- Vitamin B3 in the form of inositol hexaniacinate, 2 grams a day for at least three months. This form of B3 can help lower cholesterol and studies have shown it to be very effective for intermittent claudication. **NB Niacin produces an intense, short-term flushing of the skin, so start with 100mg daily with food and work your way up from there. It's very effective as it increases blood flow and lowers LDL, but many people are put off by the flushing effect.**
- Make sure you include a B-complex as all the B vitamins work together in the body.
- Omega-3 fish oils help to support circulation – take 2 grams daily.
- Ginger drops, taken three times daily in water, can aid circulation. Made by Metabolics – call 01380 812799 or visit www.metabolics.com.

Helpful Hints

- Discuss chelation therapy with your doctor – this involves an intravenous drip being administered by a private doctor, which over time helps to clear the arteries. There are several clinics in the UK – for details, call the Arterial Clinic on 01942 886644. Or contact Dr Wendy Denning in London on 020 7224 2423 or Dr Rodney Adeniyi-Jones, The Diagnostic Clinic, 50, New Cavendish Street, London W1G 8TL. Tel: 020 7486 6354 or log on to the website at www.thediagnosticclinic.com.
- Don't smoke, as there is known to be a strong link between smoking and the development of intermittent claudication.
- Gentle exercise is definitely beneficial, even though it may be uncomfortable. Do see your GP before starting on an exercise programme. People who exercise regularly are much less likely to develop intermittent claudication.
- Acupuncture and reflexology (especially advanced reflexology) are great for improving circulation and reducing pain. See *Useful Information*.

IRRITABLE BOWEL SYNDROME (IBS)

(see also Colitis, Constipation, Crohn's Disease, Diverticular Disease and Leaky Gut)

Nutritional physician Dr Shamin Daya, based in Harley Street, London says: 'Virtually all the above conditions have their root cause in food intolerances and a leaky gut, and when these issues are addressed the gut can, in the majority of cases, heal itself.'

One in every 12 of us visits the doctor with a digestive complaint and irritable bowel syndrome accounts for half these visits. In fact, 20 to 25% of people in the Western world are believed to suffer from IBS – to varying degrees – and this condition is three times more common in women than in men. IBS is an umbrella term used to describe a range of gut-related symptoms, such as abdominal pain, constipation or diarrhoea – or both alternating from day to day. Bloating, wind, headaches, nausea, blood/and or mucous or undigested food in the stool, anxiety, cramps and depression are also often associated with IBS.

The most commonly offending foods known to trigger IBS and all gut problems are gluten, wheat, dairy from animal sources, refined carbohydrates (white foods full of refined sugar), coffee, alcohol, tea and citrus foods – although an intolerance can be present to the most innocuous of foods that you would never suspect.

Stress is a major factor in gut problems, as the digestion shuts down during stressful times. These digestive juices then don't get to do their job properly, which leaves incompletely digested particles of food to irritate the gut. A lack of digestive enzymes and stomach acid (see *Acid Stomach* and *Low Stomach Acid*) can also lead to incompletely digested food irritating the gut.

Parasites are a growing and often overlooked factor: 20% of all people tested have parasites, and 49% of people with IBS are known to have the parasite *Blastocystis hominis*, and 20% of people with IBS have the parasite *Dientamoeba fragilis*. If you have ever travelled abroad or had a bout of food poisoning, either while on holiday or in the UK, or if you allow pets to walk on food-preparation surfaces, eat raw fish (sushi) or insufficiently cooked meats, or store meat above vegetables in your fridge, then parasites could be a factor.

You and your doctor should also consider dysbiosis – an imbalance of good to bad bacteria in the gut. Any yeasts, such as candida (see *Candida*), parasites and bad bacteria present in the bowel upset this delicate balance and can cause symptoms of IBS. This imbalance of bacteria can also be triggered by a poor diet that has insufficient fibre, and is high in alcohol, fatty foods and/or sugar. Antibiotics will also upset this balance.

Occasionally, the symptoms of IBS can reflect a more serious underlying condition, so it is very important to see your doctor in case you have Crohn's disease, ulcerative colitis, or diverticulitis, which are often mistaken for IBS. People with IBS need to support their liver by watching their intake of fats, caffeine and alcohol. See also *Liver Problems*.

Foods to Avoid
- Refined carbohydrates are generally high in gluten – therefore avoid wheat, barley, oats and rye and look for gluten- and wheat-free foods.
- Avoid yeasts, vinegar, mushrooms and refined sugars. Also most fruits other than berries, mango and papaya ferment easily – see *Candida*.
- All dairy products from animal sources including milk, chocolate, cheese, cream, ice cream and yoghurt should be avoided.
- Soya and corn (maize) can be a problem for some people. Keep a food diary so that you can note when symptoms are worse. Have an intolerance test – see page 257 for details.
- Other problem foods are often eggs and citrus fruits, especially oranges; and foods with a high tyramine content, such as cheese, port, red wine and sherry, beef, liver, herring, sauerkraut and yeast extracts.
- If you suspect candida, see *Foods to Avoid* under *Candida*.
- Melted cheese is very hard for the body to digest – avoid at all costs.
- Refined foods – white rice and pasta, as well as cakes and pastries – alcohol, fried foods, high-sugar foods, and those foods high in saturated animal fat (found in meat and dairy) all deplete good bacteria in the gut and help feed the bad guys.
- Avoid heavy, rich meals, and especially avoid fried foods.

Friendly Foods
- There are plenty of alternatives to wheat and gluten. Ask at your health shop for wheat-free breads such as Genius, and use millet, buckwheat, quinoa and/or corn-based crisp breads, and rice and corn cakes.
- You can now buy lentil, corn, millet, rice, buckwheat and potato-based pastas and/or noodles.

- Try organic rice, almond or quinoa milk.
- Eat more brown rice as this is cleansing and healing to the digestive tract, as well as potatoes, fish, lean (preferably organic) poultry and meats, fresh fruits and vegetables.
- Peppermint, fresh mint, fennel, camomile and rosemary teas can all enhance digestion and ease discomfort.
- Instead of orange juice, try low-sugar diluted apple, pear or pineapple juice.
- Add more ginger to your food, which soothes your gut and has anti-parasitic properties. This is why Japanese sushi – raw fish, which can contain parasites – is often served with ginger. (See also *Leaky Gut*.)
- Pumpkin seeds have anti-parasitic action, so munch on some daily.
- Eating pineapple, which contains bromelain, helps to digest protein. Eat pineapple in between meals.
- In order to make stomach acid for efficient digestion, you need vitamin B6 and the mineral zinc. These are found in sunflower seeds, soya beans, walnuts, lentils and lima beans, peas, buckwheat flour (this is a grass and is not related to wheat), avocados and chestnuts, brown rice, lentils, pumpkin and sesame seeds, almonds and cooked tofu.
- Eat lighter meals: soup and fish-based meals are easier on the digestion than a pizza with melted cheese! Avoid rich sauces.

Useful Remedies

- See all remedies under *Leaky Gut*.
- Take 1 acidophilus or bifidus capsule twice a day to replace healthy bacteria in the gut and improve digestion. BioCare's Bio Acidophillus is shown to survive stomach acid and make it to the gut where it needs to do its job. **BC**
- Take a high-strength B-complex to make sure you have all the nutrients necessary to digest carbohydrates, proteins and fats. Look for 50mg of most of the B-vitamins.
- Aloe vera juice, 20ml taken before meals, has helped a lot of people, as it helps increase stool bulk, enhances digestion, and eases the discomfort of IBS. Aloe Pura make a good stomach formula. Available from good chemists and health stores.
- Take 1–3 dessertspoons of organic linseeds (flax seeds) daily, providing 10–20 grams of linseeds; build up slowly, a teaspoon at a time. The mixture of soluble and insoluble fibres in linseeds helps to stimulate the bowel gently, while providing stool bulk, thus enabling the bowel to function normally and comfortably. Linseeds have also been successful in alleviating both constipation and diarrhoea, but they must be taken with plenty of water. Generally, soak the linseeds overnight in cold water, drain and use on cereals, in porridge or in smoothies. Or use a ready-cracked variety.
- See remedies under *Constipation* and *Diarrhoea* if either is your main problem.
- As absorption of nutrients is often a problem in IBS and you may be low in stomach acid (see *Low Stomach Acid*), dilute 1 teaspoon of apple cider vinegar in water and drink with each meal. If symptoms persist, instead try taking one Nutri's Nutrigest available from www.positivenutrition.co.uk along with meals. This contains some stomach acid mixed with digestive enzymes. Take it after the first few mouthfuls, do not chew it, and never take it on an empty stomach. **NB Avoid all of these remedies if you have active stomach ulcers, or if they create a feeling of warmth in your stomach. Instead take a pancreatic digestive enzyme formula that is free from HCl, which can irritate the gut.**
- Zinc helps the body to produce it's own stomach acid, so if you know that you are suffering from low stomach acid, take 30–60mg zinc daily with food.
- Try a combination of cayenne capsules (which help stop any bleeding), pure slippery elm tea (which soothes and heals the gut), and Colit capsules, containing wild yam (an anti-

spasmodic), plus bayberry and agrimony, which tighten and heal the tissues. Take 3–9 capsules daily depending on severity of symptoms. **SHS**

Helpful Hints

■ Chew, chew, chew and chew again, As you chew you send signals to the digestive system to produce its digestive enzymes, and thoroughly chewed food also gives the enzymes less to do, making them more effective.

■ Drink more alkaline waters as the gut heals more quickly if more alkaline. Water Filter Man supply alkalizing filters for your home. Call 0844 8733148 or log on to their website at www.waterfilterman.co.uk.

■ Consider using Kangen Water – a water system unit that attaches to your kitchen tap that ionizes and greatly alkalizes water – as the gut heals more quickly in an alkaline environment. It's used in Japanese hospitals with highly beneficial health results. For full details, call 020 7580 7537 or visit www.kangenmiraclewater.co.uk.

■ Oil of peppermint has anti-spasmodic properties – massage it on your abdomen and drink peppermint tea after meals. Fennel tea is another herb that aids digestion.

■ Gentle exercise on a regular basis enhances bowel function. Yoga, Pilates, swimming and walking are all good forms of exercise that do not overtax the system and enhance relaxation.

■ Remember to eat in a relaxed fashion; being stressed while you eat makes it very difficult for normal digestive function to work at its best. Sitting down for 10 minutes either side of a meal is advised. Try to avoid eating food on the run.

■ Remember, if you have an intolerance to one food, you are actually likely to be intolerant to more than one. Very few of us react to just one food, and in most cases we react to four or five. Genova Diagnostics do a thorough food-intolerance test and can be contacted on 020 8336 7750. Website: www.gdx.uk.net

■ Another excellent method is the Bio Meridian Test for food intolerance and leaky gut, where the practitioner measures your reactions, via electrodes, to a huge list of foods and substances. For practitioners, see www.biomeridian.com or call Sheila Partridge on 020 7580 7537.

■ Professor Roland Valori, a gastroenterologist at Gloucester Royal Hospital, found that 90 out of 100 of his patients who were treated by hypnotherapy experienced significant improvements. See *Useful Information*.

■ Call Smart Nutrition who offer help to IBS sufferers and can test for levels of good and bad bacteria, candida and parasites. Call 01273 775480, or check out their website at www.smartnutrition.co.uk.

■ Check out www.theguttrust.org for more information.

J

JET LAG
(see also Deep Vein Thrombosis)

Jet lag is a disturbance of the natural sleep–wake cycle triggered by air travel across time zones and has become a part of modern living. It's obvious that if you travel for many hours across varying time zones, your whole system is going to be affected. Usually, the more time zones you cross, the worse the symptoms. These symptoms include difficulty falling asleep at the 'new' local bedtime, and sleepiness and fatigue during the day. In addition, your circulation can become sluggish triggering problems such as leg, ankle and foot-swelling, or in extreme cases DVT – see *Deep Vein Thrombosis*.

Also, as you are breathing recycled air, along with myriad bacteria and viruses, you are at risk of contracting a whole host of diseases from a simple cold to something more serious such as tuberculosis, which has made a comeback. You are also exposed to considerable amounts of radiation, which can lower immune function; your pineal gland can become confused, thus affecting melatonin production (the hormone that controls the sleep–wake cycle), which plays havoc with your internal body clock.

Scientist Roger Coghill says: 'Because you are moving between local magnetic fields, while your body adjusts, you can feel very disorientated indeed.' See *Helpful Hints* for more on magnetic fields. Children under the age of 3 seem to suffer little jet lag, as they are not set in their ways, and so are more adaptable. Also the less rigid you are in your everyday life, the less likely you are to suffer jet lag.

Foods to Avoid
- On long flights, eat smaller meals and reduce your intake of caffeinated teas, coffee, alcohol and cola-type fizzy drinks, which all dehydrate the body. Caffeine can contribute to poor sleep patterns, so ask for decaffeinated varieties.
- Sugar depletes minerals and lowers immune function, which can be a real problem in the airless cabins where bacteria and viruses spread so quickly. See *Immune Function*.
- Alcohol is 2–3 times more potent when you drink it in the air.
- See also this section under *Circulation*.

Friendly Foods
- Try to eat light and healthy foods the day prior to travel, and drink plenty of water. I realize that airline food can leave a lot to be desired, but eat at regular intervals on the flight to help balance blood sugar levels.
- Foods that help to calm you down and aid restful sleep are turkey, cottage cheese, avocados, pasta, bananas and skimmed milk.
- Camomile, lemon balm or passiflora teas are all great for relaxation. Take a few tea bags with you.
- Ask the cabin crew to give you a few bottles of mineral water and keep drinking it throughout the flight.
- Eat more garlic during the week or so before flying – it's anti-bacterial and anti-viral, and thins the blood naturally.

Useful Remedies

- Take one gram of vitamin C with bioflavonoids every 2–3 hours with meals.
- Take a high-strength multi-vitamin and mineral.
- Try Emergen C, a powdered vitamin C and electrolyte formula that helps replenish depleted minerals. Sold at all good health stores and pharmacies.
- The amino acid L-theanine (extracted from green tea) helps the brain to produce more alpha waves and helps you relax without making you groggy (see under *Insomnia*).
- Melatonin produced in the pineal gland at night has proven highly effective for reducing jet lag. However bio-electromagnetics scientist Roger Coghill says: 'When you take melatonin supplements that you can buy online and in the States, most synthetic tablets contain thousands of times the natural dose that your pineal gland normally produces. If you only take small amounts for jet lag this should be fine; 0.5mg taken as you get off the plane and one more at bedtime in the short term would be fine.'
- Roger has developed a supplement called Asphalia, extracted from certain grasses, that contains natural melatonin, which mimics the normal dose made by your pineal gland at night, rather than the larger dose which you get in mass-produced tablets. Take 1–2 capsules 30 minutes before bed. Roger has permission from the MHRA (Medical Healthcare Regulatory Authority) to sell this food supplement in the UK. For more details or to find your nearest supplier, log on to www.asphalia.co.uk or call 01495 752122.
  NB Asphalia should not be taken by severe asthmatics, children under one or pregnant women in their third trimester.
- A homeopathic mixture called Jet Lag, containing arnica and cocculus, reduces symptoms of jet lag by helping the body to readjust to local time. OP

Helpful Hints

- Get a good night's sleep before your flight, which will help reduce jet lag. When you arrive, if practical, take some exercise, such as a walk or a swim.
- Try to stay up until the local time to go to bed. When I travel west to the US, I usually manage to stay up until the local bedtime (around 8pm), but if I'm going east I find this harder, and often take a nap. Basically, the sooner you get on to local time the better. Get as much sunlight as you can as soon as you arrive by going for a walk, which helps to reset your body clock.
- Also, to help reset your body clock, attach a Super Magnet to the top of your head for 15 minutes before landing. One of the reasons you get jet lag is because your body clock is trying to adjust to the new magnetic field. By using the magnet you can reset your body clock to the local magnetic field. To order a Super Magnet, call Coghill Research on 01495 752122.
- If you have a long wait for connections, try to have a shower, which will help relax your muscles and get your circulation moving again.
- Walk and stretch as much as you can on board and during transit.
- Have a light, healthy snack when you arrive to help you to sleep, otherwise low blood sugar can cause you to wake in the middle of the night.

KIDNEY STONES
(see also Acid–Alkaline Balance)

Your kidneys filter the plasma of your blood and extract all the waste and unwanted toxins, which are then excreted in the urine (a sterile liquid). Also, the residues of antibiotics, prescription drugs and hormones, and vitamins and minerals are excreted in the urine. The kidneys maintain the acid–alkaline balance of your blood within very narrow limits, and if the blood becomes too acid or too alkaline, life is not possible. Without functioning kidneys you would not survive for very long.

These remarkable organs weigh just a few ounces each and yet, if they cease to function (which is known as kidney failure), they must be replaced with a dialysis machine. Two of the main threats to our kidneys are high blood pressure and toxins. If you tend to have a poor diet, or if you take little or no exercise, it's likely that you may develop hypertension, which, sooner or later, plays havoc with the kidneys (see also *High Blood Pressure*). Other toxins that affect the kidneys are found in our air, water and food. Mercury, arsenic, pesticides and a huge amount of chemical pollutants all pose potential problems to the kidneys. Cadmium, from cigarette smoke, is a major kidney poison, and the accumulation of this metal in the kidneys is one of the key reasons why smokers often succumb to illness sooner than non-smokers do – they are simply unable to clear their blood stream of the harmful waste products as efficiently as non-smokers. If the kidneys have to work harder, they may weaken under the strain.

If over time we eat a poor diet, kidney stones can start to form as miniscule crystals that look like gravel, which can damage the delicate tubules in the kidneys and impede proper urine flow. Kidney stone episodes are more common in the summer, when urine becomes more concentrated as we tend to sweat more. The stones are generally made from minerals, such as calcium, phosphates and deposits of uric acid, the most common component of which is calcium oxalate. Kidney stones can cause excruciating pain as they try to move out of the kidneys and into the bladder. Passing a kidney stone is one of the worst pains in all of medicine. So, try to make sure this never happens to you.

Vegetarians have a 40–60% lower chance of developing stones than meat-eaters; and voracious meat-eaters tend to suffer more stones because of their higher uric acid production. Having kidney stones in the body also makes bladder infections much more likely. If you ever pass blood in your urine or have persistent back pain, then it's very important that you see your GP. People with high homocysteine levels also tend to suffer more kidney problems (see *Cholesterol* and *Heart Disease*). You can lower homocysteine levels through your diet and by taking B-vitamins.

Foods to Avoid
- Refined sugar is the worst food for your kidneys, as it stimulates the release of insulin from the pancreas, which in turn stimulates calcium excretion through the urine. Over time, this can increase the risk of kidney stones.
- If you tend to eat a lot of foods high in oxalic acid, such as chocolate, cocoa, tea, spinach, rhubarb and chard, don't eat these foods too regularly.

- Beetroot, instant coffee, grapefruit, oranges, gooseberries, peanuts and strawberries also contain oxalic acid – reduce your intake of these foods if you suffer from kidney stones.
- Also reduce or avoid high acid-forming foods, such as red meat, full-fat dairy products, refined sugar and sweet foods.
- Cut down on all fizzy canned drinks and reduce alcohol and caffeinated drinks.
- Antacids, excessive animal-based milks and carbonated drinks, such as soda water and fizzy water, can all add to the problem.
- Avoid sodium-based salts. Ask at your health shop for magnesium and potassium-based sea salts instead, and use them sparingly.
- See also *Gout*, as you also need to avoid high purine foods.

Friendly Foods
- Add cranberry juice, parsley tea, dandelion leaf tea, mullein tea and barley water, which all help to break down any stone formation.
- Drink plenty of plain, pure water, and increase to 8 glasses daily in summer. Distilled water works best for removing and preventing kidney stones – this is one of the single most important things you can do to avoid developing stones and/or breaking down stones.
- Eat black cherries, which help to remove uric acid crystals out of the body.
- Drink carrot, celery and parsley juice, or make 'smoothies' with these ingredients. Celery does contain a little oxalic acid, but makes a great kidney cleanser as it is rich in potassium, which helps to flush the kidneys.
- Eat plenty of garlic, horseradish, asparagus, parsley, watermelon, apples, cucumber, kale, parsnips, turnip greens and mango, which are all great kidney foods.
- All magnesium- and calcium-rich foods help you to avoid kidney stones and encourage healthier kidneys. Try green leafy vegetables plus apricots, blackstrap molasses, raw honey, curried vegetables, watercress, soya flour, yoghurt, muesli and sesame seeds. Raw wheat germ is high in magnesium and vitamin E.
- Asparagus is great for breaking down kidney stones.
- Try rice, oat, almond, quinoa or coconut milks as non-dairy alternatives to cow's milk.
- Use organic, unrefined olive, walnut or linseed (flax seed) oils in salad dressings.
- Use olive and coconut oils for cooking.
- Vegetable-source proteins are less likely to trigger this problem. Try tofu, quinoa, beans, lentils, peas or hemp seed protein powders.
- If you like animal protein, choose white fish in preference to meat.
- Sprinkle non-GM lecithin granules over your food. These help to emulsify saturated fats that can contribute to stone formation. Lecithin also contains choline and helps to protect the kidneys from the damage of arteriosclerosis and hypertension. Take 2 tablespoons a day. See under *General Health Hints* for a healthy breakfast smoothie.
- Kelp and all seaweeds are a great source of calcium, magnesium and trace minerals. Use nori flakes as a healthy salt substitute.
- Try spelt, amaranth or millet breads and crackers, since spelt, millet and amaranth are all alkaline foods.
- Eat more barley and lentil-based dishes.

Useful Remedies
- A great remedy for kidney stones is hydrangea root, made into a herbal drink with water, and consumed over the course of one day. Often one treatment can make a big difference. **SHS**
- Take a high-strength B-complex – especially if you are under stress. These are usually in any good multi-vitamin/mineral formula, which you also need.
- Vitamin C – 2 grams daily with food – is a good detoxifier.

- Take vitamin D3 in a halibut-liver oil capsule. **NC**
- Choline protects the kidneys from inflammation. It is available as the amino acids methionine and S-Adenosyl methionine (SAMe), which is super-strength methionine. Take 500mg a day of methionine, by Allergy Research or 50g of SAMe. **NC**
- Drink more organic green or white tea, which helps to re-alkalize the system.
- New Era tissue salts, silica, and calcium fluoride help to break down kidney stones. Take 4 of each daily.
- The herb horsetail acts as a diuretic, which promotes kidney function. It can be taken either as capsules or as a tincture to help reduce stones, but do not use it if your kidneys are already damaged.
- Take 1 cup of nettle tea 3 times a day. It is best made with the dried herbs available in tea bags or as loose tea from good health stores.
- Include either a liquid multi-mineral, such as Ultratrace, available from Higher Nature, or a multi-mineral tablet in your regimen. **HN**
- Take calcium citrate, 500mg, with each meal as the calcium binds to the oxalate and reduces the likelihood of kidney stones forming.
- The amino acid lysine helps decrease urinary calcium. Take 500mg twice daily before meals. **HN**
- Magnesium citrate helps keep calcium in the bones and out of the arteries. Take 600mg daily in divided doses.

Helpful Hints

- Lemon juice (citric acid) helps to break down stones and also smooth out irregular stones. Take 1 teaspoon of neat lemon juice every half an hour during the day for two days, away from food.
- Reflexology, massage, manual lymph drainage and other therapies that encourage toxins to move out of the tissues can temporarily overload the kidneys. Warn your therapist to be gentle if you have a kidney problem. Drink plenty of distilled water afterwards.
- Skin-brushing and lymphatic drainage massage also help remove toxins.
- If you need painkillers, avoid paracetamol, which has a negative effect on the kidneys.
- Some homeopathic remedies are excellent for strengthening kidney function. Populus and Solidago are well-known kidney remedies. HEEL also do Mucosa compositum, which helps the healing process. **OP**
- Avoid excess sweating, which may mean moderating your exercise routine and staying out of the midday sun. Do not consume strong (concentrated) drinks, which means no sodas, carbonated pops or alco-pops. If you do take alcohol, make sure that you swallow plenty of water with it. Remember that salty food is also proportionately deficient in water; take less salt. Avoid dehydration at all costs.
- Stress can make you produce more sweat, too! Stay calm.

L

LEAKY GUT

(see also Adrenal Exhaustion, Allergies, Candida, Eczema, Irritable Bowel Syndrome,
Low Stomach Acid and Lupus)

If you have a leaky gut you are unlikely to absorb sufficient essential nutrients from your food, which your body needs for good health. If the leaky gut is not healed, then the long-term implications for your health are serious indeed.

Thanks to many people's stressed lifestyles, eating too many of the wrong foods, often in a hurry, leaky gut syndrome has now reached epidemic proportions. Dr Shamin Daya, a nutritional physician based at the Wholistic Medical Centre in Harley Street, London, says: 'In my clinical experience, leaky gut is a major contributing factor in all autoimmune conditions. This is because the gut lining is an important defence mechanism within the body that protects the internal organs against pathogens and undigested food particles. Once the gut becomes leaky, not only are you not absorbing sufficient essential nutrients, but the body is then compromised and at risk from fungus and other infections, which in turn triggers inflammation elsewhere in the body, thus self-perpetuating the autoimmune process.

'Osteoporosis, recurrent candida, IBS, colitis, Crohn's, eczema and even autism are in my opinion all linked to chronic malabsorption problems.'

At any age the small villi (small finger-like protrusions) in the small intestine can become irritated or eroded, which allows larger, undigested food molecules and toxins to pass through our gut wall into the blood stream, affecting both the liver and the lymphatic system and also placing a greater strain on our immune system. These undigested food molecules are treated as foreign invaders and provoke an immune reaction. Our bodies then begin reacting to food as though it were an infection entering our system and send out antibodies to fight it. Leaky gut is now recognized as a major trigger for most food intolerances and allergies and, in some people, migraines.

Various toxins accumulate in our body, especially in the small intestine (gut) and large bowel. The accumulation tends to be a combination of undigested food, impacted faeces, bacteria, fungi, parasites and dead cells. As the toxins build up, the gut wall can become irritated and damaged, which enables partly digested food molecules to cross it and make their way into the blood stream.

Generally, if you suffer bloating, constipation and/or diarrhoea, crave sugary, refined foods, feel tired all the time, and/or notice that your food comes out the other end looking fairly much the same as it went in, you may well have a leaky gut. You may also have unexplained weight loss, skin rashes and if the leaky gut is chronic, then you may also suffer conditions such as rheumatoid arthritis or lupus. Candida, a yeast fungal overgrowth, is also a common cause of, or results from, a leaky gut – see also *Candida*. Most people with a leaky gut also tend to have low zinc levels.

Foods to Avoid

- Avoid gluten found in wheat, rye, spelt, oats and barley, as it hugely contributes to a leaky gut and triggers bloating. Eating gluten- and wheat-free foods should make a big difference.

- Refined sugar encourages fermentation and growth of unfriendly bacteria in the bowel, so keep refined sugary foods and drinks to an absolute minimum.
- If you tend to bloat a lot after meals, avoid eating fruit directly after a large protein meal, as fruit likes a quick passage through the gut. If it gets stuck behind proteins, such as meat, the fruit will ferment, which adds to the problem. Alcohol, vinegar and most pickled foods contribute to fermentation.
- Any foods to which you have an intolerance will only aggravate the problem, the most common being wheat, citrus fruits and also cow's milk and products. Chocolate should also be avoided.
- Melon is particularly bad for a leaky gut – this should only ever be eaten on its own.
- Generally fruits such as apples, grapes, bananas, pears can cause bloating because they ferment readily. Cut down or eliminate them if you suffer bloating after these fruits. Keep a food diary and note when symptoms are worse.
- Avoid heavy, fatty, large meals, which place a strain on the digestive system and the liver.
- Cut down on low-fibre foods, such as jellies, ice cream, burgers, biscuits, cakes, pies, pastries and so on.

Friendly Foods

- As an alternative to refined sugars, use a little xylitol, sold as ZyloSweet (**HN**), which contains 40% less calories than refined sugar and only has a minimal impact on blood sugar levels. You can also use small amounts of organic agave or brown rice syrup.
- Pineapple and papaya are rich in enzymes, which improve protein digestion, making it less likely that undigested proteins end up in the bowel. Eat before or in between meals.
- Mango, papaya, pineapple, pomegranate and berries do not tend to ferment as readily as most other fruits. Eat between meals.
- Try almond, rice, quinoa or coconut milk as non-dairy alternatives.
- Beetroots, Jerusalem artichokes, peas, radishes, celeriac and dandelion are all good liver-cleansers, which also improve digestion. Beans, pulses and lentils are all good gut foods. They contain inulin, which helps encourage the growth of bifidus within the large bowel. This helps to reduce the load on the liver in the long term (see *Liver Problems*).
- Unsalted sunflower, pumpkin and sesame seeds, linseeds (flax seeds soaked overnight in cold water, then drained and eaten), plus nuts are all rich sources of fibre. A great way to get more nuts and seeds into your diet is to place 1 tablespoon each of sunflower, pumpkin, hemp, sesame seeds and walnuts, hazel or Brazil nuts in a coffee grinder or food mixer and pulse for a few seconds. Keep them in a screw-top jar in the fridge and sprinkle over cereals, salads, desserts, fruit, yoghurts and so on. The mixture will stay fresh for about a week.
- Drink plenty of water – at least 6–8 glasses a day.
- Garlic and onions help to fight infections and encourage the growth of friendly bacteria in the bowel.
- Organic-source chlorella is a great way to detoxify the system. Stir into smoothies or juices, or sprinkle over cereals and fruit salads.
- Use fresh root ginger in your cooking, which soothes and heals the gut.
- Green cabbage is rich in the amino acid L-glutamine, which helps heal a leaky gut. Eat more raw or steamed cabbage, and use the liquid from the cooking to make gravy and sauces.
- Eat plenty of fresh vegetables; and if you eat fruit, eat it between meals or for breakfast.
- Try quinoa, buckwheat, millet and plenty of brown rice.
- Most health shops sell pastas made from soya, millet, buckwheat, amaranth or rice flour.
- Sprinkle rice bran over cereals.
- Drink more organic green and white teas, high in antioxidants.

- Try Genius or Village Bakery breads that are wheat- and gluten- free, and all health stores now sell wheat- and gluten-free crackers and biscuits.
- Amaranth crackers or rice cakes should be fine.

Useful Remedies

- Take a digestive enzyme capsule with meals, such as Polyzyme Forte. **BC**
- Multi formulas designed specifically to heal a leaky gut are Gastro ULC, Repairvite or LGSZyme. Call the Wholistic Medical Centre for details on 020 7580 7537.
- L-glutamine, the amino acid, helps to heal a leaky gut. Take between 1 and 4 grams a day, on an empty stomach, for the first month and then reduce to 1 gram daily. Children can take Colostrum – a quarter teaspoon twice daily on an empty stomach (see *Allergies* for more details). **NC**
- Take a high-strength, easily absorbable multi-vitamin and mineral supplement daily. BioCare make liquid multis. **BC**
- Add 1–3 dessertspoons of raw, ready-cracked linseeds (flax seeds) to your cereals or yoghurts every day. Keep the seeds in the fridge. Otherwise soak a tablespoon of golden linseeds overnight in cold water, drain and use in a breakfast smoothie. See under *General Health Hints* for a breakfast smoothie recipe.
- Use a good green powder daily in smoothies to help alkalize your system, as the gut heals faster when it's more alkaline. Green Magic Powder – containing Hawaiian spirulina, chlorella, lecithin, barley and wheat grass, kamut, pectin apple fibre, kelp and wheat sprouts, CoQ10, royal jelly, artichoke powder and lactobacillus acidophilus is a great all-round way to ingest good nutrients, healthy bacteria, keep the body more alkaline and help keep you regular. Details can be found on www.itsgreenmagic.com or call Helen Cruikshank on 08453 279688.
- Half a teaspoon of bicarbonate of soda twice daily in warm water, well away from food, will really help to re-alkalize the body and therefore help it to heal faster.
- After taking these supplements for 3 months and changing your diet, your gut should be in better shape and you could then reduce this regimen to a good multi-vitamin and mineral, plus a digestive enzyme daily.

Helpful Hints

- A urine test via Genova can detect a leaky gut – see below. Called a Gut Permeability Test.
- It is really important to have an allergy test to find foods that are a problem. One of the best I have found is available from the York Test Laboratories. Tel: 0800 458 2052 or log on to www.yorktest.com; or Genova Diagnostics do a FACT test which looks for inflammatory markers indicating that the body is reacting to certain substances. Tel: 020 8336 7750. Website: www.gdx.uk.net
- Another excellent method is the Bio Meridian Test for food intolerance and leaky gut, in which the practitioner measures your reactions, via electrodes, to a huge list of foods and substances. For practitioners, see www.biomeridian.com or call Sheila Partridge on 0207 580 7537.
- It is vital that you chew food thoroughly and more slowly, which helps break down the food more effectively. Many people with a leaky gut swallow large food particles in a hurry, which places a great strain on an already labouring digestive tract.
- Smoking increases the toxic load on the body and can make the situation worse.
- Make sure you get plenty of regular exercise and always walk for at least 15 minutes after a meal to aid digestion.
- Lower your stress levels (see *Stress*). Eat only light meals when stressed. Stress greatly contributes to a leaky gut – see under *Adrenal Exhaustion*.
- Drink more alkaline waters, as the gut heals faster if more alkaline. Water Filter Man supplies alkalizing filters for your home. Call 0844 8733148 or visit www.waterfilterman.co.uk.

■ Remember not to eat on the move – as much as possible eat in a relaxed, comfortable situation. At the very least, sit down to eat.

LEG ULCERS   (see also Cholesterol, Circulation and Diabetes)

This is a very common problem in the over-60s, and is caused by restricted circulation, and a lack of oxygen and nutrients reaching the skin. Leg and foot ulcers are more common in diabetics because of changes in circulation and the nerve-endings near the skin. As leg ulcers can be related to diabetes – ask your doctor for a blood test to rule this out.

Foods to Avoid
■ Avoid foods that impede circulation including animal fats, especially red meats, sausages, meat pies, burgers, full-fat cheeses and dairy produce, as well as hard margarines made from refined vegetable oils.
■ Avoid all fried foods and don't use mass-produced vegetable oils.
■ Cut down on alcohol, and on low-fibre foods, such as jelly and ice cream, white breads, mass-produced pies and cakes.
■ See dietary advice in *Circulation* and *Cholesterol*.

Friendly Foods

■ Eat more leafy green vegetables, especially cabbage, kale, celery, pak choy, spinach and broccoli, which contain high levels of carotenes and minerals.
■ Eat more salads and sprinkle sunflower, pumpkin and sesame seeds over them, as these seeds are high in essential fatty acids, minerals and fibre.
■ Oily fish are rich in omega-3 fats, which thin the blood naturally and aid healing.
■ Cook with a little organic butter, olive oil, ghee or coconut oil. Never heat oil to smoking, which will turn it rancid – coconut oil, ghee and butter are more stable at higher temperatures.
■ Sprinkle wheat germ and lecithin granules over breakfast cereals to lower 'bad' cholesterol.
■ Add almonds, Brazil nuts, hazelnuts and walnuts to fruit dips as they are all high in zinc, which aids skin healing.
■ High-protein foods, such as hemp seed or whey protein, are a very rich source of glutamine, which speeds the healing process. You can buy these at all health shops.
■ Eat more garlic and onions, which are anti-bacterial.
■ Drink more organic green or white teas to help boost your immune system. They are delicious with a small amounts of organic agave syrup or xylitol, instead of refined sugars. **HN**

Useful Remedies
■ Take zinc, 30mg, 1–2 times a day with meals. This is absolutely essential if you are suffering from slow wound healing.
■ Take gotu kola, 500mg, 3 times a day with meals. This herb has been used historically for wound healing and when combined with zinc can be very successful. It helps increase circulation in lower limbs and can have a slight laxative effect – for many people, this is a bonus!
■ Vitamin C, 2 grams daily in divided doses with food, is essential for healing connective tissue.
■ If the ulcers are superficial and not too deep, aloe vera gel applied topically can speed healing, ease the discomfort and protect from infection.
■ Many elderly people cannot be bothered to cook proper meals, so if this is the case make sure you take an easily absorbed, high-quality multi-vitamin and mineral.

- Try Solgar's horse chestnut seed extract. It contains the active ingredient aescin, which has been shown to be effective in supporting venous problems, and has the ability to strengthen capillaries and enhance circulation. **SVHC**

Helpful Hints

- Try Bach Rescue Remedy cream, once the skin starts to heal, which is available from good health stores.
- V-Nal Cream (from Bional) contains a combination that includes horse chestnut, butcher's broom (an anti-inflammatory), elderflower, and soothing aloe and witch hazel. It is recommended for circulation in the legs and feet.
- Place raw manuka honey on the site of the ulcer, which will speed the healing process. You can also buy manuka honey dressings (made by Comvita), which are easier to use.
- Raise your legs above hip level when resting, and move your feet backwards and forwards slowly to increase the circulation in your lower legs. Try to walk for at least 15 minutes twice a day.
- Regular acupuncture and reflexology will both greatly help to improve your circulation (see *Useful Information*).
- Magnopulse in the UK make magnet-filled dressings to place directly over wounds, which have been shown to heal faster with the magnet therapy. For details, call Magnopulse on 0800 977 5070 or visit www.magnopulse.com.

LIBIDO PROBLEMS (see also Adrenal Exhaustion, Impotence and Stress) L

It is important to remember that everyone has different appetites and you should not assume that you have a 'libido problem' just because you do not want sex as often as your friends or as people in the media. Moreover, it is quite normal to experience a decline in desire as the years go by. Other pleasures shared with your partner, which are equally fulfilling, may take the place of sex, which then occasionally surfaces at moments of great tenderness, romance or nostalgia.

Libido is only a problem, as such, when an otherwise harmonious couple have sexual needs that are wildly different. As always, a compromise is a good solution – one partner trying harder to get in the mood and the other trying to reduce high demands.

Impotence in men and frigidity in women are extreme cases of lowered libido, where one or other partner cannot or does not wish to perform.

Dr Keith Scott-Mumby, a British doctor living in Los Angeles, says: 'Without doubt, the single biggest factor that impairs sexual performance is poor general health. Conditions as varied as obesity, hypertension, stress, digestive disorders, depression and alcoholism will all result in lessened interest in sex. The number one turn-off for everyone is stress. Living a life full of worry, with an uncertain or threatening future, is bound to result in lowered libido.'

Certain prescription drugs such as statins and high blood pressure drugs are also known to affect libido. Dr Mumby also points to the natural age-related decline in sexual function: 'Hormone levels fall off slowly at first, but by the fifth decade this natural slow-down process accelerates. Women experience a dramatic shift at the menopause. Men suffer a more gradual process that is widely overlooked, known as the andropause. Beyond the menopause, lowered oestrogen levels for women may result in vaginal dryness and soreness. This obviously interferes with sexual desire and performance. The onset of andropause for men is an indicator of diminishing testosterone levels and this leads to loss of libido – interestingly, healthy women also need low levels of natural testosterone that drives their libido.'

Foods to Avoid

- If you have become overweight, make an effort to lose weight, as it helps men and women feel sexier and look better. See *Weight Problems*.
- Avoid refined carbohydrates, refined sugars, high sodium salt foods, and the saturated fats found in red meat, full-fat dairy produce, sausages, chocolates, meat pies and other manufactured and pre-packaged foods.
- Eliminate caffeine and drink only organic de-caff or, better still, herbal teas, and low-sugar or diluted fruit juices.
- Reduce your alcohol intake to around 20 units a week or less (for men, 14 for women) . Remember Shakespeare's words: 'Alcohol promotes the desire but takes away the performance.' See *Alcohol*.

Friendly Foods

- Pumpkin and sunflower seeds, Brazil nuts, linseeds and oysters are rich in zinc, which is vital for a healthy sex life.
- Include garlic and onions in your diet to improve circulation and lower LDL, the 'bad' cholesterol.
- Sprinkle cayenne pepper and turmeric over your food to add spice to your life; you can also take them in tincture or capsule form.
- Eat more fresh fruits and vegetables and replace red meat with fresh fish and chicken.
- See *General Health Hints*.

Useful Remedies

- Pycnogenol – pine bark extract – (take 80mg daily) plus the amino acid arginine (take 500mg twice daily away from food); both encourage nitrous oxide production that relaxes blood vessels, thereby improving blood flow to the reproductive organs. **NB If you suffer from regular cold sores, the arginine may trigger an attack.**
- The above formula if taken over time acts as a natural form of Viagra. Prelox from Pharma Nord contains both. **PN**
- Korean ginseng – take 500–1000mg a day – helps to reduce the underlying stress that is often linked to this problem. This is shown to be more effective when taken for a month, then stopped for a month and so on. See *Stress*.
- Pukka Herbs make Ashwagandha Plus, which contains 9 herbs known to help libido. **NC**
- Damiana, a herb from Mexico and India, is a natural aphrodisiac for men and women. Planetary Formulas make a Damiana Male Potential, a formula containing damiana, sasparilla and ginseng, among other things. **NC**
- Stress reduces B-vitamins in the body – therefore also include a good-quality multi-vitamin and mineral for men, which includes a full range of B-vitamins.
- Zinc and magnesium are often low in young men with libido problems.
- Muira puama, a South-American herb, is considered nature's most potent viagra. A daily dose of 1 gram of a standardized extract has been shown to be effective as it raises testosterone levels. In one study of 100 men with impotence problems, 66% had increased frequency of intercourse, while 70% reported intensification of libido. The stability of the erection was restored in 55% of the patients and 66% reported a reduction in fatigue. The herb is suitable for both men and women. **NC**
- The herb maca has been found to improve libido in men and women as it helps to balance hormones, so if the problem is hormonal, try 1 capsule 3 times daily (500mg). **NC**

Helpful Hints

- Measures to alleviate stress are often very effective. Take regular exercise and learn to laugh more. This releases natural endorphins, which lower stress levels and help you to feel more positive. Learn to breathe more deeply.

- If there is a problem, you must discuss matters openly with your significant other. If one partner's needs are not being met, it can lead to frustration and even hostility. It is unfair to put your partner in a position where they have no ethical means of satisfying their physical desires.
- Quit smoking. Smoking has been linked with reduced ability to maintain an erection, because it constricts the blood flow that is essential for erectile function.
- Ylang ylang, rose and jasmine therapeutic oils applied to the lower abdomen area can help revive a flagging sex drive in men and women.
- Men who use a large amount of marijuana or take steroids may also find their erectile function diminished.
- By constantly worrying about your lack of sex drive, you often make the situation worse. Studies show that a lack of vitamins C, E, A, B and the minerals zinc and selenium can cause a low sperm count and lack of sex drive. Anyone taking regular antidepressants or sleeping pills may be lacking in these nutrients.
- Have your hormone levels checked via blood or saliva tests – testosterone patches are known to help increase libido in both sexes. Once hormones are restored often sex drive returns (see also *Menopause*).
- If the condition continues, or you are worried about infertility as well as impotency, see a doctor who is also a nutritionist (see *Useful Information*).
- For help with hormones, contact Dr Malcolm Carruthers at the Andropause Centre in Harley Street, London – call 020 7636 8283, or log on to www.centreformenshealth.co.uk.
- Acupuncture can help with poor libido by unblocking energy channels within the body, which helps increase blood flow (see *Useful Information*).
- Discuss whatever turns you on with your partner. If you find that difficult, discuss sex in general until you are more comfortable with this topic. To help get you in the mood, try watching a sexy movie, which works for many people!
- Try reading *His Needs Her Needs – Building an Affair-proof Marriage* by Willard F Harley, Jr (Monarch Books); or take a look at the website at www.marriagebuilders.com.
- You could also try reading *Maximize Your Vitality and Potency: For Men Over 40* by Jonathan V. Wright, MD (Smart Publications); or visit the website at www.tahoma-clinic.com.
- All of these books can be ordered from the Nutri Centre Bookshop on 020 7323 2382.

LICHEN PLANUS (see under Immune Function)

Lichen planus is a chronic condition of the skin and mucous membranes, typically the lining of the mouth. This is thought to be caused by a virus and has some features in common with other skin problems, such as eczema and psoriasis. Sores on the skin are often localized on the wrist and ankles, but they can be widespread. Basically, the more you can support your immune system, the less likely you are to suffer this problem.

Foods to Avoid
- Anything that weakens the immune system, such as concentrated sugars, refined carbohydrates, even concentrated fruit juices, and any food to which you have an intolerance.
- Foods that are a problem for many sufferers are tomatoes, pineapples, mushrooms, coffee, red meat, chocolate and ice cream. Keep a food diary and note when symptoms are worse, so that you can identify and remove those foods from your diet.
- Alcohol, vinegars and oily, spicy foods can make the problem worse   avoid them.

- Avoid dairy produce from cows, as much as possible, as this can create an inflammatory response in the gut because it's hard to digest.

Friendly Foods
- Eat more fresh fish of any kind, but try to make it oily fish, such as organic-farmed salmon, black cod, pilchards, sardines or mackerel. Oily fish are rich in omega-3 essential fats and vitamin A. Aim for twice a week.
- Natural-source beta-carotene converts naturally to vitamin A in the body and aids soft tissue healing. Therefore, eat plenty of carrots, green vegetables, French beans, watercress, spinach, cantaloupe melons, spring greens, sweet potatoes, papaya, apricots (fresh and dried), pumpkin, butternut squash, parsley and mangoes. A little butter is also fine as it is rich in vitamin A – organic is best.
- Organic unrefined and unsalted nuts and seeds, such as sunflower, pumpkin, sesame, linseeds (flax seeds), and Brazil nuts and walnuts, are high in zinc, which can speed up healing.

Useful Remedies
- Take vitamin A, 20,000iu a day for up to 1 month, as there is speculation that lichen planus is due to a vitamin-A deficiency. **NB If you are pregnant or planning a pregnancy, only take 3000iu daily.** After this time change to a natural-source carotene supplement that is non-toxic and will convert naturally in the body. Solgar/Viridian make a high-quality carotene complex. Take as directed.
- Take a good-quality multi-vitamin and mineral.
- Olive leaf extract is anti viral and boosts immunity. Take 500mg twice daily with food.
- Take 30mg of zinc in addition to the multi once a day. Zinc and vitamin A are complementary in their action. Zinc is essential for wound healing and a healthy immune system.
- Organic aloe vera juice – taken before every meal – speeds healing and reduces discomfort as well as boosting the immune system.
- Anti-viral herbs are echinacea, liquorice and St John's wort.

Helpful Hints
- Try to rest as much as possible. Don't overwork and don't over-stress your system, as it is much harder for the body to heal.
- Use washing powders and detergents suitable for sensitive skin.
- Ultraviolet light often brings relief, but try this only under proper supervision.
- Moderate amounts of sunshine can help too, but avoid sunbathing between 11am and 3pm.
- Chickweed ointment has been useful to some people.
- Homeopathy has helped many sufferers (see *Useful Information*).

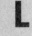

LIVER PROBLEMS

Your liver is the most overworked organ in the body, having to break down all the increasing toxins found in our environment (including our air and water) and our food. It is, in essence, the chemical factory of your body that builds or recycles substances you need for good health and breaks down those you don't. If your liver isn't functioning properly, toxins that would normally be filtered by the liver accumulate in the body. Most people's livers work only at around 35–40% of their potential capacity, because of the large amount of toxins we ingest. When it's working properly, the liver can clean up to 99% of bacteria and toxins from the blood. Around 2.25 litres (4 pints) of blood pass through the liver every minute for detoxification, and every day the liver manufactures about 1 litre (2 pints) of bile, which helps carry away toxins via the bowel.

The liver's capacity to eliminate toxins effectively varies widely between individuals. Part of this may be genetic, or linked to exposure to a wide range of pollutants, viruses and parasites – the rest is lifestyle and diet.

Typical symptoms of a sluggish liver are feeling constantly tired even though you have slept, nausea (especially after a fatty meal or alcohol), skin disorders such as acne, eczema and psoriasis, muscle and joint pain, age spots on the skin, and/ or regular infections. Also, most people don't associate being constipated with poor liver function, but blood from the bowel goes first to the liver, via the portal venous system, hence a bowel loaded with rubbish is going to overwork the liver.

Other symptoms of poor liver function can include yellowing of the whites of the eyes, yellow-looking skin, fever, nausea, difficulty digesting fatty foods, and an increased sensitivity to cigarette smoke, strong perfume, petrol and other chemicals.

Because the brain is unable to disarm a wide range of toxins, it relies on the liver to clean the blood before it gets there. So, over the long term, an under-performing liver can have dire consequences for the brain and nervous system, including memory loss, Parkinson's disease and Alzheimer's disease.

While detoxification is the key function of the liver, it also produces bile to aid fat digestion (as well as eliminate toxins); manufactures and balances hormones; stores various vitamins and minerals; assembles amino acids; makes cholesterol; controls glucose and fat supplies; and plays a key role in immunity.

Your digestive system is closely involved in the health of your liver, as the blood from your digestive system, where nutrients are absorbed from your food, goes directly to the liver for filtering before it goes anywhere else in the body. If your diet is good and your digestion and absorption are working well, then the nutrients needed for good health will make it to the liver and then on into the body. However if your digestive system is generally toxic, thanks to a poor, low-nutrient, high-fat diet, constipation, poor gut flora, a leaky gut and so on, these toxins and any others you ingest will similarly be delivered directly to your liver, which adds to the liver's workload.

The good news is that the liver is capable of regenerating itself, so with a good diet and lifestyle and the right supplements, there's no reason why you can't maintain liver function at an optimal level at any age. And if you look after your liver, your skin literally glows with health.

Begin by eliminating as many unnatural chemicals as possible from your home and environment. Keep in mind that many man-made chemicals (especially in plastics and pesticides) have a hormone-like effect within the body – therefore the incidence of hormone-related cancers (including breast, ovarian, testicular and prostate cancer) are all increasing. These chemicals are commonly found in plastic food packaging, non-organic food, plastics and laminates, synthetic fabrics (clothes, carpets, furniture), dry-cleaning chemicals, air 'fresheners' (a misnomer, most of them poison the air), cosmetics, paints, glues, food additives, medicines, household cleaning products and wallpaper… but the list is virtually endless, and they are all around us.

You could drive yourself crazy trying to avoid all these things, but you would be surprised at how many healthier, safer alternatives to all the above are available if you are willing to seek them out.

Foods to Avoid

- Avoid excess alcohol, which is a liver toxin. One to two units per day are generally considered not harmful, although the best gauge is how you feel afterwards or the next day. If you feel worse than you should, your liver is probably struggling to detoxify the alcohol.

- Reduce your consumption of non-organic food as much as possible, as certain foods such as lettuces are often sprayed up to 11 times with pesticides and/or fungicides before they are harvested.
- When you can't avoid non-organic fruits and vegetables, wash them thoroughly.
- If you're trying to detox or suspect your liver is under-functioning, avoid eating or drinking grapefruit. It contains naringenin, a compound known to slow liver detoxification. A glass of grapefruit juice can significantly affect the action of some medications, which explains why some very expensive medications are prescribed with grapefruit juice: it slows down the body's ability to remove the drug, thus increasing its efficacy.
- Avoid eating excessive protein, as protein metabolism gives the liver a lot of work to do. Generally reduce your animal-protein (meat, chicken, dairy) intake, and increase the amount of vegetable protein in your diet from beans, lentils, nuts, seeds, fermented soya products, such as tempeh or miso, plus whole grains, such as brown rice.
- Reduce your intake of saturated fats, especially hydrogenated or trans-fats, fried and highly processed foods. Don't avoid all fat: essential fats from oily fish and seeds are vital for proper liver function (see *Fats You Need To Eat*).
- Refined foods that contain fructose should be avoided.
- Caffeine, paracetamol, aspirin and most other medications place a strain on the liver. A good alternative to coffee is dandelion coffee, available in health food stores.
- Melted cheese is very difficult for the liver to process – avoid as much as possible. Pizza should be avoided.
- Eggs are an excellent source of nutrients – but for anyone with liver problems, they are hard to digest. Keep it down to two a week.
- Avoid heavy meals taken with alcohol/and or fried foods at all costs.

Friendly Foods
- Increase your intake of all fruit and vegetables, especially those rich in antioxidants, such as organic carrots, sweet potato, pumpkin, papaya, mangoes, alfalfa sprouts and watercress.
- Eat more berries, grapes, Brussels sprouts and kale. Aim for 40% of your diet to be raw in summer. This is not nearly as hard as it sounds if you eat plenty of fresh fruit and salads.
- Eat more globe artichokes, radicchio, black cherries, pears and celeriac, all of which help support the liver.
- Eat more beetroot, raw or cooked – it's one of the best vegetables for the liver because it aids digestion, improves liver function and reduces constipation.
- Also include sulphur-rich foods in your diet, such as garlic, onions, leeks, asparagus, cabbage and broccoli.
- Sprinkle a dessertspoon of lecithin granules over breakfast cereals, fruits and yoghurts, as lecithin helps the body to digest fats, which eases the burden on the liver.
- If you know that your liver is a problem, eat lighter meals regularly and avoid heavy, rich meals. If you eat too much in one sitting, especially fatty or fried foods and alcohol, then you place an enormous burden on the digestion and liver, which could make you feel nauseous.
- Foods that naturally raise glutathione levels (see below) in the body are fresh asparagus, avocado and walnuts. Spinach and tomatoes are also great foods for raising glutathione – but they need to be eaten raw.
- Curcumin, the pigment that gives the spice turmeric its yellow colour, has shown a great ability to increase glutathione production. Found in curries and mustards, curcumin also has anti-inflammatory properties. For the best effect, toast the curcumin seeds and then lightly grind them before adding them to foods. Otherwise take pure curcumin capsules. **SHS** or see www.lef.org. Curcumin may reduce effectiveness of Phase 1 of liver detoxification processes

in some people – if you are unsure, have a urine/saliva Sensitive Liver Pathway Test via Genova Diagnostics. Tel: 020 8336 7750. Website: www.gdx.uk.net.

■ Eat organically produced food as much as possible. The Food Standards Agency in the UK acknowledges that pesticide residues are likely to be considerably lower in organic food than in conventional produce.

Useful Remedies

■ As always, start with a good-quality multi-vitamin/mineral, which provides a baseline of nutrients you can then add to. Make sure it contains 15–30mg of zinc, which is needed to make liver enzymes. Many multi-vitamins now also contain most of the nutrients below.

■ Take 1 gram of vitamin C plus bioflavonoids daily.

■ Take a 1-gram fish oil capsule or 1 linseed (flax seed) oil capsule daily. Make sure the fish oil you buy is free of toxins such as PCBs and dioxins.

■ Magnesium is required by literally hundreds of enzymes throughout the body, many of which have a detoxifying function. Take at least 500mg daily in divided doses; twice that if you have backache, twitching and/or can't sleep.

■ The best-known remedy for the liver is the herb milk thistle, which contains the bioflavonoid silymarin. This promotes cell regeneration in the liver, increases levels of glutathione, and has been shown to repair liver damage from alcohol. For optimum effects, you need 600mg of standardized extract daily in divided doses with food.

■ The most powerful antioxidant and detoxifying compound in the liver is glutathione, a naturally occurring amino acid combination. Unfortunately, it is not particularly well absorbed via capsules; however, by taking alpha-lipoic acid (50–100mg a day) and N-acetyl cysteine (500 mg a day in between meals), you can help increase production of glutathione in the liver. Within the body you also need B-vitamins and selenium to make glutathione.

■ Another key nutrient needed by the liver is sulphur. It can be supplemented as MSM or the amino acids cysteine and methionine. Take 500mg of all three daily. Also include sulphur-rich foods in your diet, such as garlic, onions, leeks, asparagus, cabbage and broccoli.

■ The B-group vitamins, choline and inositol, prevent the accumulation of fat in the liver, thereby enhancing general liver function; take 300–400mg of each, 1–3 times per day.

Helpful Hints

■ Standard tests for liver function (see above under Genova Tests) involve measuring levels of key enzymes. If they are raised, it means that your liver is struggling. This indicates a chronic problem and, while it's useful in indicating a problem exists, it doesn't tell you the best way to help recovery. A better, non-invasive test that is available through nutritionists is a comprehensive Liver Detoxification Profile. This urine test tells you exactly which detox phases and pathways in the liver are under-performing and you can then be advised which nutrients are needed to restore normal function. To find a qualified nutritionist, see under *Useful Information* at the back of the book.

■ Stop smoking and reduce the amount of time you spend in traffic; there can be more pollution inside your car than outside! If you are walking or cycling, avoid busy roads where possible.

■ Indoor air pollution is now recognized as a real problem, and the availability of more natural household cleaning products, paints and fibres has improved dramatically in recent years. Visit your local health food store for natural cleaning products such as Ecover.

■ Use a water filter to remove unwanted chemicals from your drinking supply. Reverse osmosis (RO) filters remove 99.999% of all known chemicals. RO water will even filter anthrax spores. For details of RO water, contact the Pure H2O Company on 01784 221188 or visit www.pureh2o.co.uk. Or contact the Fresh Water Filter Company on 0845 177 0896 or log on to www.freshwaterfilter.com.

- Otherwise, consider using Kangen Water – a filtering device that attaches to your kitchen tap and ionizes and greatly alkalizes water. It's used in Japanese hospitals and produces highly beneficial health results. For full details, call 020 7580 7537 or log on to www.kangenmiraclewater.co.uk.
- Another good option is simply to drink bottled still, natural mineral water – Volvic and Fiji or Belgian Spa Water are the preferred choice of many nutritionists. A filter jug containing a simple carbon filter is the bare minimum, but you must always remember to change the cartridges regularly.
- Because the liver is responsible for balancing hormones, if it's not working efficiently, hormones can accumulate inappropriately or become unbalanced, triggering problems such as facial hair. Also many women who take the pill and orthodox HRT put on weight – this could be because these hormones place a greater strain on the liver.
- According to traditional Chinese medicine, the liver does most work between 1 and 3am in the morning. Liver dysfunction will often wake a person up at these times.
- The liver detoxes more efficiently when we are lying down and relaxed, so make sure you are getting sufficient sleep.
- Do not eat large meals late at night or drink alcohol after 11pm if you're aware that your liver is in trouble.
- Repressed anger and resentments affect liver function, so deal with any stress-type issues.
- Coffee enemas have long been known to stimulate liver function as they increase bile flow from the liver and gall bladder and aid detoxification. A great book to read is *Tired or Toxic?* by Sherry Rogers (Prestige Publishing).

LOW BLOOD PRESSURE (HYPOTENSION)

(see also Adrenal Exhaustion, Low Blood Sugar, Panic Attacks and Stress)

The most classic symptom of low blood pressure is a feeling of light headedness on standing, especially from the ground up. It is more common in women. It may be triggered by hereditary factors whereby the blood vessels may have lost integrity – this is basically the opposite of high blood pressure, in which the arteries are stiff.

Orthodox doctors in the UK do not think of low blood pressure as a problem, but in certain European countries the condition is often treated. Because the blood is responsible for carrying oxygen and nutrients to the body's tissues and organs, low blood pressure can often trigger problems with energy levels and mental function. The condition is frequently a sign of weakness in the adrenal glands (see under *Adrenal Exhaustion*). These glands sit on top of your kidneys and have an important role to play in your hormonal system. Adrenal weakness is often a result of overworking and excessive stresses, compounded by dietary deficiencies. Far too many of us have a lifestyle that over-stresses our adrenal glands. We work too many hours, don't get sufficient sleep and tend to rely on coffee, sugar and refined carbohydrates to get us through the day or to pick us up when our energy levels drop. In the long term, all these factors weaken adrenal function.

One of the most common complaints received by staff in health food shops these days is that of feeling tired all the time. The first question you need to ask yourself is, do you start the day with a good breakfast or find that you can't face breakfast and the only thing that gets you going is two or three cups of tea or coffee? What you are doing is putting a stimulant into your body that adds more stress on your adrenal glands.

Foods to Avoid

- Caffeine and refined sugar in any form will particularly deplete the adrenal glands. Remember that tea, coffee, chocolate and cola all contain caffeine. You might remember not to put sugar in your tea or coffee, but are you having several biscuits with it?
- Refined foods such as mass-produced breads, biscuits, cakes, pizza, burgers and pies all deplete the body of the B-vitamins necessary to keep the adrenal glands in good shape.

Friendly Foods

- Eat more quality protein, such as fresh fish, chicken, lentils, beans, pulses and tempeh. Protein helps to normalize blood sugar, which will in turn help stabilize blood pressure – see under *Adrenal Exhaustion*.
- Hemp seed proteins or whey protein are useful sources of quality protein – see under *General Health Hints* for a great smoothie breakfast recipe.
- Whole grains, which include brown rice, quinoa, spelt, buckwheat, millet and amaranth, are highly nutritious.
- Eat plenty of fresh fruit and vegetables, particularly fresh juices. If you are feeling low in energy, rather than reaching for a coffee, try a glass of carrot, beetroot, apple or ginger juice instead.
- Green tea has a small amount of caffeine, which will give you a boost – and contains many health benefits. Or try ginseng or liquorice teas, which will support your adrenal glands.
- Eat more avocados and wheat germ, which are rich in vitamin E.
- Use potassium- and magnesium-based salt, such as Solo Salt, in your diet. BioForce also make excellent herbal salts. Nori flakes or powdered kelp from health shops are high in easy-to-utilize minerals.
- Liquorice is one of simplest ways of restoring adrenal glands to normal function. Look for pure liquorice sweetened with molasses, sold in most health stores.

Useful Remedies

- Advanced Stress Formula by Holos Health contains five herbs including liquorice and Siberian ginseng, which can help to nourish the adrenals. Take one and a half teaspoons daily in a little water. See www.holoshealth.com.
- Take a high-potency B-complex – 1 twice daily with meals. Take B-vitamins with breakfast and lunch, not with supper, as they keep you more alert.
- Ginseng, taken as 1–3 grams a day for 60 days, helps to balance the body. If the blood pressure is low, ginseng can help to bring it back up and has the added benefit of being an excellent adrenal restorative.
- Try Dr Christopher's Blood Circulation capsules, which contain ginger, cayenne and hawthorn. These help to normalize blood pressure (high or low); 1 or 2 capsules three times daily with meals. **SHS (NB Anyone suffering from heart problems must check with a doctor before taking any supplement containing hawthorn.)**

Helpful Hints

- Take sensible amounts of exercise, but also make sure you are getting sufficient rest.
- See *General Health Hints*.
- See under *Adrenal Exhaustion* and *Stress*.

LOW BLOOD SUGAR (HYPOGLYCAEMIA)

(see also Adrenal Exhaustion, Insulin Resistance and Low Blood Pressure)

Low blood sugar, also known as hypoglycaemia, is something that 95% of us experience at some time if we go without food for too long – the most common cause is skipping breakfast. I have met a number of young women who suffer occasional blackouts, fainting spells and dizziness that their doctor is unable to explain. But when they tell me about their diet of missed meals and sugary drinks and snacks, I know almost immediately what the problem must be. As these symptoms are also common with Adrenal Exhaustion, see also this section.

The level of sugar in the blood is critical to how you feel. If it is too low, you may well feel very tired, find concentration difficult, become shaky, feel very hungry and drowsy, possibly have headaches, and feel anxious. These myriad symptoms can simply result from skipping breakfast. If you are one of those people who won't eat breakfast for the sake of an extra 15 to 20 minutes in bed, or simply can't face it in the mornings and then rush off to work, by mid-morning you are going to feel even hungrier than you did when you left the house. Most people then reach for coffee, tea, snacks and biscuits, something that will quickly raise blood sugar levels. Unfortunately, not long after consuming this type of food, our blood sugar drops even lower than it was before. This is a result of the body producing an excess of insulin to compensate for the sugar load. One of the problems with skipping breakfast is that even if your first meal of the day (lunch) is a good wholesome one, your blood sugar levels are still likely to remain erratic. This can lead you to becoming irritable with your colleagues or extremely emotional in response to even small problems.

Other people with low blood sugar will find it crucial to always have their meals at regular times. If their lunch hour is normally midday and someone asks them to leave it until 2pm, they are likely to start to feel weak or suffer memory problems, or may simply find it hard to concentrate.

The brain's only food source is pure glucose and, if you have not eaten for a while, the hypothalamus area within the brain will just demand more sugar. Basically, if your hypothalamus is not happy, no amount of willpower will stop you craving something sweet. Nutritionists have known for years that the easiest way to control blood sugar is to eat small, healthy, low-glycaemic meals more regularly, but most people don't do this. The average person in the West eats 16kg (35lb) of snacks a year, which causes weight gain and a very unstable blood sugar. The result is a huge increase in diabetes. As symptoms of low blood sugar are similar to those of high blood sugar (diabetes), have a check-up with your doctor. However, a single blood test is unlikely to show any problem with low blood sugar, because unless you are actually suffering a dip in blood sugar at the time of the test, results could be normal. See also *Insulin Resistance*.

Foods to Avoid

- Most people with low blood sugar rush from one sugar fix to the next. In extreme cases they might eat 6–8 chocolate-type snacks daily. Cravings for caffeine, sugar and refined carbohydrates, such as croissants, biscuits, pastries and pizzas, are all common. Not only do all these foods have a negative effect on blood sugar, but they are also low in fibre, vitamins and minerals.
- See under *Adrenal Exhaustion*.

Friendly Foods
- Fibre helps to slow down the release of sugars, and if absent, the sugars in any foods get into the bloodstream too quickly. Great fibres are linseeds (flax seeds soaked overnight in cold water/drained), oat or rice bran, sunflower seeds, and psyllium husks.
- Begin the day with a good breakfast, such as low-sugar muesli or cereal, porridge, eggs or beans on toast.
- Eat more raw foods because they are higher in insoluble fibre – carrots, cucumber, tomatoes, celery, fruits and so on.
- If you have time for only a small meal, try to make sure it is high in protein rather than carbohydrate, which will keep you more satisfied in the long term. See under *General Health Hints* for a delicious smoothie recipe made with hemp seed protein powder.
- If your blood sugar drops too low, not only can you feel faint, but you are also more likely to suffer panic attacks. At the very least, eat a banana with a handful of sunflower or pumpkin seeds (to slow sugar rush) and a low-fat fruit yoghurt. Carry almonds with you to munch on.
- Eat more brown rice, barley, oats, lentils, buckwheat, sweet potatoes, amaranth, spelt and wholemeal bread and pastas; also try corn, spinach and rice pastas. *The Low GL Diet Bible* by Patrick Holford (Piatkus) lists low glycaemic foods.
- Try natural alternatives to refined sugars such as raw organic manuka honey, brown rice syrup or the plant sugar xylitol (available from Higher Nature). **HN**
- Make sure you eat a portion of good-quality protein with each meal – such as fish, lean meats, chicken, turkey, cooked tofu, eggs or use whey or hemp seed protein powders.
- Eat smaller meals more regularly.
- Snack on fresh fruit such as apples, apricots, cherries, pomegranate, berries, papaya and low-sugar snack bars, available from health shops. Or use low-fat hummus, avocado or goat's cheese on a amaranth cracker or rye crisp bread.
- Drink freshly made or organic vegetable juices.
- Snack on low-fat yoghurts with added sunflower or pumpkin seeds to reduce sugar cravings.
- Have a piece of wholemeal toast or an amaranth cracker with a little low-fat spread and low-sugar jam.
- Drink more herbal teas and pure dandelion coffee. (NB: some brands contain 50% lactose, which is a form of sugar.)
- Drink more water.
- Make salad dressings with a combination of any unrefined organic oils, such as sesame, walnut, olive or sunflower.
- Essential fats help to sustain energy levels and balance blood sugar. See *Fats You Need To Eat*.

Useful Remedies
- Lipoic acid helps stabilize blood sugar while supporting brain function, which can be a problem with low blood sugar. Take 200mg daily.
- In the US, studies have shown that when people who eat a refined Western diet are given 200mcg of the mineral chromium twice daily, the incidence of late-onset diabetes is halved. Chromium is greatly depleted in the body by sugar and junk foods. Once you cut down on sugar and white carbohydrates, you may crave sweet foods. Therefore, begin taking 400mcg of chromium daily. It takes a few days to kick in, but really does help reduce cravings. After 2 weeks, reduce to 200mcg.
- Take 200–500mg magnesium spread throughout the day with food. Magnesium helps regulate blood-sugar levels.
- Take a strong B-complex with 30mg of niacinamide B3. **(NB Make sure it's a no-flush type niacin, as niacin can cause skin-flushing.)** B3 is essential for the control of blood-sugar levels.

- Take full-spectrum, natural-source vitamin E – 400iu daily – as vitamin E has been shown to help improve insulin response in the body.
- BioCare make Sucroguard, developed by nutritional physician Dr John Briffa, which contains all the above nutrients in one capsule. Take between meals. **BC**

Helpful Hints

- If you suffer acute symptoms, such as fainting fits, blackouts, extreme weakness and trembling, it is important to restore blood sugar levels as quickly as possible. In an emergency you need to get glucose into your body. While I would generally not recommend high-sugar foods and drinks, this is one occasion when you can use them. Drink Lucozade or similar, or eat a sugary biscuit. This is definitely not a long-term solution!
- Your own GP can refer you to the nearest doctor who is also a qualified nutritionist (see *Useful Information*).

LOW STOMACH ACID

(see also Acid Stomach, Indigestion and Leaky Gut Syndrome)

When we eat food, particularly protein-based foods, our stomachs should produce a lot of gastric juice in response. This juice is a mixture of mucous, which protects the stomach lining, and a very strong acid, hydrochloric acid. High levels of hydrochloric acid are needed for the production of pepsin, which is necessary for proper digestion before the food moves into the small intestine and the nutrients start to be absorbed. Due to various aspects of our diet, lifestyle and age, the amount of acid we produce over time tends to decline. Low levels of stomach acid are associated with poor digestion and, more importantly, the poor absorption of the nutrients we need for good health.

Conditions strongly linked with low stomach-acid levels are asthma, allergies, leaky gut and gall stones, and can be a factor in stomach ulcers. Many people feel they make too much stomach acid, whereas in reality they often produce too little. A lot of people will take an antacid, which neutralizes what little acid was available, making digestion even harder. Undigested foods can end up leaking into the blood stream, causing food allergies. Undigested food can rot in the bowel causing wind, bloating, and overgrowth of unhealthy organisms such as candida (see *Candida*).

An easy way to find out if you have low stomach acid is to take a level teaspoon of bicarbonate of soda and dissolve it in some lukewarm water well away from food. If sufficient quantities of acid are present in the stomach, the bicarb mixture is converted into gas, producing significant bloating and belching within 5–10 minutes of drinking the mix. Little or no belching denotes low stomach acid.

Foods to Avoid

- Cut down on alcohol, sugar, caffeinated foods and drinks and cow's dairy products, which can all cause an acid reflux.
- Don't eat in a rush and keep heavy, rich meals containing red meat and creamy sauces to a minimum.
- Avoid all fried foods, which are hard to digest.
- Avoid eating proteins, such as fish or meat, with carbohydrates, such as potatoes, rice or pasta, because the body uses different enzymes for each food group.
- Avoid eating fat and protein together – such as fish and chips – as the fat slows protein digestion, which is the problem with low stomach acid.

- Stop chewing gum – this makes the stomach think that food is about to arrive, which triggers stomach-acid production.
- Avoid eating large amounts of fruit directly after a large meal.
- **Friendly Foods**
- Eat fruit generally between meals or include a little papaya and pineapple with meals, which are packed with digestive enzymes.
- Bitter-tasting vegetables are great for stimulating digestion – eat more rocket, artichoke, radicchio and celeriac, as well as ginger. These foods encourage gastric-juice production.

Useful Remedies

- As levels of stomach acid production tend to drop as we age or when we are under prolonged negative stress, take 1 betaine hydrochloride (stomach acid) capsule with a glass of water just before your main meals. If you have active stomach ulcers or this causes you any discomfort, use a good-quality digestive enzyme that is free from hydrochloric acid instead, such as bromelain 500mg a few minutes before main meals.
- Try Peppermint Formula; take 10–20 drops before a meal. If you suffer with symptoms of overeating, and/or feeling bloated and uncomfortable take 10–20 drops after a meal. **FSC**
- Acidophilus and bifidus are the healthy bacteria that help to regulate digestion. Take 1 capsule of Jarro-Dophilus EPS, made by Jarrow, daily at the end of your main meal. **NC**
- B vitamins and zinc are needed to help the body naturally produce more stomach acid. Take a multi-vitamin/mineral formula daily for your age and gender that contains at least 30mg of zinc.

Helpful Hints

- Chewing food thoroughly really helps to improve the digestive process. Don't eat on the run.
- Some people have found separating proteins and carbohydrates at one meal has improved their digestion no end.
- Eat small meals regularly; try 4 snack-type meals daily. Avoid eating when stressed.
- If you have pronounced longitudinal ridges in your nails, this is a common sign of poor absorption often due to low stomach acid.
- Drink mint or peppermint, fennel or fresh mint herbal teas to aid digestion.
- The herb meadowsweet helps to regulate low stomach acid. **SHS**
- Walking for 30 minutes each day aids digestion.

LUPUS

(see also Adrenal Exhaustion, Leaky Gut Syndrome, Sjogren's Syndrome and Stress)

Lupus is an autoimmune condition that triggers inflammation in multiple sites around the body. This condition can take years to manifest and is often missed until symptoms become more apparent. Typical symptoms might include arthritis-type joint pains, skin rashes (especially a 'butterfly'-type rash on the face around the nose and cheeks that comes and goes), lowered immune function, or a low white/and or red blood cell count. There can be incidence of flare-ups of inflammation in tissues surrounding the heart and lungs and there are hugely varying degrees of lupus. A blood test should confirm this. The most common and most serious form is systemic lupus erythematosus (SLE). Symptoms can come and go and are hugely dependent on levels of stress in the patient. Osteoporosis is also seen as a result of lupus and can be further exacerbated by steroid therapy, one of the most common forms of orthodox medical treatment. Fatigue, depression, low-level fever, eye or gut problems may also be involved. Some people also develop Raynaud's syndrome – see under *Raynaud's*. An attack can be precipitated by overexposure to ultraviolet light and also upon exposure to certain chemicals such as those found in hair dyes.

Lupus requires specialist help from a nutritional physician. However, there are many things you can do to help yourself. As this is a highly multi-factorial condition, it is more than likely that for years you have eaten foods to which you have intolerances that triggered the initial inflammatory responses. See *Candida* and *Leaky Gut*.

If this situation continues in tandem with an on-going high stressed lifestyle (or personality type that reacts negatively to stress), then the stress hormones cortisol and adrenalin over time will add to the inflammatory burden on the body and contribute to the osteoporosis. Eventually, a combination of these situations could cause the immune system to start attacking itself and conditions such as lupus can arise.

Foods to Avoid
- The most likely triggers for your food intolerances are any foods containing gluten – but in some people it may be cow's milk.
- Oranges and orange juice and tomatoes may also be a problem.
- Avoid foods high in saturated fats from animal sources.
- If you tend to eat lots of 'white' refined foods high in sugar, cut them down to a minimum as sugar triggers inflammation in the body.
- Alfalfa sprouts and mushrooms are a known trigger for some people.
- Avoid refined sugars in any form, including maltose, dextrose and fructose found in mass-produced biscuits, cakes, pies and so on.
- As your immune system and your gut work more efficiently in an alkaline environment, you need to alkalize your system. See under *Acid–Alkaline Balance*.
- Certain foods are high in arachidonic acids, which tend to increase inflammation in the body – such as meat, eggs and dairy produce from animals.
- Cut down on alcohol and caffeine, which encourage cortisol production.

Friendly Foods
- Generally, eat more oily fish that is anti-inflammatory, such as organic-farmed salmon, sardines, pilchards, mackerel, anchovies, and black cod.
- Eat more vegetable-based proteins, such as lentils, quinoa, organic tofu, peas, beans, pulses.
- Use organic-sourced hemp seed protein powders.
- Eat more brown rice, buckwheat and non-wheat-based pastas.
- Try non-dairy sources of milks, such as almond, quinoa, rice and coconut.
- Try avoiding all foods containing wheat and gluten for a month and I'll bet symptoms will begin to subside. Many supermarkets and health shops now sell gluten- and wheat-free foods.
- Use a little organic agave or brown rice syrup, which have a lower glycaemic index, or use xylitol sugar such as ZyloSweet, available from Higher Nature. **HN**
- Eat more foods rich in carotenes needed for tissue healing – pumpkin, watercress, papaya, sweet potato, apricots, mango, spinach, all green vegetables and carrots.
- White fish, chicken or turkey are preferable to red meats.
- Eat more nuts and seeds high in omega-6 and -3 fats, such as linseeds, sunflower, pumpkin, hemp seeds, and use their unrefined oils for salad dressings.
- Drink more green and white teas rich in antioxidants

Useful remedies
- As high levels of C-reactive protein tend to be found in lupus sufferers, quercetin, a polyphenol found in garlic, has shown great promise for reducing chronic inflammation. Take 250mg twice daily with food.

- Gamma-linolenic acid (GLA) is found in evening primrose and borage oil. Take 2–4 500mg capsules daily. **BC**
- Fish oils are essential to dampen inflammation – take 2–3 grams of omega-3 fish oil daily
- Take 400iu of full-spectrum, natural-source vitamin E to help neutralize free radical damage caused by the inflammation.
- If you have long-term adrenal exhaustion, you most probably need supplementation of the hormone DHEA. A blood test will confirm this; ask your doctor how much you would need. In the UK you need a prescription, or order via www.lef.org.
- A high-strength multi-vitamin/mineral for your age and gender that includes a full spectrum of the B group vitamins to support your nerves.
- You will also need a multiple bone support formula that contains calcium, magnesium, D3, boron, K2 and silica. **NC**
- To help re-alkalize your body try Green Magic Powder – containing Hawaiian spirulina, chlorella, lecithin, barley and wheat grass, kamut, pectin, apple fibre, kelp and wheat sprouts, CoQ10, royal jelly, artichoke powder and lactobacillus acidophilus is a great all round way to ingest good nutrients, healthy bacteria, keep the body more alkaline and help keep you regular. Details on www.itsgreenmagic.com or call Helen Cruikshank on 07798 873266. Use in your breakfast smoothie or just take in water. See *General Health Hints* for a healthy smoothie recipe.
- L-theanine, which is found in green tea, really helps to reduce feelings of stress. See under *Adrenal Exhaustion*.
- Co-enzyme Q10 will help to raise energy levels. Take 100–200mg daily with breakfast and/or with lunch.
- Healthy bacteria known as probiotics help to keep the immune system strong and help keep candida in check. Take one Jarro-Dophilus EPS daily after a meal. Made by Jarrow. **NC**
- In numerous studies from the US, Hungary, Israel and Russia, a fermented wheat germ extract known as Avemar, sold in more than 10 countries, has demonstrated remarkably beneficial immune-modulating effects. Take one sachet daily in water at least one hour before breakfast. Must be kept refrigerated. Also available in capsules, but you would need quite a few, therefore powder is easier to take once a day. Details can be found on www.avemar.com. Available to buy in UK and Europe from the Nutri Centre. **NC**
- A high-strength antioxidant formula that contains vitamin C, carotenes and bioflavonoids.
- Collagen is a vital component of healthy joints, skin, hair, nails, cartilage, ligaments and tendons – which also improves bone strength. It is the most widely distributed protein in the body and helps signal the body to reduce inflammation. Take daily in a glass of water or diluted juice 30 minutes before a main meal. Super Strength Collagen Drink from Higher Nature. **HN**

Helpful Hints
- A urine test via Genova Diagnostics can detect a leaky gut, see below - it is called a Gut Permeability Test.
- It is really important to have an allergy test to find foods/substances that are a problem. Try the York Test Laboratories. Call 0800 458 2052 or log on to www.yorktest.com. Or Genova Diagnostics do a FACT test that looks for inflammatory markers indicating that the body is reacting to certain substances. Call 020 8336 7750 or log on to www.gdx.uk.net.
- Exercise is important, but don't exercise if you are truly exhausted as this can be counterproductive. Gentle walking is fine.
- Get some sleep, and go to bed before 10pm. Sleep is the best way to heal the body.

- Deal with negative long-term stress and your reaction to it. See *Stress*.
- Be sensible when it comes to sun exposure.
- Have your hormones checked, as you may also need progesterone, oestrogen and testosterone as well as DHEA. See under *Menopause*.
- See also *Osteoporosis*.

MACULAR DEGENERATION *(see also Eye Problems)*

Macular degeneration (also known as AMD – aged-related macular degeneration) is the slow deterioration of cells in the macula, a tiny yellowish area in the central part of the retina, which is responsible for visual sharpness. Around 240,000 people in the UK are affected. Macular degeneration is now the leading cause of blindness in people over the age of 55, and 30% of people in the West over the age of 70 have symptoms of AMD – symptoms that increase over time, thus affecting your ability to read, write, drive and so on.

There are two types of macular degeneration: wet and dry. Ninety percent of people with macular degeneration have the dry type, in which small, yellow spots, called drusens, form underneath the macular. Drusens are waste products that accumulate because of lack of antioxidants to clear them from the eyes. The drusens slowly break down the cells in the macular, causing distorted vision. In the wet type, abnormal blood vessels begin to grow toward the macular, causing rapid and severe vision loss.

Scientists believe that AMD is triggered by oxidative stress, caused by free radical reactions in the body – especially in the retina, because of its high consumption of oxygen. Free radical reactions occur as the normal by-products of living, eating and breathing, but also from over-exposure to ultra-violet radiation, smoking, a poor diet and a compromised immune system. This condition is also linked to the hardening of the arteries and poor circulation (see under *Atherosclerosis*, *High Blood Pressure* and *Circulation*).

People with a high homocysteine (see under *High Blood Pressure*) level and low B vitamin intake are associated with an increased risk for AMD and women with light-coloured irises are more at risk.

Foods to Avoid
- Full-fat dairy foods, plus meats, hamburgers, mass-produced pies, sausages, cheeses, chocolates and sugary, fatty foods – all the usual suspects.
- Definitely avoid too many fried foods and hydrogenated or trans- fats, which are found in most margarines and mass-produced vegetable oils. See *Fats You Need To Eat*.
- Cut down or eliminate sodium-based salt; instead use a natural mineral-based salt, which is available from all good health stores.
- Avoid monosodium glutamate (MSG), which is a potential retinal toxin.
- Avoid excessive alcohol, but the occasional glass of wine is fine. Too much alcohol interferes with liver function, and reduces protective glutathione levels in the eyes. (As glutathione is so important, see *Liver Problems* for more details.)
- At all costs, avoid foods and drinks containing the artificial sweetener aspartame.

Friendly Foods

- The most important foods for reducing and preventing AMD are carotenes (especially lutein and zeaxanthin). Lutein is found in all dark green leafy vegetables, such as spinach (raw is best), kale, broccoli, spring greens, watercress, cabbage and so on.
- Zeaxanthin is found in yellow and orange fruits and vegetables, such as carrots, peaches, persimmons, pumpkins, sweet potatoes, mangoes, apricots and cantaloupe melons.
- Saffron is also wonderful as it is high in zeaxanthin – eat curries.
- Other great eye foods are onions, apples, green tea, cherries, pears, grapes, cranberries, red onions, garlic, mustard greens, alfalfa sprouts, asparagus and butternut squash.
- Generally, eat more wholefoods, such as stone-ground wholemeal bread, brown rice, quinoa and buckwheat.
- Eat oily fish and white fish in preference to meats.
- Eat more blueberries, bilberries and blackcurrants.
- In addition, green drinks made from organic grasses, blue-green and sea algae, herbs and other nutrients are very helpful. Most health shops sell excellent organic green food-based powders.
- Vitamin-E-rich foods help to reduce the risk of developing AMD. These include hazelnuts, almonds, cod liver oil, raw wheat germ, avocado and tomato purée.
- Chicken and turkey (the dark parts of the meat) are high in the amino acid taurine, which is good for the eyes.

Useful Remedies

- Take a high-strength multi-vitamin and mineral daily as a base. Make sure your multi contains a full spectrum of B vitamins to control high homocysteine levels, 200mcg of selenium, 30mg of zinc, 100iu of full-spectrum vitamin E, and at least 100mg of vitamin C.
- Vitamin C helps to make collagen, which strengthens the capillaries that nourish the retina and protects against UV light. The eye contains the second-highest concentration of vitamin C in the body next to the adrenal glands. Take 1 gram daily in an ascorbate form with food.
- Bilberry has been called the vision herb for its powerful effect on all types of visual disorders. British Royal Air Force pilots during World War II reported improved night-time vision after consuming bilberry. The fruit supports the structural integrity of the tiny capillaries that deliver oxygen and nutrients to the eyes. Take 200–300mg daily.
- Bioflavonoids, such as quercetin and rutin, are plant pigments, rich in antioxidants that protect the eyes from sunlight damage. Take 1000mg daily of a mixed bioflavonoid supplement.
- Glutathione is essential for vision. This is an antioxidant found in large concentrations in the eye; if you take 200mg of lipoic acid twice daily, this helps to raise levels of glutathione.
- Cysteine is important for a healthy retina. Taken as N-acetyl cysteine (NAC), it also increases production of glutathione. Take 500mg daily half an hour before a meal.
- Taurine is another potent antioxidant that is highly concentrated within the eye, normally found in the retina. A deficiency of this amino acid alters the structure and function of the retina. Taurine also helps to prevent cataracts. Take 500mg daily.
- If you don't eat plenty of carotene-rich foods, you definitely need to take a high-strength, natural-source carotene complex.
- Most of the companies listed on pages 15–16 make all-in-one eye formulae that contain most of the above.
- Macushield contains good levels of natural-source carotenoids from marigold known to support eye health. Call 01564 711154 or log on to www.macushield.co.uk.

Helpful Hints

- Make sure you get sufficient exercise, which helps increase circulation.

- Acupuncture can help increase circulation to the eye area, as can Advanced Reflexology. For a therapist near you, log on to www.artreflex.com.
- Wear a hat or cap at all times and good sunglasses, preferably wraparound, in bright sunlight – even when young.
- Don't smoke, as this can increase the likelihood of developing AMD by more than two and a half times.

ME (MYALGIC ENCEPHALOMYELITIS)

(see also Adrenal Exhaustion, Candida, Leaky Gut and Low Blood Sugar)

Around 250,000 people in Britain are recognized as having chronic fatigue or ME, but I, and my fellow co-authors, believe that hundreds of thousands more go undiagnosed. Many people feel tired all the time and just struggle on, but only when the crushing exhaustion becomes incapacitating do people seek medical help.

Symptoms range from chronic, debilitating tiredness to depression, muscle and joint pain, headaches and decreased concentration, poor sleep quality, low blood pressure, low blood sugar, food cravings, bloating, chemical sensitivities and night sweats, to name but a few. In writing this book I now firmly believe that virtually all ME-type symptoms are linked either to a severe leaky gut and candida or adrenal exhaustion. If you read these three sections, you will be left in no doubt as to why they appear to mirror virtually all the symptoms associated with ME. And once these issues are addressed, the ME is often alleviated. Also, if you have suffered a viral illness, such as flu, herpes or glandular fever, are exposed to a lot of electrical equipment, or have running water under your home, any, or all these factors may play a part. ME is also linked to heavy metal toxicity (especially mercury), liver congestion, food intolerances and deficiencies in minerals such as magnesium; there are also possible parasite links.

What helps one person may not work for another, but without doubt eating the right diet and taking the right supplements will make a difference. If you contract a viral infection, you must give your body a chance to rest and recover, which gives you more chance of avoiding long-term illness.

Foods to Avoid

- Avoid any foods and drinks containing caffeine, refined sugar and alcohol – all of which lower immune function, weaken the adrenal system, and play havoc with blood sugar levels. Also most pre-packaged foods high in sugar are also high in saturated fats, salt, additives and preservatives.
- Most mass-produced, tinned foods and takeaways (unless they are freshly made) are lacking in magnesium. Forty percent of ME patients have low levels of this vital mineral.
- Some people mistakenly use guarana (or drinks such as Red Bull) as an energy source when they are very low in energy. Unfortunately, the primary reason they give you energy is the caffeine content, which will only serve to weaken your adrenals in the long term. Never mix Red Bull with alcohol.
- If you find yourself constantly craving foods such as wheat, sugar and snacks, are bloated, have an urgency to urinate, suffer mood swings and are always tired, you may well have candida (see *Foods to Avoid* under *Candida*).
- Almost everyone with chronic fatigue will have multiple food intolerances, the most common being gluten from wheat and dairy produce from cow's milk. See under *Allergies*.

Friendly Foods

- See also *Insulin Resistance*.
- Essential fats are vital as they support the endocrine system, boost immunity, and help balance blood sugar. Eat more organic sunflower, hemp and pumpkin seeds and linseeds (flax seeds). See *Fats You Need To Eat*.
- It is vital that you eat good-quality protein, such as organic lean meat, chicken, fresh fish, or beans, at least twice a day. Protein helps to balance blood sugar for longer periods.
- Also try organic hemp seed proteins, which are easy to absorb.
- Include plenty of vegetables and fruits in the diet, but do not eat too much fruit if you also have candida.
- Generally eat more low glycaemic foods, such as lentils, beans, pulses, millet, quinoa, barley, gluten-free porridge, buckwheat and sweet potato. Nutritionist Patrick Holford's book *The Low GL Diet Bible* (Piatkus) offers good lists of low GI foods.
- Replace animal milks with organic almond, rice, oat, quinoa, pea or coconut milk.
- Remember to include plenty of leafy greens, such as cabbage, kale, watercress, spring greens, pak choy, broccoli, celery, wheat germ, Brazil nuts, walnuts, almonds, curries, black strap molasses, unprocessed honey and beans in your diet, as they are rich in magnesium.
- Drink plenty of pure water, even if you are not thirsty, to help detoxify your system.
- Eat sunflower, linseeds, pumpkin, hemp and sesame seeds, which are packed with essential fats and fibre, and use extra-virgin unrefined olive or sunflower oils for salad dressings.
- Add coriander over your foods, which really helps to detoxify heavy metals from the body, as does chlorella.
- Green tea is high in L-theanine, which helps you to relax, so drink de-caffeinated organic green teas.
- Replace refined sugars with organic agave syrup or xylitol, which have only a minimal impact on blood sugar levels. **HN**

Useful Remedies

- L-carnitine – an amino acid – has been shown to help reduce symptoms of chronic fatigue. Take 500mg twice daily before food spread throughout the day.
- L-carnitine works well with the antioxidant lipoic acid to raise energy levels in the body. Take 200mg of lipoic acid daily.
- Advanced Stress Formula contains liquorice, Siberian ginseng, ashwagandha and gotu kola, a blend of herbs for the adrenal system. Take one and a half teaspoons twice daily in water. Available from www.holoshealth.com. **NB Not for children or pregnant women, or if breast feeding, or those with high blood pressure.**
- Take magnesium citrate, 600–1000mg per day, which helps to reduce muscle soreness. Take in divided doses throughout the day and take the last 200mg before bed.
- Take a high-strength multi-vitamin and mineral twice daily.
- Beta Glucans 1–3, 1–6, derived from yeast cell walls, are proven to strengthen the body's innate immune system (the immune system you are born with), making it more resistant to pathogens from food and air. Take 250–500mg daily. It can also be taken by children and reduces the likelihood of food intolerances triggered by a weakened immune system. Dr Paul Clayton, based in the UK and US, is a medical pharmacologist. His website research on Beta Glucans is well worth a look. Find him at www.healthdefence.com. Glucosan, developed by Dr Clayton, is available from Vitalize Health products on 0870 042 8423 or www.vitalizeshop.co.uk.
- As the body heals more quickly if it is alkaline, take an organic-source green food powder daily, such as Viridian 100% Organic Green Food Blend Powder. Available from health shops. **VN** See under *General Health Hints* for a delicious smoothie.

- A vitamin-like substance that we make naturally in the liver, Co-enzyme Q10 is often depleted in ME patients. Take 100–200mg with breakfast or lunch for extra energy. **SVHC, PN**

Helpful Hints

- Get some quality rest; it's nature's way of healing. Go to bed by 10pm.
- Take some gentle exercise. One study found that people were able to walk for 3 minutes, then rest for 3 minutes, until they had done a total of 30 minutes' walking, without any negative effect on chronic fatigue.
- Try a gentle stretching programme to tone the muscles gradually and help drain the lymph system, which is often overloaded.
- Learn to relax. Meditation is a great way to give the body and brain a complete rest.
- If you want more information on being checked for parasites, which are often linked to ME, then see all details of Genova Labs under *Irritable Bowel Syndrome*.
- Have a friend massage your aching muscles with a mix of the essential oils of thyme and lemongrass. To help lift depression, try a mix of neroli and rose in a good base oil.
- For a free information pack or for more help, contact Action for ME, Action for ME, PO Box 2778, Bristol BS1 9DJ or telephone 0845 123 2314. Website: www.afme.org.uk. Email: admin@afme.org.uk.
- If your symptoms persist, try having your house dowsed for electrical or geopathic stress. To find a dowser, call British Society of Dowsers. Tel: 01684 576969. Website: www.britishdowsers.org.
- Cranial osteopathy has helped many people with ME, as it frees up nerve endings, which releases energy in the body. See *Useful Information*.
- Hands-on healing, such as Reiki, has proven very successful for many ME patients – for more details of healers who work with ME, see under *Healing*.
- With ME, it is best to consult a doctor who is also a qualified nutritionist, as you may need injections of magnesium and B12 (see *Useful Information*).

MEMORY

(see also Alzheimer's Disease, Atherosclerosis, Circulation, Parkinson's Disease and Stress)

At the age of 61 I regularly forget people's names and where I left certain objects – we all do. And just because you forget a few things, it doesn't automatically mean that you have Alzheimer's or dementia, so don't panic. Most people think that once a brain cell dies, it's gone for ever, but it's now known that brain cells can and do regenerate. Just like our muscles, the brain needs regular use – and if you don't use it, you lose it. The secret to improving your memory is to keep your brain active and eat less junk food and more super-brain foods. However, your brain also requires quality and sufficient sleep in order to function at an optimal level. Anyone who experiences jet lag or loses a night's sleep knows how this can affect one's ability to stay sharp.

There really is no need for your memory or brain function to decline with age. My mother-in-law died at 95 and her brain was as sharp as a razor, as she had spent 30 years regularly completing crosswords.

Temporary memory loss is not uncommon after drinking alcohol; if your blood sugar level is low; after a high fever; following surgery; after an epileptic fit; or, when you are under stress. Depression and acute anxiety can also cause temporary memory loss. More serious memory loss can occur after an accident, brain injury or stroke. Senile dementia involves pro-gressive loss of short-term memory until the individual is unable to remember what they did or saw only a few moments before. Many prescription drugs, such as long-term use of statins or sleeping pills, and/or the long-term use of drug 'cocktails' (as in people who might be taking pills for high blood pressure, cholesterol, and so on), affect memory. External influences, such as poor eyesight and hearing, can also inhibit our ability to learn – thus affecting memory.

However, the vast majority of cases of poor memory are caused by years of eating too many of the wrong foods, especially saturated fats, which clog the arteries until the small capillaries are affected, preventing sufficient fresh, red blood reaching the brain and depriving it of oxygen. Simply taking a deep breath more regularly, every 20 minutes or so, can help improve brain function.

Lead is well known to affect memory, which is why lead-free petrol was introduced on both environmental and health grounds. Mercury fillings are also linked to memory loss (see *Mercury Fillings*). A high level of homocysteine, a by-product of protein metabolism, can trigger memory loss-type problems. See under *Alzheimer's Disease* for full details.

Foods to Avoid
- If you want to keep your memory sharp, you need to cut down on high-fat foods, such as meat and full-fat dairy foods. Also avoid mass-produced pies, cakes, biscuits, white bread, pizzas, burgers and so on, which not only deplete nutrients, but also contribute to clogging your arteries. Research shows that people who eat high-fat, nutrient-poor foods, such as burgers and chips, are less intelligent and have poorer memories than those who eat a low-fat, nutrient-dense diet. See under *Atherosclerosis*.
- Alcohol depletes the body of vital nutrients.
- Avoid excess sodium-based table salt, and don't add salt to food once it has been cooked.
- In some people excess wheat triggers 'brain fog'. This is usually the gluten content, although any food to which you are intolerant can trigger this problem. See under *Allergies*.
- Avoid too much refined sugar, which ages your brain.
- Avoid aspartame and monosodium glutamate (MSG), as they are brain toxins.

Friendly Foods
- Always eat breakfast. Low-sugar cereals, such as muesli or porridge, as they are rich in B-vitamins, which are often lacking in dementia patients (especially B12).
- Low blood sugar levels can easily trigger 'foggy-brain' symptoms, such as memory loss. Make sure you eat small meals regularly to balance blood sugar (see *Low Blood Sugar*).
- Omega-3 essential fats, rich in EPA and DHA, are vital brain nutrients. They are found in oily fish, salmon, sardines, pilchards, black cod, herrings and mackerel.
- Use unrefined, preferably organic, olive oil and sunflower, walnut and sesame oils for salad dressings and to drizzle over cooked foods (see *Fats You Need To Eat*).
- Fresh coffee is often criticized, but in terms of memory function it seems to help it, particularly in the elderly. Two cups a day is fine.
- Green leafy vegetables, particularly spinach, watercress, cabbage, pak choy, celery, broccoli and spring greens, as well as red and purple fruits such as strawberries, pomegranate, blueberries, blackberries and cherries, all rich in antioxidants, which will help to slow memory decline.
- Eat more apples, papaya, pineapple, grapes, prunes and raisins.
- Eat more wholegrain foods, such as brown pasta and rice, and wholemeal bread and flour, and barley and buckwheat.
- For those with a sweet tooth, use a little unprocessed honey, brown rice syrup, organic agave syrup or xylitol, such as XyloSweet. HN

- Phosphatidylcholine is a vital brain nutrient that is found in egg yolks and fish, especially sardines.
- Take non-GM lecithin granules, a brain food that also reduces the amounts of LDL, the 'bad' cholesterol, in your body. Taking this brain nutrient during pregnancy can result in brainier children. Sprinkle a tablespoon of the granules over your breakfast cereal, or into salads or yoghurts. Available from all health stores.
- Eat more ginger and live, low-fat yoghurt to aid digestion.
- Add freshly chopped sage to your salads and meals, as it has been shown to improve memory and brain function.

Useful Remedies
- Take a high-strength multi-vitamin, mineral or antioxidants formula that is suitable for your age and gender.
- Make sure that you include a vitamin B-complex, as B-vitamins are essential for normal brain function and they keep homocysteine levels in check. (These should already be in your multi.)
- The herb ginkgo biloba is proven to increase memory as it improves blood flow to the brain. **SHS**
- An extract of the periwinkle called Vinpocetine by Life Extension, like ginkgo, is a herb that helps improve circulation. It is especially useful when blood flow to the brain is diminished, as in the hardening of the arteries or minor strokes, and it also helps some people with tinnitus (ringing in the ears). Take 20–40mg daily. **NC**

- Phosphatidyl serine – take 100mg up to 3 times a day – has been shown to improve mental function. Take early in the day, as at night this can increase dreaming.
- Co-enzyme Q10, 100mg a day, can improve energy production within the brain.
- The amino acid L-glutamine also makes a great brain food, as it is the most abundant amino acid in the fluid that surrounds the brain. Take 250mg twice daily on an empty stomach 30 minutes before food.
- Acetyl L-carnitine, an amino acid, helps slow progression of early dementia and slows deterioration in the brain. Take 500mg x 3 times daily before meals.
- Glutathione is a vital brain nutrient. See *Liver Problems*.
- Research over 15 years from Dr Hirokazu Kawagishi of Shizoka University in Japan has demonstrated that a pure extract of the Lion's Mane Mushroom has a remarkable ability to increase Nerve Growth Factor (NGF) in the brain, which in turn helps make more neurons. Take daily for at least 3 months, as nerves do not grow overnight! Scientist Roger Coghill, based in the UK, supplies a pure extract of the Lion's Mane. For details or to find your nearest supplier, log on to www.asphalia.co.uk or call 01495 752122.

Helpful Hints
- Regular exercise is vital for aiding memory: the more oxygen you get to the brain, the less likely you are to lose your memory.
- Make sure you are getting sufficient quality sleep.
- Common sage contains thujone (a naturally occurring substance that gives sage its flavour), which if used as sage essential oil can trigger fits in sensitive individuals. However, Spanish sage contains almost no thujone. Regular head massage with Spanish sage essential oil (diluted in a base oil) has been shown by Dr John Wilkinson at Middlesex University to increase memory functioning.
- Rubbing the essential oil of basil and/or rosemary, diluted in a base of almond oil, into the scalp will help to increase circulation to the scalp and clear your mind, thus aiding concentration.

- Chelation therapy helps to unclog your arteries, which increases the amount of blood and oxygen that reaches the brain. Chelation therapy helps to remove deadly metal toxins from the body. I give full details of this treatment in my book *500 of the Most Important Ways to Stay Younger Longer* (CICO Books). There are several chelation clinics in the UK. For details on chelation therapy, call the Arterial Disease Clinic on 01942 886644 or call Dr Wendy Denning on 020 7224 2423.
- Play more word games and complete crosswords. During car journeys, when on a train or queuing in a supermarket, add or multiply varying numbers in your head.
- Minimize aluminium exposure – this includes many deodorants, cooking pans, some cheeses and so on (see *Alzheimer's Disease*).
- Meditation helps to improve memory.
- Minimize exposure to mercury (see *Mercury Fillings*).
- Avoid using a mobile phone for more than 10 minutes at a time. You should also avoid using them in cars and trains, because this amplifies the negative effects of them. (See under *Electrical Pollution*.)
- Stop smoking, as smoking narrows blood vessels thus depleting the brain of much-needed oxygen.
- If, after trying these remedies for three months, you are still experiencing memory problems, consult a nutritionist who is also a doctor (see also *Helpful Hints* in *Alzheimer's Disease*).
- For further help read *New Optimum Nutrition for the Mind* by Patrick Holford (Piatkus).

MÉNIÈRE'S SYNDROME *(see also Tinnitus and Vertigo)*

This is a little-understood problem of the inner ear, which causes recurrent attacks of vertigo, nausea and ringing in the ears and progressive deafness. People with this problem tend to feel unsteady and to suffer from headaches and neck pains. Causes are suggested as being linked to salt retention, food intolerances, nutritional deficiency as a result of poor absorption, or even a spasm in the walls of small blood vessels. If you have food intolerances, this can trigger leaky gut syndrome when toxins leak through the gut wall into the body, which could trigger these types of symptoms. See under *Leaky Gut*.

In Chinese medicine the ears are linked to the kidney/adrenal area, which is why stress can greatly exacerbate this problem.

Foods to Avoid
- Many people with this problem react to soya, wheat (the gluten is usually the culprit), corn and yeast-based foods.
- Avoid sodium-based salt.
- Generally avoid any foods containing gluten, salt, caffeine, fried foods and alcohol.
- Reduce full-fat milk and dairy produce from all animal sources.
- See also *General Health Hints*.

Friendly Foods
- Eat more ginger, garlic, leeks and onions, which are very cleansing.
- Papaya and pineapple contain digestive enzymes, which aid absorption of nutrients from your food.
- Add 2 teaspoons of organic apple cider vinegar to water and sip – the mixture is rich in potassium, which may be low in this condition.
- See *Friendly Foods* under *Leaky Gut* and *Vertigo*.

- Cherries, blueberries, blackberries and plums are all rich in flavenoids, which help to support ear function.
- Eat more wheat germ, pecan and Brazil nuts, almonds, buckwheat, spinach, peas and beans, which are rich in manganese, as a lack of this mineral is linked to this condition.

Useful Remedies
- Take a high-strength multi-vitamin and mineral.
- The herb ginkgo biloba helps to increase circulation in the ears.
- Take a digestive enzyme capsule with main meals. **BC**
- 5–10mg of manganese may be useful. A deficiency in this mineral has been linked to Ménière's Syndrome. Most multi-formulas will contain this amount.

Helpful Hints
- It is important to consult a chiropractor or cranial osteopath, who can check for any cranial, spinal or neck misalignments.
- Acupuncture has shown to be very useful for this condition (see *Useful Information*), because it helps to increase circulation to the ears.

MENOPAUSE *(see also Adrenal Exhaustion, Low Blood Sugar and Osteoporosis)*

As a woman in her early sixties, I am writing this section from a place of experience. Many women believe that the menopause is an illness for which you need a drug (orthodox HRT) – it's not. The menopause is part of the normal cycle of a woman's hormonal life when the menstrual cycles cease and it is a time of great potential.

The menopause generally occurs between the ages of 45 and 55, although it can occur as early as 35 or as late as 65 years of age. Chemotherapy and excess exposure to hormone-altering chemicals, such as pesticides and herbicides, can also trigger an early menopause.

Dr Marilyn Glenville, a UK-based expert on the menopause, says: 'At the time of menopause, a woman still produces oestrogen but not sufficient to prepare her womb for pregnancy. Levels of progesterone plummet or disappear completely. The ovaries continue to produce small quantities of oestrogen for at least 12 years after the onset of the menopause.'

For most women, the menopause happens in three phases. First comes peri-menopause, when you still have periods, but they may become heavier or lighter, and symptoms such as hot flushes can appear. Then comes the menopause, when ovarian function declines and periods stop. The last phase is called post-menopause, which begins 12 months after your last period.

Throughout this time, many signs associated with ageing can appear, as the hormonal balance alters with the drop in oestrogen and progesterone levels. Skin is more likely to wrinkle, there can be an increased growth of facial hair, and a thinning of hair in the temple region. Muscles lose some strength and tone, and many women suffer hot flushes and insomnia. Your joints may begin to ache and bones can become more brittle, increasing the risk of osteoporosis. Vaginal dryness often results from these hormonal changes. The vaginal wall also becomes thinner and blood flow is restricted. Dryness can make sexual intercourse painful or uncomfortable and can lead to irritation and increased risk of infection. You will be happy to note that regular sexual intercourse increases blood flow into the vagina.

Loss of bladder tone, which can result in stress incontinence (leaking urine when you cough, sneeze, laugh or exercise), can also result (see *Incontinence*). Orthodox chemical-based HRT has now been linked to an increase in urinary incontinence, and studies have shown that conditions such as Alzheimer's and memory loss may also be speeded up by orthodox HRT.

You may also experience a whole host of emotional ups and downs – one minute feeling on top of the world and the next in the pits of despair. The good news is that by eating the right diet and taking the right supplements, and through exercise and using natural hormone replacements, virtually all the symptoms of the menopause can be avoided or alleviated.

I do not advocate taking orthodox HRT because of the increased risk of high blood pressure, blood clots, weight gain, and gall-bladder and liver problems, not to mention breast and endometrial (uterine) cancers. The increased health risks of orthodox HRT have now been shown to far outweigh the benefits. Yes, it slows the rate of bone loss, but only while you are taking it. Also, if you are under a lot of stress at this time, adrenal function is greatly affected. And if you are stressed, then your adrenal glands are kept busy pumping out the stress hormone cortisol, and the endocrine system is then disrupted, which means that oestrogen levels from the ovaries can fluctuate.

I had a hysterectomy at the age of 31 and at that time no one warned me that I might need more oestrogen to protect my bones. If you keep your ovaries after surgery, you will produce some oestrogen for a time, but often not enough to prevent osteoporosis, which crippled my mother. I have always taken bone supplements, but these alone could never make up for the years of insufficient oestrogen – which is why I now have osteoporosis. Therefore, if you have an early menopause, which is becoming more common thanks to our stressful and toxic environment – or, you have a hysterectomy (even if you keep your ovaries), **please** make sure that your hormone levels are checked every year.... otherwise you could end up like me!

Also, on the subject of oestrogen, few women are aware of the condition known as oestrogen dominance This is when the amount of oestrogen in the body is not balanced by the proper amount of progesterone. This can occur from failed ovulations or from over-exposure to environmental chemicals found in herbicides, pesticides and plastics, called 'xenoestrogens', which have an oestrogen-like 'building' effect within the body. These chemicals accumulate in our fatty tissue and greatly increase the risk for hormonal cancers.

When you have too much oestrogen activity compared to progesterone, you can suffer symptoms such as water retention, bloating, and menstrual irregularities. Globally we are living in a dangerous ocean of hormone-disrupting chemicals, which are triggering lowered sperm counts and causing animals and fish to change sex – and we, too, are now seeing sexual mutations.

One problem with conventional HRT is that it does not contain natural progesterone, but synthetic hormone-like substances called progestins (or progestogen) – essentially, these are artificial hormones. These have side effects such as irritability, liver dysfunction, vaginal bleeding, blood clots and so on, and they reverse the positive effects of oestrogens on the heart. Conventional HRT also uses much higher levels of oestrogen than bio-identical HRT. For this reason, I prefer to use natural HRT – see below for details.

If you have had a partial hysterectomy (that is, your ovaries are remaining) before menopause, you will still have hormonal changes similar to the normal menstrual cycle. If you need supplemental hormones and are told that you need only oestrogen because you do not have a uterus, you should also take a bio-identical (natural) progesterone with any oestrogen supplementation. If you have had a total hysterectomy and need HRT, use the lowest dose of oestrogen possible for you, and always use bio-identical (natural) progesterone with it.

Some women go through early menopause, which can happen for many reasons, ranging from oestrogen-like chemicals in the environment to smoking, drinking heavily or being severely malnourished. Whatever the cause, it is very important to make sure that the bones remain healthy. So it is important to have a bone scan periodically and a urine –

M

deoxypyridinoline – test to measure bone breakdown. If bone loss is occurring then you need to take the appropriate measures (see *Osteoporosis*).

Also, nutritional scientist and naturopath Robert Jacobs at the Society for Complementary medicine in London says: 'Many women younger than 50 may not yet have gone through their menopause and therefore may still have high levels of oestrogen in their blood that is thought to be heart protective. After menopause, oestrogen levels drop and can thus contribute to an increased risk for heart disease – which is why balancing one's hormones is really important after the menopause, as well as living a healthy lifestyle.'

Foods to Avoid

- Make the effort to cut down on 'white' foods – cakes, biscuits, breads, pastries – plus pre-packaged refined foods, full-fat dairy from animal sources and fatty meats. Although dairy foods from animals contain calcium, they are also proteins that have often been exposed to hormones and pesticides.
- Avoid chemicals that mimic oestrogens (xenoestrogens) found in pesticides or herbicides by eating more organic foods.
- Minimize your exposure to foods stored in plastic containers and never heat or microwave food in plastic containers – the containers will leach xenoestrogens into your food.
- Cut down on caffeine, fizzy cola-type drinks, refined sugar and chocolate, and avoid drinking too much alcohol, which all act as stimulants and trigger blood sugar problems. Caffeine and/or alcohol can trigger a hot flush on their own. See under *Low Blood Sugar*.

Friendly Foods

- Increase your intake of fresh, locally grown and preferably organic fruits and vegetables.
- Fermented soya-based foods are truly one of the best foods for managing the symptoms associated with the menopause. Soya contains isoflavones (phyto-oestrogens), which have oestrogen-like effects on the body and block the harmful effects of oestrogens and xenoestrogens. But there has been much misinformation written about about soya, and Dr Glenville says: 'Soya foods in their traditional forms of miso, soya sauce and tempeh (a fermented form of soya) and natto are all rich in isoflavones, which have been proven to reduce the risk of developing cancers. But they are best eaten cooked.'
- Isoflavones are also found in chickpeas, soya beans, lentils, alfalfa, fennel, kidney beans, and sunflower, pumpkin, hemp and sesame seeds, Brazil nuts, walnuts and linseeds (flax seeds). All seeds and their unrefined oils are rich in essential fatty acids, which also help to reduce joint pain and risk of heart disease, and help to lubricate the vagina (see *Fats You Need To Eat*). For a great breakfast smoothie recipe, see under *General Health Hints*.
- Brazil nuts and sesame seeds are good sources of calcium.
- Foods from the brassica vegetable family help to protect against oestrogen-sensitive cancers (including breast cancer and cancer of the cervix), balance hormones, and can greatly alleviate menopausal symptoms. These include cabbage, watercress, broccoli, pak choy, Brussels sprouts, cauliflower, kale, mustard, rutabaga and turnips.
- Live, low-fat yoghurt increases healthy bacteria in the gut, which aids absorption of nutrients from your diet.
- Vitamin B12 has been shown to reduce the irritability, bloating and headaches associated with the menopause and is found in oily fish, eggs and lean meats.
- Potassium and pantothenic acid (vitamin B5) help support adrenal function – they are found in whole grains such as brown rice, amaranth, buckwheat, kelp, raisins, wheat germ, barley and quinoa, as well as salmon, peanuts, mushrooms, sweet potatoes, tomatoes, broccoli, cauliflower, avocados, dried apricots, banana, cantaloupe melon, oranges and fish.

- Use dried seaweeds, such as kombu, in your cooking (particularly in stir-fries), as seaweed is rich in iodine (which supports the thyroid) and calcium (see also *Thyroid*). Try nori seaweed flakes or kelp flakes instead of salt – available from health shops.
- Eat organic foods, including lean meat, chicken, vegetables and fruits, to avoid ingesting too many toxins from herbicides and pesticides.
- Folic acid, found in wheat germ, eggs, leafy greens, calves' and chicken liver, dried yeast and beetroot, is very important during the menopause to protect the bones.
- Include garlic, onions and leeks in your diet, which help to keep cholesterol levels in check.
- Sprinkle lecithin granules over cereals and into smoothies to nourish your brain and lower LDL cholesterol.
- Drink more spring water, which helps to regulate body temperature.
- Avoid very hot drinks and hot spicy foods.
- If you have trouble sleeping, try valerian and passionflower teas (and see under *Insomnia* for some great natural sleep aids).
- Drink more organic de-caffeinated green teas, which contain L-theanine – an amino acid that helps increase alpha wave activity in the brain, helping to induce feelings of calmness – or take L-theanine capsules. **NC, HN, SVHC**
- Try organic almond, oat, rice and quinoa milks as non-dairy alternatives to animal-based dairy products.

Useful Remedies

- As cruciferous vegetables help to regulate oestrogen in the body and help the liver to remove potentially harmful by-products of excess oestrogens, take one Triple Action Cruciferous Vegetable Extract daily. Available rom the Life Extension Foundation on www.lef.org or contact the Nutri Centre. **NC**
- Try the Menopause Programme, which includes herbs such as blessed thistle, squaw vine, Siberian ginseng, cramp bark and raspberry leaf, which all help to cleanse the reproductive organs and balance hormones. **SHS**
- If you dislike soya foods, then take a soya isoflavone capsule daily. Try Superpotency Soyagen. **HN**
- Take a woman's multi-vitamin and mineral such as BioCare's FemGuard or Lambert's Gynovite. Dr Glenville also has her own formula especially for before and after the menopause. For details call The Natural Health Practice on 01892 515905. Any women's multi that you choose should contain boron, vitamin K, selenium, folic acid, vitamin D, vitamin E, calcium and magnesium to support you through the menopause.
- Vitamin B-complex will help to relieve stress, depression and mood disorders, and is needed for energy production. (This should be included in your multi.)
- A remedy extracted from a Peruvian root vegetable called maca has been used for centuries to help alleviate hormonal-type symptoms. Research shows that maca helps to stimulate the pituitary gland into producing hormone precursors, which eventually raises oestrogen and progesterone levels naturally, as well as balancing the adrenal glands, the thyroid and the pancreas. Taken regularly, this root has been shown to reduce the hot flushes and symptoms associated with menopause. **NC**
- Full-spectrum, natural-source vitamin E – 400iu per day – can help to reduce hot flushes.
- Take an EFA formula containing omega-3 and -6 oils; take at least 1 gram daily. See *Fats You Need To Eat*.
- Vitamin K2 x 100mcg per day can reduce the heavy menstrual bleeding that is common in the peri-menopausal years. It is also needed to keep calcium in the bones and out of the arteries. **NB Avoid K2 if you are on blood-thinning drugs.**

- Black cohosh can relieve hot flushes and other menopausal symptoms after 4 weeks of use. Other herbs for reducing menopausal symptoms include agnus castus, hops, liquorice root, dong quai and wild yam. These herbs can be taken individually or in combination formulas. Dr Glenville provides an excellent organic formula that contains all these herbs. One teaspoonful can be taken twice daily. Call 0845 8800915 for details or log on to www.marilynglenville.com.
- As sleep can be a problem for many women, try a natural-source melatonin supplement each night before bed. It really helps. For details of Asphalia, see under *Insomnia*.
- Omega-7 fats from sea buckthorn have been found highly effective for supporting mucosal membranes; take daily to reduce a dry vagina. **PN**
- **See also details of the bio-identical hormones progesterone and oestrogen plus DHEA, below.**

Helpful Hints
- If your doctor suggests that you use orthodox pessaries for a dry vagina, then avoid ones containing oestradiol, which is a stronger oestrogen and can increase the risk factors for hormone-related cancers. Ask for oestriol-based creams and pessaries, which are a weaker form of oestrogen.
- If you are suffering heavy bleeding, you must have this checked by your doctor or gynaecologist.
- Regular weight-bearing exercise not only helps raise levels of DHEA, a vital anti-ageing hormone (see below), but also reduces stress, which makes symptoms and hormone imbalances worse. Also in mid-life our waistlines tend to expand. Exercise keeps you trim and increases bone density. It also makes you feel more positive and cheerful about life, and women who exercise regularly tend to suffer fewer hot flushes.
- Use relaxation techniques, such as meditation or yoga.
- Add essential oils of geranium, chamomile and jasmine to your bath to aid relaxation.
- If you suffer from night sweats, wear loose-fitting cotton nightwear and have a change of nightwear ready. Use cotton blankets and keep the room cool.
- Homeopathic Sepia 30c x 1 taken daily for a week helps to reduce hot flushes.
- To further help prevent vaginal dryness and painful intercourse, avoid using deodorant soaps or scented products in the vaginal area.
- Dr Glenville recommends a vaginal lubricant called Yes, which contains aloe vera. It is available on online from www.naturalhealthpractice.com. Or try a soya pessary from Arkopharma, which can be inserted to help lubrication. There are many creams containing wild yam available in health food stores, which can be used topically as a vaginal lubricant. Contact The Perfect Woman range for wild Mexican yam via their website at www.natural-woman.com.
- Read *Natural Alternatives to HRT* and *Healthy Eating for the Menopause*, both by Dr Marilyn Glenville (Kyle Cathie), available from www.naturalhealthpractice.com.
- Marilyn's website (www.marilynglenville.com) is packed with useful information; or to visit her practice, call 08705 329 244 for further details. You can also email the practice on health@marilynglenville.com.
- If you require further information on natural progesterone and a list of doctors who use it, send £1 in stamps plus a large SAE to The Natural Progesterone Information Service (NPIS), PO Box 24, Buxton SK17 9FB. Tel: 07000 784849. Website: www.npis.info/contactus.htm.

Hormones associated with the menopause

Don't use hormones in any form unless blood/and/or saliva tests show that you need them. If you have no hormonal-type symptoms and good bone density, there should be no need for extra hormones.

- **Progesterone** Natural (bio-identical) progesterone is made from an extract of wild yams and then converted to the bio-identical hormone progesterone that you made in your body prior to the menopause – which is often needed to balance excess oestrogen activity that is linked to hormonal cancers. Natural progesterone can greatly reduce or alleviate many of the side effects associated with the menopause. The natural progesterone most often comes as a cream that you rub on the skin; Pharm West's is called Pro Body Cream. **PW**

  Many women believe that if they have gone through the menopause they need only oestrogen and not progesterone, but Robert Jacobs says: 'The latest breakthroughs have shown that progesterone and oestrogen need to be balanced in the body, and oestrogen alone, unopposed by progesterone, increases the risk for hormonal-type cancers.'

- **Natural oestrogens** are synthesized from soya beans and are identical to the oestrogen that you make in your body. If you have mood swings, depression, bone thinning or insomnia you may, as well as the natural progesterone, also need natural oestrogens. Many companies now make these in a duo formula. PharmWest make a duo formula called Phyto-Oestrogen. Call 001 310 301 4015 between 6 and 8pm, Monday–Fridays. **PN**

  These creams can be applied to the inner arms or thighs, to the stomach, breasts or face. Regularly change the areas on which you apply the cream, otherwise tissues can become saturated, thus affecting absorption.

- **Cortisol** You can find out more about this stress-related hormone and how it affects the menopause and hugely contributes to osteoporosis under *Adrenal Exhaustion* and *Osteoporosis*.

- **DHEA** Around the time of menopause, women often undergo rapid age-transformation and, while most doctors suggest some kind of HRT, very few prescribe DHEA. DHEA helps reverse many of the unfavourable effects of excess cortisol. If your DHEA levels are low, you are likely to feel permanently tired all the time, have 'brain fog' and PMT-type symptoms, and your skin will age faster. Lack of DHEA can also be a factor in some autoimmune conditions, such as lupus.

  This hormone is produced by the adrenal glands and is the most abundant steroid hormone in the body. It is made from cholesterol and can be converted into oestrogen or testosterone. By the age of 65, we make only 10–20% of the amount of DHEA we made at 20. One 20-year study found that DHEA levels were far lower in men who died of heart disease than in healthier men. Low levels of DHEA have also been found in Alzheimer's patients. In fact, there is now little doubt that DHEA may help prevent the ravages of brain-ageing. It protects against Alzheimer's and dementia and increases a sense of wellbeing, which scientists have identified as being due to increased levels of endorphins (the chemicals we make naturally when we are happy and during exercise). Tests have also shown that DHEA can help prevent some cancers, heart disease, and bone and skin degeneration. It helps maintain brain function and gives powerful support to the immune system. In addition, it helps protect against infections, autoimmune disorders, obesity, diabetes and stress.

  DHEA has also been shown in numerous studies to improve mood and energy levels in both men and women, and is therefore a valid treatment for depression and long-term negative stress. This effect was found to be particularly noticeable for post-menopausal women. One German study showed that DHEA considerably increased the libido and sexual satisfaction in the women taking part.

DHEA is easy to supplement in tablet or liquid form and serum levels can be controlled with ease. But, as always, before you begin taking hormones, have a blood, saliva or urine test and find out if your hormone levels are depleted. In women, anything more than modest dosages may trigger increased facial hair growth, spots or in some cases greasy skin.

NB Because DHEA can be metabolized into testosterone and oestrogen, DHEA use should be avoided by anyone who currently has prostate cancer or breast cancer. Also do not take this hormone if you are pregnant, nursing, or have prior ovarian, adrenal or thyroid tumours. Women should avoid DHEA just prior to menopause, because their levels typically increase around that time anyway.

Where to buy DHEA

DHEA is not available over the counter in health stores in the UK, although it is freely available in the US via companies such as the Life Extension Foundation via: www.lef.org.

Numerous nutritional physicians, health professionals and doctors work with DHEA and other natural hormones. I can only offer a few such contacts, such as:

- Dr Shamin Daya at the Wholistic Medical Centre, 57 Harley Street, London. Tel: 020 7580 7537. Website: www.wholsticmedicalcentre.co.uk. **WMC**
- HB Health of Harley Street in London; for details, call Maria Somers on 07973 173478.
- You can purchase it for your own use from Pharm West.
- Dr Marilyn Glenville's practice – to visit, call 08705 329 244 or log on to the website at www.marilynglenville.com.

For more information, read *DHEA – Unlocking the Secrets to the Fountain of Youth* by Ley and Ash (BL Publications). To order from The Nutri Centre Bookshop, log on to www.nutricentre.com or email bookshop@nutricentre.com.

- **Testosterone** If levels of this hormone are low, extra testosterone may be prescribed for men to restore libido and endurance; in women, small amounts may also be required – not only to help restore libido but also for healthy bones. Women who tend to suffer very dry eyes after the menopause often need small amounts of this hormone. Again it is available in creams – but you should only use testosterone creams under the guidance of your health professional or GP.

MERCURY FILLINGS

There is now a huge body of evidence to show that mercury fillings are detrimental to health. Mercury is one of the most toxic substances known to man and is an accumulative poison. Originally, it was thought that the mercury vapour could not escape as it was locked into solid metal fillings, but we now know this is not the case. Mercury vapour is now proven to pass through the blood–brain barrier; it deposits in the brain, affecting structure and function. The British Dental Association state that about 3% of the population are estimated to suffer from mercury sensitivity (when the same ratio of people have, say, flu, this is considered to have reached epidemic proportions) – that is, around 2 million people. Yet amalgam fillings are still widely used in the UK and the US.

There is now good evidence from research at the University of Calgary in Canada showing that mercury causes brain cell degeneration. This research and many more facts on mercury are available via www.iaomt.org – The International Academy of Oral Medicine and

Toxicology. Over 14,000 papers have been published suggesting that mercury is toxic and should not be used in fillings.

Even the UK Department of Health advises all dentists not to remove or replace amalgam fillings in pregnant women. Now why do you think that is, if mercury fillings are not dangerous? Dr Jack Levenson, a dental surgeon who has passed away, spent almost 20 years investigating the effects of the potential dangers of dental amalgam, and told me a few years ago: 'Eighty percent of the mercury vapour that we inhale from mercury filling enters our blood stream and there is a strong body of research linking mercury toxicity to heart disease, Alzheimer's, Parkinson's, multiple sclerosis, motor neurone disease, thyroid problems, migraines, chronic fatigue, digestive disorders, infertility in men and women, antibiotic resistance, joint and muscle pain, impaired immune function, autoimmune diseases, hair loss and excessive hair growth, visual disturbances, numbness, tingling and tremors.'

Are you nervous? When Jack tested my teeth, two of my amalgam fillings were 10 times over the supposed safe limit of mercury emissions. I had them removed on the spot. It would seem that the government continues to refuse NHS patients safer, composite white fillings in order to save millions of pounds. If they were to admit that amalgam has poisoned millions of people, the litigation bill would be huge and health insurance companies would then be forced to pay for the fillings' removal and replacement. Money, not health, it seems is the bottom line here.

Mercury fillings are banned in Japan, Norway and Sweden and are not allowed in women and children in Austria and Germany. The US is considering a ban on amalgam fillings.

Many people suffering mercury toxicity have been found to have candida as well – see under *Candida*.

M

Foods to Avoid
- If you have mercury fillings, avoid Spanish- or Gulf-sourced mackerel, marlin, shark, swordfish, Chilean sea bass, tuna and swordfish, which often contain high quantities of mercury. (Around 20 tons of mercury plus lead, cadmium and copper is dumped into the North Sea alone, from industry every year.)
- As this list is large and is subject to change, for the most up-to-date list of which fish are high, medium or low risk of mercury, log on to the natural Resources Defense Council on www.nrdc.org.

Friendly Foods
- Generally eat more organic vegetables, fruits and grains, as mass-produced fruits, grains and vegetables are often treated with a mercury-based fungicide.
- Coriander and chlorella detoxify mercury from the body.
- Generally drink more pure filtered water.
- Currently (2010) low levels of mercury are in anchovies, catfish, clams, domestic crab, crayfish, Atlantic haddock, hake, North Atlantic mackerel, plaice, pollock, fresh salmon, sardines, scallops, tilapia, freshwater trout and whiting.

Useful Remedies
- If you have mercury fillings, take a good-quality multi-vitamin and mineral to help support your immune system.
- You need a full spectrum of B vitamins (these should be in your multi).
- Mercury depletes the mineral selenium, which is known to reduce the incidence of cancer and heart disease. Take between 100 and 200mcg of selenium daily.
- Vitamin E increases the effectiveness of the selenium – take 200iu of full-spectrum, natural-source vitamin E daily.

- Lipoic acid, an important antioxidant, helps eliminate mercury from the body. Take 200mg daily.
- Vitamin C – take 2 grams daily with food in divided doses.
- N-acetyl cysteine (NAC), an amino acid, really helps to detoxify the liver. Take 500mg twice daily, 30 minutes before food.
- Pure Encapsulations make a HM Chelate Formula, containing Vitamin C, chlorella, zinc, selenium, lipoic acid, NAC and pectin. Take 3–6 daily away from food for optimum results.
- Take any organic-based chlorella green food powder daily, such as Green Magic Powder – containing Hawaiian spirulina, chlorella, lecithin, barley and wheat grass, kamut, pectin apple fibre, kelp and wheat sprouts, CoQ10, royal jelly, artichoke powder and lactobacillus acidophilus, it is a great all-round way to ingest good nutrients, healthy bacteria, keep the body more alkaline and help keep you regular. And the more regular you are, the less toxins such as mercury you will store in your body. Details on www.itsgreenmagic.com or call Helen Cruikshank on 07798 873266.

Helpful Hints
- Many vaccines use mercury as a preservative.
- To find a list of dentists in the UK who specialize in safe removal of amalgam fillings, visit www.mercuryfreedentistry.org.uk, or write to The British Society for Mercury-Free Dentistry, The Weathervane, 22a Moorend Park Road, Cheltenham GL53 0JY. Or call their helpline on 01242 226918.
- Contact IAOMT – The International Academy of Oral Medicine and Toxicology – at 30 Bournemouth Road, Lower Park Stone, Poole BH14 OES. Tel: 01202 741622. Visit their website to view the latest research on mercury: www.iaomt.org. The Academy gives lots of information on mercury fillings and holistic dentistry.
- For a list of mercury-free dentists in your area, you can also contact Patients Against Mercury Amalgam on www.pamshelpline.com.
- www.melisa.org also carry the latest research into links between mercury and Parkinson's and mercury and multiple sclerosis.
- The Henry Spink Foundation at www.henryspink.org contains great fact sheets about mercury.
- Read *Toxic Bite* by Bill Kellner-Read (Credence) or *The Toxic Time Bomb* by Sam Ziff (Aurora).

MIGRAINE   (see also Allergies, Leaky Gut, Liver Problems and Low Blood Sugar)

One in every 10 people in the UK suffers regular migraines, but twice as many women are affected as men. However, as many as 60% never consult their doctor as to what might be causing their migraines. Sufferers on average experience around thirteen attacks annually and over 10% of school children suffer migraines that occur equally in both sexes up until the age of 12.

In Britain alone, the cost of migraines is more than £1 billion a year, which is why prevention is always preferable to cure. Migraines usually occur on one side, at the back or front of the head, and an attack can be precipitated by flashing lights or partial blindness. Some people suffer tingling sensations, sensitivity to light or noise, vomiting, and so on. Some people are debilitated for a few hours, others several days, and in addition an attack can often be accompanied by nausea and vomiting.

Migraines are in many cases linked to intolerances to foods such as wheat or cow's milk, internal toxicity and sometimes to the menstrual cycle. 'In fact,' says nutritionist Gareth Zeal, 'as many as 90% of migraine cases I see are linked to food intolerance.' In addition, 40% of migraine patients also have the bacterium *Helicobacter pylori* – see *Stomach Ulcers*. Migraines can also be a sign of liver congestion, so you really need to cut down on alcohol, caffeine and fats – and keep your diet clean. (See also *Leaky Gut*, *Constipation*, *Liver Problems* and *Low Blood Sugar*.)

Weather changes, negative stress and lack of sleep can also trigger migraines.

Foods to Avoid
- The foods most commonly known to trigger an attack are cheese, animal-based dairy produce, red wine, peanuts, chocolate of any type and colour, corn, coffee, wheat and citrus fruits and juices.
- Avoid refined sugars, which are found in most kinds of cakes, biscuits, pastries, snacks and fizzy drinks.
- Avoid food additives, colourings, preservatives, alcohol and caffeine, as much as possible.
- Avoid hard margarines, shortenings, and any foods containing hydrogenated fats and oils.
- Cut down on red meat, full-fat dairy produce and eggs if you know that you have an intolerance (see below). People who eat a diet low in saturated fats tend to suffer fewer migraines.
- If you are constipated on a regular basis, certain bacteria in the bowel can convert tyrosine (high in peanuts) to tyramine, which again is thought to be a trigger. Cheese is also high in tyramine.

Friendly Foods
- Eat more fresh pineapple and papaya, which aid digestion.
- Include more turmeric (curcumin) in your diet, as it has great anti-inflammatory properties. You can also take this in capsule form.
- Eat more linseeds (flax seeds can be soaked in cold water overnight/drained and eaten). Sunflower, pumpkin, hemp and sesame seeds all help to keep your bowels regular. Sprinkle them over a low-sugar breakfast cereal, or use in yoghurts, as a snack, in smoothies and in salads.
- Drink at least 6–8 glasses of water daily. Dehydration can trigger a migraine, especially in the summer.
- Eat more healthy grains, brown rice, quinoa, buckwheat, lentils and barley, and try amaranth, oat and rice crackers as a change from wheat.
- Try Genius or Village Bakery wheat-free breads.
- Eat plenty of fruits and vegetables, preferably organic.
- Make sure you eat quality protein, such as fresh chicken or cooked tofu, once a day.
- Otherwise use organic hemp seed protein in smoothies. Recipe under *General Health Hints*.
- Use unrefined walnut, sesame, avocado, sunflower and olive oils in salad dressings.
- Live, low-fat, non-dairy-based yoghurt contains healthy bacteria, which aid digestion and keep the bowel healthy.
- Oily fish is rich in omega-3 fats, which naturally thin the blood and reduce the severity of migraines. Eat more organic-farmed salmon, sardines, pilchards, anchovies, mackerel or black cod.
- Drink vervain tea to help reduce head pain, and add the essential oil to your bath.

Useful Remedies
- The mineral magnesium is often at low levels in migraine sufferers, as magnesium helps relax blood vessels so that oxygen and nutrients can get to the brain. Taking magnesium citrate, 600mg in divided doses throughout the day, should help; take the final 200mg just before bed.

- Ginkgo biloba helps to prevent the blood vessels constricting. Take 120mg of standardized extract daily.
- As all the B-vitamins are vital for preventing headaches, particularly folic acid, B2, and B6, take a high-strength B-complex daily.
- Include 1 gram of vitamin C with bioflavonoids daily. **BC**
- As digestive problems are heavily associated with migraines, take a digestive enzyme with main meals.
- If you crave sweet foods, take 200mcg of the mineral chromium for at least 1 month to reduce food cravings – see under *Low Blood Sugar*.
- Omega-3 fatty acids (fish oils) – 500mg taken twice daily – should help relieve migraine headaches.
- Migraine Relief Formula contains vitamin B6, magnesium citrate, willow bark (a natural painkiller), plus ginger and feverfew – a herbal anti-inflammatory with natural calming effects. Take 2 tablets daily. **NC**
- The herb butterbur has been shown to help reduce the duration of migraines. Take 500mg twice daily during an attack. You can also use it as a preventative.
- Co-enzyme Q10 helps to encourage energy production and has been shown in trials to help lower incidence of migraines. Take 100mg daily.
- Several studies have shown that taking small doses of melatonin, the hormone produced in the pineal gland in the brain to induce sleep, can help reduce incidents of migraine attacks and also can help treat an existing migraine. Bio-electromagnetic research scientist Roger Coghill says: 'If you take melatonin supplements that you can buy on line and in the States, most synthetic tablets contain thousands of times the natural dose that your pineal gland normally produces at night.' Roger has developed a supplement called Asphalia, containing natural melatonin extracted from certain grasses that mimics the normal dose made by your pineal gland to induce sleep at night, rather than the larger doses that are found in mass-produced tablets. Roger has permission from the MHRA (Medical Healthcare Regulatory Authority) to sell this food supplement in the UK. For more details or to find your nearest supplier, log on to www.asphalia.co.uk or call 01495 752122. Take 1 to 2 capsules 30 minutes before bed.

Helpful Hints

- Low blood sugar can trigger an attack, so eat healthy meals regularly – see under *Low Blood Sugar*.
- Migraine is often triggered by food intolerances, especially to wheat and cow's milk, liver congestion or hormonal problems, so keep a food diary to see if you can identify foods that trigger an attack.
- Have a food intolerance test to check which foods/substances are your specific triggers. Try the York Test Laboratories. Tel: 0800 458 2052 or log on to www.yorktest.com; or Genova Diagnostics do a FACT test that looks for inflammatory markers indicating that the body is reacting to certain substances. Tel: 020 8336 7750. Website: www.gdx.uk.net.
- Regular aerobic exercise has been shown to reduce migraine attacks and yoga helps to reduce stress levels.
- Taken regularly, rosemary or fresh ginger tea can help to bring relief from some of the symptoms.
- Grinding the teeth over many years often causes the jaw to slip out of alignment. This causes blood flow to the head to be restricted, triggering regular headaches and/or migraines. Problems with vertebrae in the neck can also disrupt blood flow to the brain. See a chiropractor or a cranial osteopath, who can re-align the neck and head (see *Useful Information*).

- Alternate warm and cold packs. Use for 10 minutes each on the back of neck to help to increase blood flow to the head.
- Contact The Migraine Trust Helpline. Tel: 020 7631 6970. Website: www.migrainetrust.org.
- Further information can be obtained from the Migraine Action Association. Tel: 0116 275 8317. Website: www.migraine.org.uk.

MOUTH PROBLEMS *(see also Bad Breath)*

Burning mouth syndrome

(see also Candida, Leaky Gut, Liver Problems and Low Stomach Acid)

This is most common in women, especially after the menopause, and may be triggered by decreased hormone production, nerve damage, stress, or sensitivity to certain foods. It may also be linked to digestive problems. In rare cases it can be due to a lack of vitamin B12 and folic acid. Symptoms can include a swollen tongue, metallic taste, soreness and a dry mouth and tongue, even when the tongue looks normal. It can also be triggered by low stomach acid (see *Low Stomach Acid*). If you have a cold or flu, symptoms are usually worse. This condition also denotes that your liver is under stress – see under *Liver Problems*. Excessive talking can exacerbate the problem. Conditions such as a leaky gut and candida can also trigger burning mouth syndrome, as can a lack of zinc and essential fats.

Foods to Avoid
- Burning mouth syndrome is usually made worse by highly spiced or acidic foods, such as vinegar, oranges or pineapple.
- Avoid too much alcohol, black tea and coffee, which are all acid forming in the body.
- Red meat, cheese and chocolate are especially acid forming, and could make symptoms worse.

Friendly Foods
- Keep your diet clean (see *General Health Hints*) and drink plenty of water.
- Eat more organic nuts, seeds and fish, which are high in zinc.
- Cereals, oats, alfalfa, eggs, liver, brown rice, skimmed milk and fish are all rich in B-vitamins.

Useful Remedies
- A swollen tongue can be a sign of iron deficiency, so have a blood test.
- A dry mouth is a specific sign of potassium phosphate deficiency – take 75 mg of the celloid complex daily. **BLK**
- Take vitamin C – 1 gram per day to prevent deficiency.
- Take vitamin B6 – 30mg per day.
- Take vitamin B12 – 800mcg sublingual tablet daily to prevent deficiency.
- Take folic acid – 400mcg per day.
- As all the B-vitamins work together, take the B6, B12 and folic acid in a B-complex daily.
- Take 30mg zinc per day – as lack of zinc is linked to this problem. As zinc depletes copper, make sure your zinc supplement contains about 1–2mg of copper.
- GLA is an essential fat found in evening primrose oil – take 250mg of GLA per day to prevent deficiency. **BC**
- Sea buckthorn is an omega-7 fatty acid that helps supports soft tissue, therefore take 4 capsules daily for one month and then 2 daily for maintenance. **PN**
- Bromelain extracted from pineapples will help reduce the inflammation. Take 250mg twice daily with food.

Helpful Hints
- Mouth problems are often a reflection of problems in the gut and digestive system. See a nutritionist who can re-balance your diet and suggest supplements to boost your immune system (see *Useful Information*).
- Suck ice cubes if the pain is severe.
- This problem is exacerbated by stress, so learn to meditate, and practise some form of relaxation.
- Sodium lauryl sulphate (SLS) thins the lining of the mouth, so use an SLS-free toothpaste such as those made by Jason, Green People or Waleda.
- As nitrates and other chemicals found in drinking water are known to make symptoms worse, install a water filter. Contact The Pure H2O Company on 01784 221188. Email: roger@pureh2o.co.uk. Website: www.pureh2o.co.uk.
- As an over-acid system may be triggering this condition, you may want to consider using Kangen Water – a water system unit that attaches to your kitchen tap and ionizes and greatly alkalizes water. It's used in Japanese hospitals and has been found to have highly beneficial health results. For full details on Kangen Water, call 020 7580 7537 or log on to www.kangenmiraclewater.co.uk.

Cracked lips

Lips that are sore and cracked, especially at the corners of the mouth, are usually a sign of a deficiency of B-vitamins, especially vitamin B2, which is found in milk, eggs, liver, green vegetables and most other fresh vegetables. B vitamins are also found in wholegrain rice, quinoa, buckwheat.

The problem is also linked to lack of natural-source vitamin E and essential fats found in wheat germ, avocados, oily fish, seeds and their unrefined oils.

Dehydration is also a major cause.

Very rarely, cracked lips can be a sign of vitamin-A toxicity. You would need to have taken thousands of units of vitamin A for over a month for this to happen, but nevertheless, if you have been taking extremely high doses of vitamin A, have a blood test.

Generally, eat more foods high in natural carotenes such as pumpkin, carrots, papaya, apricots and watercress.

Useful Remedies
- Take a high-strength vitamin B-complex.
- Take a multi-vitamin and mineral that contains at least 30mg of zinc, 1–2mg of copper, 200iu of full-spectrum vitamin E and 500mg of vitamin C.
- Rub pure vitamin E cream onto your lips at night.
- For 2 weeks, only take 30,000 iu of vitamin A and then switch to natural-source beta-carotenes, which naturally convert to vitamin A in the body and are non toxic. **SVHC, VN, HN**

Helpful Hints
- Use a lip balm made from vitamin E and aloe vera.
- Take homeopathic Nat Mur 6x twice daily for 3–4 days.

Dry Mouth

(see also under Sjogren's Syndrome)

If you have ever been extremely nervous, then you will have noticed that your mouth automatically goes dry. This is because saliva, which contains enzymes for digestion, is not required when we are under extreme stress. In contrast, if you are really hungry and see tempting food, you automatically produce more saliva.

You may simply be thirsty, but if the dry mouth is chronic, you may have digestive problems such as a leaky gut. Also, one of the classic symptoms of the autoimmune condition Sjogren's syndrome is an extremely dry mouth (and eyes). A consistently dry mouth can also denote a potassium phosphate deficiency.

Foods to avoid.
- Flour and dense grain-based foods tend to draw water from the body into faeces in the bowel and make you feel more thirsty. Therefore, keep breads, cereals, biscuits, cakes and 'drying' foods to sensible levels.

Friendly Foods.
- Fresh fruits are packed with easy-to-absorb minerals, which you may be lacking. Eat more melon, especially watermelon.
- Drink plenty of water.
- Essential fats found in nuts, seeds, oily fish and their unrefined oils help to nourish a dehydrated system.

Useful Remedies.

- Omega-7 fats, extracted from the sea buckthorn, really help to support soft tissue in the mouth – take 2 capsules daily for the long term. **PN**
- Take at least 1 gram of omega-3 fish oils daily.
- Include a multi-vitamin and mineral in your regimen.
- A dry mouth can denote a potassium phosphate deficiency – take 75 mg daily. **BLK**
- Xerostom products, based on olive oil, vitamin E, xylitol (to help protect the teeth) and betaine, all help to soothe and moisturize the mouth. They include mouth gels, toothpastes, capsules and chewing gum. For stockists, call Curaprox UK Ltd on 01480 862084 or visit www.curaprox.co.uk.
- Begin taking liquid hyaluronic acid (HA) daily in water. HA is a naturally occurring protein in the body that helps the body to hold more water. HA is what makes young skin look plump and supple. Unfortunately, as we age levels of HA in the body decline, resulting in dry skin and joint problems. Take 1ml daily in water on an empty stomach to help re-hydrate the body. For more details ask at your health store or call Modern Herbals on 01274 889047. Website: www.modernherbals.com.

Helpful Hints
- You need to be careful about dental hygiene, as the less saliva you make, the more likely you are to suffer plaque and various dental problems. Clean your teeth regularly and see an oral hygienist at least twice a year. If the problem becomes severe, you may need to use a toothpaste containing fluoride once daily and at other times use more natural toothpastes such as those made by Green People, Jason, Aloe Dent or Waleda.

Mouth Ulcers

(see also General Health Hints and Immune Function)

Mouth ulcers are quite common and usually occur on the inside of the cheek, tongue or gums. They denote that the body is run down or under stress, but can also be caused by accidentally biting the side of the mouth, excessive tooth brushing, eating food that is too hot, eating acidic and spicy food, or cigarette smoke. Many people suffer mouth ulcers after eating oranges, pineapple and/or tomatoes, while others find ill-fitting dentures or braces are the problem. Any chronic dental problem can trigger an outbreak. If the ulcers do not clear within 3 weeks, see your doctor.

Sodium lauryl sulfate, a foaming agent used in numerous cosmetics, particularly toothpaste, can also trigger this problem. You might also be deficient in B-vitamins and iron, so a blood test would be useful to confirm if you are low in iron.

Foods to Avoid
- Sugar, vinegars, pickles, tomatoes and tomato sauces, peanuts, strawberries, pineapple, plums, rhubarb, kiwi fruit, oranges and grapefruits are problem foods for those who suffer from mouth ulcers.
- Avoid really hot and spicy foods.
- Reduce your intake of sugary treat foods and white-flour-based breads, cakes and biscuits, all of which lower immune function.
- Avoid really salty foods such as crisps, peanuts and salted meats and fish.

Friendly Foods
- Low-sugar liquorice tablets or sticks can be chewed to speed up the healing of the ulcers. You can also drink liquorice tea.
- Eat more manuka honey with an activity level of 10+, as this honey is very healing.
- Drink more green or white teas, which help to boost immune function.

Useful Remedies
- Vitamin C and zinc are often deficient in people who suffer from mouth ulcers. Take 1 gram of vitamin C daily, plus 30mg of zinc.
- Vitamin B-complex helps to prevent and heal mouth ulcers.
- Take a good multi-vitamin and mineral (which should include all the Bs, some C and the zinc, in which case, there is no need to take extra).
- Omega-7 fats from the sea buckthorn aid healing of mucosal membranes. Take 4 capsules daily while the ulcers are acute, then 2 daily. Chew the capsules so that the oil goes directly onto the ulcers.

Helpful Hints
- Stop smoking.
- Rinse your mouth out with a warm salt solution several times a day. Add 1 teaspoon of salt to a glass of cooled, boiled water. Add a few drops of goldenseal or liquorice tincture to aid healing.
- If stress is the culprit, exercise and relaxation may be the long-term answer.
- Try a herbal mouthwash containing bee propolis, calendula and St John's wort – and the homeopathic remedy Merc Sol, all of which are great for mouth ulcers. **OP**
- Tea tree oil is a natural antiseptic and makes a marvellous mouthwash when a few drops are mixed with warm water. Some people have found they are allergic to the material that false teeth are made from. Ask your dentist to test you for an allergy – porcelain is used as an alternative material.
- I find that if I use a toothpaste containing fluoride, I get mouth ulcers. Try to avoid all fluoride.
- Mouth problems often reflect problems in the gut and digestive system. See a nutritionist who can re-balance your diet and suggest supplements to boost your immune system (see *General Health Hints*).

MRSA AND SUPERBUGS

(see also Antibiotics and Immune Function)

One of the unhealthiest places you can find yourself these days is in certain hospitals, where infectious microbes such as *Acinetobacter* are found. Around 5000 people die annually in the UK from various hospital-acquired infections, but many health professionals believe it could be as many as 20,000.

One of the most virulent and deadly infections is *Clostridium difficile*, which triggers acute diarrhoea, followed by MRSA. In recent years strains of pathogenic bacteria that are resistant to all known antibiotics, including methicillin, have given rise to the condition's technical name MRSA, standing for methicillin-resistant *Staphylococcus aureus*. The secret to avoid becoming one of the 1 in 10 patients who contract various hospital-acquired infections is to boost your immune function and take sensible precautions.

MRSA produces symptoms no different from any other type of *Staphylococcus aureus* ('Staph') infection. A patient may experience redness and inflammation around wound sites on their skin, but once it enters the body, symptoms can be more serious and include fever, lethargy, headache, urinary tract infections, pneumonia, toxic shock syndrome, and even death.

Staph infections, including MRSA, occur most frequently among people in hospitals and healthcare facilities (such as nursing homes and dialysis centres) who have weakened immune systems. In cases where the infection has been acquired by someone who has had no hospital contact or medical procedure, it is known as CA-MRSA – community-associated MRSA.

The media term 'superbug' has distracted from the fact that MRSA is a man-made problem that is avoidable. Overuse and abuse of antibiotics has led to the emergence of resistant strains. The key to fighting any infection is to support and enhance the process of natural immunity and not to rely on medication. This can be done through proper diet, supplements, and specific safe remedies, such as herbs and homeopathy. Make sure you boost your immune system before going into hospital for any reason. MRSA rarely affects really healthy individuals (see under *Antibiotics* and *Immune Function*).

M

Foods to Avoid

- Eliminate refined sugar, which has been scientifically shown to slow the performance of white cells needed to isolate and destroy the invader. This means stay off all manufactured and 'junk' foods, because sugar is often an unsuspected ingredient, and limit your intake of sweet fruit juices, and fruits such as dates and grapes.
- Also avoid artificial sweeteners, such as aspartame.
- Keep in mind that honey, brown rice syrup, and maple-type syrups are all sugar – but somewhat healthier.
- See also *Food Poisoning*.

Friendly Foods

- See also *Immune Function* and *General Health Hints*.
- Garlic is especially useful as it has anti-bacterial and anti-viral properties.
- You can eat small amounts of manuka pure honey with a UMF level of 15, which has been shown to kill MRSA bacteria. The higher the UMF, the more antiseptic the honey. If the MRSA causes open sores, then Comvita also make a high-strength manuka dressing. Available from all good pharmacies.
- Healthier forms of sugar that have a lower glycaemic index are xylitol, such as ZyloSweet, or organic agave syrup. **HN**

Useful Remedies

- See also this section under *Antibiotics* and *Immune Function*.
- Bee propolis is a substance that bees manufacture to sterilize their hives, which has been shown in three studies to kill MRSA bacteria. You would need to take 3 grams a day before any stay in hospital and for at least a month afterwards. Bee Health make a potent formula – call them on 01262 607890. Website: www.beehealth.co.uk.
  NB If you have a severe intolerance to bee stings avoid the propolis.
- *Astragalus membranaceous*, or Chinese root, is widely used throughout the Orient. Scientific studies from the University of Texas Medical Center in Houston have shown that it boosts immune performance by enhancing white-cell activity, stimulating interferon and reducing infection times (*Astragalus* could also therefore be beneficial for cancer and AIDS patients). For more details of the pure herb, contact The Specialist Herbal Supplies on 0870 774 4494. **SHS**
- Herbs such as pau d'arco and St John's wort have been shown to help destroy MRSA. You need 3–4 grams of St John's wort daily and 1–3 grams of pau d'arco. **NB If you are taking blood-thinning medication, avoid St John's wort.**
- Beta Glucans 1–3, 1–6, derived from yeast cell walls, are proven to strengthen the body's innate immune system (the immune system you are born with), making it more resistant to pathogens from food and air. Take 250–500 mg daily. Beta Glucans have been shown to reduce post-surgical infections by as much as 50% and they help the body to fight any bacterial infection.

- Dr Paul Clayton based in the UK and US is a medical pharmacologist. His web site research on Beta Glucans is well worth a look. Find him at www.healthdefence.com. Glucosan, developed by Dr Clayton, is available from Vitalize Health products on 0870 042 8423, or log on to www.vitalizeshop.co.uk.
- If you are placed on high doses of antibiotics, make sure that you take a course of healthy bacteria afterwards. See *Antibiotics*.
- Oregano is a powerful anti-bacterial and anti-viral herb – try BioCare's oregano oil capsules while you are in hospital. **BC**

Helpful Hints

- Make sure that if any nurse or doctor – or anyone else – has contact with you in hospital, ask them to thoroughly wash their hands in warm soapy water before touching you. You can also take anti-bacterial wipes with you and wear sterile gloves, available from all chemists. Keep your visitors to a minimum, and as much as possible make sure that your room or the area around your bed is cleaned really thoroughly. Ask a relative to take your towels and so on to wash in a very hot wash. Simple measures can save lives.
- You can buy oregano essential oil as a spray, or coat any surfaces with this oil, as it has potent anti-viral and anti-bacterial properties. You can also inhale steam with added oregano. Or, apply a little of the pure oil to the spine; or dilute it in a base of almond oil for massage.
- Researchers at the University of Leeds have shown that by using ionizers in wards, infections from *Acinetobacter* were greatly reduced. They believe the negative ions they emit remove bacteria from the air, thus stopping transmission of many infections. Take an ionizer into hospital with you and place it near your bed!
- If you have a severe infection, look into the possibility of having hydrochloric acid injections. In 1927, Dr Burr Ferguson, MD of Birmingham, Alabama, began injecting patients with severe infections using very dilute (1:1,000 concentration) of hydrochloric acid. This is a substance that occurs naturally in human stomachs in far higher concentrations. Ferguson's results were published in the journal *Medical World* in 1932. One of the most sensational cases was a

woman at the point of death from puerperal sepsis. William Howell, a doctor who had read Ferguson's findings, injected the woman with hydrochloric acid. Within an hour, her temperature had dropped from 106°C to 103°C and the woman said she felt much better. Save for weakness, the following day all trace of the infection had disappeared! These were dramatic pioneer days. Find more details via www.tldp.com/issue/11_00/martin.htm.

MULTIPLE SCLEROSIS (MS)

(see also Adrenal Exhaustion, Candida and Leaky Gut)

Multiple sclerosis (MS) is a chronic, progressive neurological and disabling disease that affects the central nervous system – the brain and spinal cord. Inside your brain and spinal cord there are two types of matter – grey and white, which are made up of millions of nerve cells. The white matter contains nerve fibres that are coated with myelin (similar to an electrical cable with a white outer-insulating case). The job of the myelin is to speed nerve transmission and allow the easy passage of electrical signals. When the myelin breaks down or becomes inflamed, nerve transmission is disrupted, thus resulting in the damage seen in MS.

MS is also an autoimmune disease, which means that the body's own immune system attacks the myelin. Initial symptoms may be tingling, numbness, or weakness affecting a hand, foot, or one side of the body; double vision; or a loss of sensation in various parts of the body. Difficulty in walking, slurred speech, tremors and inflammation of the optic nerve is found in around 55% of sufferers and are some of the early warning signs of MS. Also, a decline in cognitive function can be a symptom, such as not being able to find a word that you use regularly in conversation, or impaired reasoning ability. Dizziness and vertigo or feelings of light-headedness are common symptoms of this condition (see under *Adrenal Exhaustion*).

Bladder dysfunction occurs in more than 80% of cases. More women than men suffer MS, which can begin at virtually any age – but most commonly appears between the ages of 20–40. Depression is also common among MS sufferers.

MS is not a hereditary disease – although in rare cases it can strike members of the same family. People living nearer the equator suffer less MS, and in countries such as Malaysia or Ecuador, it is virtually unknown. This factor is now associated with low levels of Vitamin D – see under *Useful Remedies* below.

There are four main types of MS, but each sufferer has a unique set of symptoms and disease pattern, making it very difficult to diagnose. For this reason it may be missed by doctors for several years leading to considerable frustration for the MS sufferer.

Type 1 – Benign MS This usually starts with a small number of mild attacks followed by complete recovery. It does not worsen over time and there is no permanent disability. The first symptoms are usually sensory. It is only possible to classify people as having benign MS when they have little sign of disability 10–15 years after the onset of the disease. Around 20% of people with MS have the benign form.

Type 2 – Relapsing Remitting MS This is the most common form of MS. Periods of remission are interrupted by periods of attacks. The attacks can range from mild to quite debilitating. In the early stages of disease, complete recovery between the relapses is common, but over time remissions may result in residual symptoms caused by the damage to the myelin at the time of the attack. Around 25% of people with MS have the relapsing remitting type.

Type 3 – Secondary Progressive This type starts out as relapsing-remitting MS, but after repeated attacks the remissions stop and the condition moves into a progressive stage. The time it takes to move into the progressive phase varies, but it usually happens within 15–20 years from the first onset of MS.

Type 4 – Primary Progressive Some people with MS have no distinct relapses and periods of remission. From the beginning they experience steadily worsening symptoms and progressive disability. This may level off at any one time, or may continue to get worse. Around 15% of people with MS have this type, which is also known as 'chronic progressive'.

The onset of MS has been attributed to viruses and having a weak nervous system that is then aggravated by trauma, shock, infection, or toxic metals, especially mercury. Dr Patrick Kingsley, who before he retired was one of Britain's leading alternative nutritional physicians specializing in cancer and MS, told me: 'Many of my patients had high levels of mercury in their spinal fluid, and the first thing I recommend is that they have the emissions measured from any mercury fillings.' Dr Kingsley also says that, 'MS symptoms can also mimic those of candida, so this possibility plus a leaky gut would also need to be eliminated.' Parasites are another consideration. (See also *Candida* and *Leaky Gut*.)

Up to 70% of people with MS have problems absorbing nutrients properly so deficiencies are common, especially of B-vitamins, vitamin D, and the essential fats (EFAs) that are needed to make up myelin. EFAs play a critical role in MS (see the 'Swank' diet below); for this reason, therapeutic doses of some supplements are needed. Many patients also have multiple sensitivities to certain foods, the most common being cow's milk and products, plus gluten. In fact, these foods are now considered a major trigger. However, individual patients may react to almost any food, which needs to be identified on a personal basis. Many patients benefit when they follow a proper anti-candida and gluten-free diet. (See also *Allergies*.)

Exciting work is being carried on by Dr Paolo Zamboni in Italy, who has found that most MS patients have a narrowing or twisting in the veins in the neck (known as CCSVI), which prevents blood in the brain from draining properly and 'refluxing' back up into the brain, thus triggering a host of problems. By surgically unblocking these veins many MS patients are experiencing less MS-type symptoms. Contact Dr Zamboni via the Department of Surgery at the University of Ferrara in Italy – email: zmp@unife.it.

Trials at Georgetown University and the University of Buffalo have left little doubt that CCSVI is a causal factor in MS in the majority of, but not all, cases. And if CCSVI is detected after a scan, researchers recommend this should be treated as soon as possible.

Meanwhile, other research is also ongoing using stem cells to help MS (and cancer) sufferers. Professor Shimon Slavin is one of the world's leading experts in this field and runs a state-of-the-art-centre that people attend from all over the world for treatment. Contact him via The International Center for Cell Therapy and Cancer Immunotherapy, Tel Aviv Medical Center, 14 Weizman Street, Tel Aviv 64239, Israel. Email him via slavin@CTCIcenter.com.

Nutrition is a very important factor in managing MS. The most common diets used are:

The Swank low-saturated-fat diet Professor Swank started his research in the 1940s in North America. He noticed that MS was higher in countries in which the diet was rich in animal fats and where lots of dairy products were consumed. Therefore, he recommended a low-saturated-fat diet that is high in essential fats from fish oils – DHA & EPA – and GLA found in evening primrose oil. See under *Fats You Need To Eat*.

Stone Age Best-Bet Diet Research done by Canadian scientist Dr Ashton Embry has resulted in the Best Bet Diet. The thinking behind this diet is that certain people are especially sensitive to 'modern' foods, so he came up with a Stone Age diet that excludes all 'new' foods, or foods that may have been around during the Stone Age, but have changed significantly. For example, modern wheat is bred to increase its gluten capacity so that cakes, breads and pastries can gain added structure, thereby increasing their appearance and shelf life. The Best Bet Diet excludes all gluten grains, animal dairy produce, beans and legumes, eggs, margarine, refined oils, yeasts, refined sugar and saturated fat. Embry has an excellent website at www.direct-ms.org.

Foods to Avoid
- Cut down on saturated fats. Especially reduce or avoid those from animal origin – meats, and all full-fat dairy produce (butter, cheese, milk, chocolates and cream). Be careful of curries, as these are generally cooked using ghee, a clarified butter. Especially avoid cow's milk, yoghurt and even quark.
- Avoid all hydrogenated and trans-fats and oils, found in many meat-substitute meals, margarines, biscuits, cakes, pastries and most mass produced vegetable oils. (See *Fats You Need To Eat*.)
- Avoid fried food, crisps, chips, samosas, onion bhajis, burgers and so on, as this can lead to inflammation. Instead grill, stew, poach, steam and bake.
- Avoid all refined carbohydrates and any foods containing gluten, such as white bread and rice, pies, pastries, pizza, cakes and biscuits.
- As refined sugar also triggers inflammation in the body, avoid it as much as you can.
- Avoid caffeine, which is found in tea, coffee, colas, chocolates, some pain killers and many energy drinks.

- Avoid alfalfa sprouts. Although these are an excellent food source for most people, they should be avoided by those with autoimmune diseases.
- Avoid alcohol, which can cause nerve damage and depletes essential B-vitamins known to help MS.
- It's crucial that you identify and eliminate any food intolerances – see under *Allergies*.

Friendly Foods
- Great alternatives to caffeine drinks are herbal and fruit teas, diluted organic fruit and vegetable juices. Home-made is best. Drink immediately after juicing for optimum results.
- Instead of cow's milk try oat, rice, quinoa, almond or skimmed coconut milk such as kara (www.karadairyfree.com). All are widely available from health stores and some supermarkets.
- Juices, soups and stews are easy-to-absorb, nutritious foods.
- Eat plenty of oily fish – organic salmon, mackerel, herring, sardines and anchovies (see under *Mercury Fillings* for which fish should be avoided that are high in mercury). Fish oils reduce inflammation and also provide the raw materials for making myelin.
- Eat plenty of fresh and preferably organic leafy green vegetables, full of B-vitamins and antioxidants, which help to protect the good fats from damage.
- Gamma-linolenic acid (GLA) is found in sunflower seeds and safflower oil and helps to nourish the nerve endings. Use unrefined, organic seeds and oils. Keep them in the fridge.
- Pumpkin, sunflower and sesame seeds and linseeds (flax seeds) and their unrefined oils are all rich in essential fats that are vital for people with MS.
- Eat organic food as much as possible.
- People on vegan or gluten-free diets often experience some relief from symptoms – but the diet would need to be kept up for at least two years. Vegan diets are rich in essential fats needed for nerve function and low in saturated fat.
- Eat more brown rice, quinoa, kamut, lentils, barley and whole grains.

- Eat seaweeds that are rich in minerals such as nori seaweed flakes (instead of sodium salts), available from all health shops.
- Eat plenty of GM-free, organic lecithin granules, which are very important for the structure of the myelin sheath.
- Blueberries are a particularly good source of antioxidants, which protect myelin from free-radical damage. Eat daily.
- Add more curcumin – from the spice turmeric – to foods. This helps to slow the erosion of the myelin sheath. In countries where people eat plenty of curcumin, MS is very rare.

Useful Remedies
- Take a good-quality multi-vitamin and mineral to cover your basic needs.
- A full-spectrum beta-carotene complex. **SVHC, VN**
- Take 100mg of vitamin B1 (thiamine) daily, which is an essential component of myelin; as is vitamin B12 – take 1000mcg per day. Also take 50mg of vitamin B6.
- If you prefer not to take 3 pills, as the B group vitamins work together, instead take a high-strength B-complex daily.
- You can take up to 3 grams of vitamin C daily. Take it with meals in an ascorbate formula spread throughout the day.
- If muscle aches are a problem, take 200–600mg of magnesium spread throughout the day to help relax muscles.
- Omega-3-rich fish oils help to support nerve endings and are needed for normal functioning of the brain and nervous system, and the production of myelin. Take around 2–4 grams daily and more on days when you don't eat oily fish.
- GLA (as above) – around 2 grams daily to help suppress autoimmune reactions and help provide building blocks to rebuild the myelin sheath.
- Take a digestive enzyme with main meals to help increase the absorption of nutrients from your food.
- Co-enzyme Q10, a vitamin-like substance, is a potent protective antioxidant and also plays an important part in energy production. Take 100–200mg daily in divided doses with breakfast and lunch. **SVHC, PN**
- Take a probiotic (healthy bacteria) supplement daily to help keep digestion and bowel in top condition. Try Nutri's Ultraprobioplex. **NC**
- Studies have shown the amino acid acetyl L-carnitine to be more effective and better tolerated than the medication Amatadine, which is given to improve energy. Take 1000mg twice a day 30 minutes before meals.
- Lipoic acid is a major antioxidant that helps protect the myelin sheath. Take up to 400mg twice daily.
- Vitamin D regulates immune function. Countries with the lowest level of vitamin D have the highest levels of MS. During a day in the sun your body can make 20,000iu therefore with your doctor's permission take 5000iu of vitamin D3 daily for a month and then stay on a maintenance dose of 600-800iu daily. **Only take higher levels of D3 under the guidance of a health professional and/or doctor.**
- In numerous studies from the US, Hungary, Israel and Russia, a fermented wheat germ extract known as Avemar, sold in more than 10 countries, has demonstrated remarkably beneficial immune-modulating effects in the case of autoimmune conditions. Take one sachet daily in water at least one hour before breakfast. Keep refrigerated. Also available in capsules, but you would need quite a few, therefore powder is easier to take once a day. Research available via www.avemar.com It is available to buy in the UK and Europe from Nutri Centre on 0845 602 6744. **NC**

Helpful Hints

- To discover which foods you are intolerant to, contact Genova Diagnostics via 08704 190435 or check out their website at www.gdx.uk.net.
- Vitamin D helps to regulate immune function and lift mood. Ask your GP to run a 25 (OHD) test to look at your levels. Optimal levels are 45–50 ng/ml or 115–128 nmol/l. If your levels are out of this range, contact a nutritional therapist who can help you to address this. Any levels below 20 ng/ml are considered serious-deficiency states and will increase the risk of autoimmune diseases.
- Check the possibility of excess mercury in your diet or environment.
- Consider having a hair mineral analysis to check your body levels of mercury. This is a non-invasive test that requires a small sample of hair. Contact The Analytical Research Laboratories on 0131 229 1077 for details.
- Vitamin-B12 injections may help some patients.
- Take three, 10–20 minute rest periods every day, spaced throughout the day, and do some form of exercise every day, such as walking, press-ups or weight-lifting. Start slowly and build up gradually.
- Cranial osteopathy is a whole-body treatment that works with the central nervous system and the rhythmic pulsation that it produces. It has been very beneficial for some people with MS. Find a practitioner at www.cranial.org.uk.
- Have a look at www.melisa.org – a medical network that gives the latest research linking mercury fillings to MS (see also *Mercury Fillings*).
- *New Pathways* is a magazine that provides information on all aspects of complementary and orthodox therapies found to be useful in MS. Subscriptions to *New Pathways* are £10 a year, available from The Multiple Sclerosis Resource Centre, which also has an excellent website: www.msrc.co.uk. Their information line and 24-hour telephone counselling service is on 0800 783 0518.
- The Multiple Sclerosis Society also has a helpline on 0808 800 8000. Their website is at www.mssociety.org.uk.
- Under Pressure is the UK's leading MS Clinic, giving advice and treatment for all levels of MS. Susie Cornell, sufferer and author of the book *The Complete MS Body Manual* (Under Pressure Publications), is the director of the clinic. Susie leads the field with a revolutionary approach in the natural treatment of MS. For more information telephone 01245 268098 or visit www.susiecornell.com.
- For more help, read *Multiple Sclerosis* by Judy Graham (Thorsons), the founder of the Multiple Sclerosis Resource Centre. She has also written a very informative book called *Multiple Sclerosis and Having a Baby* (Healing Arts Press).

N

NAIL PROBLEMS *(see also Absorption, Leaky Gut and Low Stomach Acid)*

Nails are made up mostly from keratin, a protein-like substance also found in your hair. There are fat and water molecules in between the keratin, which help to keep nails healthy and supple.

Your nails are a great barometer of your health. For example, if you are stressed or have poor digestion, then stomach acid levels often fall, in which case you may experience longitudinal ridges in your nails, which denotes low stomach acid. Ridges across the nails (from side to side) can denote a lack of calcium and/or magnesium, and stress. White spots can show that you are either ingesting too much sugar, alcohol, and junk foods, or have insufficient zinc in your body.

Brittle, transparent and flat-looking nails that curl up at the edges are a common problem associated with low iron levels. However, as excessive iron after the age of 50 is linked to heart disease, don't take too much iron unless a blood test shows that you need it. Brittle, splitting nails are a sign of silica deficiency; while soft peeling nails often indicate a calcium deficiency. Excessively curved nails (like an upside-down spoon) can indicate a potassium deficiency.

Anyone who has their hands in water for long periods usually has weaker nails; and biting the nails is an obvious cause for poor nails. Fungal infections turn the nails white, or at the very least they cause a discolouration and deformity in the nails. Nails can thicken if you eat too much protein or when the immune system is at a low ebb. If your nail beds are red, your liver may be congested from too much fat and alcohol and you should have your cholesterol levels checked.

Foods to Avoid
- Avoid junk foods, fizzy drinks, white bread, biscuits and pastries – all these foods deplete the body of nutrients, especially B-vitamins.
- Reduce your intake of caffeine and alcohol.
- Keep sugar to a minimum.
- Hard, thick nails can denote that you are eating too much fat and excess protein. Avoid hydrogenated or trans-fats, and avoid too much fat from animal sources, including from full-fat milk, cheeses, chocolates, pies, desserts and so on.

Friendly Foods
- Make sure that you eat good-quality protein at least once a day, as nails are made from protein. Try chicken, fish, quinoa, cooked tofu, or a little organic lean red meat.
- Eggs, blackstrap molasses, almonds, red meats and spinach are rich in iron.
- Oily fish, and unrefined nuts and seeds (especially hazelnuts, Brazil nuts and walnuts, and sunflower, pumpkin and sesame seeds, and linseeds/flax seeds) are rich in zinc and essential fats. Use their unrefined oils over salads and cooked foods to nourish your nails.
- Drink plenty of fluids.
- Eat more pumpkin, apricots, papaya, green leafy vegetables (especially kale, watercress and spinach) plus cantaloupe melons and sweet potatoes for their vitamin-A content.

- Cereals, brown rice, buckwheat, amaranth, oats, organ meats, eggs, lentils, peas, nuts and leafy green organic vegetables are all rich in B-vitamins, which are vital for healthy nails.
- Eating a small amount of pineapple and papaya before or after meals aids digestion.
- Eat one avocado a week and sprinkle organic wheat germ over cereals and desserts, as they are rich in vitamin E.
- Silica-rich foods are lettuce, green and red peppers, cucumber, bean sprouts, asparagus and all high-fibre foods, vegetables and whole grains.

Useful Remedies

- Take a comprehensive multi-nutrient vitamin and mineral formula that includes essential fats – all of the companies listed on pages 15–16 have in-house nutritionists who can help you choose the right multi for your age and gender.
- Take a B-complex plus 2.5mg of biotin, a lack of which is linked to brittle nails. Vegetarians and vegans often also have low levels of B12, which is found in meat, fish and eggs, therefore make sure that your B-complex contains at least 50mcg of B12. (Most multi formulas will include all the B-group.)
- The mineral silica is important for healthy nails. Take 75mg daily.
- If you have fungal infections, as well as following a low-sugar diet, the herbs pau d'arco (2 x 500mg capsules twice daily) and cat's claw (2 x 500mg capsules twice daily) will reduce fungus in the body and nails.
- New Era Tissue Salt Combination K helps reduce brittle nails, and Combination L helps reduce fungal problems.
- MSM, an organic form of sulphur, helps to strengthen nails. Take 1000mg daily.
- White blobs (more than tiny spots) on the nails can denote a lack of selenium. Take 200mcg daily.
- Collagen is a vital component of healthy joints, cartilage, ligaments and tendons, and it also helps nails. Take daily in a glass of water or diluted fruit juice 30 minutes before a main meal. Super Strength Collagen Drink is available from Higher Nature. **HN**

Helpful Hints

- Massage jojoba, neem and lemon oil into your nails to nourish and prevent splitting. **OP**
- Nail-polish remover contains solvents, which are notorious for drying out nails and making them more brittle. Most nail salons and beauty counters sell oils specifically for the nails, which can be used after polishing. Always use a base coat.
- To remove yellow stains from nails, soak them in a cup of warm water that contains the juice of 1 lemon for 15 minutes daily.
- Massage your nails regularly with jojoba, olive or almond oil.
- If you have a fungal infection, soak your nails in white distilled vinegar for at least 10 minutes twice a day. You can also use diluted tee tree oil or neem oil on the nails. The Organic Pharmacy makes a neem and tea tree cream, which can be used on hands and nails. **OP**
- Bacteria, viruses and superbugs can breed under the nails and being in close contact with someone who has dirty nails is a great way to pass on infections. Also if you shake hands with someone who has a cold, this too will spread the virus. Keep your nails clean.
- If your nails are constantly in water, then wear surgical or rubber gloves. Wear gloves when gardening.
- Only use nail salons that keep their instruments scrupulously clean.

NAUSEA (see Vomiting)

NUMBNESS/TINGLING SENSATIONS

FINGERS AND TOES

These types of symptoms are usually a sign of poor circulation (see *Circulation*, *Diabetes* and *Raynaud's Disease*), but can be caused by pressure on a nerve. These sensations are common if you sleep or sit in an awkward position, but may also be a symptom of cervical spondylosis (pressure on nerves in the neck, causing numbness in the hands, a stiff neck, or headaches) or carpal tunnel syndrome (numbness in the thumb-side of the hand, and sharp pain at night). If you suffer continually with really cold fingers and toes during the winter, you may well be suffering from Raynaud's Disease (see *Raynaud's Disease*). Any conditions that reduce circulation to the nerves in the skin will produce these types of symptoms. If symptoms continue have a check-up, as numbness is also linked to multiple sclerosis, ME and Sjogren's syndrome.

Foods to Avoid
- See this section under *Atherosclerosis* and *Circulation*.
- Generally avoid caffeine, animal fats and smoking.

Friendly Foods
- See also *Circulation*.

- You are likely to be lacking in essential fats, which are found in oily fish, linseeds (flax seeds), and sunflower and pumpkin seeds and their unrefined oils. See also *Fats You Need To Eat*.
- Eat more blueberries, blackberries, sweet potatoes, cherries, apricots, spinach, watercress, kale and all leafy green vegetables. These are all rich in flavonoids, which help strengthen capillaries.
- Wheat germ and avocados are rich in vitamin E, which thin the blood naturally.
- Garlic is great for circulation, while ginger will warm you.
- Lecithin granules aid repair of the nerve endings – sprinkle them on breakfast cereal or in yoghurts.

Useful Remedies
- Take a high-strength vitamin B-complex daily. A deficiency of B-vitamins can cause tingling in the nerve endings.
- Older people may also benefit from a B12 injection or a 1mg B12 tablet; a lack of this vitamin is linked to tingling in the extremities.
- Take 1–2 grams of vitamin C with bioflavonoids daily, spread throughout the day with meals, to help repair nerve endings.
- Lipoic acid – a major antioxidant has been shown to improve diabetic neuropathy, it is also a great nutrient for the brain and helps balance blood sugar levels. Take 200mg daily with food.
- Essential fats are needed for good circulation and well-toned blood vessels. Omega-3s (found in fish oils) have been shown to reduce blood-vessel spasms; omega-6s (in nuts and seeds) inhibit blood-vessel constriction.
- Fish oil is a great source of omega-3 fatty acids (EPA and DHA). A pure fish oil such as Krill Oil (made by Cardio-Red, tel: 07797 887372) would be more beneficial than linseed (flax seed) oil. Omega-6 fatty acids (GLAs) are found in evening primrose and borage (starflower) oils. See *Fats You Need To Eat*.
- As this problem can denote a deficiency of calcium, take 600mg of calcium daily, plus a multi-mineral that includes 400mg of magnesium.
- The herb gotu kola taken over time (3 months) helps to increase circulation to the extremities. 500mg twice daily.

Helpful Hints

- If, after taking these supplements for 6 weeks, you still have numb and tingling fingers or toes, see your GP.
- Walking for half an hour each day, or skipping, rebounding and swinging your arms full circle regularly, will help to get your circulation moving.
- It is also helpful to massage your hands and feet. Obviously, it is easy to massage one's own hands, however if you find it difficult to massage your feet, ask your partner, a relative or a friend to do it for you. Use essential oils of geranium, ginger, black pepper and lavender in a base oil. If you have no one to massage your feet, pop a few drops of the oils in the bath and soak your feet for 10 minutes.
- Reflexology and acupuncture often help reduce or eliminate this type of problem (see *Useful Information*).
- You may have a trapped nerve, in which case consult a chiropractor or osteopath.

OBESITY
(see Weight Problems)

O

OSTEOARTHRITIS
(see Arthritis)

OSTEOPOROSIS

(see also Acid–Alkaline Balance, Adrenal Exhaustion, Leaky Gut, Menopause and Stress)

Osteoporosis silently threatens men and women – and, thanks to our high-stressed lifestyles, over-consumption of sugary refined foods and a host of other factors – we are now at huge risk from a health time bomb. More than 1.14 million post-menopausal women in the UK alone have been diagnosed with osteoporosis. Hip fractures cause more than 1150 premature deaths every month and the combined costs of hospital and social care for patients with hip fractures amounts to more £2.3 billion annually. One in two women and 1 in five men over the age of 50 will break a bone through osteoporosis.

Your bone mass peaks in your mid-twenties, but, if you live a fast-paced lifestyle and tend to become stressed easily by releasing plenty of the stress hormones adrenalin and cortisol, then you seriously need to start looking after your bones now. Excess production of stress hormones can hugely deplete minerals from your bones. In addition, if you also tend to eat in a hurry, eat plenty of refined sugary or pre-packaged foods and may also have taken antibiotics, then you may have a leaky gut. This is an often overlooked problem that also contributes to your risk of developing osteoporosis and a host of other health problems in later life, because you may not be absorbing sufficient nutrients from your diet. Therefore, before reading on, please read the *Absorption, Acid-Alkaline Balance, Adrenal Exhaustion* and *Leaky Gut* sections.

Although osteoporosis still tends to be thought of as a disease of old age, there is now no doubt that its roots lie in adolescence. Many young people love fizzy drinks, high in the industrialized-altered version of the mineral phosphorous, and too much can deplete bone. I reiterate that junk foods, alcohol, too much caffeine and refined sugar also deplete minerals – so does stress.

Other hormones besides cortisol and adrenalin, along with genetics also play an important role. For example, when I was in my early thirties I had a hysterectomy and at that time no one warned me that I might need to use prescribed oestrogen to protect my bones. If you keep your ovaries after surgery, you will produce some oestrogen for a time, but often not enough to prevent osteoporosis that crippled my mother. I have always taken bone supplements and done plenty of weight-bearing exercise, but these alone I now know did not compensate for the years of insufficient oestrogen – which is why I now have osteoporosis. My Type A personality, of always being in a rush and having plenty of stress in my life, which at times I did not deal with effectively, plus antibiotics in my teens and twenties, which at times have triggered leaky gut issues, have also contributed to my osteoporosis.

Therefore, if you have an early menopause, which is becoming more common thanks to our stressful and toxic environment, or you have a hysterectomy (even if you keep your ovaries), please make sure that your hormone levels are checked every year – otherwise you could end up like me. Make no mistake, osteoporosis can kill you. I beg of you to take heed – prevention is absolutely better than cure.

Osteoporosis is also associated with a lack of weight-bearing exercise, excess animal protein in the diet, low body weight and lack of skin exposure to sunshine (being out in the daylight increases vitamin-D levels in the body). My mother undoubtedly suffered osteoporosis partly due to her poor diet, but also, she never exposed her skin to the sun. When she died at 78, her skin was amazingly wrinkle free but her bones were in a dreadful state. Hence I firmly believe that women who are fanatical about staying out of the sun would definitely benefit from exposing their skin regularly to 15 minutes of early morning or late-afternoon sun to boost their vitamin-D levels – and everyone, including children, should now also supplement extra vitamin D3.

Other risk factors are a family history of osteoporosis, premature menopause, some cancers and long-term use of certain drugs, such as tranquillizers and steroids, a thin body-frame (which I have) and smoking. Women who suffered anorexia when they were younger, and those who exercise to the point where their periods stop, are also at risk because of lowered hormone levels. As always, a sensible balance is needed.

Traditionally, osteoporosis is prevented and treated by hormone replacement therapy (HRT). But nutritional scientist and naturopath Bob Jacobs says: 'Women who have taken orthodox HRT for 10 years or more may have a greater bone density than those who have not taken it, but they lose any increased bone density rapidly when the HRT is stopped, and end up with only 3.2% higher bone density than women who took nothing. When women exercise regularly, eat a healthy diet and take the right vitamins and minerals, bone density can be maintained and even increased, without having to endure the potential side effects of conventional HRT, which are an increased risk of breast and endometrial (womb) cancers, thrombosis and strokes. If extra hormones are required, it is far better to use bio-identical hormone therapy.' (See *Useful Remedies*, below.)

Other hormones, such as DHEA and testosterone, also play a part in good bone health.

My co-author, naturopath Stephen Langley, adds: 'Calcium is relatively easy to get (and absorb) in our diet, as it is abundant in so many foods – the problem is not that you aren't getting enough calcium in your bones, but keeping it in your bones. To do that you need other nutrients, particularly magnesium, otherwise all the calcium you eat will end up in your tissues and will then be excreted. This is why, rather than loading up on dairy foods (which are acid forming and thus deplete minerals from your body), women would be better advised to eat far more magnesium-rich foods, such as green leafy vegetables, to buffer excess acidity.'

Foods to Avoid

- Generally cut down on caffeine-based foods and drinks. More than 3 cups of strong coffee a day can increase your risk of developing osteoporosis by as much as 80%.
- Our Western diets tend to be very high in acid-forming foods, which cause calcium to be leached from the bones. These include all 'white' foods: breads, cakes, croissants, biscuits, refined sugars, white pasta and rice and so on (see *Acid–Alkaline Balance* for more information).
- Gluten sensitivity can be an issue (see under *Allergies*) as coeliacs, for instance, suffer more osteoporosis due to poor calcium absorption.
- Some people eat too much animal protein, which increases acidity of the blood and promotes calcium loss from the bones.
- Avoid fizzy drinks, because the artificial carbonation creates carbonic acid, which dissolves bone, and the excess phosphates force more calcium to be excreted.
- Avoid excess alcohol. Consuming more than 2 alcoholic drinks daily decreases calcium absorption from your diet. It also interferes with the synthesis of vitamin D, which helps the bones absorb calcium.
- All dairy foods from animal sources increase calcium loss, but also provide calcium – eating 100g (4oz) of kale or spring greens will have at least as much beneficial effect on calcium balance as 200g (8oz) of milk or 100g (4oz) of Cheddar cheese.
- Avoid fluoride as much as you can, which is also linked to bone loss – see under *Fluoride*.

Friendly Foods

- Vegetarians tend to suffer less osteoporosis, as their diet usually contains far more vegetables, pulses, grains and fruits.
- Foods that are high in calcium and magnesium and will help reduce calcium loss from bones are green leafy vegetables, such as kale, alfalfa, watercress, kelp, broccoli, cabbage and spring greens.
- Fish and sesame seeds contain as much calcium as many animal- based milks.
- Eat more fermented soya-based foods, such as tempeh and natto, which are high in phyto-oestrogens (isoflavones). See this section under *Menopause*.
- Magnesium is found in brown rice, buckwheat, lentils, peas, corn, almonds, cashew and Brazil nuts, sunflower, sesame and pumpkin seeds, wheat germ and wholegrain cereals.
- Vitamin D is found in egg yolks, oily fish, organ meats and milk. It allows the body to absorb the calcium and phosphorous needed for healthy bones.
- Vitamin K is vital for healthy bones, as it keeps calcium in the bones and out of the arteries, where calcium deposits add to arterial plaque. Vitamin K is found in broccoli, green cabbage, lettuce and especially kale.
- As low stomach acid is often a factor in osteoporosis, eat more pineapple or papaya before meals to aid absorption – see *Low Stomach Acid*.
- Silica is another important mineral for healthy bones, found in lettuce, celery, cucumber, green and red peppers, bean sprouts, asparagus, millet, oats and parsnips.
- Boron is a trace mineral needed for healthy bones. It is found in raisins, prunes, nuts, non-citrus fruits and vegetables.
- Add 1 tablespoon of organic cider vinegar and honey to a glass of warm water daily. Sip throughout the day. This helps the body to assimilate more calcium.
- Drink mineral waters in preference to tap water. Fiji water is rich in silica.

- Otherwise, try Kangen Water – a water system unit that ionizes and greatly alkalizes water thus supporting your bones. It's used in Japanese hospitals with highly beneficial health results. For full details contact the Wholistic Medical Centre in London Tel: 020 7580 7537 or have a look at www.kangenmiraclewater.co.uk

Useful Remedies

- Natural plant phyto-oestrogens and soya-based oestrogen supplements (isoflavones) promote a positive calcium balance, help make bone more resistant to releasing calcium, and reduce urinary calcium loss. Oestrogen levels decline with age in both men and women, with a particularly dramatic drop in women at menopause. **HN**
- Natural phyto-oestrogen cream contains bio-identical (meaning the exact molecule that is found in the human body) progesterone made from wild yam and oestrogen from soya beans, which helps to prevent osteoporosis and can, in tandem with proper nutrition, help increase bone density. To find out if you are at risk of osteoporosis, have a bone-density scan via your doctor and also ask for a urine DPD test to show if you are currently losing bone. If the bone scan is OK and the urine test shows no bone loss, then you don't need extra hormones. But if your density is low and the urine test shows excessive bone breakdown, then the use of natural hormones, the right diet, supplements, and exercise can be very useful. For a free information sheet on phyto-oestrogen cream call 001 310 301 4015 (6-8pm Mondays to Fridays or log on to www.pharmwest.com See also under *Menopause* for a full list of bio-identical hormones and where to source them.

- With regard to your needs for magnesium and calcium as part of an overall program – an optimum dose **for anyone with osteoporosis** would be 600mg of magnesium and 500mg of calcium daily, taken in a chelated (or citrate) form, as they are more easily utilized. They should be taken in divided doses throughout the day, with the final dose taken just before bedtime – as these mineral are known as nature's tranquillizers.
- To **prevent** osteoporosis, start taking around 300mg of calcium citrate and 400mg magnesium citrate daily from your early 40s.
- Vitamin K2 x 100mcg daily is very important for gluing the calcium into your bone matrix. Research has shown that vitamin K2 can reduce fracture risk by 65%. Most bone multi formulas contain some vitamin K2.
  NB If you are taking blood-thinning drugs, then check with your doctor before taking any vitamin K.
- Vitamin C – 1–2 grams taken daily with meals in an ascorbate form – promotes the formation of proteins required in bone and is also involved in the synthesis and repair of all collagen, including cartilage and matrix of bone.
- Collagen is a vital component of healthy joints, cartilage, ligaments and tendons and also improves bone strength. It is the most widely distributed protein in the body and we lose about 1.5% annually after the age of 30. Take daily in a glass of water or diluted juice 30 minutes before a main meal to support your bones. Try Super Strength Collagen Drink from Higher Nature. **HN**
- Zinc – 15mg per day – is necessary for bone building. This should be in any multi-vitamin/mineral.
- Vitamin D3 , 1000iu daily is **essential** for calcium and phosphorus absorption. Lack of vitamin D is now linked to more than 17 major diseases associated with ageing.
- Boron, 3mg per day, is necessary for the conversion of vitamin D into its active forms. It also helps the body produce natural oestrogen. This mineral is vital for healthy bones.
- Vitamin B6, taken as 100mg per day, is a necessary co-factor for many enzyme reactions involved in bone-building.

- All the companies listed on pages 15–16 make multi-vitamin/mineral and bone formulas that contain a balanced supply of most of these nutrients, which also includes hydrochloric acid (stomach acid) to aid absorption. Don't be afraid to call and ask a nutritionist for help.
- The mineral strontium (citrate) has the unique ability to bind calcium into the bone and thus increase bone density. Take 200mg a day – but must be taken 12 hours away from calcium supplements.

Helpful Hints

- With such fast-paced lifestyles, our tissues tend to be more acid – thus causing calcium to be leached from our bones and magnesium from the muscles, and these are the minerals that help to re-alkalize our bodies. Therefore, learn to deal with stress in your life and your reaction to it. Basically, the more stressed you become, the more damage in the long term you are causing to your bones.
- After the age of 50, or before if you have surgery or go through an early menopause, have a bone scan every two years and have all hormone levels checked.
- Do not smoke. Women who smoke generally experience menopause up to a year and a half earlier than non-smokers, and thus face a longer period of oestrogen deficiency and accompanying bone loss. Smoking also hampers efficient processing of calcium. Smokers have a higher rate of spinal fractures than non-smokers.
- Osteoporosis is a largely preventable disease and there are some commonsense things you can do to reduce the risk. As well as keeping your hormones balanced, another important preventative is weight-bearing exercise. Swimming and cycling are great exercises, but they don't increase bone density as they are not weight-bearing. Skipping, jogging, walking, using weights, aerobics and rebounding (mini-trampolines) are great exercises to beat osteoporosis. Tennis players have a 30% higher bone density in their serving arm compared with their non-serving arm. For anyone already suffering osteoporosis, join a local gym and begin exercising with a professional. In an ideal world, begin weight training in your 20s and 30s before your bones start to thin – but it is never too late.
- Sunlight is needed to make active vitamin D in the body, so even if you are not a keen sunbather, then at least expose your skin to 15 minutes of sun regularly – but not between 11am and 3pm.
- Dr Marilyn Glenville is one of the UK's leading experts on natural ways to cope with the menopause and osteoporosis. She has also written an excellent book: *Osteoporosis, The Silent Epidemic* (Kyle Cathie). For more information log on to: www.marilynglenville.com

PALPITATIONS

(see also Adrenal Exhaustion, Heart Disease, Low Blood Sugar, Stress and Tachycardia)

This is a fairly common problem that just about everyone experiences at one time or another. If you are under stress or have suffered a shock or are anxious or even over-excited, then as the stress hormones adrenalin and cortisol are released, your heart automatically responds by beating faster. Once the anxiety has passed, your heart rate should calm down, but if it doesn't, then you have a problem. Palpitations occur when the heart beats irregularly; it can skip a beat or feel like a fluttering in the chest. If you find that you regularly suffer any of these symptoms and they do not recede when you are calm, or if you are regularly short of breath, then you definitely need to see your doctor. Palpitations can also indicate that there is some problem with the electrical circuitry in the heart.

Not only does over-production of the stress 'fight-or-flight hormones' adrenaline and cortisol trigger palpitations, but food sensitivities can also be a factor. Low blood sugar can also contribute to palpitations and panic attacks – see *Low Blood Sugar*.

A lack of iron or imbalanced hormone levels, especially the thyroid and/or progesterone levels, can also be potential factors. A blood or saliva test via your GP should indicate if hormonal imbalances are the culprit.

Also, in highly sensitive individuals, electro-pollution from mobile phones, digital cordless phones and WIFI is known to trigger palpitations. See under *Electrical Pollution*.

Foods to Avoid
- Avoid heavy alcohol intake, which can damage the heart muscle.
- Caffeine found in teas, coffee, all chocolates (pure dark chocolate has the highest concentration of caffeine), fizzy drinks and anything containing caffeine, as it stimulates the release of adrenaline into the blood stream. I know of several people, including relatives of mine, who suffered this problem if they touched **any** caffeine; once caffeine was eliminated, their palpitations disappeared.
- Too much refined sugar, stress and caffeine deplete magnesium from the body, the very mineral the body needs to stay calm.
- Food additives can trigger an attack in sensitive individuals.
- Generally, don't eat large, heavy meals, which place an added strain on the body.
- Avoid any energy drinks containing the plant extract guarana, which is basically neat caffeine. Same for drinks like Red Bull.
- Any foods to which you are intolerant may also cause palpitations. The most common are wheat, eggs, dairy produce from cows and citrus fruits.
- Avoid eating large meals if you are anxious.

Friendly Foods.
- See *Angina*, *Atherosclerosis*, *Stress* and *General Health Hints*.
- Drink more passiflora or camomile tea to help calm you down.
- Use small amounts of brown rice syrup, organic agave syrup, stevia or xylitol instead of refined sugar. Available from all health stores.
- Make sure you drink plenty of water, as dehydration can also be a contributing factor in palpitations.

Useful Remedies
- A pinch of cayenne pepper swallowed with a little water in most cases helps regulate the heartbeat very quickly.
- An irregular heartbeat is also linked to an electrolyte imbalance, including calcium, magnesium, potassium and even sodium. Take 99mg of potassium daily for 1 month. SVHC. Also take a calcium/magnesium formula containing 100–400mg of magnesium and 200mg of calcium twice daily – in divided doses, taking the final dose at bedtime. (Your doctor can do a blood test to see if you are lacking in potassium, sodium or calcium.)
- Folic acid – 600 mcg daily – helps to stabilize the heartbeat. Sometimes a high homocysteine level can contribute to this problem – see under *High Blood Pressure* for details.

- Vitamin B5 (pantothenic acid) helps to combat feelings of stress – take 100–500mg daily. Also take a B-complex, as all the B-group vitamins work together to calm the nerves.
- Take a good-quality multi-vitamin and mineral containing 400iu of natural-source vitamin E. This helps the heart muscle to receive more oxygen.
- Co-enzyme Q10, a vitamin-like substance made in the body that helps to regulate heartbeat. As we age we manufacture less, so try 60mg daily – and then increase to 100mg daily. **PN**
- Vitamin D3 has been shown to help alleviate arrhythmia – take 1000iu daily.
- Cortisol manager tablets contain ashwagandha, phosphatdlyserine and L-theanine (an extract of green tea). This combination is excellent for reducing cortisol production and calming you down. If you are a Type-A person who rushes around all day, feels stressed and needs to 'slow down', then try taking one of these tablets when the adrenaline starts 'pumping', thus triggering palpitations, and also take one or two before bed. I have found them marvellous for reducing the 'fight-or-flight'-type symptoms and they help me to get a better night's sleep. However, if you are at a point of total and utter exhaustion, then read the *Adrenal Exhaustion* section, because if your body is not producing sufficient cortisol, there is no benefit in taking this formula.
- Otherwise try plain L-theanine capsules. Take 100mg, 3 times daily spread throughout the day. If you drink green tea, look for the decaffeinated brands.

Helpful Hints

- As palpitations can be linked to an overactive thyroid, ask your doctor to do a blood test to check for thyroid and other hormone imbalances.
- Learn to meditate, which reduces stress, as worrying about this condition can precipitate an attack. See under *Adrenal Exhaustion* and *Stress*.
- To combat worrying, which only exacerbates the condition, learn how to breathe properly by taking yoga lessons.
- Take a calm, deep breathe every 20 minutes.
- Essential oils of lavender and ylang ylang have a calming effect – try a few drops in your bath. You can also inhale the ylang ylang directly from the bottle to help slow your breathing. Try regular aromatherapy massage, which is very relaxing.
- Go for leisurely walks, breathing slowly and deeply.

PANIC ATTACKS

(see also Adrenal Exhaustion, Low Blood Sugar, Palpitations, Phobias and Stress)

Panic attacks occur during periods of acute anxiety and in Britain there are approximately 10 million sufferers. Feelings of intense panic induce hyperventilating (breathing too fast), which can cause light-headedness and tingling in the fingers and toes caused by a reduction in carbon dioxide in the blood. Panic attacks have a huge variety of causes, most of them based on fears or phobias. Obviously, if a loved one dies suddenly, for example, in a car accident, and you are with them, a panic attack would be triggered by acute shock. Some people have panic attacks if they see spiders; or, if a person has had one heart attack or stroke, he or she may panic at the least sensation of pain, believing another attack is imminent. During 1998, following a near-death experience, for almost two months I suffered panic attacks – and believe me if someone tells you to pull yourself together, they are wasting their time. Reassurance and patience are what are needed. Panic attacks are hugely linked to adrenal exhaustion and low blood sugar. See these sections.

Foods to Avoid

- Avoid stimulants, especially caffeine, refined sugar and alcohol, which can all trigger severe mood swings and disrupt blood sugar levels.
- Sugar substitutes such as aspartame should also be avoided.
- Tinned and pre-packaged foods are high in salt. Combine this with a panic attack and your blood pressure can rise.
- People who tend to eat too many starchy foods, such as breads, potatoes, croissants, bananas, coffee and so on, are more likely to suffer panic attacks, as blood sugar is greatly affected by these types of foods.

Friendly Foods

- Protein, fibre and healthier fats such as eggs, fish, quinoa, amaranth, sunflower, pumpkin, flax or hemp seeds, plus protein powders will help balance blood sugar and reduce the likelihood of a panic attack. Eat small amounts of protein, fibres and fats with every meal.
- Eat more calming foods (with some added protein) that will also help to balance your blood sugar, such as brown rice, buckwheat, couscous, wholewheat noodles, sweet potatoes, porridge, quinoa, wholemeal bread and pastas, lentils, beans, and rice and corn pastas. These slower-release carbohydrates are essential for stabilizing blood sugar levels – often a factor in panic attacks.
- Eat small meals regularly. Don't skip meals.
- Snack on organic nuts, seeds and low-fat yoghurts. Health shops now sell numerous low-sugar seed/protein bars.

- Cut down on sodium-based salts; use a magnesium/potassium-based salt. Try Himalayan crystal seas salt, or use nori seaweed salt flakes, which are high in minerals.
- Generally, include more beans, pulses, fruits and vegetables in your diet.
- Eat more oily fish rich in omega-3 fats, and seeds such as sunflower, sesame and pumpkin, as well as walnuts, almonds and Brazil nuts, linseeds and hemp seeds, which are all rich in omega-6 essential fats. (See *Fats You Need To Eat*.)
- Low levels of serotonin are linked to feelings of depression. Serotonin is made from a constituent of protein called tryptophan. Fish, turkey, chicken, cottage cheese, beans, wheat germ, avocados and bananas are all rich in tryptophan, which helps to keep you calm. If you tend to eat lots of bananas, then eat with a few sunflower seeds or an oat cake to slow the fast-releasing sugars from the banana.
- Sprinkle wheat germ over a low-sugar breakfast cereal. Nature's Path make cereals from amaranth, quinoa and kamut, which are sweetened with apple juice. Available worldwide. Cereals are rich in B-vitamins, which help to keep you calm.
- Porridge is a very calming food. Use a few raisins or xylitol to sweeten. Add fresh fruit for added fibre.
- Eat more lettuce, mushrooms, peppers and root vegetables, which are also calming foods.
- Use small amounts of brown rice syrup, organic agave syrup, stevia or xylitol instead of refined sugars, which have a much lower glycaemic index than refined sugars. Available from health stores.

Useful Remedies

- Homeopathic Argent Nit, Gelsemium and Aconite taken in a combination help reduce anxiety. These are very potent – the Organic Pharmacy make them in one mixture. Take one pill as soon as you feel onset of symptoms. **OP**
- Take a good high-strength B-complex daily to help support your nerves.
- Inositol, one of the B-group vitamins, has been shown to reduce panic attacks. A good source is lecithin granules. Sprinkle liberally over yoghurts, fruit and so on.

- Take up to 2 grams of vitamin C daily with meals, as mild to moderate deficiency is associated with nervousness.
- Take 400mg of calcium and 600mg of magnesium daily. Many people who suffer panic attacks are lacking in these minerals. Take in divided doses throughout the day.
- Take potassium – 99mg per day. Low levels can increase susceptibility to anxiety. **SVHC**
- Take tryptophan – 250–500mg per day. This is the precursor to serotonin, which is called the 'happy brain neurotransmitter'. Panic attacks can be reduced by increasing serotonin levels in the brain. Take 1 in the morning and 1 if needed in the evening. **HN, VN**

Helpful Hints

- Bach Flower Remedies are helpful for reducing panic attacks. Try Star of Bethlehem, Rescue Remedy, or Jan de Vries Emergency Essence, and if you feel an attack coming on, treat the flower remedy as your medicine. Say to yourself as you place it under your tongue, 'This will calm me down in under 3 minutes.' Keep repeating this phrase and it will help.
- Regular exercise reduces stress and builds confidence. A regular aromatherapy massage with lavender oil helps you to stay calm and balances the emotions. A warm, relaxing bath and sound, restful sleep do wonders to ease stress.
- Learn how to control the attacks; fighting them will make them only worse. Tell yourself that this is just the body's way of getting you to take care of yourself. Speak to yourself gently, as you would to comfort a child.
- Hypnotherapy and self-hypnosis called Neuro-Linguistic Programming have proven very successful for reducing panic attacks and phobias. See *Useful Information*.
- If you suffer regularly from panic-type attacks, carry a large paper bag with you and, if you begin hyperventilating, immediately blow into the bag slowly and calmly, which should help calm you down and stop you from fainting.
- Carry homeopathic Aconite 200c, and take at the onset of an attack, as it is a great remedy if you have intense fear.
- First Steps to Freedom, a self-help group, have a helpline for people with phobias. Fact sheets, self-help booklets, audio/video tapes, books and online support groups are available. For further information write to First Steps to Freedom, PO Box 476, Newquay, TR7 1WQ. Tel: 0845 120 2916. The helpline is open 10.00am–10.00pm every day. Website: www.first-steps.org. Email: first.steps@btconnect.com

PARASITES
(see under Irritable Bowel Syndrome)

PARKINSON'S DISEASE *(see also Leaky Gut and Mercury Fillings)*

Parkinson's Disease (PD) is a degenerative disorder of the central nervous system that becomes more common with increasing age. Men tend to be more affected than women and around five in every 1000 people in their 60s, and 40 in every 1000 in their 80s have Parkinson's. Although Parkinson's tends mainly to affect people over 50, it sometimes occurs in younger people if they have suffered any type of brain inflammation, carbon-monoxide poisoning, long-term over-exposure to toxic metals and pesticides, or certain drugs. People who use a cocktail of pesticides in their homes have been found to be at twice the risk of developing Parkinson's.

This condition triggers deterioration of the nerve centres in a small part of the brain called the substantia nigra, which is responsible for sending messages down the nerves in the spinal cord to control muscles in the body. These messages are passed between brain cells, nerves and muscles by neurotransmitters, and dopamine is the main neurotransmitter produced within the substantia nigra. In PD patients, a number of these cells die and the amount of dopamine produced is therefore reduced.

As these events occur, a PD sufferer will generally find walking or getting out of a chair more of an effort. Muscles can stiffen and feel generally more tense. It's common for patients to experience tremors, rigidity and muscular spasms in different limbs to varying degrees. Other symptoms can include unsteadiness, chronic constipation, bladder problems, insomnia, difficulty swallowing, depression, weight loss, impulsive behaviour, impaired speech, a fixed facial expression and a shuffling gait. The person knows what they want the muscle to do, but the messages received by the muscle group are not properly co-ordinated to allow smooth movement.

People with PD also tend to suffer more melanoma skin cancer – which is why any PD sufferer should use organic, high-factor sun creams and wear a hat.

No single cause has yet been proven but nutrient deficiencies, heavy metal toxicity (especially from mercury and aluminium), exposure to pesticides, over-consumption of the artificial sweetener aspartame, viruses and carbon-monoxide poisoning are all linked to neurological conditions.

Children and adults should keep away from anything containing aluminium and mercury if they have had a recent vaccination, as many vaccinations often contain heavy metals that could potentially trigger neurological and other disorders in later years – see under *Mercury Fillings*.

Some prescription drugs can cause Parkinson-like symptoms. In addition, patients with Parkinson's have been found to have high levels of iron in the substantia nigra area of the brain, which can produce reactions that destroy dopamine-producing cells.

To replace dopamine most patients take a synthetic form of the amino acid levodopa (L-dopa), which the body then makes into dopamine, helping to restore brain function. Nutritional physician Dr Shamin Daya, based at the Wholistic Medical Centre in Harley Street, London, says: 'The main problem for these people is that they often lack the important co-factors of nutrients, such as zinc, magnesium, sometimes B1 or/and a type of activated vitamin B6 known as pyridoxal 5 phosphate (P5P), which are required to convert L-dopa to dopamine.'

Many of the drugs used to treat Parkinson's can cause lethargy and extreme mental confusion, or completely uncontrolled jerky movements if there is too much L-dopa in the body. As every case is unique, I strongly recommend that anyone with Parkinson's consults a nutritional physician, as this condition needs specialized care. Your doctor should be able to refer you to a nutritional physician if you are willing to pay privately.

Anyone with PD also needs to take care of their liver function and to make sure that they do not have a leaky gut. The gut is known as our 'second brain' by nutritional physicians, and if it is not working properly, you may not be absorbing sufficient nutrients from your diet and also suffer food intolerances. See under *Leaky Gut* and *Liver Problems*.

Foods to Avoid
- As much as possible, only eat organic-source foods and never use chemical-based spray pesticides in or near your home.
- Avoid foods cooked in aluminium or iron pots.
- Reduce stimulants such as coffee, colas, tea and alcohol, as these foods can affect tremors.
- Cut down on animal fats, especially red meat, cow's milk and cheese, which impair the metabolism of essential fats (see *Fats You Need To Eat*).

- Avoid refined sugars, in any form, that are found in highly refined and processed foods, such as mass-produced cakes, sugary drinks, refined breakfast cereals and bars, biscuits, pies and pre-packaged meals.
- Especially avoid additives and preservatives such as monosodium glutamate and aspartame, because of their negative effect on the brain.
- With professional guidance you may also need to eliminate gluten found in grains such as wheat, rye, oats and barley, as the gluten can prevent the absorption of nutrients and medication in some people.
- Don't fry food and avoid all hydrogenated and trans-fats, often found in margarines and pre-prepared foods. Frying foods causes more oxidation in the brain, which basically means more damage. These fats are also found in most mass-produced cakes, biscuits, pies and so on. Always check labels. Avoid all mass-produced vegetable oils.
- Protein foods sometimes interfere with the absorption of L-dopa, therefore only eat protein such as fish, organic chicken or lean meats in the evening after the final dose of L-dopa has been taken.

Friendly Foods

- Ensure an adequate dietary intake. Because chewing can become difficult, loss of appetite is common and nutrient deficiencies can speed the progression of the disease. Foods can be liquidized or meal replacements used.
- As much as possible eat only organic foods, which contain fewer pesticides and herbicides. A University of Miami post-mortem study in 1994 found pesticides more commonly in those who had died of Parkinson's Disease.
- Research has shown that restricting protein intake is helpful and that 90% of the daily intake should be eaten with the evening meal, when you are not having your L-dopa medication. This is extremely important advice not always given to patients on L-dopa. Protein competes for absorption with the L-dopa, so eating protein during the day, when most sufferers take their medication, can block the efficacy of the medication.
- Protein can be found in organic lean meats such as turkey plus fresh fish, eggs, beans, quinoa, lentils, nuts and seeds, fermented soya foods and wholegrains. The best sources of protein for Parkinson's sufferers are small amounts of soya, egg yolks, oily and white fish and poultry. You can also add organic hemp seed protein or whey protein to breakfast smoothies. See under *General Health Hints* for a great recipe.
- Generally, eat more beans and pulses rather than gluten-based foods such as breads. You can buy gluten- and wheat-free breads in most supermarkets and health stores.
- Include apples, pears, papaya, pumpkin, mangoes, cabbage, kale, watercress, cauliflower, carrots and broccoli in your diet.
- Root vegetables tend to be sprayed less, so eat more red beets and their tops, green beans, turnips, spinach and pumpkin.
- Use unrefined, organic sunflower, sesame (seeds) and olive oils for salad dressings and to drizzle over cooked foods such as brown rice or quinoa. These oils are rich in essential fats, which are vital for healthy brain function, as they enhance brain cell wall stability (see *Fats You Need To Eat*).
- Get into the habit of juicing. Use organic carrots, beetroots and artichokes, which are high in vitamins and minerals and help to cleanse the liver (see *Liver Problems*).
- If you have mercury fillings, use nori seaweed salt flakes, chlorella, apples and coriander, which detoxify metals from the body. See under *Mercury Fillings*.
- Dried or ready-to-eat organic fruits, such as prunes, figs and apricots, help to ease or prevent constipation, as does drinking at least 6 glasses of water daily.

P

- Black and purple grapes, blackberries and blueberries are high in antioxidants to help support the brain.
- Linseeds are high in omega-6 and omega-3 fats and really help to ease constipation. Soak a tablespoon of linseeds (flax) in cold water overnight, drain next morning and eat over low-sugar cereals, porridge or in smoothies.
- Begin drinking green or white teas, which are rich in antioxidants.
- Eat low-fat, live probiotic yoghurts to ensure there are plenty of friendly bacteria in the bowel.

Useful Remedies

- It is vital to take various nutrients in specific amounts for each individual case, and the supplements you take also depend on the time of day and which medication you are taking. Again, I strongly recommend that you see a qualified nutritionist or nutritional physician who can devise a programme specifically for you. Your own GP will need to refer you to a nutritional physician.
- Studies from the Birkmayer Institute for Parkinson's in Vienna has shown that NADH, a co-enzyme form of vitamin B3, can help increase energy levels, reduce depression and stimulate the body to produce more L-dopa. 5mg should be taken on an empty stomach at least 40 minutes before food. Professor Birkmayer's highly absorbable NADH is called Springfield Enada and is available worldwide. **NC. NB Anyone who is very stressed and suffers from palpitations should avoid this supplement. However, in some cases the intravenous form of this nutrient is more effective in Parkinson's – speak to your doctor about the intravenous form.**

- L-methionine – an essential sulphur amino acid, which readily crosses the blood-brain barrier where it can be converted into the vital nutrient S-Adenosyl methionine (SAMe). L-dopa supplementation reduces brain SAMe levels. Try L-methionine 500mg twice daily, 30 minutes before meals. **NC**
- Taking a full-spectrum antioxidant formula, such as vitamin C in combination with other antioxidants, vitamin E for example, helps to counteract the negative side effects of L-dopa. **NC, HN**
- The amino acids tyrosine and phenylalanine help to ensure that the brain has sufficient raw materials for the synthesis of dopamine. Dosages need to be set by a qualified doctor or nutritionist.
- The amino acid acetyl L-carnitine is very important, as it helps protect the brain and improves memory. One to one and a half grams daily in divided doses 30 minutes before meals.
- Lipoic acid is a major antioxidant to support brain function and removes heavy metals. Take 200mg three times daily.
- When we are young, the body makes a vitamin-like substance called Co-enzyme Q10, but as we age, levels fall. Parkinson's patients have been found to have 35% less CoQ10 than healthy people – it is needed to protect neurons in the brain. Under medical supervision, take around 200–400mg daily with a small amount of fat (such as olive oil or butter). **PN**
- Chlorella helps to rid the body of unwanted heavy metals – take 500mg twice daily. Otherwise use Green Magic Powder in smoothies or simply drink with a little water – containing Hawaiian spirulina, chlorella, lecithin, barley and wheat grass, kamut, pectin apple fibre, kelp and wheat sprouts, CoQ10, royal jelly, artichoke powder and lactobacillus acidophilus, it is a great all-round way to ingest good nutrients, encourage healthy bacteria, keep the body more alkaline and help keep you regular. Details on www.itsgreenmagic.com or call Helen Cruikshank on 07798 873266.
- Melatonin produced in the pineal gland at night is a very important antioxidant for the brain, as it induces natural sleep. Many PD patients experience sleep problems and Bio-

electromagnetics scientist Roger Coghill says: 'When you take melatonin supplements that you can buy on line and in the States, most synthetic tablets contain thousands of times the natural dose that your pineal gland normally produces.' Therefore, Roger has developed a supplement called Asphalia, extracted from certain grasses that contain natural melatonin, which mimic the normal dose made by your pineal gland at night, rather than the larger dose which you get in mass-produced tablets. Take 1–2 capsules 30 minutes before bed. Roger has permission from the MHRA (Medical Healthcare Regulatory Authority) to sell this food supplement in the UK. For more details or to find your nearest supplier, log on to www.asphalia.co.uk or tel: 01495 752122. **NB Asphalia should not be taken by severe asthmatics, children under one and by pregnant women in their third trimester.**

■ If you have mercury fillings, also see this section under *Mercury Fillings*.

Helpful Hints

■ As mercury fillings are linked to Parkinson's, have them checked by a holistic dentist and removed if necessary (with all the necessary protection during removal – otherwise you can become even more contaminated). See *Mercury Fillings*.

■ As many of the world's oceans are heavily polluted, high levels of mercury are also being reported in some coastal fish; see under *Mercury Fillings*.

■ There is a strong link between aluminium and mercury toxicity and PD, therefore avoid all aluminium cookware or aluminium foil. Read labels carefully, as cake mixes, antacids, buffered aspirin, self-raising flour, pickles, processed cheeses, and most deodorants and toothpastes contain aluminium.

■ Monosodium glutamate (MSG), the food additive, and aspartame, the artificial sweetener, have been linked to Parkinson's; therefore avoid all additives and preservatives whenever possible. More than 3,000 foods and drinks contain artificial sweeteners.

■ Also avoid in house 'air fresheners', many of which contain a cocktail of chemicals.

■ The anti-ageing hormone DHEA is well known to support brain function. This can easily be supplemented if you ask your doctor to test your hormone levels via a blood or saliva test. Never self-medicate with hormones.

■ See under the *Allergies* for details of the York and Genova Tests to discover any food intolerances.

■ Reduce stress. At times of stress the body uses dopamine to make the stress hormones nor-adrenaline and adrenaline, using up your already short supply. Tools for reducing stress include exercise, massage, relaxation techniques, meditation or enjoyable hobbies (see under *Stress*).

■ If tremors are worse at or after meal times, avoid protein (meat, fish, beans, nuts, seeds) at meals where you take your medication, as protein competes with the L-dopa for absorption.

■ Constipation is a major symptom that must be dealt with to ensure the proper elimination of toxins. In addition to dried fruits, linseeds (flax seeds) and water, try abdominal massage in a clockwise circular motion to massage the bowel. Take walks after meals, or supplement with magnesium (150mg x 3 times per day) to relax the bowel. See under *Constipation*.

■ As organophosphates (OPs) from pesticides and herbicides are now found in drinking water, use a good-quality water filter such as Kangen Water – an ionized, antioxidant water system that helps alkalize and rehydrate the body. As most people with Parkinson's are usually toxic, this water helps to re-balance the body. It's used in Japanese hospitals with highly beneficial health results. For full details contact the Wholistic Medical Centre on 020 7580 7537 or log on to www.kangenmiraclewater.co.uk

■ Read *Parkinson's Disease, The Way Forward* by Dr Geoffrey Leader and Lucille Leader (Bath Press). To order, call 020 7323 2382. This user-friendly book presents an integrated approach to the management of Parkinson's disease.

- Dr David Perlmutter, a neurologist in Naples, Florida, has pioneered the use of intravenous glutathione, which has had a dramatic effect on most of his Parkinson's patients. His book, *The Better Brain Book* (River Head Books) makes fascinating reading. Available from the Nutri Centre bookshop (**NC**), or log on to Dr Permutter's website: www.perlhealth.com
- Stem-cell therapy holds great promise for Parkinson's patients – for more details of where you can find cutting edge treatments, see under *Multiple Sclerosis*.
- For further help, contact The Parkinson's Disease Society. Helpline: 0808 800 0303. Website: www.parkinsons.org.uk. Or the European Parkinson's Disease Society. Tel: 01732 457683. Website: www.epda.eu.com

PCOS – Polycystic ovarian syndrome

(see also Infertility, Low Blood Sugar and Liver Problems)

One in five women who has a scan during gynaecological investigations has polycystic ovaries. About 80% of these women experience a variety of symptoms and are then classed as having PCOS. Symptoms may include irregular or no periods, erratic or no ovulation, sub-fertility, recurrent miscarriages, excess facial and body hair, fatigue, acne, weight gain that is hard to shift, hair loss, mood swings, abdominal pain, aching joints and dizziness. In the long term there is a sevenfold increase in the risk of cardiovascular problems and diabetes. Depression, anxiety, low self-esteem and possibly low iodine levels are also factors with this condition.

The job of the ovaries is to produce hormones, ripen and release eggs ready for fertilization, and prepare the lining of the womb for pregnancy. If no fertilization occurs, then the lining is shed, leading to a period. This whole process is governed by the sex hormones. Follicle-stimulating hormone (FSH) and luteinizing hormone (LH) are made by the pituitary in the brain, and in response to these hormones the ovaries then produce progesterone, testosterone and oestrogen. PCOS occurs when there is an imbalance in these hormones, namely high oestrogen, testosterone and LH. High levels of the hormone insulin needed to balance blood sugar levels are also produced. The body's insulin receptors on the surface of cells seem to switch off and stop listening to the signal from insulin, and so to compensate, the body overproduces insulin, which further disrupts the sex hormones. Research shows that by enhancing the body's ability to register the insulin, all hormone levels can become normalized.

Foods to Avoid

- Also see this section under *Low Blood Sugar*.
- Eat less red meat, beef, pork, animal-source dairy products and fried foods. Excess consumption of the wrong kinds of fat can lead to weight gain and cardiovascular problems (sufferers of PCOS have a higher risk of developing cardiovascular problems). When preparing foods grill, bake or stir-fry with olive oil. See under *Fats You Need To Eat*.
- Refined sugar in all forms, as sugar affects hormone levels in the body. Avoid it in mass-produced breakfast cereals and bars, cakes, biscuits, sweets, fizzy drinks, cordials and chocolate. Nutritionist Gareth Zeal says: 'Most women with this problem tend to be eating too many animal-based products including milk, cheese and meat, plus excessive amounts of starchy refined carbohydrate foods, such as cakes, biscuits, bread, white potatoes and so on.'
- Alcohol exerts an oestrogen-like action in the body, so it is best avoided. If you must indulge, keep to a minimum and drink red wine, as this helps to protect against cardiovascular disease.
- Cut right back on caffeine, which can disrupt hormone levels – coffee, tea, cola drinks, chocolate, energy drinks and some painkillers contain it.

Friendly Foods

- Eat small regular meals that contain complex carbohydrates – such as brown rice, pasta, rye bread, millet, sweet potatoes and quinoa – as these foods help to keep blood sugar levels in the body more even and hence reduce insulin, which disrupts hormone levels. See under *Low Blood Sugar*.
- Eating small amounts of protein with all meals and snacks helps to make insulin more effective by slowing the release of sugars into the blood. Lentils, beans, eggs, fish, lean chicken and turkey, nuts and seeds are all ideal as sources of protein.
- Foods from the brassica family – cauliflower, broccoli, watercress, cabbage and Brussels sprouts – help encourage excretion of excess hormones.
- Omega-3 essential fatty acids, found in linseeds (flax seeds), hemp seeds and oily fish (salmon, mackerel, sardines, pilchards, herring and anchovies), have an important role to play in helping to control insulin resistance and hence hormone disruption.
- Go organic, as many of the pesticides liberally sprayed onto foods can have a hormone-disrupting action
- Fibre is known to bind to excess hormones and help to remove them from the body. Eat more whole grains, brown rice, millet, beans, lentils, oats and lots of fresh fruit and vegetables.
- Eat live, sugar-free yoghurt daily to feed the good bacteria in the gut, as this helps to break down excess hormones.
- Phyto-oestrogens help to reduce high oestrogen levels. Therefore eat foods such as miso and tempeh (a fermented form of soya), plus linseeds (flax seeds), beans and lentils.
- Use organic rice or agave syrup, or xylitol instead of refined sugars, as they have a much lower glycaemic index.
- As PCOS can be related to low Iodine levels, use nori seaweed or kelp flakes as a salt substitute – or increase your intake of sea vegetables such as samphire or kelp.

Useful Remedies

- Ask at your health shop for a multi-vitamin/mineral for your age. Take daily.
- B-vitamins are essential for balancing sugar levels in the body and help with oestrogen-related hormonal problems. Most multi-vitamin and mineral formulas contain B-vitamins. Your multi should contain plenty of B-group vitamins, so there's no need to take twice.
- Agnus castus (1ml twice daily) and saw palmetto (1ml twice daily); taken together. These have been used for centuries to balance female hormones and are great for reducing PCOS symptoms.
- Methionine is an amino acid that greatly helps support liver function. Take 500mg twice daily, 30 minutes before main meals. See under *Liver Problems*.
- The mineral chromium helps to balance blood sugar, which is a major factor in PCOS. Take 100–200mcg twice daily.
- Almost all the companies featured on pages 15–16 offer brassica vegetable-extract capsules that help to balance hormones. The Life Extension Foundation make a Triple Action Cruciferous Vegetable Extract with Resveratrol (from red grapes); www.lef.org or contact the Nutri Centre on 0845 602 6744. **NC**

Helpful Hints

- If you are overweight, lose weight. Studies at St Mary's Hospital in London found that moderate weight loss helped to correct hormonal abnormalities, reduced body hair, and improved chances of conception.
- Exercise not only helps with weight loss and strengthens the heart, but also releases feel-good hormones in the body. Aim for at least three 20-minute sessions per week. Start with a brisk walk outside, as daylight is also known to lift low moods and depression.

- Use a water filter. Millions of women currently take contraceptive pills and some of the chemicals they contain inevitably find their way into the water cycle; if you drink unfiltered tap water, it may have an effect on your hormone levels.
- Food wrapped or cooked in plastic or cling film will have a negative effect on hormone balance. The risk is increased when these plastics are heated. If you do have to buy food that is wrapped in plastic, transfer these foods to a glass container as soon as you get home. Above all, never microwave food wrapped in cling film or in plastic containers.
- Women with PCOS have found acupuncture useful in helping to kick start non-existent cycles and regulating cycle length.
- Learn to relax and tackle your stresses, both physical and emotional. Stress contributes to high insulin levels and hormonal imbalances.
- Essential oils of agnus castus, geranium and rose may be beneficial to balance hormones, while sandalwood, neroli, ylang ylang and mandarin are good for relaxation. Add to a relaxing bath or use in an oil burner.
- www.verity-pcos.org.uk is a great, informative website with lots of practical information and fact sheets. They also run conferences about PCOS three times a year.

PHLEBITIS   *(see also Atherosclerosis, Circulation and Leg Ulcers)*

P

Phlebitis is caused by inflammation of the walls of the veins, usually near the surface of the skin. It is often combined with the formation of small blood clots on the area of the inflammation. It may be triggered by a sensitivity to external irritants, such as washing powders, or by food intolerances. The condition can occur after injections or intravenous infusions and is common in intravenous drug abusers. It is more common in people who have varicose veins and also in blood vessel disorders, such as Buerger's disease. Symptoms include swelling and redness along and around the affected segment of vein, which can become very tender when touched. The best way to prevent this condition is to keep your circulation in good condition by eating more of the right foods.

Foods to Avoid
- Identify and avoid foods to which you have a sensitivity, the most common being wheat and dairy produce from cows and any animal sources. (See under *Allergies* for details of the York, Genova and Bio Meridian Tests to help you find problem foods.)
- You may also be sensitive to gluten.
- Cut down on all saturated fats, found in animal produce, sausages, meat pies, full-fat cheese, milk, chocolate and hard margarines.
- Don't fry food and never use mass-produced, refined, hydrogenated oils. See *Fats You Need To Eat*.
- Reduce your intake of cakes, burgers, biscuits, highly refined breakfast cereals, mass-produced white breads and pastas.
- Many of these foods are packed with fats, salt and refined sugar. Refined sugar converts to fat in the body if it is not used up during exercise (see also *General Health Hints*).

Friendly Foods
- Increase your intake of oily fish, which is rich in the omega-3 essential fats that help to thin blood naturally.
- Sprinkle wheat germ and lecithin granules over low-sugar cereals and desserts. They help to emulsify the bad fats, which aids circulation.

- Buy a packet each of organic, unsalted walnuts, Brazil nuts, almonds, sunflower and pumpkin seeds, sesame seeds and linseeds (flax seeds), which are high in omega-6 essential fats. Whiz them all in a blender and keep in an airtight jar in the fridge. Sprinkle over any foods you like. These add healthy fats, fibre and minerals such as zinc to your diet, which are vital for skin and wound-healing.
- Eat more stone-ground wholemeal bread, pasta and noodles. Try lentil, corn and rice pastas, which are readily available in supermarkets and health shops.
- Use skimmed milk, or try non-dairy alternatives, such as rice or almond milks.
- Include garlic in your diet, which thins blood naturally.
- Olive oil and avocados are rich in mono-unsaturated fats, which are healthy and aid healing.
- Eat more fresh fruits and vegetables, especially pineapple and papaya, which are rich in digestive enzymes that aid healing. They are also anti-inflammatory.
- Eat more curries rich in turmeric, which again has anti-inflammatory properties.

Useful Remedies
- Take 400iu daily of natural-source vitamin E to help thin the blood naturally and ease discomfort. **BC**
- Take a high-strength multi-vitamin and mineral specifically for men and/or women over 50.
- Some people find relief by placing raw papaya on the affected area for an hour a day.
- Bromelain, extracted from pineapple, has good anti-inflammatory effects. Take 500mg daily.
- Use Circulation Tincture – containing witch hazel, horse chestnut, ginger and bilberry, which all help to increase circulation and reduce swelling associated with this condition. Available in one liquid formula from the Organic Pharmacy. **OP**
- Pycnogenol – pine bark extract – has been shown to reduce inflammation, ease pain, improve blood flow and help make veins more elastic. Start with 80mg twice daily and then, after a month, reduce to 40mg daily.

Helpful Hints
- Basically, you need to get moving. Begin by walking for 15 minutes daily and gradually increase over a one-month period to 1 hour a day.
- When applicable, use stairs instead of lifts.
- An extremely gentle and easy exercise regime, such as swimming, yoga, qigong or t'ai chi, would also be helpful; as would reflexology and acupuncture (see *Useful Information*). T'ai chi can be practised by people of any age – even if they are in their 80s and 90s.

PHOBIAS *(see also Adrenal Exhaustion, Low Blood Sugar and Panic Attacks)*

A phobia is an extreme or irrational fear attached to a specific object or situation that is not life-threatening – but for the person with the phobia, the fear is often overwhelming and their lives can become a nightmare. The most common phobias are a fear of confined spaces, or various animals and insects, such as birds or spiders. Certain social situations provoke anxiety in some people, who fear they will become trapped or embarrassed. As adrenal exhaustion and low blood sugar can contribute to this problem, please also read these sections.

Foods to Avoid
- See under *Low Blood Sugar* and *Insulin Resistance*.
- As much as possible, avoid stimulants such as coffee, tea, alcohol and refined sugars, and cut down or eliminate foods or drinks containing caffeine or sugar.
- See also *Panic Attacks* and *General Health Hints*.

Friendly Foods

- Low levels of serotonin are linked to feelings of depression. Serotonin is made from a constituent of protein called tryptophan, therefore include more foods such as fish, turkey, chicken, cottage cheese, beans, avocados, bananas and wheat germ in your diet to help raise your mood and keep you calmer.
- Calming foods also include brown rice and pastas, noodles, couscous, sweet potato, lettuce, mushrooms, peppers and root vegetables.
- Oats are a great food for helping to re-build nervous tissue – have oat-based porridge with a protein shake for breakfast daily.
- Sprinkle wheat germ over breakfast cereals or fruit whips. There are plenty of cereals available made from amaranth, quinoa and kamut, sweetened with a little apple juice. Cereals, including porridge, are rich in B-vitamins, which help to keep you calm.
- Drink more decaffeinated green tea and liquorice tea.

Useful Remedies

- The amino acid L-theanine – found in green tea – really helps to keep you calm without making you feel in any way sleepy. Take 100mg 4 times throughout the day. **NC**
- The herbs ashwagandha, Siberian ginseng and gotu kola are adaptogenic herbs, which help the adrenal system to normalize. These are all included in the Advanced Stress Formula by Holos Health www.holoshealth.com **NC**
- Take a high-strength vitamin B-complex daily to help support your nerves.
- 5–Hydroxytryptophan (5HTP) is a supplement that helps to raise serotonin levels in the brain naturally, helping to improve mood and calm you down. Start with 25mg and increase over 10–14 days to 75mg three times daily. **HN**

Helpful Hints

- Learn to meditate. People who practise meditation regularly have lower blood pressure than they would have otherwise, are less anxious, and are more able to cope during stressful situations.
- First Steps to Freedom, a self-help group, have a helpline for people with phobias. Fact sheets, self-help booklets, audio/video tapes, books and online support groups are also available. For further information write to First Steps to Freedom, PO Box 476, Newquay, TR7 1WQ. Tel: 0845 120 2916. The helpline is open 10.00am–10.00pm every day. Email: first.steps@btconnect.com Website: www.first-steps.org
- Hypnotherapy is an excellent way to find the root cause of your problem and to learn how to let it go so you can lead a normal life (see *Useful Information*).
- Celebrity hypnotherapist Paul McKenna has made some great self-hypnosis CDs that help to remove phobias. Website: www.paulmckenna.com
- Homeopathic Aconite 200c is a good remedy when you are experiencing intense fear or terror.
- Take some more exercise, because this helps to produce more mood-boosting chemicals in the brain.

PILES (HAEMORRHOIDS)

(see also Constipation and Varicose Veins)

Piles are basically varicose veins formed inside the anus when veins become enlarged. If you suffer chronic long-term constipation, then the veins can break through the anus and protrude externally. If you feel this happening and the vein is still soft and pliable, you can carefully ease the swollen vein back inside the anus. But if the pile becomes hardened and forms a clot and remains outside the anus, this calls for immediate medical attention. When you go to the loo, if you have piles or an anal fissure, you can often see blood in the stools and experience extreme discomfort and itching in that area. Also, if your liver is congested – which is common in this problem – it can place more pressure on your back, which in turn adds pressure to your venous system, which can make piles worse.

Other factors involved in the formation of piles are persistent coughing, pregnancy and childbirth, standing and/or sitting for long periods, overuse of laxatives, and travelling long distances while in a seated position for hours on end – all of which raise pressure in rectal veins. If you bleed from the anus at any time, you should seek medical attention immediately.

The secret to avoiding piles is to avoid constipation in the first place.

Foods to Avoid
- Generally, you need to avoid eating too many flour-based foods – cakes, mass-produced white breads, refined biscuits, pies and desserts – as flour and refined sugars gunk up the bowel. If you mix flour and water together, you get a very sticky paste and this does not change consistency in the bowel!
- Melted cheese and full-fat cheeses can also cause constipation.
- Red meat takes a long time to digest. If you must eat meat, have only small portions and no more than twice a week.
- Coffee, canned fizzy drinks and alcohol all dehydrate the bowel.
- Avoid mass-produced foods such as burgers and high-fat take-aways.
- Reduce your intake of full-fat dairy products from cows.
- Avoid sodium-based salt.
- For some people, eating citrus fruit and tomatoes makes the situation worse.

Friendly Foods
- Drink at least 6–8 glasses of water daily, even if you are not thirsty.
- Eat far more fresh, lightly cooked vegetables and salads – especially green leafy vegetables such as celery, spinach, kale, watercress, bean sprouts, spring greens and cabbage.
- Figs, prunes, apples, pineapples, apricots, bananas, mangos, papaya, avocados, grapes and melons will all help reduce the constipation. Strawberries, raspberries, peaches, sultanas, raisins and dates can be eaten regularly (unless you have blood sugar or candida-, fungal-type problems).
- Linseeds (flax) are really helpful for keeping the bowels more regular. Soak one tablespoon of linseeds in cold water overnight and then drain and add to low-sugar breakfast cereals, porridge or in smoothies. Adjust the amount to suit your individual needs.
- Eat good-quality protein, such as skinless chicken, fish, tempeh, beans, peas and pulses.
- Eat more wholemeal bread, pastas and noodles.
- Enjoy low-sugar, high-fibre cereals for breakfast. Try cereals made from quinoa, amaranth, rice or millet, which are less likely to irritate the gut than wheat bran and cereals.
- Use oat and rice brans over cereals and in smoothies.
- Try blackstrap molasses, unsweetened jams, organic agave syrup or xylitol instead of refined sugars.
- Replace cow's milk with low-fat goat's milk and organic rice, almond, quinoa or coconut milks.
- Almonds, sunflower, pumpkin and sesame seeds are all rich sources of fibre.
- Experiment with coffees made from rye and chicory or herb teas, such as rose hip, and unsweetened fruit juices.

- Use more unrefined organic olive, sunflower and walnut oils for salad dressings.
- Eat live, low-fat yoghurt, which is rich in friendly bacteria that encourage healthy bowels.

Useful Supplements

- Pine bark extract known as pycnogenol, an antioxidant, has been shown in studies at the University of Munster in Germany to help stop bleeding and significantly reduce pain from haemorrhoids if 300mg is taken daily while symptoms are acute, then reduced after four days to 150mg daily for a further 4 days. You can also use pycnogenol-based creams. **PN**
- The herb butcher's broom helps to improve circulation in the lower body and helps tone the veins. Take 500mg twice daily.
- Horse chestnut capsules help to strengthen the capillaries – take 50–75mg of standardized aescin (the active ingredient) twice daily.
- Take 2 grams of vitamin C spread throughout the day with meals, plus 1 gram of bioflavonoids and 400iu of full-spectrum, natural-source vitamin E daily to strengthen blood-vessel walls.
- Vitamin A, 20,000iu per day for a month, will help to repair tissue damage. **Take this dose for only 1 month and take no more than 3,000iu daily if you are pregnant or planning a pregnancy.** Note that liver is very rich in vitamin A; if you eat a lot, you do not then need to take extra vitamin A as a supplement. After one month, switch to a natural-source carotene complex (7mg daily), which naturally converts to vitamin A in the body and is very safe. **SVHC**
- Take a vitamin B-complex to aid digestion, which in turn aids bowel function.
- Zinc is vital for soft tissue healing; take 30mg daily with 1–2mg of copper.
- After 3 months on this regimen, switch to a good-quality multi-vitamin and mineral.
- Rutin (found in buckwheat) helps to strengthen vein walls. Take 300mg daily.
- prebiotic fibre from the agave and other plant sources helps encourage production of friendly bacteria in the bowel, which in turn aids more efficient bowel function. Try Agave Digestive Immune Support powder from The Life Extension via www.lef.org or call any of the companies mentioned on pages 15–16 and ask for their prebiotic formulas.

Helpful Hints

- Insert pilewort suppositories – which are best used before going to bed. They are made with olive oil, beeswax and pilewort, to help soften the pile and reduce any swelling. **OP**
- After you have opened your bowels, squeeze the cheeks of the bottom together several times. This action will encourage blood flow into that area, which helps stop piles forming.
- Take one or two cayenne pepper capsules with main meals to increase circulation and help to reduce any bleeding. **SHS**
- Apply combinations of zinc oxide, vitamin E, and aloe vera gel or olive oil to the affected area. This should help to soften the piles and make them less painful.
- Apply cold witch hazel lotion frequently to haemorrhoids to shrink the swollen blood vessel. The Organic Pharmacy supplies a witch hazel, bilberry and horse chestnut cream. **OP**
- In an acute situation, or if you cannot see your doctor immediately, try dissolving 1 tablespoon of Epsom salts into 6 tablespoons of lukewarm water and carefully apply with cotton wool to the affected area. This helps to reduce the swelling until you can see your GP.
- Nelson's Homeopathic Pharmacy make the remedy Haemorrhoid, which is very useful. Email: mailorder@nelsonshp.com or call 020 7079 1288.
- Homeopathic remedies, such as Staphysagria or Aesculus (horse chestnut) can also help. See a qualified homeopath for individual remedies.
- Bathing the anus in cold water every morning can help prevent recurrence of piles.
- Bowel function can be affected by drugs such as antacids, anti-depressants, excessive iron tablets and laxative abuse. If you think these may be a factor, see your doctor.

- Laxatives taken in the long term can make the bowel lazy, and can increase the need to strain.
- Squat rather than sit to open your bowels to take pressure off the lower part of the bowel.

PILL, CONTRACEPTIVE

The progestogen-only pill, or mini-pill, provides contraception by thickening the mucous in the cervix and making it impenetrable by the sperm. Progestogen is synthetic progesterone. The combined pill, which contains both oestrogen and progestogen, prevents pregnancy by thickening the mucous and suppressing ovulation. Potential side effects from taking the pill are an increased risk of cancers of the breast and cervix, blood clotting in the legs, high blood pressure, increased risk of heart disease and stroke, weight gain, fluid retention and migraines.

Women who took the pill for 10 years or more back in the sixties have a much higher risk of developing breast cancer. The pill depletes the body of vital nutrients, such as vitamins B and C, plus the minerals magnesium, calcium and zinc. I took the pill for more than 10 years from the late 1960s to early 1970s, which I believe was the root cause of my continual heavy bleeding, so that at 31 I needed an emergency hysterectomy. If you must take the pill, then have regular breaks of several months at a time. Taking the pill over long periods can increase the risk of developing candida (see *Candida*).

P

Foods to Avoid
- Greatly reduce your intake of refined sugars, too much animal protein, dairy products from cows, saturated fats found in dairy and hard margarines, cakes, pastries, burgers, sausages and so on.
- Reduce your intake of sodium-based salt, caffeine and tobacco.
- Reduce alcohol intake.
- See *General Health Hints*.

Friendly Foods
- Include organic raw wheat germ in your diet, as it is rich in vitamins B and E.
- Eat far more whole-grains, brown rice, millet, quinoa, couscous, wholemeal breads and pastas, fruits and vegetables.
- Cereals and oats are also rich in B-vitamins.
- Cherries, papaya, mango, cantaloupe melons, apricots, and most fruit and vegetables are rich sources of vitamin C.
- Eat more fish, plus sunflower, pumpkin and sesame seeds, which are high in zinc, as the pill raises copper levels which lower zinc levels.
- Eat more live, low-fat yoghurt, containing healthy bacteria, which are depleted by the pill.
- Eat more cabbage, watercress, broccoli and cauliflower, which contain a hormone-regulating substance called indole-3-carbinole.
- See also *General Health Hints*.

Useful Supplements
- Take a multi-vitamin and mineral such as Femforte 1 by BioCare. **BC**
- Make sure any supplement/multi-nutrient you take contains at least 30mg of zinc.
- Take a B-complex, as the pill depletes all the B-vitamins.
- Take vitamin C in a magnesium or calcium ascorbate form. Taking 250mg–500mg with food daily helps to prevent any deficiency caused by the pill.

- Indole-3-carbinol is an important nutrient extracted from broccoli, watercress and cabbage, which helps to regulate hormones. Take 200mg daily. From all good health stores.
- Support your liver by taking nutrients One & Two by Metabolics, which aid detoxification of excess hormones from the liver. Available from the Wholistic Medical Centre on 020 7580 7537 or via Metabolics on 01380 812799. Three capsules daily with meals.
- See also *Liver Problems*.

Helpful Hints
- Studies since the 1960s have consistently shown that women are at a greater risk of a pulmonary embolism when taking the pill – even the lower oestrogen-containing pills. If you are on the pill, you should not smoke, as this considerably increases the risk of some hazards, such as blood clots and heart disease.

POLYCYSTIC OVARIAN SYNDROME

(see PCOS – Polycystic Ovarian Syndrome)

POLYMYALGIA RHEUMATICA *(see also Fibromyalgia and Rheumatoid Arthritis)*

POST-NATAL DEPRESSION

(see also Adrenal Exhaustion and Low Blood Sugar)

Post-natal depression affects one in every 10 women following the birth of their babies. Although the birth of a child is, for most women, a time of great joy, some women feel extremely low immediately after giving birth, which in itself can be incredibly exhausting. This can be due to hormonal changes, fluctuating blood sugar levels and/or nutrient deficiencies. In naturopathic terms post-natal depression is linked to adrenal exhaustion, as hormones produced during pregnancy and the birth, such as cortisol and adrenaline, sap the adrenal glands, which can leave you feeling totally exhausted and emotionally drained. See under *Adrenal Exhaustion*.

In addition, anxiety about coping with a new baby, lack of sleep, perhaps financial problems, and, of course, the realization that life has changed for good, can all add to this condition. For a few women, the feeling of depression lasts for much longer than a few weeks, which can seriously undermine their ability to cope.

Firstly ask your doctor to test for low iron levels – an obvious factor if there was heavy blood loss during or after the birth. This condition can be greatly alleviated by taking the right supplements for a few weeks. Symptoms vary from increased or decreased appetite, a feeling that one is a failure, depression, an inability to cope, feelings of panic, and sometimes aggressive feelings towards the baby (see also *Low Blood Sugar* and *Depression*).

Nutritional physician Dr Shamin Daya says: 'Depression basically denotes an imbalance in the brain chemistry. Once the right nutrients are given in the right amounts, especially B vitamins, then the depression can easily be alleviated.'

Nutritionist Gareth Zeal adds, 'Women who take 3–4 grams of omega-3 fish oils, plus 1000iu of Vitamin D3 during and after pregnancy are dramatically less likely to suffer post-natal depression. Their children are also less likely to suffer many childhood conditions such as ADD or have poor eyesight and will be far less likely to develop depressive-type conditions in later life.'

Foods to Avoid

- Reduce stimulating foods, such as refined sugar, caffeine and alcohol, which trigger the release of more cortisol.
- See *Foods to Avoid* under *Adrenal Exhaustion* and *Low Blood Sugar*.

Friendly Foods

- See *Friendly Foods* in *Adrenal Exhaustion*, *Depression* and *Low Blood Sugar*.

Useful Remedies

- As low levels of B-vitamins are associated with this condition, take a high-strength vitamin B-complex daily for at least 2 months.
- You can take the herb agnus castus to help re-balance your hormones even if you are breast-feeding – take 5ml of the tincture daily.
- Magnesium helps induce feelings of calm. Take 1000mg daily in divided doses with food, plus 30mg of zinc (supports brain chemistry), and iron (in a formula such as Spatone, or take iron phosphate in doses based on blood tests via your GP) – 1–4 capsules daily. Taking these minerals will greatly ease symptoms after a few days.
- Take a multi-vitamin and mineral that contains at least 500mg of vitamin C and 150mcg of selenium.
- Try Femarone, a herbal formula containing raspberry leaf, squaw vine and uva ursi, which all help to balance hormones following childbirth. **SHS**
- Omega-3 fish oils; taking 4 grams daily can really help mother and baby (via breast milk).
- Take homeopathic caulophyllum, cimicifuga, pulsatilla and sepia – 1 pill, 4 times a day. This blend helps to balance the hormones and reduces feelings of doom and hopelessness, tears and so on. **OP**
- Mother can also take vitamin D3 – 1000iu daily, again to help mother and baby.

Helpful Hints

- Post-natal depression is often caused by the sudden fall in progesterone levels just before birth in women whose bodies are slow to begin making progesterone again. You can use a natural progesterone cream, which is easily absorbed and will bring your progesterone levels up again until your body takes over. If you require further information on natural progesterone and a list of doctors who use it, send a first-class stamp to The Natural Progesterone Information Service, PO Box 24, Buxton, SK17 9FB. Via blood or saliva tests your doctor can tell you if your progesterone levels need topping up.
- In Britain, natural progesterone cream is available on prescription – but overseas and in Ireland it is available over the counter and it can be ordered for your own use. For an information sheet, call Pharm West on 001 310 301 4015. **PN**
- Homeopathic Ignatia 30c, taken twice daily for up to a week, is particularly good for mothers who thought that having a baby was going to be all roses.
- And for those who feel enveloped by a black cloud, try homeopathic Cimicifuga 30c twice daily for up to a week.
- As much depression is linked to the liver, see also *Liver Problems* and *Depression*.
- Mild post-natal depression can be greatly helped by getting more sleep, and by getting out of the house and away from the baby for brief periods. Don't bottle up your feelings; talk things over with a friend or relative. Releasing your feelings really helps to put things in perspective and to realize just how many women are in a similar situation.

P

PRE-MENSTRUAL TENSION and PRE-MENSTRUAL SYNDROME (PMT/PMS)

(see also Low Blood Sugar and Liver Problems)

PMS causes a variety of physical and emotional symptoms in the days prior to menstruation. They vary from mood swings, food cravings and depression to breast tenderness and enlargement, fluid retention and bloating. Changes in hormone levels also cause some women to experience migraine-type symptoms. For one in 10 women, pre-menstrual mood changes are extreme. PMS is associated with imbalanced levels of progesterone and oestrogen (see *Menopause* for details of natural progesterone and oestrogen creams). Low blood sugar is common prior to a period and once blood sugar is balanced symptoms often disappear (see also *Low Blood Sugar*). Many women with PMS also have candida (see also *Candida*) and food intolerances mainly to wheat, caffeine, gluten and sometimes animal dairy foods. Congestion of the liver is also linked to PMS (see *Liver Problems*).

Foods to Avoid

- Generally, you need to cut down on animal fats, burgers, sausages, and heavy, rich, meat-based meals that usually contain high levels of saturated fat and salt.
- All high-salt foods, such as crisps and salted peanuts, and highly processed meat, such as salami, should be avoided, as salt will add to the water-retention problem.
- Stimulants such as alcohol, tea and coffee, caffeine in any form, fizzy and energy drinks, chocolate, snacks, cakes, biscuits and fast foods (such as croissants and Danish pastries) will all play havoc with your blood sugar.

Friendly Foods

- Starting the day with an oat-based cereal, such as porridge, with a chopped apple and a few sunflower seeds and raisins, will help to balance blood sugar until lunchtime.
- It would also be wise to eat some protein with breakfast, which really helps to balance blood sugar for longer as protein takes longer to digest. Try an omelette or poached or boiled eggs – or make a smoothie with nuts and seeds with added whey or hemp seed protein powders. See under *General Health Hints* for a recipe.
- Drink more water and try calming herbal teas such as camomile.
- Include small amounts of quality protein with each meal. Fresh fish, eggs, chicken and turkey without the skin, cottage cheese, cooked tofu, lentils, quinoa, peas, and sunflower, pumpkin and sesame seeds, plus all dried beans and pulses, are rich in fibre, protein and essential fats.
- Foods such as tempeh or miso, sweet potatoes, pumpkin, broccoli, cauliflower, and Brussels sprouts all help to balance your hormones naturally.
- Add organic sunflower and walnut oil to salad dressings.
- Snack on apples, pears and bananas, and try rice and oat cakes, spelt, amaranth crackers and wholemeal bread spread with a low-fat houmous, tahini or goat's cheese. If you tend to eat too many bananas, this can affect blood sugar, so always eat a few pumpkin or sunflower seeds at the same time to slow the sugar release.
- Many health food shops now sell low-sugar snacks. Eat these with a piece of fruit; again, this will help reduce any cravings.

Useful Remedies

To be taken all the time, not only during a period:

- B-complex containing at least 50mg of B6 per day, which is needed in the liver to process oestrogens.

- Gamma-linolenic acid (GLA) is the main ingredient in evening primrose oil, which helps to reduce breast pain. Take 100–500mg of GLA daily. **BC**
- Take 1 gram of omega-3 fish oils daily, to help reduce tender breasts and raise mood.
- Take calcium at 400mg and magnesium at 600mg per day in divided doses, to reduce the symptoms of PMS, as these minerals help keep you calm. Most companies make a two-in-one formula.
- Also take a multi-vitamin and mineral for women, which contains a further 50mg of B6 to make your total daily intake 100–150mg per day.
- If your sugar/carbohydrate cravings are acute, take 150mcg of chromium daily, which kicks in after a few days and really helps to reduce sugar cravings.
- The amino acid L-glutamine also helps to reduce sugar/starch cravings and heals any leaky gut. Take 500mg twice daily 30 minutes before food.
- Try the herbal menstrual formula Femarone, containing blessed thistle, squaw vine and barberry and cramp bark – which all help to cleanse the reproductive organs and balance hormones. **SHS**

Helpful Hints
- Dr Marilyn Glenville, a leading nutritional physician and expert in women's health problems, has formulated drops containing blue cohosh, agnus castus, lady's mantle and cramp bark that help relieve breast pain, water retention, mood swings and headaches. For more information, log on to the website: www.marilynglenville.com
- When you are stressed, you produce too much adrenaline, which eventually exhausts your endocrine (hormone) system and depletes calcium from your bones. See *Osteoporosis* and *Stress*.
- Start taking more regular exercise to reduce stress, or learn to meditate. Find some time each day to call your own, even if it's only a relaxing bath for 30 minutes.
- Treat yourself to an aromatherapy massage each month, or add essential oils of rose, ylang ylang, neroli, jasmine or geranium to your bath. Clary sage is great for reducing cramping period pains.
- If you smoke, give it up.

PRICKLY HEAT

Basically, this condition arises because the skin cannot release perspiration adequately. This irritating and unsightly condition usually affects fair-skinned people, such as myself, in tropical or sub-tropical climates. It initially appears as an itchy red, raised rash of hundreds of tiny bumps anywhere on the body. It has been linked to food intolerances (see under *Allergies*), and chemical levels in drinking water, but can just as easily be triggered by sun lotions, shower gels and soaps to which the individual becomes more sensitive in the heat and sun. I tend to suffer prickly heat on my shins if I stand for too long in tropical temperatures, which causes blood to 'pool' in my legs. Alcohol, antibiotics and aspirin can also trigger prickly heat. Many people who suffer these types of reactions have a leaky gut (see under *Leaky Gut*).

Foods to Avoid
- Try cutting out cow's milk and products, as well as wheat, peanuts, tea and coffee – although the culprits could be something quite unusual, such as radishes or orange juice. See *Allergies*.
- Avoid really hot drinks and highly spiced foods.

Friendly Foods

- Eat more foods that nourish the skin from the inside out, such as apples, carrots, spinach (best raw), watercress, broccoli, pumpkin, cantaloupe melons, apricots, mango, papaya and figs.
- Artichokes, beetroot and asparagus cleanse the liver, which in turn aids healing in the skin.
- Onion and garlic are rich sources of quercetin, which is a natural anti-histamine.
- Avocados and oily fish are fabulous for the skin.
- Include more organic sunflower and pumpkin seeds, linseeds (flax seeds), almonds and Brazil nuts in your diet; these are rich in essential fats.
- Use more organic, unrefined extra-virgin olive, walnut or sunflower oils over food and in salad dressings.
- Drink bottled or pure filtered water.
- Muesli and most cereals are high in B-vitamins, which help to prevent dry skin.
- Nettle tea will help reduce the inflammation.

Useful Remedies

- Take 2–3 grams of vitamin C in an ascorbate form with meals, as vitamin C acts like a natural anti-histamine.
- Take a natural-source carotene complex for 14 days before travel and throughout your holiday.
- Take a high-strength B-complex.
- Take a multi-vitamin and mineral formula daily for your age and gender.
- Omega-3 fish oils help protect against free radical damage in the skin from the sun, and if you are taking sufficient amounts, these fats help to reduce burning of the skin. Take 2 grams daily long term. But you still need organic sun creams!
- Take 1000iu of vitamin D3 daily throughout the year.

Helpful Hints

- If at all possible, expose your skin to sensible amounts of full-spectrum light prior to going into intense sunshine, as this helps to build more pigment in the skin. Several clinics in the UK offer Full Spectrum Real Sunlight – in which the harmful UVA and UVB rays have been greatly reduced, which enables you to make more vitamin D while encouraging production of the natural pigment. For details, call the Wholistic Medical Centre in London on 020 7580 7537 or log on to: www.realsunlight.co.uk
- In most cases, prickly heat will clear up on its own in a few days if the affected area is kept cool and dry. Take regular cool showers and allow the skin to dry naturally.
- Use a skin brush regularly to help remove dead skin cells and allow the pores to work correctly.
- Avoid using any insect repellent on the affected areas.
- Once your skin is dry, apply aloe vera gel.
- Don't use any type of oil-based product, which can block your sweat glands.
- If the prickly heat does not clear within 4–5 days and any infection sets in, you must see a doctor.
- To prevent prickly heat, avoid situations that can lead to excessive sweating, such as hot, humid environments and strenuous physical activity.
- Wear loose-fitting cotton clothes.
- Buy products in their most natural and unadulterated state. For anyone who suffers from dermatitis or skin allergies, The Green People Company makes organic skin, hair and body lotions, sunscreens and toothpaste, and they also have an advice line. Tel: 01403 740350. Email: organic@greenpeople.co.uk Website: www.greenpeople.co.uk

- Many strong antibiotics and drugs make the skin very sun-sensitive. If you are taking antibiotics, stay out of the sun.
- The herb St John's wort can also make the skin sensitive.
- Essential oils, such as lemon oil, can make your skin hyper-sensitive when exposed to sunlight; do not use such oils if you are going in the sun.
- Stay out of the midday sun and never allow your skin to go red.
- Take the homeopathic remedy Urtica 6c three times daily in between meals to reduce the redness. Discontinue once the rash begins to fade. Or try homeopathic Sol/Urtica 30c, which helps prevents prickly heat. You can also use Urtica Cream. **OP**
- Avoid hot baths and showers.

PROSTATE PROBLEMS *(see also Cholesterol)*

Approximately 60% of men aged around 60 or over have some degree of prostate enlargement. It's the most common cancer in men and is responsible for 25% of newly diagnosed cases of cancer in England and Wales. Younger men are more likely to suffer from prostatitis, which is an inflammation of the prostate gland. Symptoms of prostatitis are an urgency to urinate more regularly, which can be painful and there may be blood in the sperm. Treatment of this condition is generally by antibiotics.

The prostate is a walnut-sized gland that sits below a man's bladder. Its job is to secrete seminal fluids and to contract strongly during orgasm to cause ejaculation. As men get older it is common for the prostate gland to enlarge gradually, up to 2–4 times its normal size, to about the size of a lemon. This is largely attributable to hormonal changes associated with ageing. After the age of 50 or so, a man's levels of testosterone decrease, while the level of other hormones, including oestrogen, increase. Unfortunately, older men will have had a lifetime of exposure to plastics, petrochemicals and pesticides, which all have hormone-disrupting (oestrogen-like) effects in the body and are linked to hormonal cancers. Although testosterone levels decrease with age, some of the testosterone is converted into a far more potent form – dihydrotestosterone (DHT) – and the normal process by which it is broken down is inhibited by the excess oestrogens. The potent DHT collects in the prostate and causes the overproduction of prostate cells, which ultimately results in prostate enlargement.

Other common factors affecting the prostate are heavy metal toxicity (mercury, aluminium) and over-proliferation of fungus in the gut that overspills into the prostate.

The tube that takes urine from the bladder to the outside (the urethra) passes through the prostate, so the enlarged gland places pressure on the urethra, impeding the flow of urine and triggering the need to urinate more often. Many men get up 3 or 4 times during the course of the night. Other symptoms include difficulty in beginning urination, poor stream, dribbling at the end of urination and sometimes pain. An enlarged prostate can also trigger urinary infections, bladder stones and kidney damage.

The majority of prostate problems are a result of this gradual enlargement, termed benign prostatic hypertrophy (BPH), but occasionally the prostate can be affected by cancer. If you have blood in your urine, difficulty in passing urine or any swelling in your testicle area, please, please go to see your doctor.

Research from John Hopkins Bloomberg School of Public Health has also found, in a study involving 5000 men, that those with lower LDL cholesterol levels can potentially reduce their risk of developing high-grade prostate cancer by as much as 60%. See dietary guidelines under the *Cholesterol* section.

Foods to Avoid

- As pesticide and herbicide residues are linked to prostate cancer, avoid non-organic foods as much as possible.
- Reduce your intake of animal fats found in meat, full-fat milks and cheeses, chocolate, hard margarines and fatty take-aways. Animal-based dairy foods and too much non-organic red meat (usually high in chemical and hormone residues) increase the risk of prostate cancer.
- Don't eat processed meat pies and pastries.
- Avoid fried and barbecued foods.
- Reduce your intake of caffeine, alcohol and refined sugars.
- See also *General Health Hints*.

Friendly Foods

- The carotene lycopene is the most abundant nutrient stored in the prostate and studies have shown that men who eat 10 or more cooked tomatoes (in a little olive oil) weekly are 45% less likely to develop prostate cancer. The lycopene in tomatoes is released when they are heated in a small amount of oil. A great way to do this is to cut tomatoes in half, brush them with a little olive oil and add chopped garlic and basil. Grill or bake for a few minutes and serve. Lycopene is also found in guava, pink grapefruit and watermelon.
- Eat organic foods as much as you can to avoid pesticide residues on fresh produce and hormones used in animal production. Additionally, locally grown fruits and vegetables in season contain more nutrients than those flown thousands of miles.

- Sprinkle linseeds (flax seeds soaked overnight and drained, or use ready-cracked linseeds) over cereals and yoghurt, or add to soups and smoothies (see *General Health Hints* for a smoothie recipe). They are rich in essential fats and zinc.
- Pumpkin seeds are rich in zinc, magnesium (a muscle relaxant) and essential fats, helping reduce the conversion of testosterone to the potent DHT. Eat them raw or try lightly toasting them tossed in a little soya sauce to make a delicious and very prostate-friendly snack over salads or just on their own. Alternatively, blitz 2 tablespoons each of hemp, sunflower and linseeds (use ready-cracked flax seeds), keep them in an air-tight jar in the fridge, and sprinkle daily over cereals, salads, fruits and yoghurts.
- Eat more oily fish, which are rich in omega-3 essential fats, and use unrefined organic walnut, sesame, sunflower and olive oils for salad dressings, or drizzle over cooked foods (see *Fats You Need To Eat*).
- Include plenty of fibre in your diet from fruits and vegetables, especially broccoli, kale, cauliflower and Brussels sprouts, which help to balance hormones naturally.
- Lentils, alfalfa, tomatoes, salad leaves, yellow peppers and organic carrots, watercress and pumpkin will help protect against cancers.
- Eat more brown rice, quinoa, millet, oats, cereals and oat and rice bran. The fibre helps remove excess hormones out of the body.
- Eat more pulses, such as barley, kidney beans, soya beans, plus lentils, and corn, rice and lentil pastas.
- Have one serving of cooked tempeh (a fermented form of soya), miso or soya sauce daily.
- There is currently much discussion about soya-based foods, such as tofu and soya milk. While this argument is ongoing, it is generally accepted that fermented soya in the form of miso or tempeh is beneficial if taken in moderation. Cooked tofu is OK, but if in any doubt, avoid unfermented soya products, such as soya yoghurt and soya milk; or check with your health professional.

Useful Remedies

- The mineral zinc is more abundant in the prostate than in any other organ in the body and its supplementation has been shown to reduce prostate overgrowth and symptoms of BPH. Zinc inhibits the conversion of testosterone to DHT, the primary hormonal trigger for prostate enlargement. Zinc deficiency is common in those with prostate problems. Take 20mg zinc 2–3 times per day. As zinc depletes copper levels, take a proportionate amount of copper, approximately 1mg of copper for every 15mg of zinc.

■ The herb saw palmetto has been proven effectively to reduce enlargement of the prostate gland and dramatically improve the symptoms of BPH. Its active components reduce the production and activity of DHT. Take as capsules – 150–350mg of standardized extract twice a day. Or try Pros Formula containing saw palmetto, horsetail, couchgrass and hydrangea, which all help to normalize prostate function. Take 1 capsule 3 times daily. **SHS**

■ Another good herb for an enlarged prostate is pygeum. It is particularly good for relieving symptoms such as frequent or difficult urination and associated sexual dysfunction. Take 50–100mg of standardized extract twice daily.

■ One of the oldest remedies for enlarged prostate is nettle, taken either as a tincture or as tablets. Take 5ml of tincture, or 200–300mg of standardized extract, 2–3 times per day in capsules. You can also try nettle tea with a little honey.

■ Prosta DHT is a multi-formula containing most of the above. Take 2 daily. Call The Wholistic Medical Centre to order on 020 7580 7537. Email: info@wholisticmedical.co.uk

■ Otherwise, all companies featured on pages 15–16 have multiple prostate formulas for men.

■ The mineral selenium has been found to help prevent prostate enlargement and there is a significant inverse relationship between selenium levels in the body and prostate cancer. Taking 200mcg per day can significantly reduce your risk of either. Check your multi before taking extra selenium.

■ Essential fats, especially omega-3 fish oils, can also help prevent prostate enlargement. Take 1 gram of fish oil with 4 grams of linseed (flax seed) oil daily. **BC**
NB Diets that are too high in omega-6 fats (from refined margarines, pies etc) and saturated fats (from animal produce) are linked to an increased risk of prostate problems – see under *Fats You Need To Eat*, **whereas omega-3 fats from oily fish, linseeds and hemp seeds can help reduce the risk.**

■ Include a natural carotene-source supplement that is rich in lycopene. Take 20–40mg daily.

■ As a deficiency of Vitamin D3 is linked to prostate, colon, breast and a host of other cancers, take 1000iu every day.

■ Take 2 grams of vitamin C with added bioflavonoids daily, with food, because seminal fluid, which the prostate produces, requires vitamin C in large amounts.

Helpful Hints

■ Filter your main tap water supply before drinking. This is because hormone residues from the contraceptive pill and HRT are found in most water supplies and they have an oestrogen-like 'building' effect in the body, which in the long term can trigger hormonal cancers. Kangen Water is an ionized, antioxidant water system that helps re-alkalize the body, thereby killing fungus and other pathogens. It's used in Japanese hospitals with highly beneficial health results. For full details contact the Wholistic Medical Centre on 020 7580 7537; or log on to www.kangenmiraclewater.co.uk

■ An enlarged prostate is usually discovered via a rectal examination by a doctor. All men aged over 40 should have an annual rectal examination. Early detection greatly increases your chances of a complete cure.

■ Ask your partner to see if they can feel any abnormalities; make this a fun thing, but try doing it once a month.

■ Regular exercise is vital as it boosts immune function and also naturally reduces levels of stress hormones. However, do not cycle as this will put pressure on the prostate. Swimming and walking are great exercises.

- To help improve circulation to the area and reduce inflammation, lie on your back, bend your knees, bring the soles of the feet together and bring the feet as close to your buttocks as possible. Relax your legs, letting the knees fall outwards towards the ground. Hold this position for 5 minutes. Attempt this exercise only if you are fit and have no joint problems in your hips and legs.
- Massage essential oils of cypress, tea tree and juniper berry mixed with a little jojoba carrier oil into your lower back and groin areas to help strengthen the prostate.
- See an osteopath or chiropractor to check that the pelvis and spine are not misaligned. In certain cases a major nerve connection from the lower part of the spine to the prostate becomes trapped and once this is released water can be passed normally (see *Useful Information*).
- If you have prostate cancer; see *Useful Remedies* under *Cancer*.
- There is a test for prostate health called a PSA, or Prostate Specific Antigen, test. If your levels of PSA are elevated, it can mean that your prostate is becoming enlarged, or it may possibly be an indication of prostate cancer. This is not a test for cancer *per se*, but it indicates prostate-cell activity. Another good test is the PCA3, which is short for Prostate Cancer gene 3. Prostate cancer cells make much more of this protein than normal cells do, and when PCA3 protein is high, it leaks into the urine. Both these tests can be carried out by your doctor.
- Other factors can raise the levels of PSA – for example, ejaculation can raise it for 2 days, although, in general, the higher the level, the more likely it is to be a sign of cancer. Biopsies are needed to confirm this.

- Men who self-medicate with the anti-ageing hormone DHEA should take care, as DHEA can convert into testosterone and then further into oestrogen, a growth hormone that can trigger hormonal cancers. Always have blood and saliva tests to monitor your hormone levels before taking any hormone supplements, creams, pills or patches.
- Harvard University have published a book entitled *Testosterone for Life*, showing research that men with low testosterone levels are at a higher risk of prostate cancer. Again, have your hormones checked.
- For further help and advice contact The Prostate Help Association, Langworth, Lincoln LN3 5DF. Website: www.prostatehelp.me.uk They also have informative self-help books and CD-ROMs for sale. Otherwise, contact The Prostate Cancer Charity via their helpline, 020 8222 7666, or website www.prostatecanceruk.org
- If your prostate is enlarged, be cautious about using over-the-counter cold or allergy remedies. Many of these products contain ingredients that can inflame the condition and cause urinary retention.
- Read *Prostate Health in 90 Days* by Larry Clapp (Hay House) or *Prostate Cancer* by Philip Dunn (Ostrich Publishing), available through the Prostate Help Association website.

PSORIASIS *(see also Candida, Leaky Gut and SAD Syndrome)*

This is a chronic skin condition that can occur at any age. It is characterized by patches of red, raised and scaly skin. Once it begins scaling, the skin can take on a silvery, fish-like look. It does seem to have some hereditary links, but symptoms often don't appear until adulthood. It usually does not itch, but can cause discomfort and embarrassment. Areas most commonly affected are arms, elbows, behind the ears, scalp, back, legs and knees. Psoriasis may also be triggered by prolonged stress, a traumatic event, food intolerances, essential-fatty-acid deficiencies, low stomach-acid levels, constipation, liver congestion and vitamin B deficiency. It is also linked to a leaky gut, food intolerances and a yeast fungal overgrowth such as candida. Many people with psoriasis may have poor liver function, as skin problems can denote that the liver is under stress – in which case you need to see a qualified nutritionist, who can modify your diet to help detoxify the liver. See *Liver Problems*.

Lack of the sunshine vitamin D and lack of exposure to full-spectrum sunlight is also a factor in this condition.

Foods to Avoid
- Eliminate wheat and any food containing wheat for 1 month and see if this helps. Some people also have an intolerance to gluten (see under *Allergies* for useful tests to find culprits).
- Dairy from animal fats can be a problem – skimmed milk should be OK.
- Citrus fruits and tomatoes aggravate the problem in some sufferers.
- Cut down on saturated and hydrogenated fats, especially red meat, mass-produced vegetable oils, take-aways, mass-produced burgers, red meat, cakes, pastries, pies and full-fat dairy produce.
- It is likely that you are eating too many of the above foods, which are all acid forming in the body. See *Acid–Alkaline Balance*.
- Keep a food diary and note when symptoms become worse. It's often the foods that you eat and/or crave the most, such as starchy, sugary foods, that are the root trigger.
- As much as possible, eliminate alcohol, as it makes the liver work harder and thus affects the skin. In some people, the single biggest trigger for psoriasis is alcohol consumption.

Friendly Foods
- Most people with psoriasis are deficient in essential fats. Therefore, eat more salmon, sardines, mackerel, herring, pilchards or anchovies at least twice a week – and be sure to read *Fats You Need To Eat*.
- Eat as great a variety of fresh foods as possible.
- Eat more brown rice, millet and buckwheat, which are gluten free.
- Eat more pectin-rich foods, such as apples and carrots. Greatly increase your intake of whole fruits and vegetables.
- Figs, prunes, kiwi, spinach, watercress and papaya are all great for the skin (see under *Candida* as high-sugar-content fruits can exacerbate fungal conditions such as candida).
- Add unrefined, organic walnut, sunflower, sesame and olive oils to salad dressings and drizzle over cooked foods.
- Use organic rice or low-fat goat's milks instead of cow's milk. Otherwise try almond milk.
- Pumpkin seeds, linseeds (flax seeds) and sunflower seeds are all high in zinc and essential fats.
- Begin making fresh vegetable juices with raw beetroot, artichoke, carrots and apples or any vegetables you have to hand. Add to this a teaspoon of green food powder (see details of Green pH under *Acid–Alkaline Balance*), 20 drops of dandelion and milk thistle tincture, and half a cup of organic aloe vera juice, which all help cleanse the liver – and drink immediately upon juicing.
- Another good green food powder is Green Magic Powder – containing Hawaiian spirulina, chlorella, lecithin, barley and wheat grass, kamut, pectin apple fibre, kelp and wheat sprouts, CoQ10, royal jelly, artichoke powder and lactobacillus acidophilus. It is a great all-round way to ingest good nutrients, encourage healthy bacteria and keep the body more alkaline and the skin healthier. Details on www.itsgreenmagic.com or call Helen Cruikshank on 07798 873266.
- Celeriac, artichoke and kale are also great for the liver
- Stay hydrated – drink plenty of water and fluids.

Useful Remedies

- Evening primrose oil, 5–6 grams daily, will help to reduce the inflammation associated with psoriasis. Evening primrose oil is high in gamma-linolenic acid (GLA) – therefore if you don't want to swallow high doses of evening primrose oil, take 1–2 grams of pure GLA daily. **BC**
- Omega-3 fish oils are highly anti-inflammatory and help nourish and lubricate the skin from the inside out. Taking 3–5 grams or more daily is highly effective for this condition.
- Take a B-complex that contains 400mcg of folic acid and 100mg of B6, which are often low in people with this condition.
- B12 injections have proved helpful to many people who have low stomach acid (see *Low Stomach Acid*).
- Take vitamin C with bioflavonoids – 2 grams daily to help reduce the inflammation in divided doses with meals.
- Take a multi-vitamin and mineral that contains at least 30–40mg of zinc. A good multi should also contain a full spectrum of the B vitamins – in which case, there is no need to take both.
- Betaine hydrochloride (stomach acid) is often useful. One capsule taken with main meals aids digestion and the absorption of nutrients. If you have active stomach ulcers, take a digestive enzyme instead, which is free of betaine hydrochloride.
- Most psoriasis sufferers are very deficient in vitamin A. For 1 month take 25,000iu of vitamin A daily and then reduce to 5000iu daily (this amount should be in your multi). **NB If you are pregnant or planning a pregnancy, do not take more than 3000iu of vitamin A daily.** Liver is very high in Vitamin A – if you eat a lot of it, you may not need the supplement, but I don't know anyone who eats liver every day!
- After one month on vitamin A, switch to a daily intake of natural-source carotenes, which convert to vitamin A in the body and are non-toxic.
- There has been extensive research into the healing properties of the plant *Mahonia aquifolium* for psoriasis sufferers. It is available as cream, ointment, shampoo, conditioner, scalp oil and body lotion. For details ask at your health shop or visit Taylor Jackson Health Products at www.taylor-jackson.com
- Take at least 1000iu of vitamin D3 daily – a lack of which is linked to many skin conditions and a host of diseases.
- A highly concentrated form of whey called DermaWhey has been shown to soothe skin conditions such as psoriasis. Details from the Life Extension Foundation via www.lef.org or call the Nutri Centre on 0845 602 6744. **NC**

Helpful Hints

- Regular colonic irrigation therapies help to detox the bowel. See *Useful Information* for contact details.
- Sea bathing is beneficial for psoriasis. Many sufferers find relief after bathing in Dead Sea salt because of its high mineral contents. Add 1kg (2¼lb) to your bath and soak for 10 minutes.
- Homeopathic Ars-iod 6x taken twice daily for a few weeks is particularly good for dry, scaly, itching skin.
- Moderate sun exposure also helps psoriasis, but remember to wear a hypo-allergenic sunscreen.
- Smokers run a greater risk of developing psoriasis.
- Many people with this skin condition tend to be holding on to emotional issues, such as resentment, anger and bitterness. If emotions are repressed, the liver is affected – and in the long term, skin problems can result.
- For more help, read *Healing Psoriasis: the Natural Alternative* by Dr John Pagano (Pagano Organization).

R

RAYNAUD'S DISEASE

(see also Circulation, Sjogren's Syndrome and Stress)

Raynaud's is five times more common in women than in men – and commonly begins between the ages of 18 and 30, although it can be later.

This condition occurs when constriction occurs in the blood vessels, which triggers intermittent spasms within the smaller blood vessels – usually in the fingers and toes and occasionally in the nose and tongue. If Raynaud's-type symptoms appear alone, without any other condition being present, it's known as Raynaud's disease, but if other symptoms are apparent, such as dry mouth, eyes and nose, aching joints and/or osteoporosis, then you may have Sjogren's syndrome, an autoimmune condition. See under *Sjogren's Syndrome*.

Initially, symptoms start to occur when the extremities are exposed to cold temperatures, especially if the person is stressed. The nerve receptors in these areas become particularly sensitive to the slightest chill, and fingers and/or toes can become white, bluish or red, and tingling and numbness are common symptoms. This condition is linked to poor circulation and a diet low in essential fats and other nutrients, including iron. Another trigger for Raynaud's is smoking, which greatly affects micro-circulation. In rare cases the skin can ulcerate if it is starved of blood for too long (see also *Circulation, Fats You Need To Eat* and *Leg Ulcers*). Other factors include repetitive activities using the hands, such as typing, or using vibrating tools.

Sometimes Raynaud's remains dormant for years, but can re-surface under conditions of extreme stress, exhaustion or after an infection. Raynaud's can also affect the tissue in the lungs, in which case cold air can trigger coughing attacks.

If allowed to worsen, or if the skin ulcerates, Raynaud's can become serious and in rare cases can lead to gangrene, necessitating amputation – therefore it needs to be taken very seriously from the outset. People who tend to be stressed much of the time, are highly strung and have poor circulation are at a greater risk. Rheumatoid arthritis, lupus and some thyroid conditions may also be linked to Raynaud's-type symptoms, as well as those associated with scleroderma, a chronic connective tissue autoimmune condition in which the body accumulates too much collagen, resulting in hardening of the skin and various internal tissues. Other symptoms of scleroderma include joint pain or puffy hands and feet, gut problems, dry mucous membranes, dental and jaw problems and sometimes, as it progresses, fatigue. The earlier you can recognize such symptoms and seek medical advice and specialist help, such as consulting a rheumatologist, the better. People who suffer scleroderma are likely to also have Sjogren's syndrome. Anyone with autoimmune disease should read the section on *Leaky Gut*, which is often a major contributing factor in all autoimmune conditions.

People suffering Raynaud's are also at a much greater risk of heart disease and stroke, another reason to take this condition seriously.

As people with A and AB blood types have a propensity to clot more readily than other blood types, they are more likely to suffer from conditions relating to circulation, such as Raynaud's.

Foods to Avoid
- Cut down on saturated fats found in hard margarines, fatty meats, full-fat milk and animal-based dairy produce.
- Avoid coffee and caffeine, energy drinks, chocolate (the darker the chocolate, the more caffeine), which constricts blood vessels.
- See also *Foods to Avoid* under *Atherosclerosis* and *Circulation*.

Friendly Foods
- You need to eat more foods that are high in natural-source vitamin E, such as wheat germ, avocados, nuts and seeds.
- Rutin-rich foods help to strengthen the small blood vessels. These include buckwheat, the peel of citrus fruits, rose hips, apple peel and cabbage.
- Make stews, soups and casseroles that are full of root vegetables – sweet potatoes, carrots, pumpkin and so on – as these types of foods warm you through and are rich in minerals.
- Eat iron-rich foods: lean red meat, liver, poultry, eggs, blackstrap molasses, fish, broccoli, kale and leafy green vegetables, such as spinach and watercress.
- Magnesium is a nutritional vasodilator, so include in your diet more low-sugar cereals, oats, honey, wholemeal bread and pastas, almonds, Brazil nuts, walnuts, mustard and curry powder. All leafy green foods are rich in magnesium – and foods like chlorella and green food powders are also high in iron.
- Cook with garlic and onions, which help to thin the blood naturally, plus fresh root ginger and cayenne pepper, which warm the body.
- Eat plenty of fruit high in vitamin C, such as cherries, kiwi and blueberries. In winter, make berry-and-fruit compotes, or lightly glaze fresh fruit with a little honey and grill on kebab sticks. Serve with low-fat, live yoghurt and sprinkle with lecithin granules (which lower LDL-cholesterol levels).
- Eat more oily fish – rich in omega-3 essential fats
- Linseeds (flax seeds) are also rich in omega-3 and omega-6 fats. Soak overnight in cold water, drain and eat over cereals, fruit smoothies or in porridge daily.

Useful Remedies
- If you are not on blood-thinning drugs, take 400–600iu of natural-source full-spectrum vitamin E daily.
- Take vitamin C with bioflavonoids – 1–3 grams a day with food. These play a key role in the synthesis of collagen, which is the key component in the walls of blood vessels. Vitamin C is essential to ensure that the small arteries that supply the fingers do not become damaged during attacks.
- Take niacin (vitamin B3) in a formula that creates a flushing sensation. Start by taking around 30–50mg, 2 or 3 times daily, and gradually increase to 100–1000mg or more under medical supervision per day (in divided doses). **Beware – this vitamin really boosts circulation and for about 30–45 minutes after swallowing, it can cause a pronounced red flushing effect on the skin. Anyone suffering from liver disease should not take high doses of niacin.**
- If you take the flavonoid quercetin earlier in the day, before taking the niacin, this reduces the flushing and suppresses inflammatory responses. Take 500mg daily.
- Otherwise take a high-strength vitamin B-complex daily and if symptoms are severe ask your doctor for a B12 injection.
- Take a high-strength multi-mineral that contains 500mg of magnesium, 500mg of calcium and 20mg of potassium, plus a trace of manganese.
- Gamma-linolenic acid (GLA) is an essential fatty acid found in evening primrose, borage and

blackcurrant oils, and is important for relaxing muscles. A recent study found that 12 capsules a day of evening primrose oil dramatically decreased the number of Raynaud's attacks. But as most people don't want to swallow 12 pills and the ingredient they need is the GLA, take 2–4 Mega GLA capsules daily. **BC**

- Essential polyunsaturated fatty acids, known as omega-3 and omega-6 fatty acids, have been shown to lower the 'unhealthier' LDL fats and thin the blood naturally. Therefore you can either take 8 grams of linseed oil capsules **or** 4 grams of pure omega-3 fish oils daily. Fish oils also improve one's tolerance to cold – which is why the Inuits rarely feel the cold! See under *Fats You Need To Eat*.
- The herb gotu kola really helps to increase circulation. Take 500mg twice daily during the winter or while symptoms are acute.
- Cayenne pepper in capsules helps to improve circulation. Start on 1 capsule 3 times daily and increase if desired. Take this with food – and you should see benefits after a month.
- If the cayenne pepper causes too much warmth in the stomach, then try Bl-Circ Formula containing a small amount of cayenne with ginger, hawthorn, low-odour garlic, ginseng and parsley. **SHS**
- Add a few drops of Ginger Tincture to water and sip throughout the day – it really helps warm you right though. Call Metabolics for stockists on 01380 812799..

Helpful Hints

- If you suffer Raynaud's-type symptoms all year round, have a blood test to determine what is going on and get a proper diagnosis.
- Wear mittens, which are more effective at keeping you warm than gloves. At all costs, keep your hands and feet warm. Many stores now sell cashmere or wool hand/wrist covers, which leave fingers free to work.
- Avoid handling cold items from the fridge. Wear gloves in cool supermarkets.
- Do not clap hands together and rub them too hard, which may damage blood vessels.
- Run hands under warm (NOT hot) water – moist heat is preferable to dry heat sources.
- Otherwise place your hands under your armpits to warm them gently through.
- Take regular exercise to improve circulation. Swimming, walking while swinging your arms in circles, skipping, and rebounding on a mini-trampoline are all wonderful ways to improve circulation.
- If your feet are affected, then wear warm bed socks at night and avoid tight-fitting shoes, which restrict circulation.
- Learn to control your stress levels, as stress has a huge impact on Raynaud's. See under *Stress*.
- Make tea infusions with fresh root ginger, cinnamon twigs or angelica root.
- Try massaging hands and toes regularly with **diluted** essential oils of black pepper, rosemary, lavender or geranium, or add a few drops of each oil to your bath.
- Use a good-quality, rich hand cream, preferably organic, to help soften the skin.
- Use only pH-balanced cleansing bars rather than mass-produced soaps.
- Avoid damaging the affected fingers, especially if they are ulcerated. Wear gloves.
- Reflexology and acupuncture have helped many sufferers (see *Useful Information*).
- For further information contact Raynaud's and Scleroderma Association, 112 Crewe Road, Alsager, Cheshire ST7 2JA or call 01270 872776. Website: www.raynauds.org.uk

REPETITIVE STRAIN INJURY (RSI)

(see also Carpel Tunnel Syndrome)

Half a million people in the UK suffer from chronic pain in their wrists, elbows, shoulders or neck due to RSI. And thanks to the huge numbers of us who work on computers, numbers are on the rise. In typing this book I, too, have succumbed to RSI, but I keep it under control by wearing a wristband that goes through my thumb and around my wrist, which contains magnets. It's certainly helped me and you can find these bands in all good sports shops.

Meanwhile, an average of 4.7 million working days are lost each year to RSI, which obviously needs to be taken more seriously. Common symptoms include numbness, tingling pains, loss of grip, and restricted movement. Anyone who has a job or plays a sport regularly that involves repetitive movements is at risk of contracting RSI. The condition is basically inflammation of the tendons, known as tendonitis. Tendonitis usually heals within a few weeks, but if it becomes chronic calcium salts can deposit along the tendon fibres. The tendons most commonly affected are the Achilles, biceps, elbow, thumb, knee, inside of the foot or shoulder joint.

Foods to Avoid
- Caffeine reduces the body's ability to cope with pain.
- Cut down on refined sugars and refined junk foods, which trigger inflammation in the body.

Friendly Foods

- Eat more oily fish, rich in vitamin A, to aid tissue healing and reduce inflammation.
- Eat plenty of foods high in natural carotenes, which have anti-inflammatory properties. These include asparagus, French beans, broccoli, carrots, papaya, raw parsley, red peppers, spring greens, sweet potatoes, watercress, spinach, apricots, pumpkin, tomatoes and cantaloupe melon.
- Nuts (unsalted) and seeds, especially pumpkin, sesame, sunflower and linseeds (flax seeds), plus fish, are all high in zinc.
- Include more turmeric in food, as it has highly anti-inflammatory properties.
- Pineapple, cherries and ginger all have anti-inflammatory properties.

Useful Supplements
- Take 2 grams of vitamin C as magnesium ascorbate daily in divided doses with food, as vitamin C plays a major role in the prevention and repair of injuries. **BC**
- Natural-source beta-carotenes will help reduce inflammation and maintain tissue integrity. Take 30mg daily.
- Zinc – take 30mg per day. Zinc functions alongside vitamin A. An increased copper-to-zinc ratio is often found in individuals with chronic inflammatory conditions.
- Bioflavonoids are extremely effective in reducing inflammation. Take a 1-gram bioflavonoid-complex daily.
- Include a multi-vitamin and mineral in your regimen that includes 400iu of natural-source, full-spectrum vitamin E, 200mcg of selenium, and 100–150 mg of vitamin B6.
- Take glucosamine (1000mg daily in divided doses) and MSM (1000mg) daily. MSM is an organic form of sulphur and has proved useful for alleviating this problem. Most glucosamine supplements are derived from crab shells. If you have an intolerance to shellfish, ask for the vegetarian version made from corn. By Health Perception, available at health stores.
- Omega-3 fats have an anti-inflammatory effect on the body; take 2–4 grams daily.
- Take 600mg of magnesium daily in divided doses to help soothe the nerve endings and repair muscles.

- Collagen is a vital component of healthy joints, cartilage, ligaments and tendons. It is the most widely distributed protein in the body and we lose about 1.5% annually after the age of 30. Take daily in a glass of water or diluted juice 30 minutes before a main meal to support your tendons. Super Strength Collagen Drink from Higher Nature. **HN**

Helpful Hints
- Magnets help to increase circulation, which brings more oxygenated blood to the problem area. Have a look at www.magnetichealthcare.com or www.magnet-healing.co.uk
- Proper stretching and warming-up before exercise are important preventive measures.
- Rest the injured area as soon as it hurts to avoid further injury.
- Wrap some ice or a bag of frozen peas in a towel and apply to the painful area for 10 minutes every hour while symptoms are acute. Do not wrap so tightly that circulation is impaired.
- Compress the area with an elastic bandage to limit swelling.
- Elevate the injured body part above the level of the heart to increase drainage of fluids out of the injured area.
- You can also massage the affected areas with essential oil of wintergreen, which has anti-inflammatory properties. This really helps.
- If you sit for long hours at a desk, take regular breaks and really stretch out.
- Higher Nature makes an organic sulphur (MSM) and boswellia muscle balm that really helps to ease pain. **HN**
- The Alexander Technique helps individuals to learn about healthy posture and, therefore, how to reduce or even eliminate RSI problems. Acute problems may benefit from treatment with osteopathy, chiropractic or acupuncture (see *Useful Information*).
- If after trying all these ideas for 6 weeks you are no better, consult a specialist in sports injuries or at least have an X-ray or scan.

R

RESTLESS LEGS
(see also Circulation)

This is a very distressing yet very common condition, which causes tickling, burning, or pricking sensations, or an irresistible urge to kick the legs about with involuntary twitching in the muscles of the lower legs. Up to 10% of adults are affected – around 6 million in the UK alone! It can occur sporadically during the day, usually if you sit for long periods, but it's more likely to occur when you are resting, which is why this condition can greatly affect sleep patterns. Also known as Ekbom's syndrome, restless legs is more common in pregnant and middle-aged women, smokers, diabetics, people with low blood sugar (see *Low Blood Sugar*), and those who drink too much coffee. It could also be partly hereditary. Common factors are a lack of iron, full-spectrum vitamin E and the mineral magnesium (see also *Circulation*).

Foods to Avoid
- Cut down on your alcohol intake.
- The biggest trigger is caffeine in any form, so avoid coffee, tea and fizzy drinks. Eliminate any foods containing caffeine, including chocolate.
- Avoid too many foods containing sugar, which can cause your blood sugar to fluctuate and make symptoms worse.
- Reduce refined pastries, cakes, mass-produced pies and biscuits.
- See *General Health Hints*.

Friendly Foods

- You need to eat quality protein from chicken, fish, eggs, low-fat cheeses, pulses, beans, peas, cooked tofu and so on – at least once a day.
- Eat more brown rice, quinoa and couscous. For snacks, eat rye crisp breads, or amaranth or rice crackers, which are delicious spread with a little low-fat humous or tahini.
- Eat more leafy green vegetables (especially kale and watercress), fruits and honey, which are rich in magnesium.
- Iron-rich foods are liver, lean red meat such as venison, rabbit, free-range chicken, eggs, cereals and blackstrap molasses.
- Essential fats are vital, therefore include oily fish in your diet at least twice weekly, and sprinkle organic unsalted sunflower and pumpkin seeds over cereals and salads.
- Eat raw wheat germ and avocados, which are rich in vitamin E and healthier monounsaturated fats.
- Eat more blueberries and bilberries when in season.
- Drink calming herbal teas, such as camomile, lemon balm or vervain.
- As you need plenty of B-vitamins with this condition, eat more porridge and low-sugar oat-based cereals and oat bran.
- Invest in a low glycaemic index (GI) cookbook.

Useful Supplements

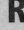

- If you are deficient in iron take a liquid formula such as Spatone that is easily absorbed and does not cause constipation. Available from health stores worldwide.
- Take a high-strength B-complex to calm the nerve endings. Folic acid (5mg) and B6 (100mg) are the most important. Take these with breakfast or lunch.
- Natural-source, full-spectrum vitamin E – 400iu daily – can be extremely effective in alleviating this condition. **NB If you are on blood-thinning drugs, vitamin E thins the blood naturally, so tell your doctor and have regular blood tests so that you can reduce your drugs.**
- The mineral magnesium is very important for relaxing muscles, so take a good-quality multi-vitamin and mineral that contains 500mg of magnesium and also 400mg calcium. Take with your evening meal.
- Cayenne pepper capsules really rev up the circulation and have an anti-cramping affect. Take 3 a day in divided doses with meals.
- See also *Useful Supplements* under *Circulation* and *Raynaud's Disease*.

Helpful Hints

- A simple blood test will tell you if you are anaemic and actually need to take extra iron (see *Anaemia*).
- Get plenty of exercise.
- Massage your legs and feet (especially before bed) with essential oils of rosemary in a carrier of almond or olive oil, using kneading movements from the ankle upwards towards the knee. The legs can be bathed in alternate hot and cold water to improve circulation.
- Use cramp bark cream before going to bed. **OP**
- Try reflexology, acupuncture or regular aromatherapy massage to rev up the circulation.
- Take all the suggested supplements for at least 3 months.
- Wearing magnets in your shoes or in bed socks greatly aids circulation, which can reduce the symptoms considerably at night. Magnets are available at all large pharmacies.
- If it's practical, go for a walk for at least 30 minutes in the evenings.

RHEUMATOID ARTHRITIS   *(see Arthritis)*

ROSACEA

(see also Candida, Leaky Gut, Low Stomach Acid, Lupus and Sjogren's Syndrome)

This is a common skin disorder in adults between the ages of 30 and 50, and women are three times more likely to be affected than men. It's thought that hormones play a role in this condition, and naturopaths state that lymphatic congestion is often a factor. Symptoms are a chronic acne-like eruption or flushing of the face, which usually affects the area around the nose and chin. Sometimes the tiny pustules are filled with sebum; with others it's just fluid.

Rosacea can be inherited, but it is more commonly associated with drinking too much alcohol, prolonged stress, coffee, tea, spicy foods, the menopause, lack of stomach acid and/or B-vitamins. It can also be triggered by food intolerances, the most common triggers being wheat, cow's milk and oranges. Many people who suffer rosacea also suffer from migraines (see *Migraine*). A leaky gut is also highly implicated in rosacea (see *Leaky Gut*) and you may also be intolerant to gluten found in wheat and grains. You also need to take care of your liver (see *Liver Problems*).

Facial butterfly-type rashes are also linked to autoimmune conditions such as lupus – see under *Lupus*.

Generally, the poorer your digestion, linked to food intolerances in combination with stress, the worse your symptoms are likely to become.

R

Foods to Avoid

- Generally, cut down on coffee, tea, alcohol, hot drinks and hot spicy foods, which increase blood flow and hence flushing.
- Minimize caffeine found in coffee, chocolate, energy drinks, colas etc
- Keep a food diary and note as the flush appears what you were eating, drinking or feeling prior to the onset of symptoms.
- Avoid heavy, rich or fried foods, which place a strain on the digestion and liver.
- Avoid eating too much food made from flour – these tend to be pies, cakes, and so on, which are often high in refined sodium-based salt, refined sugar and saturated fats.
- Avoid oily, spicy foods.

Friendly Foods

- Bitter foods, such as radicchio, fennel, chicory, celeriac and young green celery, stimulate stomach acid.
- Take a teaspoon of apple cider vinegar or lemon juice in warm water before a meal.
- Drink plenty of water, even if you are not thirsty.
- Eat more pineapple and papaya to improve your digestion.
- Eat plenty of leafy greens, especially spinach, watercress, kale, cauliflower, broccoli, cabbage and celery.
- Eat more beetroot and artichokes to help cleanse your liver.
- Include plenty of live, low-fat yoghurt to help replenish healthy bacteria in the gut.

Useful Remedies

- Prebiotics are the foods that healthy bacteria like to live on; these usually contain inulin, a compound found in chicory and artichokes. Take daily as recommended – most of the vitamin companies featured on pages 15–16 produce prebiotic capsules and powders.

- Probiotics – healthy bacteria – can also be helpful if taken for a month to restore healthy levels of bacteria in the gut, which in turn can help reduce the facial rashes. Jarro-Dophilus EPS, made by Jarrow, will help replenish gut flora; take one daily after food. They are enteric-coated, which means they can pass through stomach lining and do not need to be kept in the fridge. Available from the Nutri Centre. **NC**
- If you are not suffering from active stomach ulcers, take one betaine hydrochloride (stomach acid) capsule with main meals. If this causes a slight burning sensation, then switch to a pancreatic digestive enzyme capsule that is free from betaine hydrochloride. **BC**
- Rosacea sufferers often have a decreased secretion of the pancreatic enzyme lipase. Take 1 Lipozyme with main meals. **BC**
- As B-group vitamins are often depleted, also take a B-complex.
- There is a skin regime called Sher, which has helped many sufferers. For full details, contact The Sher System, PO Box 573, Staines, Middlesex. Tel: 01784 227805. Website: www.sher.co.uk
- Apply a cream called Rose Plus, which contains pine bark and blackcurrant leaf. It has potent anti-inflammatory properties and helps reduce redness and inflammation. **OP**
- People who take pycnogenol – pine bark extract – regularly report a great improvements after 3 months. Take 80mg twice daily. **PN**
- Try a herbal tincture made specifically for rosacea, which includes milk thistle, red clover, bilberry and gingko. **OP**
- Mix 1 teaspoon of fenugreek seeds in a cup of boiling water, allow to cool, strain and drink twice daily. This really helps to clear lymphatic congestion

Helpful Hints

- Sipping diluted lemon juice with main meals can help to treat low stomach acid, which is a factor in this condition.
- Homeopathic Arsenicum Brom 6c taken twice daily for 2 weeks helps to reduce symptoms.
- Exposure to heat and cold can trigger an attack.
- Try regular rebounding (buy a mini trampoline), which again helps clear any lymphatic congestion.
- Some women who take the hormone DHEA are affected by spots appearing on the face and forehead, which can mimic rosacea-type symptoms. Check with your health professional in case you are taking too high a dose of DHEA.

S

SAD SYNDROME – SEASONAL AFFECTIVE DISORDER

(see also Depression)

Approximately 2 million people are affected by this problem in the UK and 12 million across Northern Europe – mainly between September and April. It's far more common in women than in men and symptoms include low moods, increased appetite and food cravings (usually for starchy, sugary, fatty foods), weight gain, PMS-type symptoms, depression, loss of libido, irritability and an increased feeling of being of 'no use' to anyone. Other symptoms are difficulty concentrating, lack of energy and an increased desire to sleep during the winter months. Many people report that they feel sleepy during the day, yet cannot sleep well at night. Not everyone experiences the same symptoms.

Symptoms usually begin in late autumn or early winter and tend to disappear in late spring and early summer. Due to lack of full-spectrum light, during the winter months our pineal gland, situated in our brain, produces more melatonin, the hormone that regulates glandular function and makes us feel more sleepy.

Melatonin is crucial for controlling our biological rhythms and is secreted mainly at night, see-sawing with serotonin, its counterpart, which is secreted on exposure to bright daylight. Melatonin helps you to sleep, while serotonin raises mood and makes you feel positive. Therefore with lack of light, you make more melatonin and less serotonin. In countries where sunshine is rare during the winter months, suicide rates increase.

Foods to Avoid
- When there is insufficient light, the body naturally craves sugary carbohydrates to increase its serotonin levels, which is why many women put on weight in the winter. Do your best to reduce your intake of stimulants such as coffee, mass-produced chocolate, caffeine and refined sugary, starchy-based foods and drinks.
- Alcohol lowers brain levels of the neurotransmitter serotonin, which helps to keep us positive, so drink less of it.
- Reduce your intake of refined, sugary, starchy foods, and if you crave sugar use a little brown rice syrup, organic agave (plant-based) syrup and/or xylitol as a sweetener. HN
- See section on *Low Blood Sugar*, since this condition usually goes hand in hand with SAD syndrome.

Friendly Foods
- Eat foods that help the body to produce more serotonin – fish, turkey, chicken, cottage cheese, beans, avocados, bananas, whey protein and wheat germ.
- Sixty percent of the brain is made up of fat, so eat plenty of oily fish, which is rich in omega-3 fats. Add linseeds (flax seeds) to your breakfast cereal, as they are also rich in essential fats.
- Organic milk is also a good source of the amino acid tryptophan, which helps raise serotonin levels.
- Include more organic tempeh, miso soup and beans in your diet. Kidney, canellini and black-eyed beans are a rich source of fibre and protein to help raise your mood.
- During the winter make rich stews with plenty of green and root vegetables, and add brown rice and pastas.
- Low-sugar, oat-based muesli and cereals are rich in B-vitamins, which are great mood foods. Eat porridge for breakfast – sweeten with a chopped apple and a few raisins.
- Try dairy- and sugar-free organic chocolate made with agave syrup, goji and acai berries with blueberry and coconut oil from Glamour Food, produced by the Organic Pharmacy. For stockists of Glamour Food call 0844 800 8399. In the US call (323) 650 2201 internationally; + 44 (0)20 7351 2232. OP

Useful Remedies
- Firstly, take a good-quality multi-vitamin and mineral supplement that contains at least 200mg of magnesium plus 30mg of zinc.
- Add to this a high-strength B-complex, as lack of vitamins B3, 6, 12 and folic acid are all linked to depression. Vitamins B6, B3 and inositol are necessary to convert tryptophan into serotonin.
- Lack of vitamin D (especially D3) is hugely associated with SAD syndrome. During the winter months, take a minimum of 1000iu daily and if symptoms are acute take 2000–4000iu daily

S

for a couple of weeks. During a day in the sun, you can naturally produce as much as 20,000iu of vitamin D!

- Tryptophan, an amino acid, helps boost serotonin levels. This supplement has been shown to be as effective as orthodox antidepressants, without the negative side effects. 250mg can be taken twice daily. **VN**
- St John's wort has proven very effective and you will need 500–1000mg a day. **NB Not to be taken with blood-thinning drugs. If you are on any prescription drugs, check for contraindications with your GP.**
- Take 2 grams of omega-3 rich fish oil capsules daily, as lack of essential fats can contribute to the feelings of depression.

Helpful Hints

- Make the effort to walk in natural daylight for at least 15 minutes a day, especially when the sun is out. We need around 10,000 lux of full-spectrum light daily to maintain serotonin levels. One lux equates to the light of one small candle!
- Try using a Real Sunlight lamp, available at several specialist clinics in the UK. The harmful frequencies of UVA and UVB have been filtered out, making this sunlight safe. Developed in Sweden, these lamps have been so successful that the Swedish government are installing them in many care homes, especially those in which residents are rarely exposed to natural sunlight. The lamps are used to boost immune function and relieve the depression associated with SAD Syndrome, and they do it by increasing levels of vitamin D3 naturally. Real Sunlight lamps are available in London at The Wholistic Medical Centre, 57 Harley Street, info@wholisticmedical.co.uk Tel: 0207 580 7537. For a list of salons and clinics offering this specialist treatment, contact Real Sunlight Ltd on 08456 800 853.
- Tanning beds should not be used to treat SAD. The light sources in tanning beds are high in ultraviolet (UV) rays, which harm both your eyes and your skin. Light boxes emit full-spectrum light. Use Biolight's full-spectrum light bulbs – available from the Sensory Company. Tel: 0845 838 2233. Email: webinfo@thesensorycompany.co.uk
- Exercise as much as possible during daylight to increase the production of serotonin – the feel-good hormone.
- Take a winter holiday in the sunshine.
- The SAD Association (SADA) has a support network, and if you send a large SAE to PO Box 989, Steyning BN44 3HG, you will receive an information sheet. If you want a full SADA information pack, containing full details of SAD treatments, where to obtain light-therapy equipment, how to adapt your lifestyle, clinics, meetings and books, then send £5. Website: www.sada.org.uk
- Sad Lighting makes light boxes used specifically for SAD Syndrome. Contact them via www.sad-lighting.co.uk
- For more help contact 'Lumie' at www.lumie.com run by Angela Young – an expert on the various light therapies.

SCALP PROBLEMS

Dry, flaking, itching scalp (dandruff)

This condition occurs when the tiny cells in the outer layer of skin are shed at a faster rate than normal. Dandruff usually results from a malfunction of the sebaceous glands, affecting the amount of sebum or oils they produce. If too little sebum is secreted, the hair becomes brittle and dandruff appears. Dry skin on the scalp is also linked to eczema and psoriasis. An itchy scalp can be associated with candida (see *Candida*). Dandruff is also connected with food intolerances.

Foods to Avoid
- I'm afraid it's the usual culprits of highly refined, starchy foods that are high in animal fats, full-fat dairy products and refined sugars.
- See also *General Health Hints*.

Friendly Foods
- You need to increase your intake of essential fats found in oily fish, sunflower, pumpkin, hemp, flax and sesame seeds.
- Use organic walnut and olive oils, not only for salad dressings, but also drizzled over cooked dishes. Udo's Choice Oil is a balanced blend of omega-3 and omega-6 fats, which will help to feed the skin from the inside out. See under *Fats You Need To Eat*.
- Eat more wholefoods, brown rice and stone-ground wholemeal bread, barley, quinoa, amaranth, buckwheat, millet and pasta.
- Greatly increase your intake of fresh fruits and vegetables, especially organic carrots, spinach, watercress, papaya, apricots, cantaloupe melon, guava, mango, pumpkin, sweet potato and squash, which are all rich in natural-source carotenes.
- Eat pineapple and papaya with main meals to aid digestion.
- Include more low-fat, live yoghurt in your diet to aid digestion.
- Eat more wheat germ and avocados, which are rich in vitamin E.
- Dry skin also denotes dehydration, so drink at least 6–8 glasses of water daily.
- Use nori seaweed flakes instead of salt, as they are a rich source of minerals that help nourish the scalp. From all health shops.

Useful Remedies
- Take a good-quality multi-vitamin and mineral that contains 30mg of zinc, which is vital for skin healing.
- Take a B-complex (usually included in any multi).
- Biotin – a B vitamin. You will need an extra 2½–4mg daily, as biotin is excellent for scalp problems.
- Your multi should contain some vitamin A – but make this up to 10,000iu per day for up to 2 months. **NB If you are pregnant, take no more than 3000iu altogether. And avoid taking extra vitamin A if you eat a lot of liver.** After 2 months, start taking a natural-source carotene complex, which naturally converts to vitamin A in the body. SVHC, VN
- Most people with a dry skin or scalp are lacking in essential fats, usually omega-3 fish oils that help to nourish your skin from the inside out. Take 2 grams daily.
- The plant/herbal extract *Mahonia aquafolium*, made into a cream, really helps to moisturize the scalp. Look at www.taylor-jackson.com

Helpful Hints
- Use natural-based shampoos that contain no chemicals and colourings. Organic Pharmacy (**OP**) and Green People both make great ranges. All health shops sell ranges of organic products. To find your nearest stockist for Green People or to order, call 01403 740350. Website: www.greenpeople.co.uk
- Massage your scalp with pure rosemary oil mixed with jojoba or olive oil and leave on overnight.
- Homeopathic Arsenicum album 6x can be taken once or twice daily for a week.
- You can loosen dandruff, which sticks to the hair and scalp, by rinsing the hair with sour milk

or a mild solution of lemon juice (use 2 tablespoons of lemon juice to a little under 0.5 litre – 1 pint – of cooled boiled water).

■ Apply chickweed ointment to itchy areas.

■ For more help, see under *Hair Problems*.

Greasy scalp

Greasy hair and scalps are usually caused by overactive sebaceous glands, which produce a waxy, natural oil known as sebum that keeps hair supple. This problem is more common during the teenage years, because as we age for most people the scalp gradually becomes drier. It is far more common in men and teenagers and is linked to acne and hormonal changes. (See also *Acne*.) A greasy scalp can be aggravated by frequent washing with strong shampoos, which destroy the acid balance of the scalp. Always use a pH-balanced shampoo or add a little vinegar or lemon juice to your final rinse.

Foods to Avoid

■ Cutting down on refined carbohydrates, especially sweets, chocolates and soft drinks often helps.

■ Reduce your intake of red meats, which take a long time to digest and can putrefy in the gut.

■ Cut down on alcohol, caffeine and saturated fats, which place an extra burden on the liver. See *Liver Problems*.

■ Avoid melted cheeses, which are very difficult to digest.

Friendly Foods

■ Eat more organic tofu, broccoli, watercress, cauliflower, Brussels sprouts, lentils and beans, which help to regulate hormone levels.

■ Drink at least 6–8 glasses of water every day.

■ Drink organic beetroot juice to help cleanse the liver (see *Liver Problems*).

■ Eat more fish, especially oily fish, plus avocados, sunflower, pumpkin, hemp and sesame seeds and linseeds (flax seeds). Also use their unrefined oils for your salad dressings. See under *General Health Hints* for a great breakfast smoothie that includes plenty of seeds.

■ See also *General Health Hints*.

Useful Remedies

■ Vitamin A helps to balance oil production. Take 5000iu daily for 2 months and then switch to a natural-source carotenoid complex, which converts to Vitamin A in the body and is totally non-toxic. **NB If you are pregnant or planning a pregnancy, do not take more than 3000 IU of vitamin A daily – otherwise the natural source carotenes are safe to use.**

■ Take an essential fatty acid formula – see *Fats You Need To Eat*.

■ Take a multi-vitamin and mineral plus 2–3mg biotin, the B-vitamin that is often deficient with this problem. (Good multis should contain biotin.)

Helpful Hints

■ Wash hair regularly with mild or very dilute shampoo (try herbal shampoos, such as seaweed or rosemary).

■ Take plenty of exercise, which will help to reduce over-production of sebum.

■ Massage your scalp regularly.

■ Homeopathic Nat Mur 6x can be taken once daily for 7–10 days.

■ Consult a qualified nutritionist, who can help you to rebalance your diet. For details of a good trichologist, see *Hair Loss*.

■ Avoid hair products containing sodium lauryl sulphate, which is used for cleaning concrete!

Head lice

This is a common problem, especially in school-aged children. The most obvious symptom is a constantly itching scalp; upon examination grey-coloured insects can be seen. These are the adult lice. The lice eggs (nits) are white and stick to the hair. As the eggs have a 7–14-day incubation period, patience and regular daily treatments are necessary to get rid of them. Many orthodox treatments contain organophosphates (pesticides), which are now linked to cancers. Head lice are attracted to clean and dirty hair alike.

Foods to Avoid
See *General Health Hints*.

Friendly Foods
See *General Health Hints*.

Useful Remedies
- The spray Nice 'N' Clear contains tea tree, lavender, citronella, nettle, thyme, orange and neem oil, which help to kill the lice. For details call 0800 289515.
- Chinese Whispers is a herbal, non-chemical-based formula that has been shown in medical trials to kill the lice. For details of your nearest stockist, call Tree of Life on 01782 567100. Website: www.treeoflifeuk.com
- A Vogel make a tincture called Riddance, containing neem from the Indian neem tree – a great insect repellent.

Helpful Hints
- Comb the hair daily with a fine-toothed comb to remove the lice.
- Check the head daily as close personal head-to-head contact with someone who is infested can spread the lice.
- Wash all clothing in a really hot wash and then leave in the freezer for 2–3 days to kill any remaining lice.
- Combine 1 part lavender oil and 1 part tea tree oil to 3 parts olive oil. Massage into the head and then rinse with vinegar.

SCIATICA

Sciatica is usually a symptom of a structural problem in the lower back, where the sciatic nerve becomes trapped or pinched. The pain tends to affect the buttocks and backs of the thighs, and can travel down the back of the leg and in some cases as far as the feet. It may also cause numbness, pins and needles and/or weakness in those areas.

The most common cause is a trapped nerve, but a slipped or bulging disc in the lower back, which causes pressure on the sciatic nerve, can also trigger it. Other causes include an abscess, an inflammation of the sciatic nerve, or the after-effect of minor injury to the back – resulting, for example, from lifting too heavy a weight in the gym or sitting in an awkward position. If you suffer shingles in that area, then you may also experience post-herpetic neuralgia pain.

Foods to Avoid
- Avoid excessive consumption of foods that drain the body of thiamine (vitamin B1) and magnesium, such as coffee, tea, colas and fizzy drinks, chocolate and refined sugars, which reduce the body's ability to cope with pain. Sugar triggers inflammation in the body.

- Lack of magnesium and thiamine can also contribute to muscular pain and spasms.
- Red meats, full-fat dairy produce and cheeses are high in arachidonic acids, which exacerbate inflammation.

Friendly Foods
- Cereals, wheat germ, meats, Bovril, fresh peanuts, brewer's yeast and Brazil nuts are all rich in thiamine.
- Magnesium-rich foods are cereals, honey, wheat germ, almonds, Brazil nuts, mustard and curry powder.
- Eat plenty of green leafy vegetables, yellow peppers and fresh fruits, which are all nutrient rich, to support your nerves.
- Add more turmeric and cayenne pepper to foods, as they act like powerful anti-inflammatories.
- Ginger helps to reduce pain – add to cooking or make fresh ginger tea.
- Eating porridge for breakfast helps support the nerves. Sweeten with a chopped apple and a few organic raisins or chopped dried apricots (which are also rich in magnesium).

Useful Remedies
- Take NT188 containing B-vitamins and passiflora to help calm the nerves. **BC**
- Also try magnesium malate – 500mg twice daily – to help relax the nerve endings.
- Calcium has anti-spasmodic properties; take 400–600mg daily in divided doses.
- Take 100mg daily of thiamine (vitamin B1) to nourish the nervous system. This should be in any good high-strength vitamin B-complex. Take daily with meals.
- Vitamin B12 injections may be helpful in some cases.
- Take 200iu of natural-source, full-spectrum vitamin E twice daily, which helps to reduce any inflammation.
- Organic sulphur (MSM) plus the amino sugar glucosamine has shown great results in reducing this type of pain. Take 1000mg MSM daily, plus 500mg glucosamine twice daily, until symptoms ease. If you are highly sensitive to shellfish, then ask for the Health Perception glucosamine, which is derived from corn.
- DLPA, an amino acid, encourages the production of the body's own pain-killing chemicals. 400mg can be taken 3 times daily until symptoms ease. Also helps to lift your mood. **SVHC**
- Take 1–3 grams of vitamin C with bioflavonoids to aid tissue healing.

Helpful Hints
- To reduce pain and discomfort, use an ice pack plus a hot water bottle wrapped in towels. Place each alternately on the site of the pain for 10 minutes; try this twice daily.
- To relieve sciatica, lie down on your back with your knees bent, feet flat on the floor. Place your hands underneath your buttocks (palms down) beside the base of your spine. Close your eyes and, taking long, deep breaths, rock your knees from side to side for two minutes. Reposition your hands every few minutes to enable different parts of the buttocks' muscles to be pressed. Gently move your legs from side to side with your knees pulled into your abdomen and your feet off the floor, and support your legs by holding them with your palms just behind your upper legs.
- See a qualified osteopath or chiropractor as soon as possible and then try acupuncture, which is excellent for pain relief. See *Useful Information*.
- Many alternative practitioners have found that regular deep-tissue massage gives enormous relief to sciatica sufferers, as muscular spasms in this area can be mistaken for sciatica.
- Essential oils of wintergreen and peppermint are nature's painkillers.
- Homeopathic Lachesis is good for left-sided sciatica. Take 30c, 3–4 times daily for up to 4 days. For right-sided sciatica, try Lycopodeum 30c.

- Join a local yoga or t'ai chi class, which helps keep you supple but is very gentle exercise.
- When sleeping or resting, lie on your side with a pillow between your knees to minimize pelvic strain. If you sleep on your back, put a soft pillow under your knees.

SHINGLES (HERPES ZOSTER)

(see also Immune Function and Stress)

Shingles is caused by the same virus as chickenpox. The basic rule is that you cannot contract (or have a very low risk of contracting) shingles if you have not had chickenpox, as the virus lies dormant for many years in a nerve root in the spine. There is anecdotal evidence that a person suffering from shingles can pass the virus, especially to a young child, and give them chickenpox. Also, if a child who has chickenpox is in contact with an elderly relative who has once suffered chickenpox, the contact may reactivate the virus in the form of shingles. All people who have suffered chickenpox are at risk of contracting shingles. Someone who has never had chickenpox has a low risk of contracting shingles from someone else.

Shingles is common after the age of 50, but younger people are beginning to suffer from it, too. People infected with HIV are at a greater risk of shingles. It is unusual to suffer more than one attack, but if you do, then you need to boost your immune functioning. The virus can be activated by shock, stress, or lowered immune function. As the virus multiplies and attacks the nerve, it can cause searing pains along the nerve pathways, and is known as a post-herpetic neuralgia (PHN). After a few days, the skin erupts in itchy blisters. These generally heal within two to four weeks, but nerve pains may last for several weeks. If the blisters for any reason become infected, seek immediate medical attention.

If the facial nerves are affected (known as trigeminal neuralgia), there may be temporary paralysis, and if the optic nerve is affected, the cornea may be damaged. Shingles most commonly appears on the trunk, but can also appear on the palms, inner areas of the arms, legs or feet. See also *Herpes* and *Cold Sores*, as shingles is caused by a form of herpes virus.

In rarer cases, the person may experience middle ear and throat problems and/or a loss of taste and smell. See under *Taste and Smell (Loss of)*.

The secret to preventing shingles is to keep your immune function in good shape. See under *Immune Function*.

Foods to Avoid
- Foods that are rich in arginine, an amino acid found commonly in chocolate, carob, lentils, beans and nuts. This feeds the virus and can make symptoms worse.
- Refined sugary foods made with white flour; high-saturated-fat foods, which have a negative effect on the immune system; and sugar, which increases inflammation in the body.

Friendly Foods
- Eat good-quality protein at least once a day, such as lean meats including turkey and lean pork, plus fish, corn and tempeh, all of which are rich in lysine, an amino acid that has been shown to interfere with replication of the virus.
- Most people feel very poorly with shingles, therefore homemade vegetable soups that are easy to digest and rich in nutrients would be very beneficial.
- Add whey protein to smoothies to aid skin-healing. For a great recipe, see under *General Health Hints*.
- Live, low-fat yoghurts aid digestion and replenish the healthy bacteria in the bowel.
- See *General Health Hints*.

- Garlic and rosemary are highly anti-viral. Use in cooking daily.
- Drink plenty of organic green tea, rich in compounds that help to kill the virus.

Useful Remedies

- At the onset of symptoms, begin taking 500–1000mg of lysine daily. If you are already suffering, take up to 4 grams daily.
- Take up to 5 grams of vitamin C daily in an ascorbate form spread throughout the day with meals, while the situation is acute. This may trigger loose bowels, in which case reduce the dose by 1 gram at a time until this stops.
- Beta Glucans 1–3, 1–6, derived from yeast cell walls, are proven to strengthen the body's innate immune system (the immune system you were born with). Take 250–500mg daily while symptoms last and take daily whenever you feel 'run down'. Dr Paul Clayton, who is based in the UK and US, is a medical pharmacologist. His website research on Beta Glucans is well worth a look. Find him at www.healthdefence.com Glucosan, developed by Dr Clayton, is available from Vitalize Health products via 0870 042 8423 or www.vitalizeshop.co.uk
- Try a cream containing St John's wort and lemon balm – both are anti-viral and regular applications can help reduce pain and speed healing. **OP**
- Oregano capsules have highly anti-viral properties – take 2 daily in divided doses with meals while symptoms last. They can repeat on you somewhat, so if you have this problem, take just one capsule daily. **BC**
- Take zinc in the form of a cream and apply regularly to fight the virus. Also take 30mg daily internally in the form of a multi-vitamin and mineral.
- Liquorice can also help to kill the virus.
- Omega-3 fish oils are highly anti-inflammatory. While the condition lasts, take 3 grams daily with meals.
- Use coconut oil for cooking, as it reduces replication of the virus.
- During an attack take 30,000iu of vitamin A daily for 2 weeks only, as this will greatly aid skin healing and boost immune function. **NB If you are pregnant or planning a pregnancy, then do not take more than 3000iu of vitamin A daily**. After the 2 weeks, switch to a natural-source carotene complex that converts naturally to Vitamin A in the body and is non toxic.
- Olive leaf extract acts as an anti-viral – see *Antibiotics* for details.
- The herb St John's wort is very useful for relieving the depression and nerve pain associated with shingles. Take 500mg, 3 times daily. **NB This herb should not be taken by anyone taking blood-thinning drugs such as Warfarin. You may become sensitive to the sun while taking this herb.**

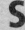

Helpful Hints

- Rest as much as possible when the attack starts and make sure you see your doctor in case of complications, such as infection.
- Make sure you change your toothbrush and face towels regularly, as these can harbour the virus.
- Calendula or melissa cream can be applied to the sores to help calm them down. **OP**
- Homeopathic Rhus Tox 6x, taken 3–4 times daily for 3 days, will help reduce the pain.
- Applying plain yoghurt mixed with a little zinc oxide cream along the path of the affected nerve 2–3 times daily can clear herpes zoster in 24–48 hours, if you start the regimen at the first sign of an outbreak.
- Hot and cold compresses help relieve nerve pain.
- Essential oils of wintergreen and peppermint are nature's painkillers.

SINUS PROBLEMS   *(see also Allergies, Allergic Rhinitis and Catarrh)*

Sinusitis is an inflammation of the mucous membranes in the sinuses. It usually occurs after a viral or bacterial infection, such as a cold or flu, which has affected another part of the respiratory system. It can also be caused by injury to the nose, dental treatment, or swimming. Common symptoms are a blocked nose and nasal-sounding speech, often accompanied by facial pain and headaches, which can be made worse by bending forward. If you suffer chronic sinus problems, they are more than likely linked to food intolerances (see under *Allergies* and *Leaky Gut*) and/or stress. Some people also have deviated septums or polyps in the nasal cavity, which can increase the likelihood of suffering chronic sinus problems.

Foods to Avoid

- At all costs, if symptoms are acute, avoid mucous-producing foods, such as full-fat animal-source milks, cheese, chocolate, white bread, croissants, pastries, cakes and anything else containing refined white flour, fat, sugar and/or milk.
- At the onset of an acute sinusitis attack, try eating really lightly. This clears the body of toxins and gives the digestive system and liver a rest, which boosts immune function.
- Avoid refined sugar in any form for at least 6 days, as sugar greatly impairs your immune functioning and encourages bacterial growth.
- Basically, avoid any foods for which you have an intolerance – the most common being wheat and dairy produce from animal sources, oranges or eggs. I have met people who suffer such symptoms after eating foods as diverse as garlic, kiwi fruit and even bananas. You need to be tested for food intolerances before cutting any large food groups from your diet. Find details of the York and Genova Tests under the *Allergies* section.

Friendly Foods

- For 3 or 4 days, live on really thick soups that are full of fresh vegetables and a little chicken, lentils, brown rice or barley.
- Eat more garlic (if you are not sensitive to garlic) and onions.
- Hot curries with cayenne pepper also help clear the sinuses as the spices dilate blood vessels and increase blood flow to the area and help clear any mucous.
- Drink plenty of freshly blended vegetable juices – especially cucumber, carrot, parsley, beetroot, kale and apple, which are very cleansing.
- Snack on fenugreek seeds and add fresh root ginger to meals.
- Drink plenty of water and elderflower tea to help to reduce congestion.
- Salads would be great with some protein, such as fresh fish or lean meats.

Useful Remedies

- The amino acid N-acetyl cysteine (NAC) really helps to support the liver and breaks down mucous to enable it to be expelled; take 500mg before meals twice daily.
- The B-group vitamins are often lacking in this condition; take a high-strength, vitamin B-complex daily with food.
- Vitamin C – take up to 3 grams daily in divided doses with meals to reduce allergic responses to foods and external allergens, as vitamin C acts like a natural anti-histamine.
- Take a multi-mineral that has 400mg of magnesium and 30mg zinc to boost immune function.
- The bioflavonoid quercetin, 400mg one to three times daily, acts as an natural anti-histamine and is highly effective.
- Echinacea and golden rod also helps to reduce mucous – it is available in tincture. Ultimate Echinacea Complex contains these herbs. Available from the Nutri Centre (**NC**) or log on to www.holoshealth.com

- Try Sin/All containing eucalyptus and golden seal, which helps to balance and tone the mucous membranes. This works well alongside Anti-Cat, which contains elderflowers, and Herbal Snuff, which was created to be sniffed up each nostril to support the mucous membranes. Power Garlic and eyebright (if the eyes are affected) are also good herbs to use for this condition. **SHS**
- Try the homeopathic remedy Kali Bich 6c three times a day in between meals until symptoms are relieved.

Helpful Hints
- Inhaling steam is another useful treatment. Add a few drops of mint or eucalyptus oil to boiling water, place a towel over your head, and inhale for 5 minutes daily.
- The Neil Med Sinus rinse is a godsend for people with sinus problems. It's a very simple "wash out" for the nose that takes less than two minutes to use. Take once or twice daily – available from Boots and all major chemists. Or log onto www.neilmed.com or www.pharmacy2u.co.uk Tel: 0845 803 9033. They also make a spray gel that helps soothe and hydrate irritated nasal passages. I was told about this range by an Ear Nose & Throat specialist and it really does help when used daily.
- Add some sea salt to tepid water and place a small amount in the palm of your hand, and inhale this mixture up each nostril. This helps to clear the nasal passages – or buy a sea salt nose spray. Available from all good chemists.
- Avoid dry atmospheres; and when the central heating is on, make sure there is a bowl of water near the radiator to keep the air moist. Blow your nose very gently as some people can suffer nosebleeds when the nasal cavity becomes infected or very dry.

S

SJOGREN'S SYNDROME

(see also Raynaud's Disease, Rheumatoid Arthritis, Leaky Gut Syndrome, Lupus, Osteoporosis and Stress)

Sjogren's syndrome is named after Henrik Sjogren, a Swedish ophthalmologist, who in 1933 noted that many of his female patients with various forms of arthritis also suffered from dry mucous membranes. Sjogren's is an autoimmune condition, in which the body's immune system turns on itself and starts attacking the moisture-producing glands, such as the eyes, nose, skin, throat, mouth and vagina, which can all become chronically dry. The dry mouth can trigger an increase in dental problems. The skin may become so dry that highly irritating skin rashes appear along with thread veins close to the skin's surface. The skin may darken and if scratched intensely, then infections can also occur. Ninety percent of sufferers are women.

There are two types of Sjogren's: primary and secondary. Primary Sjogren's patients are likely to have different antibodies circulating in their blood from those with the secondary form, which is linked to other autoimmune conditions, such as rheumatoid arthritis and lupus.

This condition often goes undiagnosed for several years, as the symptoms are so varied. As well as inflammation in the body and the dryness of mucous membranes, other symptoms can include Raynaud's Disease, osteoporosis, joint and muscle pains, a long-term low white blood cell count, fatigue, a propensity to lung problems such as bronchitis, high cortisol levels, hormone imbalances, especially around the menopause, low thyroid function and sleep problems, low levels of the hormone DHEA, and/or excess acidity in the body. Some sufferers, especially those who have previously been diagnosed with lupus (or rheumatoid arthritis), may also be highly sensitive to sun exposure and suffer rosacea-type facial rashes around the nose and chin.

Other important factors often overlooked by the orthodox medical establishment include leaky gut syndrome, in which the gut wall becomes permeable and food particles leach into the blood stream – thus triggering an autoimmune-type response. Multiple food intolerances (usually to refined sugars, wheat and/or gluten and animal-source dairy produce), in conjunction with a highly strung personality, or highly stressed lifestyle, can also over time definitely play a part in this condition. Therefore, it's really important that before reading on, you should also read the *Acid–Alkaline Balance*, *Candida*, *Leaky Gut*, *Raynaud's Disease*, *Rheumatoid Arthritis*, *Lupus* and *Stress* sections.

It's usually a rheumatologist who eventually diagnoses Sjogren's via blood tests and by taking a full medical history. The Epstein-Barr virus is also linked to this condition.

The main point to stress with Sjogren's and other autoimmune conditions is that it has most probably taken years for your symptoms to develop, and while you may feel, or be told, that such conditions are 'incurable', there is a huge amount that you can do to help yourself – but it will take time. The first step is to start thinking positively, be kind to yourself, and then find a good nutritionist who can organize the appropriate tests to discover the root factor that has contributed or triggered your condition. See *Useful Information* to source a qualified nutritionist.

It's also important to note that several prescription drugs have side effects that mimic some Sjogren's symptoms, which is another reason to investigate all symptoms thoroughly.

Foods to Avoid
- See this section under *Acid–Alkaline Balance*, *Leaky Gut* and *Rheumatoid Arthritis*. And keep in mind that it can take several months to re-alkalize your body, which has probably been too acid for many years.
- Avoid tomato juice and acid fruits (in the mouth), such as oranges and grapefruits.
- Avoid all fizzy drinks and cordials high in refined sugars.
- Cut down on diuretics, such as alcohol, coffee and excess black tea, as these can contribute to the dryness in the body.
- Cut down on all flour-based foods, because when flour and water are combined they make a sticky paste. In the bowel these types of foods draw fluids from the body in order to aid excretion and thus add to dryness.
- Generally, cut down on refined starchy, sugary foods, which can affect immune function and trigger tooth decay.
- Once you have been tested for food intolerances (see under *Allergies*), avoid the offending foods. In the meantime, greatly reduce your intake of wheat, gluten, refined sugars and animal dairy produce.

Friendly Foods
- When the body is dry it requires far more essential fats, therefore eat more oily fish, organic nuts and seeds and use walnut, olive, sesame and flax oils for salad dressings.
- Drink alkalizing water, such as Kangen Water. This is a water system that attaches to your kitchen tap, and ionizes and greatly alkalizes water, which aids healing because the tissues heal more quickly when more alkaline. The system is used in Japanese hospitals with highly beneficial health results. For full details, call 020 7580 7537 or log on to www.kangenmiraclewater.co.uk
- Green tea has antioxidant and anti-inflammatory properties. Drink regularly and use the organic decaffeinated versions. Steep for at least 5 minutes before drinking. Sweeten with a small amount of xylitol, organic agave syrup or stevia, which have a low impact on your blood sugar levels.

- Instead of wheat-based breads, try amaranth crackers or oat cakes (but avoid these if you are chronically constipated).
- Use almond, quinoa or rice milks instead of animal-based milks.
- Eat far more pulses, lentils, barley, quinoa, brown rice, plus any fresh vegetables and fruits. Please read *Leaky Gut* and *Candida* before eating huge amounts of fruit!
- Increase your intake of foods high in carotenes – watercress, pumpkin, papaya, carrots, all green leafy foods, apricots and cantaloupe melons.

Useful Remedies

- This list could go on almost to infinity – which is why it's vital for you to consult a nutritionist who can pinpoint your main triggers and then deal with the problems in order of urgency!
- Gamma-linolenic acid (GLA), the main ingredient in evening primrose oil, is very important for this condition as it helps reduce inflammation – take 2 grams daily in divided doses with meals. **BC**
- Omega-3 fish oils or linseed oil capsules (if you are a vegetarian) are important to nourish the mucous membranes and help alleviate the dryness. Take at least 2 grams daily.
- Co-enzyme Q10 helps to protect teeth and gums and also increases energy levels – take 100mg daily with breakfast or lunch.
- A good-quality multi-vitamin/mineral for your age and gender that contains at least 30mg zinc per day, as many people with this condition are often low in zinc. Try Triple Zinc formula by Metabolics (Tel: 01380 812799), which contains three types of zinc – picolinate, citrate and sulphate. These are easy to absorb and improve zinc levels quickly. To start with, take 2 capsules daily for 6 weeks, then take one a day for 6 weeks, and then just one capsule per week.
- Probiotics – healthy bacteria – are important for gut health, which is almost always an issue in autoimmune conditions. Available from all health stores. Take daily after main meal.
- Use liquid hyaluronic acid (HA), a naturally occurring protein found in all bone and cartilage structures in the body. HA provides the cushioning effect in all joints and it's the high content of HA in young people that keeps their joints so supple. HA helps relieve the dryness in tissues, due to its ability in helping maintain hydration. Take 1 sachet daily in water on an empty stomach before breakfast. For more details call Modern Herbals on 01274 889047. Website: www.modernherbals.com
- Omega-7, extracted from the sea buckthorn, is an essential fatty acid useful for helping to reduce the dry eyes, nose, vagina etc, as it also helps the body retain moisture. Take 4 capsules daily for first month and thereafter 2 daily. **PN**
- Lack of vitamin A is very much linked to dryness – take a natural-source carotene complex daily, as this converts to vitamin A naturally in the body and is totally non toxic.
- A fermented wheat germ extract known as Avemar has demonstrated remarkable immune-modulating effects, and helps restore immune systems that are overstimulated. Avemar has been shown in numerous trials to reduce the symptoms of autoimmune disease. Take one sachet daily in water at least one hour before breakfast. Avemar is also available in capsules. It must be kept refrigerated. Details on www.avemar.com Available in the UK from the Nutri Centre. **NC**

Helpful Hints

- As long-term stress of any kind is very much linked to this condition, do all you can to control your reactions to stressful situations. Regular meditation and t'ai chi (there are plenty of at home DVDs available on Amazon, such as *T'ai Chi – Exercises for Deep Relaxation* by Hun Yuan Fa Soong Gong) are both proven ways to reduce the 'fight-or-flight' stress responses that can do much damage in the body. See under *Stress*.

- As some sufferers have very dry mucous membranes in the nose, try using Naso Gel from Neil Med to keep it moist, otherwise you may suffer nose bleeds. Available from Boots and all good chemists. Alternatively, call 0845 803 9033 or log on to www.neilmed.com or www.pharmacy2u.co.uk
- Use sterile 'natural tears'-type eye drops if and when your eyes become very dry. Always use these natural tears during flights.
- Practise good dental hygiene and see an oral hygienist at least twice a year. The dry mouth can cause gums to recede more quickly and trigger dental issues.
- Curaprox make Xerostrum products including chewing gum, toothpaste, mouth wash and pastilles, especially for people with dry mouth problems, based on olive oil, xylitol and various vitamins. For details and stockists worldwide, log on to www.curaprox.co.uk or call 01480 862084.
- As lack of the hormone DHEA is linked to Sjogren's, have a blood test and supplement as needed under medical supervision.
- Have your thyroid function tested.
- Warm, moist atmospheres are preferable to dry 'desert'-like conditions.
- Use good-quality butter-type body creams to keep your skin moisturized.
- Use pH-balanced moisturizing soaps based on ingredients such as olive oil.
- Be sensible with sun exposure, as it can add to skin dryness.

SKIN CANCERS
(see under Sunburn)

S

SMOKING
(see also Bronchitis)

Smoking triggers nine out of every 10 cases of cancer, and every 15 minutes someone dies thanks to smoking. Nine and a half million people in the UK smoke and 450 children start smoking every day. Passive smoking also kills. Chronic Obstructive Pulmonary Disease (COPD) is an umbrella term for all chronic lung conditions; it can be fatal and is mainly caused by smoking. For more information on COPD, log on to www.lunguk.org

If you smoke, the best favour you can do for yourself and for those around you is to give it up. A pack a day equates to losing a month of life each year. One cigarette can increase your heart rate by 20 beats a minute and can also increase your blood pressure. Smoking one packet of cigarettes a day depletes 500mg of vitamin C from your body, yet the average daily intake is 60–100mg. Cigarettes increase carbon monoxide levels in the blood and it takes the circulatory system 6 hours to return to normal after you have smoked a cigarette. Perhaps now you understand why heart disease, cancer and strokes, as well as high blood pressure and numerous other chronic diseases, are linked to smoking. It's also worth noting that smoking ages your skin and tests have shown that the skin of a 40-year-old smoker is comparable to that of a 65-year-old non-smoker.

The more you can control your blood sugar, the easier it will be to give up smoking for good and avoid the mood swings associated with withdrawal. It may, therefore, also be useful to read the section on *Low Blood Sugar*. People with A or AB blood types tend to have stickier blood – and therefore smoking would increase their risk of heart disease and strokes even more.

Foods to Avoid

- Cut down on the foods that you have just prior to enjoying a cigarette, such as wine, beer or coffee.
- Cut down on saturated animal fats, which will harden your arteries over time.
- Cut down on caffeine, colas, refined sugary starchy foods, tea and other stimulants.
- See also *Heart Disease*.

Friendly Foods

- As smoking makes your body far more acid, eat plenty of foods that re-alkalize your body, such as fruits, vegetables, millet, buckwheat and wheat germ. See *Acid–Alkaline Balance* for a large list.
- Oats are a nerve tonic that should help reduce addictions. Have organic porridge every morning.
- Begin using unrefined walnut, sunflower and olive oils for salad dressings, and use sunflower and pumpkin seeds and linseeds (flax seeds) over breakfast cereals and salads.
- Eating more leafy greens, such as cabbage, watercress, spring greens, spinach or kale, reduces your risk of lung cancer.
- Drink organic green and white teas, which are high in antioxidants. Some researchers believe that Japanese men who smoke suffer less incidence of cancer and other lung diseases thanks to the protective effects of green tea.
- Cantaloupe melons, pumpkin, apricots, carrots, papaya, French beans, mangoes, raw parsley and watercress are all high in natural-source carotenes, which help to protect lung tissue.
- Eat more oily fish, rich in vitamin A.
- Generally, eat small meals regularly to control blood sugar (see *Friendly Foods* under *Low Blood Sugar*).
- If you eat meat, then have one portion of organic liver once a week, as it is rich in lung-protective vitamin A.

Useful Supplements

- A high-strength multi-vitamin and mineral, in a formula that includes essential fats and antioxidants, helps to give some protection.
- Make sure any multi-formula you take contains a full spectrum of B-vitamins.
- Take 2 grams of vitamin C daily in divided doses with meals.
- Natural-source beta-carotenes, 30mg daily, will help protect some of the damage done in the lungs by smoking – but it still far better to stop smoking ASAP.
- 500mg magnesium taken daily helps ease difficulties with breathing. Take before bed.
- N-acetyl cysteine – take 500mg twice daily before meals. This amino acid helps bronchial conditions, as it loosens mucous and strengthens tissue.
- 200mcg per day of the mineral chromium helps to keep your blood sugar on an even keel, as many people who stop smoking struggle to balance their blood sugar. Take between meals.
- Try a herbal extract tincture made from crushed lobelia leaves, ginger, oats, liquorice and thyme; taken twice daily it helps reduce the cravings and supports the lungs. Take with homeopathic remedies Staphysagria, Tabacum and Nux Vomica, which really help reduce withdrawal symptoms and cravings. **OP**

Helpful Hints

- Soak in an Epsom-salt or sea-salt bath, which helps remove nicotine through the pores. Accompanying this with skin brushing would be even better.
- For more help contact ASH – Action on Smoking and Health, First Floor, 144–145 Shoreditch High Street, London E1 6JE. Tel: 020 7739 5902. Website:www.ash.org.uk
- QUIT is a charity that helps people stop smoking. Tel: 0800 00 2200, www.quit.org.uk

SORE THROATS   *(see also Colds and Flu and Immune Function)*

If you tend to suffer from a persistent sore throat, it usually denotes that your immune system is struggling to cope. When I become overtired and my throat becomes sore, I know that if I were to eat any foods high in refined sugars, this could send my immune system off the deep end, thus triggering a cold or infection. I now know my limits and listen to my body. If you are at this point, never underestimate how what you eat during the next 48 hours can be the deciding factor as to whether you become ill or not. Also make sure you are getting sufficient rest, which is one of the easiest ways to help boost immune function.

Regular bouts of tonsillitis (see also *Tonsillitis*) mean that your lymphatic system is under stress and your body is telling you to detoxify. Regular sore throats are also associated with the yeast fungal overgrowth candida (see also *Candida*).

Inflammation and pain in the throat can trigger symptoms such as pain upon swallowing or speaking, a dry tickling feeling, build-up of mucous in the nose and sinuses and occasionally a husky voice or loss of your voice. These types of infections are caused by bacteria or viruses. A sore throat caused by a streptococcal infection (often called strep throat) needs to be identified and treated, or it could trigger rheumatic fever in some cases. If symptoms are severe, please see your doctor.

If I start a sore throat, I take homeopathic Streptococcus 10M immediately, along with the Wellness Formula (see below under *Useful Remedies*) and the soreness almost always disappears within a day.

S

Foods to Avoid
- Eliminate refined sugar in any form for 4 days to give your immune system a chance to fight infection.
- Greatly cut down or avoid all white-flour-based products, snacks and burger-type meals. Avoid all 'white' foods.
- Coffee, sugary drinks and alcohol dehydrate the body and act as stimulants. If your adrenal glands are exhausted, these foods will add to the problem.
- Cut down on all full-fat animal-source dairy produce, especially chocolate and full fat milks.

Friendly Foods
- Increase fluid intake: include lots of filtered water, herbal teas, especially green and white tea, diluted fruit juices, and broths.
- Sip warm water with powdered vitamin C, plus lemon, ginger and/or garlic with a little honey.
- See also *Friendly Foods* under *Colds and Flu*.

Useful Remedies
- One of the best remedies I have found for alleviating a sore throat, which usually heralds the start of a cold, is the Wellness Formula, made by Source Naturals Inc. It contains garlic, propolis, elderberry extract, olive leaf extract, vitamin C, astragalus, zinc and grapeseed extract – an excellent combination of nutrients needed to boost immunity, as they are anti-viral and bacterial. At the first sign of a sore throat or feeling that you 'have something coming', take 1 or 2 tablets, three times daily. Available at all good health stores. **NC**
- At the same time take homeopathic Streptococcus 10M as directed for 3 days – it really helps eliminate a sore throat. Available from all specialist homeopathic pharmacies, such as Nelsons (www.nelsonhomeopathy.com), Ainsworths (www.ainsworths.com) or the Organic Pharmacy via www.theorganicpharmacy.com
- Ask at your health shop for either a bee propolis (**avoid if you are highly sensitive to bee stings**) or an echinacea throat spray and use as directed.

- Try Ultimate Echinacea Complex, which also contains astragalus (which boosts the immune system). **NC**; or log on to www.holoshealth.com
- Natural-source beta-carotenes convert naturally to vitamin A in the body, which hugely supports a healthy immune system. Take up to 30mg daily when you feel poorly.
- Take at least 2–3 grams of vitamin C daily in divided doses with meals.
- Take a vitamin B-complex to support your adrenal glands along with an extra 500mg of B5.
- Low levels of selenium are linked to viral infections. Take a multi-vitamin and mineral that includes 200mcg of selenium and 30mg of zinc.
- Zinc gluconate lozenges really help reduce a sore throat, take 3–4 daily. Available at health shops and good chemists.
- If you end up taking antibiotics, make sure you replenish healthy bacteria by taking acidophilus/bifidus capsules twice daily for 6 weeks. See under *Antibiotics*.

Helpful Hints
- Crush fresh sage, make into a tea, allow to cool, and gargle. Sage is antiseptic and eases the soreness. If the throat is really sore, soak a cloth in the sage mix and apply to the throat area.
- You can also crush an onion and wrap it in a cloth and place on the throat.
- Propolis tincture can be diluted in water and used as a gargle.
- Change your toothbrush regularly.
- At the onset of a sore throat use homeopathic Aconite or Belladonna 30c – if the throat is red and worse on the right-hand side. For children's sore throats, a hacking cough and swollen tonsils, try Chamomila 30c – give 3 times daily for 2 days.

- The herb thyme is also a natural antiseptic. It can be made into a solution and used as a gargle for sore throats or sipped as a tea mixture to help relieve sore throats and coughs. Or mix oregano, thyme and basil essential oils and massage onto the throat area.
- Tea tree oil is a natural antiseptic; use diluted with a little sea salt as a gargle, **but do not swallow.** Gargle with a mixture of warm water and a quarter teaspoonful of turmeric powder and a pinch of salt.

SPIRITUAL EMERGENCY

(see also Adrenal Exhaustion, Depression, Low Blood Sugar and Panic Attacks)

This title may appear out of place in a health book, but believe me, spiritual emergency (when a spiritual awakening becomes a physical and sometimes a mental crisis) is a well-known phenomena in the East. As our interest in spiritual subjects gains pace, it is becoming far more common in the West. I have yet to meet an orthodox doctor (apart from a handful of GPs, including my own) who has heard of this condition, or recognizes any of its specific symptoms, but it definitely exists.

Most psychiatrists tend to diagnose a spiritual emergency as psychosis, depression, schizophrenia or a total nervous breakdown (which it may well be), but if this subject could receive wider attention, many people could avoid being sent to mental homes, given strong prescription drugs and labelled as being 'mentally ill'.

Of course, mental illness can have a huge range of causes, including overuse of social drugs, such as crack, LSD or cannabis, extreme and prolonged stress, which hugely alters brain chemistry, and a poor diet lacking in essential brain nutrients – but it can also be linked to a spiritual-type breakthrough.

Back in 1998 I experienced a huge spiritual emergency in which I began affecting electrical equipment, could clearly see people's energy or auric fields, became super-psychic, telepathic and could clearly 'hear' people in the spirit world. I received huge amounts of information, which placed an enormous strain on my brain and nervous system. The full story is told in my book *Divine Intervention* (Cico Books).

Symptoms of intense breakthroughs are diverse and wide-ranging; this is an abbreviated version. The body may experience muscle tremors, fever or cold. Some people hear voices or, depending on their culture and beliefs, see visions of angels, demons or archetypal animals. The person may undergo a physical near-death experience or a symbolic feeling of death and rebirth. There may also be a sense of having 'married God', or even that you are the reincarnation of Jesus, Buddha or another important spiritual figure. You may manifest objects, such as holy ash, or phenomena, such as stigmata. Can you imagine an orthodox doctor's reaction to such a list of symptoms?

And, whatever your personality is, at the time of a spiritual breakthrough it becomes hugely amplified. Feelings of humility alternate with a belief that you are a super-being; you may wonder, 'Why doesn't everyone want to listen to *me?*' You may believe that you can fly, or have a sense that you have become indestructible, or feel unconditional love interspersed with episodes of panic.

At such times people often experience various phenomena, such as seeing auras and hearing other realms, either spontaneously, as in my case, or during spiritual development courses. Also, growing numbers of people who regularly use social drugs, such as cannabis, crack or ecstasy, tend to suffer far more mental health problems.

While researching my spiritual/science books *The Evidence For the Sixth Sense* (Cico Books) and *Countdown to Coherence* (Watkins Publishing) in which I deal in depth with these types of issues, I spoke at length to Professor Frederick Travis, head of the Center for Brain, Consciousness, and Cognition at the Maharishi University in Iowa, who has studied brain function for more than 30 years.

When I asked him about the effects of dangerous social drugs, he told me: 'These types of drugs block the uptake of neurotransmitters. Within the brain you have "pleasure circuits", which fire when you eat a favourite food, such as chocolate or you see a fabulous sunset. The neurotransmitter dopamine is released and travels to the receiving part of a cell, where it is held for a moment, then "let go" and recycled and taken back up by the neuron that fired it. But if you take a drug like cocaine, it fills up the re-uptake receptors, and the dopamine just sits in the space between the two cells, so the receptors just keep firing. That is the basis of the "rush" that users experience.'

'Which causes what to happen in the long term?' I asked. 'The dopamine circuits can eventually be destroyed,' Travis told me. 'Users no longer enjoy such intense highs on a single dose, so they take more and more drugs to feel that rush again. This spiral takes them ever further away from living a stable life, as their brains suffer more and more damage which can trigger psychosis, depression, suicidal tendencies, sometimes multiple-personality disorders and schizophrenia.'

In regard to schizophrenics, Travis and others have found that they have a thinning of the brain cortex, which means they have less grey matter and fewer cortical connections. Therefore, they find it difficult to maintain a coherent sense of individualized 'self' – as they cannot integrate thinking, feeling and a sense of self at the same time – and can easily become disoriented into other levels of feeling and of reality. A shaman might term such events as a spirit 'walk-in', but Fred says that such people are 'picking up' energetic aspects of the Whole Consciousness and therefore becoming confused in their everyday reality, as their brains are flooded with information. This also helps explain phenomena such as speaking in tongues: as at times of intense religious experiences, people may link to the universal field of consciousness that contains all knowledge, and since their brains cannot process so much information, it comes out as a garbled mess!

Studies have demonstrated that if schizophrenics learn to meditate and also have counselling, over time, in conjunction with a good diet, their condition can improve.

There is not sufficient space in this type of book to deal with the huge panoply of mental health conditions, but it's important to realize that in some cases people can be helped via diet, supplements and the right specialist support.

Nevertheless these types of conditions/symptoms are in many cases linked to adrenal exhaustion and low blood sugar – see these sections before continuing.

We all have psychic abilities and are capable of miracles, but most of us don't truly comprehend this ultimate truth. When you undergo this type of experience you need to find professional help to determine the most appropriate course of action.

If, during your spiritual growth, you begin to feel ultra-special and your ego comes into play, you need to ground yourself (see below). Find your nearest spiritualist church, which will undoubtedly know of someone who can help you. Hands-on healing would definitely be of benefit during a spiritual-type emergency – see under *Healing*.

But if anyone starts to self-harm, threatens others, thinks they can fly and generally becomes a danger to themselves or others, medical help should be sought.

Foods to Avoid
- Sometimes during this type of situation you don't want food, but it is imperative that you eat to help ground yourself.
- The last thing you need is stimulants, so avoid caffeine, refined sugars (although, see below) and alcohol.

Friendly Foods
- If your brain is in absolute overdrive and feels as though it's on fire, then eat some sugary food quickly. The brain uses pure glucose as a fuel, and as you may be processing huge amounts of information, your brain will need an energy supply. It is always preferable if you can eat small healthy meals regularly, but if the situation is acute then eat sugar or a banana. Controlling your blood sugar helps to control the events and your ability to cope with them – see under *Adrenal Exhaustion* and *Low Blood Sugar*.
- Generally, eat far more 'earthy' grounding foods, such as porridge made with organic rice milk, stews and thick vegetable or grain-based soups.
- You may not want it, but you need protein, which helps balance your blood sugar levels for longer periods. Fish and animal products might repulse you, in which case eat some beans, pulses, cooked tofu and brown rice with plenty of fruits and vegetables. Otherwise, make smoothies with fruits, sunflower and pumpkin seeds and add a tablespoon of whey, hemp seed or rice-based protein powder, which is easy for the body to utilize. See under *General Health Hints* for a great smoothie recipe.
- Drink plenty of water, and calming herbal teas such as vervain, liquorice or camomile.
- Your digestion may be upset, so include fresh ginger in soups and drink ginger teas. See under *Leaky Gut* and *Stress*.

Useful Remedies
- Begin taking Bach Rescue Remedy and Star of Bethlehem immediately and then every 2 or 3 hours.
- Also begin taking homeopathic Arnica 200c every few hours to help reduce feelings of shock.
- For anyone who is quite psychic, intuitive and has a very open personality, try homeopathic Phosphorous 30c, 3 times daily, which will help to balance the energies.

- Take one homeopathic Aconite 200c daily. Taken at the onset of any symptoms, this can help to relieve some of the stress and reduce fear.
- Take a high-strength B-complex to support your nerves. Try an extra 1000mg of pantothenic acid (vitamin B5) daily to support your adrenal glands, which are most probably working overtime.
- Take a multi-vitamin and mineral formula daily.
- The brain is made up of 60% fats, so take 3–4 grams of fish oil daily. If you are vegan or vegetarian, then take linseed oil instead.

Helpful Hints

- Contact the Spiritual Crisis Network, a charity formed by clinical psychologist Isabel Clarke and her colleagues, plus Catherine Lucas (www.breathworks-mindfullness.co.uk), who went through a profound spiritual emergency. For help contact them via info@SpiritualCrisisNetwork.org.uk). Website www.SpiritualCrisisNetwork.org.uk
- Ask your health professional to read *Madness, Mystery and the Survival of God* or *Psychosis and Spirituality* by Dr Isabel Clarke www.o-books.net Her latest book (Ed.) is *Psychosis and Spirituality: consolidating the new paradigm* (Wiley-Blackwell).
- In London, the College of Psychic Studies takes students from all over the world and helps them to integrate their newly found gifts and knowledge in a balanced and safe environment. Tel: 020 7589 3292. Website: www.collegeofpsychicstudies.co.uk
- At this time you need all the support and patience friends and family can provide, as you may say and do many things – such as levitate or produce ash – which can initially be very frightening. You may also experience periods of complete and utter bliss. I beg of you to write any insights or channelling down – don't try sharing them with everyone you know, which can elicit negative responses. At such times a person can also easily be persuaded to join cults.
- Avoid negative thoughts as much as you can. For every negative thought, try to replace it with a positive one.
- Try not to panic – the experience will pass, it just takes time. See also *Panic Attacks* and *Stress*.
- Read *Spiritual Emergency* by Stanislav and Christina Grof MD. To order in the UK, call 020 7323 2382. This book really helps when personal transformation becomes a crisis. So would my books *The Evidence For The Sixth Sense* (CICO Books) and *Countdown to Coherence* (Watkins Publishing).

STITCH

This is a sudden, sharp pain in the side or abdomen, which usually wears off after a few minutes when we rest. The pain is almost certainly caused by a spasm in the gut wall, for example, after eating a large meal when blood has been diverted from muscles momentarily to aid digestion. If we then do some physical exercise, the stitch will come on. Therefore, it makes sense not to exercise until at least an hour after eating. A stitch is the body's way of telling you that it needs more oxygen, so should you get it, stand still and breathe deeply.

People who tend to be sedentary, eat insufficient fresh fruit and vegetables and too much sugar, caffeine and animal protein, are often lacking in calcium and magnesium, which causes a build-up of lactic acid, resulting in regular attacks of muscle cramps or a stitch. Basically, a stitch is triggered by an over-acidic environment – therefore see under *Acid–Alkaline Balance* section.

Foods to Avoid
- Generally, cut down on refined sugar/starchy foods, such as croissants, biscuits, cakes, pizza and white-flour-based foods.
- Any foods that remove the mineral magnesium from the body, which is needed to alleviate stitch. Magnesium is particularly depleted by too much alcohol and caffeine.

Friendly Foods
- Magnesium-rich foods, such as green leafy vegetables, fruits plus brown rice, barley, lentils and whole grains rich in fibre will give you more protection in the long term. Blackstrap molasses are rich in magnesium and calcium.
- Honey and dried apricots are also high in magnesium.
- Include good-quality protein in the diet, such as fresh fish, eggs, cooked tofu and lean meats, at least once a day.

Useful Remedies
- Take a high-strength vitamin B-complex daily.
- Calcium 400mg and 600mg of magnesium to help reduce spasm and relax the muscles. Take in divided doses with food.
- Take Emergen-C or electrolyte sachets, which are high in vitamin C and minerals. Take one sachet before exercising to help reduce any chance of stitch. Available from all chemists.

Helpful Hints
- If you can, bend down and touch your toes to relieve a stitch; or take a deep breath and have a good stretch.
- A stitch is more likely to occur if you exercise while food is still digesting in the gut. Avoid strenuous exercise for an hour after a substantial amount of food.
- Generally, take regular exercise to avoid lactic acid accumulation in the body.
- Before doing heavy exercise, especially jogging/running, take a quarter of a teaspoon of bicarbonate of soda in a small glass of diluted fruit juice, as this helps delay the onset of lactic acid build-up and should help you to avoid developing a stitch.
- A stitch generally occurs when you have not warmed up properly before exercise.
- Do not sit for long periods without going for a walk or a good stretch.
- Breathe deeply more often.

STOMACH AND DUODENAL ULCERS

(see also Acid–Alkaline Balance, Acid Stomach, Low Stomach Acid and Stress)

Stomach ulcers are small raw areas on the walls of the stomach where the protective mucous coating has worn away. This may be due to the mucous lining being insufficient to start with, and so being affected by factors such as stress, smoking, alcohol, excess caffeine intake, erratic eating habits, over-consumption of refined starchy foods and so on.

Duodenal ulcers are small raw spots in the lining of the duodenum, and tend to be smaller than stomach ulcers. They are predominantly caused by stomach acid infiltrating the sphincter muscle and getting into the small intestine. This is why having too much stomach acid (which tends to affect Type O blood types) can be a problem. The condition is also exacerbated by smoking and alcohol, which both relax the pyloric sphincter muscle, thereby allowing acids to escape on to the walls of the small intestine, which lacks the same protection as the stomach.

A bacterium called *Helicobacter pylori* has been found in over 90% of duodenal ulcers and 80% of gastric ulcers. This bacterium is also linked to stomach cancers, low energy levels, and skin conditions such as rosacea and urticaria. Inflammatory conditions, such as migraines, are also linked to *Helicobacter pylori*. Treatment with high-dose antibiotics usually kills the bacterium – however it commonly recurs.

Stomach ulcers are more common in Type A blood groups and tend to affect older people whose protective stomach lining has been eroded. There is a link between stomach ulcers and cancer. The pain of a stomach ulcer often becomes worse after eating. Duodenal ulcers are more common in Type O blood types and tend to affect younger people. They generally do not progress to cancers and the pain of duodenal ulcers is usually relieved by food.

Stress is a major factor in any type of ulcer, because when you are stressed the body produces more stomach acid. Intolerances to foods such as wheat, cow's milk (animal dairy in general) and prescription drugs, plus long-term use of aspirin, steroids and non-steroidal anti-inflammatory drugs, such as ibuprofen, can also be contributory factors in ulcers. See under *Leaky Gut*. Nutritionist Gareth Zeal says: 'In clinical practice I have found that if people take an omega-7 essential fat known as sea buckthorn with a meal at the same time as using aspirin (if this has been prescribed), the omega-7 helps to reduce the risk of internal bleeds.'

Foods to Avoid
- There is a proven link between over-consumption of caffeine and ulcers, so avoid or greatly reduce coffee and colas. Organic decaffeinated coffee is usually tolerated in small amounts.
- Eliminate all dairy produce from any animal source for at least one month.
- Alcohol irritates the gut wall – keep to a minimum or eliminate for a while.
- Don't eat too much refined sugar and too many rich fatty foods, which again tend to hugely irritate the gut.
- Avoid spicy foods, which can aggravate the gut lining.
- Avoid eating late at night, which places a great strain on your digestive system and liver.
- Avoid citrus fruits (especially oranges and grapefruit), raw tomatoes, rhubarb, plums and pineapple. The concentrated juices seem to cause the most problems.
- Avoid all refined white-flour-based foods.
- Avoid thermally hot or cold foods and drinks.
- Avoid high animal proteins, such as beef and pork, as these increase stomach acid production.
- Eliminate cola-type drinks, which play havoc with gut lining.

Friendly Foods
- Eat lots more fresh cabbage, which is rich in the amino acid L-glutamine, known to heal the gut. Eat it raw or add to fresh vegetable juices. If you cook the cabbage, then use the cooking water for gravy or drink once it has cooled.
- Replace cow's milk with organic rice or almond milk.
- Eat plenty of vegetables and fruits, such as bananas, figs, lychees or pears. Before eating lots of fruit, read the *Candida* section, as ulcers are often linked to fungal overgrowth.
- Include barley, brown rice and wholemeal bread, pastas and noodles plus lentils, millet, amaranth, quinoa and couscous in your diet.
- Eat more jacket potatoes, sweet potatoes, peas, corn and apples, which are high in fibre.
- Mashed pumpkin is great for healing the gut, as is papaya.
- Add seaweed, such as kombu, to your bean dishes as it contains healing properties. Seaweed aids healing of ulcers.
- Use seaweed nori flakes instead of salt, as they are high in minerals and are delicious.

S

- Fish, nuts and seeds (linseeds/flax seeds, and sunflower, pumpkin and sesame seeds) are high in zinc, which aids tissue healing. See under *General Health Hints* for a delicious smoothie recipe that includes hemp seed protein.
- Eat more live, low-fat yoghurt, manuka honey and liquorice, which all help to heal the gut and kill the *Helicobacter pylori*.
- Add cinnamon to fruit dishes.
- Slippery elm – preferably in a tea – helps to soothe and heal the whole digestive tract, including the stomach and duodenum. Sip throughout the day in between meals. **SHS**
- Drink more green and white organic teas.

Useful Remedies
- Ulc-Dig capsules contain marshmallow, barberry, pau d'arco and poke root, which help to promote healing in the gut. **SHS**
- Chew 1 to 2 tablets of deglycyrrhized liquorice 20 minutes before food. This encourages healing of the stomach lining and helps to eradicate the *Helicobacter* if this is present.
- Take Gastro ULC – a formula designed to help heal gastric ulcers and leaky gut. Take one with each main meal. Made by Apex Energetics (www.apexenergetics.com). To order call the Wholistic Medical Centre on 0207 580 7537.
- Vitamin A is vital for the stomach lining to be able to heal. Take 20,000iu daily for the first month and then reduce to 10,000iu for another month. **NB If you are pregnant or planning a pregnancy, then take no more than 3000iu of vitamin A daily.**

- After two months take a carotene complex daily for on-going maintenance, as it naturally converts to vitamin A in the body and is totally non toxic.
- B-vitamins aid digestion and reduce the risk of ulcers. Take a B-complex daily.
- Take vitamin C as magnesium or potassium ascorbate, 500 mg before meals and at bedtime, as most ulcer patients are lacking this vital vitamin. **BC**
- Mastica is a resin from a plant found in the Aegean sea. Taking 500–1000mg per day for two weeks has been shown to rapidly heal gastric ulcers. It also helps to remove any *Helicobacter*.
- Taking L-glutamine (2–4 grams twice daily) 30 minutes before meals (for one month, then half dose) really helps heal the gut. **HN**
- Omega-7 essential fats from the sea buckthorn help rebuild mucosal tissue. Take 2 grams daily for 3 months – after this reduce to 1 gram daily with meals. **PN**
- NAC (N-acetyl cysteine) is an amino acid derivative that can inhibit the growth of *Helicobacter pylori* if taken regularly. Take 600mg twice daily in between meals. This is also a great supplement to support liver function.

Helpful Hints
- Chew food thoroughly. Never rush a meal, as digestion is made difficult when you are stressed or in a hurry.
- Don't drink too much liquid with meals, as this dilutes digestive juices.
- Ulcers can be encouraged to heal by eating only small quantities of food at a time.
- Avoid stress and rushing as much as possible, as stress over a prolonged period can cause great harm to our digestive system.
- Smoking greatly increases the risk of ulcers.
- Drinking 75ml of concentrated aloe vera juice 20 minutes before meals also helps to soothe the digestive tract. Aloe Pura make a good Digestive Aid Juice, which greatly soothes the stomach lining. It contains aloe vera, papaya, peppermint oil, camomile and slippery elm. Available from good health stores and larger chemists. www.optimah.com
- Homeopathic Mercuricus corrosivus or Argentum nitricum 6c can be taken 3 times daily for a week.

STRESS
(see also Adrenal Exhaustion, Depression and Immune Function)

More than 7 million working days are lost in the UK every year through stress-related conditions and it is a major contributing factor for a host of health problems. Not all stress is bad – it can help to keep you sharp and alert – but in the longer term how your body copes depends on your *reaction* to the stress.

Aeons ago when our ancestors were faced with life-and-death situations, the hormones adrenaline and cortisol were released from the endocrine system, which incorporates the pancreas, thyroid and pituitary, plus the adrenal glands, which are situated just above the kidneys. The released hormones made the heart pump faster, giving an instant energy boost to the body and brain. Muscles tensed, cholesterol production increased and enzymes in the blood caused the blood to thicken, so that if our ancestor was injured, then their blood clotted more easily. Blood vessels would constrict; endorphins, the body's own painkillers, would be released; and oxygen consumption increased. Known as the 'fight-or-flight' reaction, these responses saved many lives back when our ancestors fought off marauding animals and invaders.

Today, our automatic physical responses to stress remain the same, but unfortunately these days they tend to trigger heart attacks, strokes, cancers, stomach ulcers and even Alzheimer's disease. Why? Because if we don't disperse this constant stream of stress hormone production through regular exercise and relaxation, then, in the longer term, excess fight-or-flight hormones become highly toxic to every major organ and set up inflammatory responses in the body. It's like putting rocket fuel in a scooter: you eventually burn out the engine.

For the most part these days instead of going for a walk, breathing deeply and calming down, we tend to head for the coffee/cola machine or eat another refined sugary 'treat' to keep us going, which triggers even more adrenaline to be released, thus exacerbating the situation. Make no mistake, prolonged chronic, relentless stress can kill you.

The first signs of stress usually show up in behavioural changes, such as feeling constantly irritable, having sense-of-humour failures and feeling suppressed anger. You try to do more than one job at once and begin to feel that you cannot cope, or you may break down in tears, and/or you are tired yet 'wired'.

Then come the physical symptoms: palpitations and headaches, lack of appetite/or cravings for refined sugary, starchy foods, insomnia, poor digestion, muscle cramps, frequent urination, constipation and/or diarrhoea, a dry mouth, constant thirst, feeling clammy or cold or too hot.

Also, your brain doesn't work properly and you forget simple words or names. That's because stress creates more free radicals, and research at Stanford University has shown that raised cortisol levels damage the connections between brain cells, affecting brain functions. Luckily, if you stop the stress, the connections can grow back. Long-term stress also makes the body far more acid and vital minerals are then leached from the bones and muscles to re-alkalize the body (see *Acid–Alkaline Balance*). Long-term stress and the over-acidity it triggers can be an important factor in *Leaky Gut* and all its consequences, including autoimmune conditions, skin conditions such as eczema and psoriasis, and eventually osteoporosis.

If any or all of these symptoms sound familiar, you need to **stop and rest,** because the next stage could be a total burn-out, possible mental health problems, a heart attack or a stroke. Whether your stress comes from a bad relationship, work, children, illness, lack of money – whatever it is, if possible make a space and time between what is stressing you and your reactions to it. Talk to someone and tell him or her how you are feeling; ask your doctor to send you for counselling. If more people could do this, thousands of lives could be saved.

S

Additionally, research from Glostrup University Hospital in Denmark on women who have high-stress jobs has found that they are more than twice as likely to develop heart disease in later life – you have been warned.

Research has also demonstrated that if you think negatively, tend to be angry a lot of the time, and are under long-term negative stress, especially after 50, then you are more likely to suffer heart and arterial disease. This is because so many of us hold in emotions that we should literally 'get off our chest'. Remember, the more indirect you are, the more stressed you become. Emotions held in for long periods will eventually cause a fuse to blow.

There are also those infuriating (but wise) souls, who are always positive; they love stress and positively thrive on it. However, we are all unique and you need to learn your limits and listen to your body. There are many things you can do to reduce the negative effects of stress on your body, which can help you to stay healthier.

Foods to Avoid
- Never underestimate just how much your diet can affect your stress levels and your ability to cope with it. Avoid any foods and drinks containing alcohol, caffeine, refined sugar and artificial sweeteners, especially aspartame, which are all stimulants that cause the adrenal glands to overwork .
- Reduce refined (white) and processed foods: they're high in additives/preservatives and sugar, and usually low in nutrients. The more refined and processed food you eat, the more stress you place on your liver, digestive system and ultimately your adrenal glands.
- Cut down on heavy meals, especially red meat, which is hard to digest, and when you are stressed, digestion is one of the first things to be affected.
- Don't eat in a rush.

Friendly Foods
- When you are stressed, it's vital to eat small, balanced meals regularly, which help control your blood sugar and thus support your adrenal glands. See under *Low Blood Sugar*.
- Stress breaks down protein in the body quickly, which is why most people who are stressed tend to lose weight. Make sure that you eat around 100–175g (4–6oz) of quality protein daily, preferably at breakfast and lunch, as it helps to balance blood sugar levels. Eat protein such as eggs, fish, lean organic meats, tofu, cheese, amaranth, quinoa, peas, lentils, beans and pulses.
- Whey is an easily absorbed form of protein. If you don't have a problem with cow's milk, then try Solgar's Whey to Go; otherwise, use organic-sourced hemp seed, pea, rice or soya protein powders. See under *General Health Hints* for a great smoothie recipe.
- Eat oily fish and unrefined sunflower, pumpkin and hemp seeds – all rich in essential fats that reduce inflammation triggered by stress hormones (see *Fats You Need To Eat*).
- Liquorice tea helps to support adrenal function and echinacea tea will help to support your immune system, which is greatly affected by stress. Valerian and camomile teas with a little honey help to calm you down.
- Green tea contains L-theanine – an amino acid that encourages production of alpha waves, the brainwaves you produce during relaxation. Use a decaffeinated green tea.
- Make sure you eat breakfast – a low-sugar muesli, eggs, protein powder or wholemeal toast would be fine. Try oats, especially porridge made with rice milk, as oats are a rich source of B vitamins, which help you to stay calm.
- Wholewheat pasta, noodles and breads, couscous, quinoa, amaranth or oat crackers, lentils, brown rice and barley are all calming foods.
- Avocados, turkey, cottage cheese, bananas, potatoes, ginger, yoghurt, leafy green vegetables, lettuce and low-fat milks will also help to de-stress you.

- Generally, increase your intake of easy-to-digest food, such as homemade vegetable soups, mashed sweet potatoes, poached fish, stewed fruits and so on, which helps take some of the burden off your digestive system.
- See also *General Health Hints*.

Useful Remedies

- If the stress has been induced by shock or trauma, use homeopathic Aconite 30c, and take it every hour in between meals for a few days. Give the shocked person some sweet tea, as at times of shock the brain uses more glucose.
- Take a high-strength multi-nutrient formula containing vitamins, minerals, antioxidants and essential fats, because your body needs more nutrients when under stress. Ask any of the companies featured on pages 15–16 to recommend a formula to suit your age and gender.
- If you are not taking a high-strength multi-vitamin/mineral, then begin taking at least a high-strength B-complex daily with breakfast to support your nerves.
- Urinary excretion of vitamin C increases with stress, so take 1–2 grams of vitamin C in divided doses with meals, plus 400iu of natural-source, full-spectrum vitamin E to thin your blood naturally, as stress also thickens the blood. **NB Avoid the vitamin E if you are on blood-thinning drugs such as Warfarin.**
- BioCare's AD206 contains vitamins C and B5, and Siberian ginseng and other nutrients involved in the support of the adrenals in one convenient capsule to be taken 3 times per day. **BC**
- You need additional calming minerals, so take 400mg of calcium and 600mg of magnesium, which are known as nature's tranquillizers, in divided doses, with the last dose at bedtime (they should be in any good multi).
- Take a high-strength fish oil (1 gram) containing EPA and DHA essential fats. These thin the blood naturally and help keep blood pressure down.
- To calm anxiety, try a herbal formula called Advanced Stress Formula, containing the herbs ashwagandha, gotu kola, liquorice and Siberian ginseng. **NC**; or log on to www.holoshealth.com
- L-theanine is an amino acid found in green tea, which helps increase alpha wave production, the brainwaves you produce when you are calm, and which help you to feel more relaxed without inducing drowsiness. These are available in capsule form. Take as needed. **SVHC, NC**
- If you are a Type-A person who rushes around all day, you will also feel stressed and need to 'slow down'. Try taking Cortisol Manager tablets, which contain ashwagandha, phosphatidyl serine and L-theanine. Take one of these tablets when the adrenaline starts 'pumping' and a further one or two before bed. They are excellent for reducing cortisol production and calming you down. I have found them marvellous for reducing 'fight-or-flight'-type symptoms, and they really help me to get to sleep. However, if you are at the point of total and utter exhaustion, then your body may not be producing sufficient cortisol – in which case there would be no benefit in taking this formula. See under *Adrenal Exhaustion* and *Low Blood Sugar*.

Helpful Hints

- Do all you can to change your reaction to stressful situations, as long-term chronic stress makes your whole body **far** too acidic, which can trigger or exacerbate a huge range of conditions, from eczema and arthritis to cancers and heart disease. The easiest way to do this is to practise regular meditation or t'ai chi, which are proven over time to reduce the release of stress hormones and help you cope more positively in stressful situations.

- Learn how to relax! Have a weekly massage, play soothing music, walk in the park breathing deeply and slowly, have a long bath – anything that gives your body real space and time to relax.
- Make sure you get sufficient sleep, about 6–8 hours. Sleep deprivation is a major stress in itself and lowers your tolerance to other stresses.
- Numerous validated studies carried out at the Institute of HeartMath in Boulder Creek, California, have demonstrated that once you learn how to entrain your heart and mind as one, then production of the anti-aging hormone DHEA is increased, while cortisol production linked to stress decreases. You can literally entrain your alpha-brain activity, produced during relaxation, to synchronize with your heart rate. Your heart can influence your brain and thus reduce your stress levels. By attaching a small sensor to a fingertip, you can watch your heart rhythms in real time on your computer screen – and then experience how your thoughts can change its beating. The Institute of HeartMath offers software, devices and downloadable books that can help you develop heart/brain coherence. Find them at www.heartmath.org.
- Apply pure rosemary, nutmeg and clove oils directly to the adrenal area – around your waist area at the back – which will support adrenal function and help you to feel more positive.
- If you tend to wake regularly between 3am and 5am, this is a sign that your adrenal glands are struggling – see under *Adrenal Exhaustion*.
- Take stock of your life. An important first step is to identify sources of stress. Keep a diary and write down the things that are winding you up. After a month you will see that it's most probably the same things over and over again. Take steps (if possible or practical) to remove what stresses you from your life. Change your attitude from being negative to positive.
- Laughter releases stress – learn to lighten up and don't take life too seriously.
- I know it's hard, but as much as you can stop worrying so much. Dale Carnegie once said that 85% of the things we worry about never actually happen – trust that things will turn out for the best.
- Keep a pet. Studies with cat and dog owners have shown the considerable stress-reducing abilities of a furry companion. When cats purr they produce calming alpha waves, so stroke your cat and de-stress!
- Concentrate on what you can change in your life and let go of the things over which you have no control.
- Doctors agree that if we could all practise a pleasurable hobby that requires a fair amount of concentration, it would take our minds off what is stressing us and so reduce the release of stress hormones and help calm us down. At the very least, watch a movie that makes you laugh.
- Avoid obvious pressures, such as taking on too many commitments and deadlines. Learn to see when a problem is somebody else's responsibility, and refuse to take it on.
- Learn to say no and mean it – stop feeling guilty.
- If you are in a very stressful situation, if possible walk away. Go for a walk, take some slow deep breaths, calm down and then go back. If you do this, you will feel more able to cope.
- Get plenty of exercise, as relaxed muscles mean relaxed nerves that reduce stress. A brisk walk or vigorous exercise session is good instant first aid for feelings of stress. If this is impossible, you will still benefit from regular exercise.
- Take a deeper breath every 20 minutes; this helps to re-alkalize the body and slows the release of stress hormones.
- Try a simple progressive muscle relaxation exercise to free the body of physical tensions and distract the mind. Lying down flat on the floor with your palms up, breathe into your tummy.

Then, beginning with your feet and calves, tense the muscles as hard as you can and then relax. Work your way up your body, tensing and releasing each muscle group in turn, finishing with your head and face. Then just relax and stay there for 5 minutes, imagining that you are simply empty space; and just let go.

- Have a regular massage using essential oils of lavender, valerian, frankincense, neroli, jasmine or ylang ylang, which will all help to calm you down. The oils are absorbed into the body, so leave them on overnight to increase their effectiveness.
- Hypnotherapy on a weekly basis will really help to calm you down (see *Useful Information*).
- If you have an emotional problem that you cannot solve or if you can't handle the stresses in your life, seek outside help and advice. Simply talking with a trusted friend can be very beneficial, although it is often better to find a professional counsellor, who can both help you to handle your problems and teach you effective stress-reduction techniques.

Cortisol and Stress

Cortisol is a steroid hormone made by the adrenal glands and is produced in response to any stressful 'fight-or-flight' situation. Aeons ago this perfectly normal and natural response gave us the extra energy boost and mental sharpness either to run from our attacker or stand our ground and fight. Either way, our bodies would utilize the cortisol and levels would then return to normal.

Cortisol is both good and bad. It is needed to help regulate blood pressure and cardio-vascular function, as well as to regulate the body's use of proteins, carbohydrates and fats. It is also released during times of infections, trauma, fatigue, temperature extremes, and crucially when you worry too much. Basically, cortisol signals the liver to release stored sugars (glycogen) to fuel the brain and muscles – if this continues unabated, it can lead to *Insulin Resistance*. See this section. In the short term, cortisol is a good guy, but if levels circulating in your body become, and remain, too high – that is, chronically elevated – then cortisol damages tissues and organs, and greatly affects memory and brain functioning. And stress hormones in the long term deplete bone. Other common symptoms include palpitations, depression, sleep disorders, high blood pressure, anorexia, low blood sugar, insulin resistance, thyroid problems, menstrual disorders, osteoporosis and obesity (when combined with high insulin levels). You get the picture. Too much stress and cortisol can kill you. Think of Pacific salmon: after spawning, this fish undergoes rapid cortisol-induced ageing, and death follows in a matter of days. You should also be aware that oestrogen replacement from orthodox HRT can increase cortisol levels.

One of the best methods for measuring cortisol levels is an adrenal stress index saliva test. This test measures cortisol levels from early morning to midnight. The results are plotted on a graph and compared with a normal daily output of cortisol. This test is available via Genova Diagnostics. Tel: 020 8836 7750, or contact your health practitioner.

STROKE

(see also Angina, Atherosclerosis, High Blood Pressure, Heart Disease and Stress)

Strokes are the third most common cause of death in the West and account for the disability and dementia of approximately 150,000 people every year in the UK alone. Sixty thousand of these patients die as a result of a stroke. Children and young people can suffer a stroke, but nine out of every 10 cases occur in the over 55s – and the risk for stroke increases with age.

Anyone diagnosed with Raynaud's Disease, or who suffers from an overactive thyroid, especially before the age of 45, or is Asian, African or Afro-Caribbean, is also at an increased risk.

A stroke occurs when there is a loss of blood supply to the brain, which damages or destroys an area of brain tissue. Depending on the part of the brain affected, there may be sudden loss of speech or movement, heaviness in the limbs, numbness, blurred vision, confusion, dizziness, loss of consciousness or even coma. Stroke often causes weakness and paralysis on one side of the body, involving the arm and/or leg and face. Symptoms can last for several hours or for the rest of the affected person's life, depending on the severity of the stroke. 'Mini' strokes may even go unnoticed and can contribute to subtle reductions in mental function.

Many people who suffer a stroke go on to make a partial or even complete recovery. Over time, arteries gradually narrow owing to a build-up of sticky cholesterol-like substances. Arterial blockages cause nine out of 10 strokes (called ischaemic strokes). The blockages may be the result of thickening of the arteries (atherosclerosis). Sometimes blood clots travel from another part of the body, such as the heart or neck, to the brain, causing a cerebral embolism. The other 10% of strokes (called haemorrhagic strokes) are caused by bleeding into the brain from a ruptured blood vessel, which is most commonly caused by high blood pressure.

The risk of having a stroke is higher among people with an unhealthy lifestyle – smoking, eating too much salt and too much saturated fat, high oestrogen levels, prolonged stress, high LDL (bad)-cholesterol levels, and being overweight all contribute. People who tend to be angry or aggressive a lot of the time are also at a far higher risk, as stress and anger raise LDL-cholesterol levels, which thickens the blood. People with Type A or AB blood are also at a higher risk, as they tend to have stickier blood.

The first step toward heart disease and stroke is damage to the delicate inner lining of your arteries; this leads to the development of plaque, which thickens the arteries and poses the eventual risk of a total blockage. See under *Atherosclerosis*.

A lack of vitamin C weakens the matrix of the artery wall, making it more prone to damage. Free radicals from smoking, eating excessive fried foods and high-fat foods, plus prolonged stress, can lead to increased arterial damage, especially if the person is deficient in antioxidants, such as vitamins C and E. But there is another factor produced by the body that many nutritional doctors believe is equally as dangerous as having high cholesterol – it's called homocysteine.

High levels of homocysteine, a toxic by-product of the metabolism of proteins, are known to damage arteries. Researchers have found that a high level of homocysteine in the blood is as great a risk factor for cardiovascular disease as smoking or having a high blood cholesterol level. The good news is that if you have sufficient vitamin B6, B12 and folic acid, your body will convert homocysteine into less toxic substances. Studies have confirmed that the less vitamin B6 and folic acid in your blood, the higher your levels of homocysteine. This is why taking a high-strength vitamin B-complex daily could save your life.

At times, symptoms of stroke are not obvious. If you suspect that someone may have recently had a stroke, ask all the following questions ASAP – it could save his or her life:

   * Ask the person to smile.
   * Ask the person to raise both arms at the same time.
   * Ask the person to speak a simple sentence, such as, 'It's sunny outside today.'
   * Ask the person to stick out their tongue.

If the person you are testing has trouble with any of these four tasks, take him or her to hospital or call for **immediate** medical assistance. The faster anyone who has suffered a stroke can be treated, the less damage will be done to the brain. **Stroke sufferers need urgent medical attention within 3 hours.**

As an over-acid system is also linked to strokes – see under *Acid–Alkaline Balance*.

Foods to Avoid

- Avoid mass-produced refined white foods. Replace refined grains (white bread, pasta, rice, cakes and biscuits) with wholegrains, such as brown rice, wholegrain breads and pastas, quinoa and oats. Wholegrains contain more vitamin B, which has often been removed in processed 'white' products.
- Reduce your intake of saturated fats from red meats, full-fat dairy produce, cheese and high sugar and saturated fat mass-produced chocolate.
- Avoid fried foods or hydrogenated margarines. Those most at risk of having high homocysteine levels are high-protein (meat) eaters with a poor dietary intake of vitamin B6, B12 and folic acid. See also *Fats You Need To Eat*.
- Reduce your intake of animal-based dairy products – they're associated with an increase in cardiovascular disease, especially strokes. There are two possible reasons for this – first, while high in calcium (which is often poorly absorbed), dairy foods are relatively low in magnesium. Calcium requires adequate magnesium to be deposited in the bones, otherwise it is usually deposited in soft tissues, including joints and arteries. Second, dairy foods are often high in fat and protein, which can raise homocysteine levels, but lack adequate levels of the B-vitamins needed to process it into less toxic substances.
- Avoid all fizzy drinks because of the sugar content that causes damage to the circulatory system and leads to an increase risk of strokes.
- Caffeine can drive up blood pressure. Cut down on coffee, tea, cola and other caffeine-based energy-type drinks and foods. Good alternatives include green or white tea, peppermint tea, fruit teas, or diluted fruit juices.
- Cut down on wines and beer – but an occasional small whisky at night is fine.
- Eliminate sodium-based salts from your diet because of the effects on blood pressure. Replace them with magnesium- or potassium-based salt, such as Solo salt, or sprinkle powdered kelp or nori seaweed flakes (available from all health shops) on to food.
- Avoid all highly preserved meats, such as bacon and salami, salted nuts and smoked foods.

Friendly Foods

- Eat plenty of fresh fruits and vegetables and their freshly made juices for the vitamin C and the other protective antioxidants they contain.
- Eat more beta-carotene-rich foods, such as carrots, sweet potatoes, papaya, spinach, watercress, spring greens, mangoes, cabbage, broccoli, cantaloupe melon, pumpkin and tomatoes. In the Nurses' Health Study, which monitored 121,000 US female nurses aged 30–55 over a 20-year period beginning in 1988, those who consumed more than 15–20mg of beta-carotene a day had a 40% lower risk of stroke than women who reported eating less than 6mg a day.
- Potassium-rich foods help prevent strokes and a recent study showed that a low potassium intake can increase the risk of stroke by 50% in the over-65s. Therefore, eat more potassium-rich foods. Bananas, low-fat yoghurt, baked potatoes with the skin, prune juice, tomato juice, Swiss chard, spinach and all leafy greens, squash, asparagus, dried apricots, oranges, kidney beans and lentils are all rich in potassium. **NB If you have kidney disease or take a diuretic medication to lower blood pressure, check with your doctor before taking any extra potassium.**
- Vitamin B6 and folic acid are found in oranges, lemons, bananas, tomatoes, green leafy

vegetables, beans, nuts, seeds and wholegrain products. Many breakfast cereals are fortified with additional folic acid. Enjoy organic porridge oats for breakfast made with half skimmed milk and half water; add a chopped apple plus a few raisins for sweetness, plus some wheatgerm for its vitamin E.

- Make sure you eat a serving of greens, especially dark green leafy vegetables, every day. Spinach, cabbage, lettuce, spring greens, kale, chard, broccoli, peas and watercress are all good.
- Eat more foods rich in essential fats, such as oily fish, and use unrefined olive, walnut and sunflower oils for salad dressings. Include more raw, unsalted nuts and seeds – especially linseeds (flax seeds), pumpkin and sunflower seeds – in your diet. The easiest way to get seeds in your diet is to sprinkle them, whole or freshly ground, on your breakfast every morning (see *Fats You Need To Eat*).
- Trials at Johns Hopkins University School of Medicine in Baltimore have found that resveratrol, a phytopolyphenol compound found in red wine, red grapes, raspberries, blueberries and cranberries, contains a protective enzyme, which in the event of a stroke, helps shield oxygen-starved cells from death. Therefore it makes sense to increase your intake of these foods.
- Garlic and onions help to thin the blood naturally.
- People who drink at least 3 cups of green or black tea daily can reduce their risk of stroke.
- Dark chocolate contains a compound called epicatechin, which was found in research from Johns Hopkins University School of Medicine, in Baltimore, to help protect the brain against damage done by strokes, as it 'shields' the brain cells. One or two squares a day of organic dark chocolate should be fine. Otherwise, try small amounts of Glamour Food dairy- and sugar-free organic chocolate made with agave syrup, goji and acai berries with blueberry and coconut oil. For stockists of Glamour Food call 0844 800 8399. In the US call (323) 650 2201 internationally; + 44 (0)20 7351 2232. **OP**. These epicatechin nutrients are also found in green tea.
- Magnesium-rich foods include honey, kelp, raw wheat germ, dates, almonds, Brazil nuts and curry powder.
- Cayenne pepper is a powerful heart and circulation tonic and has been known to reverse plaque formation on the arterial walls.

Useful Remedies

- Magnesium relaxes constricted arteries and reduces the risk of a blockage. Take 400–600mg per day in divided doses. Many doctors have found that anyone who has suffered a stroke caused by a clot in the brain should be given intravenous magnesium as soon as possible after the stroke. Magnesium has a powerful dilatory action on the arteries and helps restore blood flow to the damaged tissue.
- Take a high-strength vitamin B-complex to help lower homocysteine.
- Fish oils, take 1–3 grams daily, to thin the blood naturally. If you're a vegetarian, then take linseed oil capsules instead.
- Take 1 gram of vitamin C, plus 400iu of natural-source vitamin E, which protect against clotting. **NB If you are on blood-thinning medication, check with your doctor before taking vitamin E as it naturally thins the blood.**
- Co-enzyme Q10 – 100mg per day helps to strengthen the heart muscle. People who have adequate levels of CoQ10 are less prone to strokes.
- Bioflavonoids – taking 1 gram daily helps to strengthen capillaries.
- Take a good-quality antioxidant formula that contains at least 200mcg of selenium.

Helpful Hints

- Research shows that people living in soft-water areas are more prone to high blood pressure, which can lead to strokes, as soft water is low in minerals, including magnesium. Therefore, if you live in an area of soft water, supplement around 400–600mg of magnesium daily – take in divided doses. Avoid drinking artificially softened water, which uses sodium.

- Stop smoking, which doubles your stroke risk.
- Certain types of combined oral contraceptives can make the blood stickier, which increases the risk of clotting. Orthodox HRT is also linked to an increased risk (see under *Menopause*).
- Control your blood pressure (see under *High Blood Pressure*).
- Take regular exercise, which makes the heart stronger and improves circulation. It also helps control weight. Being overweight increases the chance of high blood pressure, atherosclerosis, heart disease, and adult-onset (Type II) diabetes (see *Weight Problems*). Brisk walking alone for a total of 2 to 3 hours a week has been shown to reduce risk of strokes in women by up to a third. Also, cycling, and swimming lower the risk of both stroke and heart disease. Remember to start gently if you've not exercised for some time, and if you have heart or circulation problems, consult your doctor before starting any exercise regime.
- Homeopathic Aconite 30c – taken 3 times daily between meals for 3 weeks – helps to reduce the effects of shock on the body.
- Read *Put Your Heart In Your Mouth* by Natasha Campbell-McBride, available from the Nutri Centre. **NC**
- Read *Heart and Blood Circulatory Problems* by Jan de Vries (Mainstream Publishing).
- For more help, contact the Stroke Association at www.stroke.org.uk

SUNBURN

(see also Age Spots and Ageing)

S

The sun has had such a bad press over the years, and skin cancer rates are rising, as a result of which we are all supposed to have become more sensible in the sun. But most people haven't changed a bit. No matter where I am in the world, I see fair Europeans of all ages literally cooking their skin, as I once did. A few wise people stay out of the midday sun, but I still see far too many young children with no hats, sunglasses or tee shirts out in the midday sun. Parents are often nearby, doing the same thing.

At the opposite end of the spectrum you have people such as the actress Nicole Kidman, who never sunbathes – so I hope she takes plenty of vitamin D3!

Sunshine gives off a cocktail of frequencies, but principally ultraviolet (UV) radiation. The UVA rays are the ageing rays; UVB are the burning; and UVC are the most dangerous. Both UVB and UVC are mostly absorbed by the ozone layer (what's left of it); UVA can penetrate deeper into the skin than UVB or C, and UVA causes damage down into the fat layer of your skin – 2.5mm (¼in) into the dermis. To try to protect itself, your skin begins to thicken and it turns brown. We all know that too much sun accelerates ageing – in fact, 80% of age-related skin damage comes from too much sun exposure.

Yet the slower you can tan, the more you reduce the sun's ageing effects on your skin. When the skin turns red in the sun, it is the red-blood-cells' response to the heat that is being generated on the skin. Your blood is basically trying to cool your skin.

Black and Asian skins contain more melanin, the thick treacle-like substance that resides in your epidermis. The darker the skin, the more melanin it contains and the more easily it can reflect UV rays. Also, darker skin is able to resist the penetration of the sun's rays down to the dermis – five times more effectively than white skin. People with greasy skin make more sebum, which helps to block the UV rays, hence people with dark and oilier skins are able to tan better and suffer less wrinkling. Basically, the fairer you are the more easily you will burn, the faster your skin will age, and the greater your risk of developing skin cancers. But sunshine on your skin makes you feel so good. If you don't expose your skin to sufficient sunlight, then you can become depleted in vitamin D – especially D3, which is vital for healthy bones, teeth and immune functioning. Lack of sunshine and full-spectrum light can also trigger SAD Syndrome (see page 354), as the body produces less serotonin – the feel-good hormone. Full-spectrum light is vital for good health and your state of mind. Modest sunbathing helps to lower cholesterol and increases hair and nail growth, but too much will lower your immune function. People who live in colder climates and have little sun tend to suffer a higher incidence of internal cancers. What we need to do, as always, is to find a healthier compromise. For example, if you expose your skin to just 15 minutes of sun a day, then you can produce several days' supply of vitamin D.

See under *Helpful Hints* for details of how to recognize various types of skin cancers.

Foods to Avoid
- Avoid foods and drinks that will trigger dehydration, such as alcohol, caffeine and too many fizzy drinks.

Friendly Foods
- Obviously, if you are out in the hot sun, you will sweat more and you can quickly dehydrate, which can lead to low blood pressure, which in turn can trigger a fainting episode. Drink plenty of water and if it's really hot, then add a little extra sea salt to your food. Or use an electrolyte mixture (available from all chemists) to replenish lost minerals.

- The most important foods you need to eat more of to help protect your skin from the inside out (at any age) are essential fats and carotenes. Carotenes are found in carrots, sweet potatoes, tomatoes and tomato purée, asparagus, mustard and cress, raw parsley, red peppers, steamed spinach, apricots, pumpkin, papaya, spring greens, watercress, mangoes and cantaloupe melon.
- Essential fats are found in sunflower, pumpkin, sesame and hemp seeds and linseeds (flax seeds). Use their unrefined oils in salad dressings and drizzle over cooked foods (for more details see under *Fats You Need To Eat*).
- When you are in the sun, eat plenty of grilled oily fish and enjoy avocado and olive salads.

Useful Remedies
- Take a high-strength multi-vitamin and mineral, and an antioxidant formula that contains at least 100mcg of selenium (known to reduce incidence of skin cancers).
- Taking 3000–5000iu of vitamin D3 daily for 2 months prior to your holiday should help you reduce the risk of burning. But please be sensible in the sun.
- Take 30mg of natural-source carotene complex for six weeks before and a month after your holiday in the sun, as research in Germany has found that if you take carotenes for around 10 weeks or more, this helps to protect your skin from the ravages of sunburn.
- Take 2 grams of omega-3 fish oils daily, as essential fats nourish your skin from the inside out. Vegetarians can use linseed oil capsules.
- People who take 2 grams of vitamin C daily, along with 400iu of full-spectrum, natural-source vitamin E, appear to have added sun protection. But obviously also with a sunscreen!
- Melanin is made up from the amino acid L-tyrosine. Try taking 1000mg daily 30 minutes before meals to help the body tan naturally. Start taking a week or so before you go away.
- Pine bark extract, known as pycnogenol, has been proven to reduce inflammation on the skin triggered by UV radiation and reduces the likelihood of cell abnormalities – but again be sensible in the sun. Take one or 2 capsules daily. **PN**
- Try Urtica cream, which reduces the stinging and inflammation of sunburn. From any homeo-pathic pharmacy; or via the Organic Pharmacy. **OP**

Helpful Hints

- Skin cancers are on the increase, especially in countries and latitudes that enjoy hot sunshine all year round. And as the ozone holes become larger and more widespread, skin cancers are increasing proportionately, especially after the age of 50. The most dangerous type is malignant melanoma, which is a tumour of the melanocyte (the melanin-producing cells). This is usually pigmented either black or brown and can evolve from an existing mole, or simply appear. It begins to itch, grows larger, and the skin can break down around the 'mole'. The secret to surviving melanoma is to consult a doctor, dermatologist or oncologist as fast as you can. If caught before the cancer spreads internally, it can be treated successfully. The good news is that if you have reached your 60s and have no skin cancer, the incidence of melanoma reduces. Taking 200mcg of selenium daily plus natural-source carotenes can help reduce the likelihood of you developing malignant skin cancers. If you have a malignant cancer, see *Cancer* section.
- You may see small skin ulcers, tiny flaking patches, or small areas of skin that start to bleed, keep scaling and won't heal. This could be a squamous or basal cell carcinoma. These are not so dangerous, but again they need prompt checking and treatment.
- If you are using rejuvenating creams based upon Retin A, glycolic acids, AHAs etc, then wear a higher-factor sunscreen and be really careful not to let your skin go red. Use these types of creams in the winter months – more details under *Ageing*.
- Don't allow your skin to go really red. This can trigger skin cancers and cause broken and unsightly capillaries.
- If you suffer skin conditions such as eczema or psoriasis, moderate sunbathing and seawater will help your skin.
- No matter how much people tell you that sun beds are safe, they are not, and continued use greatly increases the risk of skin and other cancers.
- Real Sunlight lamps, available at several specialist clinics in the UK, are safer than sun beds, as the harmful frequencies of UVA and UVB have been filtered out. Developed in Sweden, they can relieve the depression associated with conditions such as SAD syndrome. They have been so successful that the Swedish government are installing them in care homes where residents are rarely exposed to natural sunlight. These lamps increase levels of vitamin D3 naturally, boost immune function and reduce depression. Real Sunlight lamps are available in London at The Wholistic Medical Centre, 57 Harley Street, info@wholisticmedical.co.uk Tel: 0207 580 7537. For a list of salons and clinics offering this specialist treatment, contact Real Sunlight Ltd on 08456 800 853.
- If you carry the herpes simplex virus, too much sun can trigger an attack of cold sores. See under *Cold Sores*.
- Lupus sufferers must be careful in the sun – see under *Lupus*.
- Many scientists now believe that chemical-based sunscreens (containing ingredients such as sodium lauryl/laureth sulphate, octyl methoxycinnamate (OMC), benzophenones, synthetic fragrances and colourants) may do more harm than good. Certain preservatives in sunscreens, such as parabens, mimic the affect of oestrogens, which can disrupt hormones and are linked to hormonal cancers. If you develop a rash after sun exposure, check the ingredient list in the cream. PABA (a constituent of folic acid and a member of the B-vitamin family) can trigger skin reactions in some people.
- Try Green People's organic sunscreens. The UV protection comes from titanium dioxide and extract of cinnamon. These sunscreens contain edelweiss, from the Alps, which helps protect against skin cancers and is high in antioxidants. They also contain green-tea extract, avocado oil, echinacea, myrrh and calendula, which help soothe the skin. They are available

S

in 15, 22 or 25 protection factor. Sold in good health shops and department stores, or order via www.greenpeople.co.uk.
- Other good makes are Curasol by Curaderm (www.curadermbec5global.com), Caudalie (www.caudalie.com) and Dr Hauschka sun products (www.drhauschka.co.uk).
- During tests it was found that the amount of sun cream you put on your body can be crucial in protecting your skin. Most people only apply sufficient to achieve 20% of the sun protection factor on the bottle. Apply protection regularly.
- To help avoid cataracts and ageing eyes, wear good wrap-around sunglasses that block 99–100% of the UVA rays.
- Wear a hat, which greatly reduces the UV radiation to the eyes.
- Avoid the sun between 11am and 3pm in an English summer – and make that 11am and 4pm in hotter climates.
- Please try to be sensible – wear a light wrap or tee shirt in the heat of the day and always re-apply the creams after swimming.
- Certain antibiotics, arthritis drugs, diuretic drugs and antihistamines (such as Benadryl) can trigger extreme reactions. If you are taking any such drugs and you are going away to the sun, check with your doctor.
- The herb St John's wort is also known to trigger sun sensitivity in some people. Large amounts of the herb gotu kola can do the same in some people.

SUPERBUGS
(see MRSA)

SWOLLEN FEET AND ANKLES
(see Foot Problems and Water Retention)

TACHYCARDIA (RAPID HEART BEAT)
(see also Adrenal Exhaustion, Panic Attacks, Palpitations and Stress)

Tachycardia is a sudden increase in heart rate to over 100 beats per minute in an adult. It occurs in healthy people during exercise, but if tachycardia occurs when you are resting, then you should consult a doctor as a matter of urgency. Symptoms may include palpitations, breathlessness and light-headedness, sweating and/or dizziness. These types of symptoms may also denote extremes in blood sugar levels or blood pressure levels. Low or especially high (hyperthyroidism) thyroid function can also be a factor in some people. A low iron level or low levels of the hormone progesterone may also need to be considered. Food intolerances are well known to trigger tachycardia and should be investigated. See under *Allergies*. Keep a food diary and note which foods trigger the symptoms – if, for instance, you suffer a rapid heartbeat within 10 minutes of eating wheat. Whatever the trigger, this condition needs thorough investigation by your health professional or doctor.

Foods to Avoid
- Drinking too much alcohol, which can damage the heart muscle.
- Caffeine, as it triggers the release of adrenaline into the bloodstream, thus precipitating an attack.
- At all costs, avoid high-energy drinks, full of refined sugars and caffeine.

Friendly Foods
- As dehydration can also be a factor in these types of symptoms, make sure you are taking sufficient fluids.
- Eat more potassium-rich foods. These include all leafy green vegetables, bananas, fresh and dried fruits, nuts, fish and sunflower seeds.
- See *Friendly Foods* under *Heart Disease*.
- Eat more garlic, onions and pomegranate, which are heart-healthy foods.

Useful Remedies
- Take a high-strength multi-vitamin and mineral for your age and gender that contains a full spectrum of B-vitamins. See pages 15–16 for a list of companies that would be happy to help you.
- Co-enzyme Q10, a vitamin-like substance manufactured by the body – as we age, production slows. Taking 100mg daily helps strengthen the heart muscle and increases energy levels.
- Natural-source, full-spectrum vitamin E helps the heart muscle receive more oxygen and naturally thins the blood. Take 400iu daily. **NB If you are on blood-thinning medication, such as Warfarin, avoid the vitamin E until you have spoken to your doctor.**
- The mineral magnesium, which helps to regulate the heartbeat, is often deficient. Take 300–600mg daily in divided doses with meals.
- L-theanine (extracted from green tea) really helps to keep you calm. Try 50–100mg two or three times daily. **NC**
- A pinch of cayenne pepper under the tongue can help normalize your heartbeat.

Helpful Hints
- As palpitations may be linked to an overactive thyroid or low iron levels, ask your doctor to do a blood test.
- To combat worrying, which only exacerbates the condition, learn how to breathe properly by taking yoga, t'ai chi or relaxation lessons.
- Practise meditation regularly, as this helps you to cope with stressful situations in a calmer way. If you feel an attack beginning, splash your face with cold water, then lie down, close your eyes and breathe deeply and slowly for a few minutes until the attack passes.
- Essential oil of lavender or ylang ylang has a calming effect, so add a few drops to your bath. Try regular aromatherapy massage, which is very calming.
- Go for leisurely walks, breathing deeply.

TASTE AND SMELL, LOSS OF

In young people this condition can occur after a cold or with blocked sinuses, but as we get older and our immune system weakens, loss of taste and smell is very common. If the nose becomes too dry and 'stuffed up', then the sense of smell can quickly be impaired. When you have a cold, your ability to taste and smell can be reduced by up to 80%. Hayfever, allergic rhinitis, nasal polyps and smoking can all interfere with taste and smell. A lack of zinc is often the culprit in this condition, as many people do not absorb sufficient zinc from their diets. Certain heart and prescription drugs can also cause a loss of taste and smell. It is generally easier to smell and taste in warm, moist atmospheres than in cold, dry ones.

Babies have many taste buds in their mouths – including the cheeks. Once we become adults, the sensitivity of all our taste buds is diminished and in old age it is greatly diminished.

Your tongue is covered with tiny projections called papillae, inside which are the sensory nerves that enable you to taste. Saliva is needed for taste and without it our diet would be virtually tasteless.

The average nose can detect approximately 4,000 different odours, while an especially sensitive one can recognize around 10,000. Inside the nose we have two small receptor sites, which are yellow-brown patches of mucous-covered membrane found in the roof of the nasal cavities. They are covered in millions of hair-like antennae. As we age, these antennae become less effective.

Foods to Avoid
- Generally, you need to avoid mucous-forming foods, such as full-fat milk, chocolate, cheeses and animal-source dairy produce. Soya milk can also be a problem for some people.
- Sugary, fatty, starchy white foods will also make the situation worse.
- See *Foods to Avoid* under *Colds and Flu*.

Friendly Foods
- Keep your diet clean, with plenty of fresh fruits and vegetables.
- Eat more brown rice, quinoa, barley, lentils, cereals, oats and wholemeal bread and pastas.
- Zinc-rich foods include lean steak, lamb and beef, calves' liver, raw oysters, fresh (preferably organic) peanuts, hazelnuts, Brazil nuts, ground ginger and dry mustard.
- Sunflower, pumpkin and sesame seeds and linseeds (flax seeds) contain fair amounts of zinc.
- Try organic-source rice, almond or coconut milk as a non-dairy substitute.
- Eat more garlic and onions, which are anti-bacterial and anti-viral.

Useful Remedies
- Take 15–30mg of chelated zinc or zinc picolinate, which can be useful in helping to restore the sense of smell. For best results take on its own at night before bed. Otherwise take Triple Zinc by Metabolics (tel: 01380 812799), which contains three types of zinc – picolinate, citrate and sulphate. These are easy to absorb and improve zinc levels quickly. Taking 1 to 3 capsules daily for 6 weeks should be fine; then one capsule daily for a further 6 weeks and then just one capsule a week.
- If an infection triggers a loss of taste and smell, take 10,000iu of vitamin A for a month, which helps support the upper respiratory tract. After the month, switch to a natural-source beta-carotene supplement, such as one of those made by Solgar, which naturally converts to vitamin A in the body and is non-toxic. **NB Anyone planning a pregnancy, or who is pregnant, should take no more than 3000iu of pure vitamin A daily. The carotenes are safe and non-toxic. SVHC**
- Include a high-strength multi-vitamin and mineral, plus 1 gram of vitamin C daily in your regimen.
- If the problem is linked to a cold or sinus infection, then see these sections under *Colds and Flu*, *Sinus Problems* and *Immune Function*.

Helpful Hints
- Homeopathic Nat Mur, Silica or Pulsatilla are also very useful for loss of taste; Belladonna or Hyos are useful for loss of smell.
- Tap water is often contaminated by chemicals, which can exacerbate this problem. Invest in a

reverse-osmosis water-filter system, which is more effective than over-the-counter carbon filters. For details contact The Pure H2O Company on 01784 221188. Email: roger@pureh2o.co.uk Website: www.pureh2o.co.uk
■ See a qualified nutritionist, who will help rebalance and detoxify your system.

TENNIS ELBOW

(see Bursitis and Carpal Tunnel Syndrome)

THROAT PROBLEMS

(see Sore Throat)

THRUSH

(see also Candida and Cystitis)

Vaginal thrush is caused by the same fungus, *Candida albicans*, that causes oral thrush. Infections develop when the bacteria in the vagina are destroyed. This happens if we take too many antibiotics, eat too much refined sugar, or starchy mass-produced junk-type foods, become very run down, or continue to use highly perfumed soaps and deodorants and so on.

Symptoms can include itchiness or general soreness of the vagina, and sometimes the vulva swells and is accompanied by a thick, whitish discharge, which smells rather yeasty. You may feel the need to urinate more regularly and there could be some slight stinging when you pass urine. If the infection takes hold, the lymph glands in the groin can swell. If this happens, you must see a doctor (see also *Candida*). If you suffer cystitis regularly, then you may be very run down – this can lead to thrush. If this is the case, then avoid sexual intercourse for at least a week to help ease symptoms. As chronic thrush is also linked to diabetes, see your doctor.

Foods to Avoid
■ See *Foods to Avoid* under *Candida*.
■ As the body needs to be kept more alkaline, see the dietary advice in *Acid–Alkaline Balance*.
■ Totally avoid pistachio nuts and peanuts, which harbour moulds that can add to the problem.
■ Avoid all blue cheeses.
■ Avoid all refined sugary foods as the fungus feeds off sugar.

Friendly Foods
■ Eating 250ml of plain, live yoghurt daily helps to clear thrush.
■ See *Friendly Foods* under *Acid–Alkaline Balance* and *Candida*.

Useful Remedies
■ Take 1000mg twice daily of the herb pau d'arco, which has anti-fungal properties.
■ Grapefruit seed extract (use 800–1200mg daily) is anti-fungal. It also acts like a natural antibiotic.
■ Take a course of acidophilus/bifidus – healthy bacteria, which help to kill the yeast overgrowth. **BC**
■ Thyme and rose essential oils – use a few drops diluted in a douche of lukewarm water twice daily to help kill the bacteria.
■ Douche with yoghurt (1 pot natural live yoghurt to 1.75 litres/3 pints of boiled, cooled water); or use apple cider vinegar diluted into water (4 tablespoons to 1 litre/¾ pint of boiled, cooled water). This helps to re-acidify the area, as the good bacteria prefer a slightly acid

environment in the vaginal area. You could also try douching in lukewarm water with a few drops of tea tree oil, a crushed garlic clove and a little organic cider vinegar added.
- Include a high-strength multi-vitamin and mineral in your regimen.
- Eat more garlic, which is highly anti-fungal.

Helpful Hints
- While an attack lasts avoid sexual intercourse, which could be very painful. Your partner will also need to be treated for any candida, as you are probably passing the problem back and forth.
- Try lavender and tea tree pessaries until symptoms ease. Never use tea tree oil directly onto any affected area. Always dilute in luke warm water.
- In conjunction with the above, you can also take pau d'arco and powdered or garlic oil capsules as directed until the condition eases, as they are highly anti fungal. **SHS**
- Wear cotton underwear and change it every day.
- Avoid vaginal deodorants, perfumed bath salts and talcum powder.
- Only use pH-balanced soaps.
- Vitamin E or calendula cream may relieve itching.
- Homeopathic Lycopodium 6c or Kali Mur 6c – take 2–3 times daily for up to a week to help to reduce symptoms.
- For oral thrush use Borax 6c twice daily for up to a week.

T THYROID, UNDERACTIVE AND OVERACTIVE *(see under Adrenal Exhaustion and Fluoride)*

Undiagnosed thyroid problems have reached epidemic proportions, as symptoms can vary so hugely. Your thyroid is often the most ignored gland in your body. It is situated in your neck, just below the Adam's apple, and produces hormones that affect every major organ and the metabolism and repair of every single cell, and it has a major influence on hormonal function. Every drop of our 4.5–5.5 litres (8–10 pints) or so of blood circulates through our thyroid every hour, bringing with it the substances the thyroid needs to do its work. Thyroxine (also known as T4) is the main hormone produced by the thyroid gland, and is converted by the liver to T3 (tri-iodothyronine), which is the active form of the hormone. Basically, the more T3 you produce, the faster your metabolism. If you don't produce sufficient T3 hormones, many systems in your body begin to slow down – heartbeat, circulation, blood pressure, energy levels, metabolism and temperature. A slower metabolism means that you don't burn calories as efficiently as you could, so you gain weight more easily. Also, when the body slows down, its ability to detoxify is impaired.

Up to 20% of the population are probably suffering from some degree of hypothyroidism (underactive thyroid) and the older you get the more prone you are to this condition. But it needn't be that way. Symptoms that should make you investigate whether your thyroid may be underactive include persistent low energy levels, mental 'fogginess', depression, cold hands and feet, weight gain even with a poor appetite, high cholesterol even if you eat sensibly, a slow pulse, low blood sugar (see *Low Blood Sugar*), headaches, infertility, dry and sometimes puffy skin, brittle nails, poor vision and memory, constipation, sore throat, nasal congestion, thinning hair, low libido and heavy periods.

Your ability to metabolize beta-carotene (from foods such as sweet potatoes, papaya and carrots) needed for optimum immune function and tissue repair, can be decreased if you have an underactive thyroid.

An underactive thyroid is seven times more common in women than in men, especially in women with low levels of the hormone DHEA. Unfortunately, because some of the symptoms associated with an underactive thyroid are often attributed to the menopause, thousands of women go undiagnosed or are offered orthodox HRT as a one-stop cure-all. Yet there is much you can do to help yourself.

If you have your thyroid tested, make sure they test your TSH, T4, T3 and thyroid antibodies. Ask your health professional to organize a Total Thyroid Profile (a blood test) by Genova Diagnostics (tel: 020 8336 7750; website: www.gdx.uk.net).

Otherwise you can try a temperature test developed by Broda Barnes that's used by some nutritionists. Here's how it works. Shake out a thermometer and keep it by your bed. When you wake up in the morning and before getting up, put the thermometer under your arm and lie there for 10 minutes. Your temperature should be 36.5–36.7°C (97.7–98°F). Do this for at least 2 days. (Women should do this test on days 2 and 3 of their period, as body temperature fluctuates during the cycle.) If either of your temperature readings is below 36.5°C (97.7°F), take it again over a longer period, say a week, to see if it is low on a fairly regular basis. If it is, you're probably hypothyroid – your thyroid gland is under-functioning. For more help log on to www.brodabarnes.org

In many cases a low temperature will not necessarily indicate a condition that would be medically diagnosed as an underactive thyroid (and treated with synthetic thyroid hormones), but nevertheless you could benefit from the following guidelines.

If you take steps to improve your thyroid efficiency, check your early-morning temperature again for a couple of mornings every month or so. As it starts to increase, you should find that some of your symptoms also start to improve.

An overactive thyroid (excess T3 production) is known as hyperthyroidism and is relatively rare. In this condition the thyroid produces too many hormones, which can trigger symptoms such as goitre – when the thyroid becomes more prominent and the eyes bulge. Other common symptoms are anxiety, insomnia, an inability to relax, shakiness, excessive sweating, feeling warm even on cold days, rapid heartbeat, palpitations, breathlessness, and weight loss even with a hearty appetite. If you are diagnosed with an overactive thyroid, you need the help of a competent physician or nutritional practitioner.

Long-term adrenal exhaustion can disrupt many processes in the body, including the thyroid – see under *Adrenal Exhaustion*.

Foods to Avoid – for an underactive thyroid

- Certain foods are known to inhibit thyroid function. These includes soya (soya milk, tofu and so on), apples, pine nuts, cruciferous vegetables (such as cabbage, broccoli and kale), spinach, peaches, pears and turnips. Also avoid walnuts, pine nuts, peanuts, mustard and millet. These foods are generally good for you, but avoid them until the thyroid has stabilized. This is more of a problem if you aim to eat these foods raw; once cooked, they can be eaten in moderation.
- Avoid all foods and drinks containing caffeine, which stimulate the release of adrenaline, which can affect the thyroid.
- Avoid fluoride as it interferes with thyroid function – see under *Fluoride*.

Friendly Foods – for an underactive thyroid

- Iodine (an element) and the amino acid tyrosine are the two nutrients the body uses to make thyroid hormones. Iodine can be found in seafood and seaweed (for example kelp, nori and arame), mushrooms, Swiss chard, butter beans, pumpkin seeds, and sesame seeds (tahini), egg yolk, lecithin, minced beef, artichokes, onions, leeks and garlic. **NB Those suffering** from autoimmune thyroid disease such as Hashimoto's or Graves disease would not be helped by extra iodine.

- Use organic sea salt or sprinkle powdered kelp or nori flakes over meals.
- The amino acid tyrosine is in all protein-rich foods, especially fish, butter beans, pumpkin seeds, bananas and avocados. If you have adequate protein in your diet you should be getting enough tyrosine.
- Essential fatty acids are vital for proper thyroid function, so include oily fish, seeds and cold-pressed oils in your regular diet. See *Fats You Need To Eat*.
- Eat more radishes, watercress, wheat germ, brewer's yeast, mushrooms, tropical fruits, watermelon, seeds and sprouted foods such as alfalfa. Make your own watermelon juice and add aloe vera juice, a great thyroid blend.
- Use organic-source coconut oil for cooking and for flapjacks – it helps to stimulate the thyroid. Higher Nature also make an organic coconut butter. **HN**
- The trace mineral manganese is also important for thyroid function – therefore eat more pecans, almonds, Brazil nuts, rye, barley and buckwheat.
- As low selenium is also linked to low thyroid function, eat more asparagus and garlic.

Useful Remedies – for an underactive thyroid

- A high-strength multi-vitamin and mineral complex taken every day provides a baseline of nutrients for the body to work with.
- Inflammation and oxidation within the body can trigger problems in manufacturing certain enzymes necessary for proper thyroid function. Therefore, take a broad-spectrum antioxidant formula.
- Selenium is needed for the manufacture of thyroid hormones. Take 200mcg daily. Selenium levels are low in soil in many countries and if the minerals are not in the soil, they won't be in your food!
- Kelp tablets contain iodine, follow the directions on the label, aiming for around 150mcg of iodine a day. **NB Don't take more than 500mcg of iodine a day, unless under your doctor's instruction, as too much iodine can upset thyroid balance. Do not take iodine if you have Graves or Hashimoto's disease.**
- The body makes thyroxine from the amino acid L-tyrosine, so take 500mg twice daily on an empty stomach (plus 50mg of B6 and 100mg of vitamin C to aid absorption).
- Siberian ginseng – take 1–3 grams (or 2–6ml of tincture) daily for a month, then stop and start again a month later. This can help reduce the effects of stress on your adrenal glands, your thyroid and your health in general. **NB Avoid Korean ginseng if you suffer from high blood pressure.**
- 1 gram of vitamin C with food, as well as 100mg of CoQ10 taken early in the day, can help raise energy levels.
- Thyro Complex is a formulation by naturopath Martin Budd, an established authority on thyroid health. He spent 15 years researching nutritional support required for healthy thyroid function. Take 1–3 tablets daily 30 minutes before food. **NC**
- Essential fats are crucial for helping to normalize thyroid function. Take 4-6 grams of fish oil daily with food until you note an improvement, and if you are vegetarian, then take linseed oil 40-60 ml (just over a tablespoon) per day stirred into vegetable juices until your condition improves. **Then reduce to 2 grams of omega-3 a day, or a dessertspoon of linseed oil.**

Helpful Hints

- As well as checking your thyroid hormone levels, ask your doctor to check levels of DHEA, which can easily be supplemented if low.
- Stop smoking – smoking is known to make an underactive thyroid worse. Cigarettes aren't an

easy addiction to give up, but worth the effort. For smokers, the number one thing they can do to improve their health and healthy lifespan is to quit smoking.

■ Managing stress is often the key – learn to relax, ensure you have 'down time' regularly, try yoga, t'ai chi, massage or meditation, and exercise regularly (see *Stress*).

■ Support your digestion. It is well established that our digestive capacity declines with age or when you are under stress at any age. Tyrosine, needed to make thyroid hormone, is a component of protein. Protein is relatively difficult to digest, so less digestion means less tyrosine and therefore less thyroid hormones. The answer is to chew well, relax over meals, and ensure you have an optimum level of nutrients in your diet to support digestion. If you have low stomach acid (needed to digest protein), you'll find that eating beetroot gives you pink urine, which doesn't normally happen, so this can be used as a simple test at home. Both digestive enzymes and betaine hydrochloride (stomach acid) capsules may be needed in the short term until your digestion becomes more efficient. See under *Low Stomach Acid*.

■ Consider food intolerances. Dr James Braly reports in his book, *Dangerous Grains* (Avery Publishing) a correlation between wheat (gluten) intolerances and thyroid problems. You can test for food intolerances with an at-home blood test from York Laboratories; call 0800 458 2052.

■ Exercise regularly. Exercise stimulates thyroid function – 30 minutes of aerobic exercise at least 3 times per week. If you are just starting an exercise programme, start gently and build up.

■ Avoid fluoride (in toothpaste) and chlorine (in tap water) as they are both chemically similar to iodine and block the iodine receptors in the thyroid. Consider putting in a good water filter.

■ If an underactive thyroid is diagnosed early enough and the patient is otherwise energetic, homeopathic thyroid treatment can be very useful. One such product called Thyroidea Compositum, made by the German company HEEL, is one of the most useful non-drug substances. Available from homeopathic pharmacies. **OP**

■ Read *Hypothyroidism, the Unsuspected Illness* by Broda O'Barnes and Lawrence Galton (Harper and Row); or *Why Am I So Tired – Is Your Thyroid Making You Ill?* by Martin Budd (Thorsons). For further details or to order Broda's book, log on to www.brodabarnes.org

TINNITUS

Tinnitus is a chronic and distressing condition in which the patient suffers a ringing, buzzing or humming in one or both ears. This condition can have a variety of causes, which include high blood pressure, exposure to loud noise or an explosion, long-term use of aspirin, use of beta blockers and antibiotics, compacted ear wax, spinal or cranial misalignment (which can reduce circulation to the ears) and food intolerances. Low zinc levels can be a major contributing factor in this condition. Tinnitus is more common in older people, but is appearing in younger people who are exposed to excessively loud music. Ageing rock stars, who are exposed to loud music over many years, often suffer from tinnitus. In Chinese medicine, adrenal and kidney function are linked to ear problems – therefore if you are totally exhausted and/or stressed, this could also trigger tinnitus or make any existing problem worse. This condition can also be linked to a congested liver. See *Liver Problems*.

Foods to Avoid
■ Avoid alcohol, smoking and caffeine, all of which may aggravate the condition.
■ Cut down on sodium-based salt, which can increase a build-up of fluid in the ear or raise blood pressure.

- Avoid all full-fat cow's milk and products for 2 weeks as they are mucous-forming, which can block the ears and sinuses. See under *Sinus Problems*.
- Generally, cut down on saturated fats, such as red meat, cheese, chocolate, highly refined, white-flour-based foods, pies, pastries, biscuits and so on.
- Yeast-based foods such as Marmite, Bovril and yeasty breads can also make this problem worse.
- Don't use hard margarines or highly refined cooking oils and eliminate fried foods.
- Read labels carefully and avoid any foods containing hydrogenated or trans-fats. See *Fats You Need To Eat*.

Friendly Foods
- Eat plenty of garlic and onions, which are very cleansing.
- Choose low-fat dairy options, such as fully skimmed milk or cottage cheeses.
- Use organic rice milk for making porridge and with cereals, and try live, low-fat yoghurts in desserts instead of creams.
- Try organic-source almond or coconut milks.
- Generally, increase fruits and fresh vegetables, and include more nutritious foods, such as lentils, barley and corn, rice and spinach-based pastas, in your diet.
- Jacket potatoes are a wonderful food, add a little yoghurt or use a non-hydrogenated spread such as Vitaquell, Biona or Olivia. Higher Nature also make organic walnut, pumpkin and hemp seed or coconut butters. **HN**

- Add more cayenne pepper to foods to help increase circulation.

Useful Remedies
- For 1 month take 25,000iu of vitamin A to nourish the inner ear nerve cells. (If you are pregnant or eat lots of liver, which is high in vitamin A, then limit your intake to 3000iu a day.) After the month, switch to natural-source carotenes daily, which convert to vitamin A in the body. These are safe and non-toxic. Take one to 2 capsules daily. **SVHC, VN**
- Take 30mg of zinc in a multi-vitamin and mineral supplement, as lack of zinc is greatly associated with tinnitus. For the first month take an extra 30mg of zinc three times daily before bed to aid absorption until symptoms ease. Otherwise take Triple Zinc by Metabolics (tel: 01380 812799), which contains three types of zinc – picolinate, citrate and sulphate. These are easy to absorb and improve zinc levels quickly. Taking 1 to 3 capsules daily for 6 weeks should be fine; then one capsule daily for a further 6 weeks and then just one capsule a week.
- Taking vitamin B12 – 1000 mcg a day – helps reduce noise-induced tinnitus as it nourishes nerve endings.
- As all the B-vitamins work together, also take a high-strength B-complex.
- Taking ginkgo biloba, 120–240mg of standardized extract daily, helps increase circulation to the ear, which should help if poor circulation is the underlying cause.
- Try garlic and horseradish tablets or tincture, which act as decongestants.
- Herbs such as gotu kola, cayenne pepper and prickly ash will all help to increase circulation to the head. Have a word with the herbalist at Specialist Herbal Supplies and find out which herb may help you most effectively. **SHS**

Helpful Hints
- Recordings of soothing music or sounds help mask the unwanted noise, especially when you are trying to get to sleep.
- Regular exercise may provide relief by increasing blood circulation to the head.
- Practise relaxation techniques such as Mindful Meditation – which has been proven to help tinnitus sufferers and is becoming more widely available on the NHS.

- Cranial osteopathy or chiropractic can release built-up tensions in the head and neck, which can trigger tinnitus.
- Acupuncture has proved very beneficial for some sufferers (see *Useful Information*).
- You can call the Tinnitus Helpline for up-to-date research. Freephone 0808 808 6666, www.tuneouttinnitus.org.uk
- Impacted wisdom teeth and tooth decay can cause this problem. When we grind our teeth over many years, the jaw can be misaligned. This is known as TMJS (temporomandibular joint syndrome). Dentists who specialize in treating TMJ problems (or any good dentist) can make a small brace to be worn at night that holds the jaw in its correct position, which often alleviates tinnitus. There is a craniofacial pain clinic in Great Bookham near Leatherhead, Surrey, which is dedicated to the treatment of head, neck and facial pain; call AJ Hedger and Associates on 01372 457959; www.revahealth.com/dentists/uk/surrey

TONGUE PROBLEMS

The tongue is a great indicator of your overall health and mirrors the levels of toxicity in the body. A healthy tongue should be pink, moist and clean, with little or no coating. A white coating usually denotes the digestive system is not working as it should; liver and bowels are sluggish; and you are eating too many mucous-forming foods, such as full-fat, animal dairy-based foods, refined sugary, starchy foods and red meat. Smokers are more likely to have a coated tongue. Candida, the yeast, fungal overgrowth can cause a thick, white coating on the tongue (see also *Candida*). If you have a heavily coated tongue, this can also contribute to bad breath, so buy a tongue scraper from any large chemist's and use daily.

A swollen tongue can denote dehydration, therefore drink plenty of fluids – or, it may be linked to an iron deficiency (have a blood test to check). If your tongue swells suddenly, this can be an acute allergic reaction (this can be triggered by nuts, shellfish or anything to which you have a severe intolerance) and you would need to seek immediate medical attention.

Naturopath and Chinese doctor Stephen Langley says: 'By looking at a person's tongue, I can easily determine the overall state of that person's health. For example, if the coating is yellow, this indicates excessive heat in the body associated with constipation, over-acidity or pain and inflammation. If the tongue is "scalloped" looking, as though it is indented with teeth marks along the sides (which is very common), this can indicate either poor absorption and assimilation in the gut or exhaustion of the adrenal glands.'

Foods to Avoid
- Red meat, full-fat, animal-source dairy produce and most starchy foods made with mass-produced, highly refined white flour can add to the mucous load in the body and slow digestion.
- Reduce your intake of alcohol, caffeine, fried foods and junk-type take-aways, which place a strain on the liver. See *Liver Problems*.
- See also *General Health Hints*.

Friendly Foods
- To clear the coating, you need to keep your diet really clean for 7–10 days.
- During any detoxification process the tongue is likely to become even more furred as the body begins eliminating acidity.
- Drink plenty of fresh vegetable juices made with garlic, ginger and any fresh vegetables you have to hand. Celery, artichoke, chicory, celeriac, kale and beetroot are great liver cleansers.

- See *Friendly Foods* under *Constipation*.
- Eat more pineapple and papaya, which greatly aid digestion.

Useful Remedies
- Take the healthy bacteria acidophilus/bifidus daily for 6 weeks to replenish healthy bacteria in the bowel. **BC**
- Prebiotics are plant compounds that encourage the growth of healthy bacteria in the bowel. Try Agave Digestive Immune Support. One scoop daily with breakfast really helps to keep you regular. Log on to www.lef.org or call the Nutri Centre. **NC**
- Take a digestive enzyme with main meals.
- The herb milk thistle will help to improve liver function. Take 500mg 3 times daily.
- The celloid mineral sodium phosphate – 600mg daily – helps to reduce a creamy coating. **BLK**

Geographical tongue

In this condition, the tongue often resembles a map, when discolouration forms irregular shapes on the surface. Usually it disappears of its own accord, but sensitivity to certain foods can exacerbate the problem (see *Allergies*). I have had letters from pregnant women whose geographical tongue disappeared once the baby was born. It is also linked to iron and/or vitamin-B deficiencies. The patches can also be caused by infection or irritants, such as vinegar.

Foods to Avoid
- Cut down on caffeine, highly spiced foods, vinegar, pickles, pineapple and plums.
- Refined orange juice may also be a problem for some people.
- Alcohol will also irritate the delicate tissues in the mouth.

Friendly Foods
- Include more ginger and live, low-fat yoghurt in your diet, which is very soothing.
- Garlic and onions are very cleansing.
- Drink plenty of water.
- Eat more foods containing B-vitamins, such as wholegrains, oat bran, wheat germ, quinoa, amaranth, brown rice, organic muesli, oats, lecithin granules and brewer's yeast. Liver is also high in B-vitamins and vitamin A – but only eat once a week and make it organic.
- Eat plenty of fresh fruits and vegetables.
- See also *General Health Hints*.

Useful Remedies
- CT 241 is a formula of herbs, such as horsetail, and silica, kelp, vitamin C, boron and digestive enzymes, which improve absorption of nutrients from food and encourage soft tissue healing. **BC**
- Take a high-strength B-complex daily with breakfast or lunch.
- Take a multi-vitamin and mineral suitable for your age and gender that contains around 30mg of zinc, as low zinc levels are linked to this problem.
- Ask your doctor to check if you are low in iron, in which case take a liquid formula, such as Spatone, which will not cause constipation.
- Take New Era calcium fluoride tissue salts 4 times a day.

Helpful Hints
- Tea tree oil can be diluted in warm water and used as a mouthwash as well as 1% hydrogen peroxide in water.
- Some sufferers report an improvement after taking a garlic capsule daily.

TONSILLITIS
(see also Immune Function and Sore Throat)

A nasty sore throat, accompanied by difficulty swallowing and ear pain, are the most common symptoms of tonsillitis. It makes you feel dreadfully low and symptoms may also include fever, nausea, headache and swollen, painful lymph glands in the neck. Tonsillitis is especially common among children. Antibiotics are not necessarily needed as more often than not tonsillitis is caused by a virus, which is not killed off by antibiotics – and it is only if a secondary bacterial infection occurs that antibiotics are warranted. Recurrent infections indicate that the immune system is struggling or that food intolerances, especially to animal-source dairy, are involved (see *Immune Function*).

Foods to Avoid
- While an infection is present, anything that increases mucous production needs to be avoided. This includes dairy produce (most especially from cows) – cheese, milk, full-fat yoghurts, chocolates, cream and butter – along with eggs, soya milk and nut butters.
- Toast, crisps and spicy foods can cause discomfort to an inflamed throat.
- Fizzy drinks and other refined sugary/fatty foods and drinks will greatly lower immune function.
- Caffeine, found in tea, coffee, chocolate and colas, adds stress to the immune system and is best avoided.
- Once the infection is over, if you suspect that dairy foods are causing a problem, continue to keep them out of the diet. Keep calcium levels high by eating lots of sesame seeds or tahini (ground sesame seeds), almonds and Brazil nuts, bony fish, such as sardines and pilchards, plus dark green leafy vegetables, including kelp, broccoli, cabbage and watercress.
- Reduce packaged and processed foods high in hydrogenated and trans-fats, artificial flavourings, colourings, preservatives and sweeteners.

Friendly Foods
- Freeze low-sugar, diluted fruit juices by making them into ice lollies. This is a great way to help soothe a sore throat while an infection is present – blackcurrant and apple are particularly good.
- Vegetable soups and chicken broths are full of healing nutrients that will boost the immune system and are easier to swallow than regular food. Use plenty of sweet potatoes, cabbage, squash, pumpkin, carrots, broccoli plus lentils or brown rice – with a little chicken or lamb.
- To tempt a child with a low appetite, put lots of different colours on the plate – oranges, reds, purples, blues, yellows and greens. Colourful foods contain bioflavonoids, which have many immune-boosting and protective properties. A bowl full of blueberries, blackberries, cherries, plums, apricots, papaya and oranges will give any child lots of nutrients. Or blend these fruits with a small amount of rice milk to make a nutritious smoothie. For a recipe, see under *General Health Hints*.
- When your child is ready to return to solid foods, begin with light, easily digested meals, as the digestive system is taxed during an infection. Go for thicker stews and lightly steamed vegetables with chicken or fish.
- Increase all fresh fruits and vegetables and wholegrains, as these will help supply the immune system with the raw ingredients it needs in order to function well.
- Include more vitamin-C-rich foods, such as strawberries, kiwi, sweet potatoes, blackberries, red and yellow peppers, broccoli and peas.

Useful Remedies
- Try Sambucol, an extract of elderberries, which has proven anti-viral action and tastes great,

too. Children can have 2 teaspoons twice a day and adults a dessertspoon 4 times a day. It also comes as a lozenge – adults should have 1 lozenge 4 times a day.

- Vitamin A is known to help heal inflamed mucous membranes and boost immune function. During an infection children over the age of 5 can have 10,000iu for 2 days then reduce to 2,500iu daily; and for 7–10-year-olds – 10,000iu for just 2 days and then 3,500iu daily until symptoms ease. After this time, you can switch the child to a beta-carotene capsule daily, which is totally safe. Watercress, pumpkin, papaya, carrots and watermelon are all rich in carotenes. **NB Anyone planning a pregnancy, or who is pregnant, cannot take more than 3000 iu of vitamin A daily, but carotenes, which naturally convert to vitamin A in the body, are fine.**
- Holos Health make an Ultimate Echinacea Formula, which contains phytolacca, a herb that specifically helps alleviate the symptoms of tonsillitis, plus echinacea, golden rod, wild indigo and astragalus – all known to boost immune function. Available from the Nutri Centre or log on to www.holoshealth.com **NC**
- Applying a little neat tea tree oil externally to the painful area on the throat should help ease the pain.
- Suck zinc lozenges 3 times a day, as zinc aids the immune system and has been shown to reduce the duration of a sore throat.
- During an infection add 4 grams of powdered vitamin C to water and sip throughout the day. This will keep levels boosted and help the immune system to fight the infection. BioCare makes a good non-acidic one called magnesium ascorbate. **BC**

- Beta Glucans 1–3, 1–6, derived from yeast cell walls, are proven to strengthen the body's innate immune system (the immune system you are born with), making it more resistant to pathogens from food and air. Take 250–500 mg daily. It can also be taken by children and reduces the likelihood of food intolerances triggered by a weakened immune system. Dr Paul Clayton based in the UK and US is a medical pharmacologist. His website research on Beta Glucans is well worth a look. Find him at www.healthdefence.com. Glucosan, developed by Dr Clayton, is available from Vitalize Health products on 0870 042 8423. Website: www.vitalizeshop.co.uk

Helpful Hints

- Add manuka honey and root ginger to hot water for a soothing drink. The ginger is full of zinc, which is healing, and the manuka honey has strong anti-bacterial action.
- Gargling with salty water, or red sage and echinacea – used 4 times daily – really helps. **SHS**
- Slice an onion, wrap it in an old cloth, and wrap it around the throat. Replenish every 3 hours. This can really help to clear congestion from the lymph glands in the neck.
- Get lots of rest and maintain a high fluid intake.
- Humidifiers can help to keep a dry throat moist and ease discomfort.
- If the tonsils become infected and antibiotics are necessary, then follow them up with a probiotic. These are healthy bacteria needed by the gut, which are killed along with the infection by the antibiotics. See under *Antibiotics*.

TRAVEL SICKNESS

This is extremely common, especially in children and older people. Just worrying about a journey can be sufficient to trigger symptoms in a sensitive individual. Eating a large meal prior to travelling and stuffy atmospheres can also make symptoms worse. Some people can read while moving, but for others trying to focus on something stationary while in a moving vehicle can disturb the balance in the inner ear, resulting in nausea. Also, if anyone who suffers from travel sickness notices the scenery flashing by – such as on a train – often this makes symptoms worse, because the balance of the inner ears is linked to the receptors in the eyes. Symptoms include looking pale, feeling clammy and sometimes nausea, vomiting and, in extreme cases, fainting.

Food to Avoid
- On short trips, avoid eating and drinking anything immediately prior to your journey.

Friendly Foods
- On the day prior to travel, eat lighter foods, salads, fish, tofu and fresh fruit compotes; or grilled fruits, soups and low-fat yoghurt.
- If you are on a long trip and can face food, eat really light, low-fat foods, such as rice or oat cakes. Otherwise, try dry toast or a cheese biscuit.
- Sip small amounts of fresh lemon or lime juice in warm water.
- Peppermint and ginger herbal teas can also be sipped to calm the digestive tract and stomach.
- Recently on a cruise I suffered sea sickness and was told that if I ate a green apple very slowly it would help – and it did.

Useful Remedies
- Magnesium is nature's tranquillizer. If you tend to start feeling nervous the day before your trip, begin taking 200mg of magnesium 3 times a day for a couple of days prior to travelling.
- Ginger is really successful at reducing the feelings of nausea and you can take 4 ginger capsules 2 hours prior to travel – but it is often more effective when you can taste the ginger.
- Make tea with a small piece of fresh root ginger and a little honey and take in a flask to sip during your journey; or take 1–2ml of the tincture in a little water.
- Take a high-strength vitamin B-complex daily with meals to support your nerves.

Helpful Hints
- Stay fairly still and breathe calmly. Look ahead to the horizon and not downwards to help keep the fluid in the ears balanced.
- Try to sit at the front of any vehicle.
- If possible, open a window.
- Avoid the company of people eating strong-smelling foods.
- A drop of peppermint oil on the tongue helps reduce feelings of nausea.
- You can even simply inhale the aroma of peppermint oil, as it has been shown to reduce feelings of nausea and subsequent vomiting.
- Acupressure can help control motion sickness. Press the point that is approximately 5cm (2in) up from the centre of your wrist on the underside of your arm – it's the point between 2 tendons. Press for 20 seconds every half or so to reduce symptoms; or wear Sea Bands, which work on a similar principle. Available from most large chemist's.
- Try homeopathic Cocculus 30c – take 1 pillule before travelling and 1 every few hours during the journey.

TREMORS   *(see under Alzheimer's Disease and Parkinson's Disease)*

This problem can be triggered by a huge variety of causes, such as extreme nervousness, excessive consumption of caffeine or alcohol, and/or an overactive thyroid gland. Recovering alcoholics and drug addicts often suffer tremors. If the tremors occur when resting or you suffer involuntary jerking, this may be associated with conditions such as Parkinson's disease and rheumatic fever. On rare occasions, tremors can be inherited. Mercury and heavy-metal toxicity are linked to tremors (if you have mercury amalgam fillings, see *Mercury Fillings*); cigarettes are high in cadmium and nickel, so stop smoking. If you suffer blood-sugar problems, this could make symptoms worse (see *Low Blood Sugar*).

As certain prescription drugs are also known to have a side effect of tremors, check with your doctor. If the adrenal glands are totally exhausted, then tremors may result – see under *Adrenal Exhaustion*.

Foods to Avoid

- Any foods or drinks containing aluminium (see *Alzheimer's Disease*).
- Greatly reduce any foods or drinks containing caffeine; this includes chocolate, fizzy canned drinks, guarana, coffee and strong tea.
- Avoid alcohol and spicy foods, which are stimulants.
- Don't eat too many highly sugary, starchy foods, which can make you feel even more nervous.
- Avoid preservatives and additives.

Friendly Foods

- Generally, you need calming foods, such as sweet potatoes, pasta, wholemeal bread, brown rice, lentils, barley, cereals and oats.
- Porridge made with organic rice milk, and a chopped raw apple or banana, plus a little manuka honey to sweeten, makes a very calming breakfast or supper.
- Turkey, chicken, cooked tofu, bananas, wheat germ, avocados, sunflower seeds, pumpkin seeds, linseeds (flax seeds) and oily fish are all calming foods as they nourish the nerves.
- Almonds, dates, Brazil nuts, mustard, curry powder and all green leafy vegetables are a good source of magnesium, which calms the muscles.
- Drink more water.
- Drink more green or white tea, which contains L-theanine, an amino acid that helps to calm you down. Avoid at night, as these teas contain some caffeine, or ask for decaffeinated versions. Otherwise, you can take 100mg of L-theanine twice daily in between meals.

Useful Remedies

- Include a multi-vitamin and mineral supplement that contains a full spectrum of B-vitamins to nourish your nerves and also contains at least 30mg of zinc. (Often when we are falling off to sleep our bodies jerk; this is often due to lack of zinc.)
- Calcium and magnesium help to reduce muscle spasms. Take 400mg of calcium with 600mg of magnesium in divided doses, the final dose before going to bed.
- Either take 4 evening primrose oil capsules daily or 400mg of gamma-linolenic acid (GLA – a fatty acid found in evening primrose oil that helps to reduce tremors). **BC**

ULCERS, DUODENAL AND STOMACH

(see Stomach Ulcers)

V

VARICOSE VEINS *(see also Circulation, Constipation and Piles)*

Varicose veins are caused by long-term poor circulation and weakened valves in the veins, which allow blood to accumulate, thus stretching the vein walls. The most commonly affected areas are the legs, where eventually the veins can be clearly seen on the skin's surface. Over time they bulge, become bluish and lumpy looking, and can become painful.

If they are not treated, they can also ulcerate, especially in older people. Anything that slows the return of the blood from the legs to the heart will aggravate varicose veins.

This condition is closely linked to constipation and if you strain when you go to the toilet, then blood is forced into your lower body, which makes the problem worse. Vein problems are also linked to standing or sitting for long hours, being overweight, pregnancy and crossing your legs too much. Perhaps most frightening of all, vascular surgeons are seeing children as young as 11 with problems, who are 'couch potatoes' and sit at computers or watch TV all day – see also under *Diabetes* and *Deep Vein Thrombosis*.

Another common condition, known as thread or spider veins, involves chronically dilated and overly permeable capillaries near the surface of the skin. Whilst they are harmless and rarely cause any problems, they can be distressing for cosmetic reasons. You can prevent them developing or worsening with much of the same advice below (see also *Helpful Hints*).

When I became pregnant at 18, after working long hours standing in a supermarket, I developed varicose veins. In my 20s these were made worse when I worked for 9 years as an air stewardess and often had to be on my feet for 15 hours at a stretch. Today, I tend to sit at a desk for lengthy spans, which greatly restricts my circulation. My mother and father both had vein problems. Yes, you can inherit a tendency for veins, but if I had known then what I know now, I could definitely have prevented their onset. In my 40s I had some veins stripped, but the problem has returned. However, today, thanks to more efficient diagnostic techniques and improved surgical procedures, you can in many cases eliminate varicose veins – but it is much better to prevent them in the first place.

Foods to Avoid
- Cut down on heavy meals, red meat and cheeses, as they're low in fibre and take a long time to pass through the bowel, potentially contributing to constipation. Furthermore, saturated, fried and hydrogenated fats thicken the blood, which make it travel more slowly through your veins and arteries, increasing the risk of vascular problems.
- Foods made with flour from any source tend to block the bowels; therefore reduce your intake of flour-based foods, especially croissants, meat pies, pizzas, cakes, biscuits and so on. Choose grains that are easier to digest, meaning low in gluten, such as wholemeal spelt breads or 100% rye breads, and eat more brown rice, rolled oats, quinoa and barley.
- Coffee, tea, colas and especially alcohol will dehydrate the bowel.
- See also *Constipation* and *Circulation*.

Friendly Foods
- Bilberries, blueberries, blackberries, sweet potatoes, pumpkin, squash, cherries, apricots, spinach, spring greens and cabbage. In addition, eat more citrus fruits, broccoli, red grapes, papaya, tomatoes, tea and red wine, which are all rich sources of flavonoids and vitamin C

powerful antioxidants that help to strengthen capillaries and reduce the risk of haemorrhoids, thrombosis and bruises.

■ Rose hips (try rose hip tea), buckwheat and apple peel contain the bioflavonoid rutin, which also helps to strengthen your veins. Buckwheat makes great pancakes and can also be added to breads and biscuits. You can buy organic buckwheat pancake mixes from most health stores.

■ Avocados, sprouted seeds such as alfalfa, plus eggs, raw wheat germ and unprocessed nuts are rich in vitamin E, which reduces stickiness in the blood.

■ Garlic, onions, ginger and cayenne pepper all aid circulation.

■ Eat plenty of fish, especially oily fish. The essential fatty acids (EFAs) they contain reduce pain and keep blood vessels soft and pliable. Aim for 2–3 portions per week. Eat more unrefined, preferably organic, sunflower, hemp, pumpkin and sesame seeds and linseeds (flax seeds), which are all high in essential fats and fibre (see *Fats You Need To Eat*).

■ Drink more water, 6–8 glasses a day of bottled or filtered water. Water maintains blood pressure and helps reduce constipation.

■ Make sure that your diet contains plenty of fibre to prevent constipation. Fruits, vegetables, whole grains such as brown rice and quinoa, beans and lentils are your best sources. If you feel you need more than you're getting in your diet, skip the bran – a harsh, insoluble fibre – and use instead soluble fibre-rich (cracked) linseeds (flax seeds), such as Linusit Gold or psyllium husks, both available in your local health food store.

■ Sprinkle oat bran over cereals and into smoothies – see under *General Health Hints* for a good basic recipe.

■ If constipation is a real problem for you, in addition to the fibre, water and exercise recommended above and below, eat 4 prunes prior to each meal.

Useful Remedies

■ For centuries plant extracts such as butcher's broom and horse chestnut seeds (commonly known as conkers) have been used to reduce inflammation and swelling associated with leg problems, and science has now validated these age-old remedies. Dr John Wilkinson, a scientist who specializes in plant research, says: 'We have found that saponins, a group of active agents found in the roots and seeds of these plants, constrict and strengthen veins, have anti-inflammatory properties, and reduce swelling, thus making venous return to the heart more efficient. The compounds in these plants are safe and can be taken internally in capsule form daily (but not during the first 3 months of pregnancy, or by people on blood-thinning drugs). Plant extracts can also be used topically in a cream or gel. We have found that butcher's broom is highly effective when taken in isolation, but its effects appear to be amplified when combined with horse chestnut, vitamin C and the flavonoid rutin.'

■ Most health shops sell butcher's broom, which also reduces heaviness, tingling and cramping associated with varicose veins. Take 100–300mg standardized extract 2–3 times daily, or try V-Nal combination capsules made by Bional, available at most chemists and health shops worldwide.

■ Horse chestnut seed extract can also be taken either as a combination or on its own. Clinical trials have confirmed its ability to aid vein contraction, reduce vein fragility and permeability and significantly reduce lower-limb swelling. You need 50–75mg of aescin twice daily (aescin is the active ingredient in horse chestnut). If you prefer a tincture, take 1–4ml twice a day.

■ Another herb, gotu kola, has also shown impressive clinical results in treating both varicose veins and varicose ulcers by improving circulation in the lower limbs and stimulating connective tissue repair. Try 500mg twice daily with meals.

■ Pycnogenol – pine bark extract – improves the elasticity of vein walls and reduces inflammation. Initially take 80mg twice daily for a month and then reduce to 80mg daily. **PN**

- Silica is an excellent mineral for toughening up veins. Take 200mg of silica compound daily. **BLK**
- An antioxidant complex containing vitamins A, C and E, selenium and Co-enzyme Q10 helps prevent free-radical damage to the blood vessels, as well as aiding in connective tissue repair. Take 1–2 grams of vitamin C daily with meals and 400iu of natural-source full-spectrum vitamin E, which also enhances circulation through its anti-clotting effects.
- If veins are sore and swollen, buy some witch hazel in tincture or cream form and apply directly to the veins. Witch hazel in capsules and tincture can also be taken internally to reduce the swelling. **OP**
- Apply a little vitamin-E cream mixed with 2 drops of juniper oil topically where the skin is sore.
- If you have facial thread veins, try Jason Vitamin K Cream for the face, which contains bioflavonoids, ginkgo biloba and calendula. It is available from most good health and department stores worldwide. For your nearest stockists, call Kinetic on 0845 0725825 or log on to www.kinetic4health.co.uk.

Helpful Hints

- If the veins are swollen, itchy and painful, soak a bandage in cold witch hazel, apply to affected area and wrap firmly for 30 minutes with the leg elevated. This should help reduce the swelling.
- For those on their feet all day, physiotherapist Geraldine Watkins recommends lying on the floor, bending the knees and placing the lower legs on a chair or bed for 15 minutes daily to give the leg valves a rest and encourage excess fluid to be absorbed back into the system. If the legs are swollen, then a cold compress should be applied.

- It's vital for your overall health that you stay active. Even brisk walking for 45 minutes to an hour a day will help. Otherwise, rebounding, skipping, playing tennis, jogging and dancing are all wonderful exercises for supporting veins. And if your legs ache, no matter what your job, swimming is the best all-round exercise for keeping legs healthy.
- Also, if you stand a lot all day, wear insoles to support your arches – these are available from John Bell and Croyden in London on 020 7935 5555, or any good chemist or back shop. Avoid heels over 5cm (2 in), and at the first sign of vein problems, start wearing support tights or socks.
- If you are at a desk for much of the day, take regular breaks, look for some stairs and climb them! Make sure you move for at least 30 minutes a day. But whilst seated use a D-shaped foot rest, available from chemists such as John Bell and Croyden in London, as bending and circling the feet keeps circulation moving. When at your desk, make sure your knees are lower than your hips, which reduces compression in the arteries and veins in the groin area. Also avoid wearing tight-fitting trousers, which adds to compression in the groin and the back-of-knee areas when seated for long periods.
- Avoid crossing your legs, doing heavy lifting or putting any kind of unnecessary pressure on your legs.
- Reflexology, acupuncture and a firm massage can all help to increase circulation (see *Useful Information*).
- If the veins are sore and throbbing, make a warm-water compress with added cypress and geranium essential oils. Use cold compresses to reduce any swelling.
- Avoiding constipation and/or straining to pass stools is essential for preventing varicose veins. Continually straining to go to the toilet forces blood into your lower body, which makes the problem worse. Haemorrhoids are similar to varicose veins of the anus – see also *Constipation* and *Piles*.

- Facial thread veins can be treated using a fine needle, often called Red Vein. The needle is quickly inserted into each end of the vein and a current passes through the needle, which cauterizes the tiny capillary, then the needle is quickly injected down the length of the vein, which makes the vein disappear. Available at most beauty salons. Costs around £35 for 15 minutes. You then need to keep the treated areas dry for several days.
- You can also have thread veins lasered, which I found more effective. The laser literally 'smashes' the thread vein and, although you may have some bruising for a few days, it works very well. For details, contact Skin Clinics, who have several clinics around the UK. Call 0800 028 7222 or visit www.sknclinics.co.uk.
- To avoid facial thread veins in the first place, avoid very hot or very cold water on your face, as any extremes can cause delicate veins to rupture.
- Avoid strong winds, and if you are out on a boat or skiing, wear really thick protective creams.
- Avoid too much sunbathing.
- Finally, get a proper diagnosis, says Mr John Scurr, a consultant vascular surgeon based at the Middlesex Hospital in London. 'Many people believe there is little point in having veins, haemorrhoids and so on treated, thinking they will return. But these days newer diagnostic and treatment techniques are giving good long-term, and in many cases permanent, relief.' For any further queries on all aspects of vein problems, log on to Dr Scurr's website: www.jscurr.com.

V

VEGETARIANISM

This subject is obviously not a health condition, but as I receive numerous letters from parents who are concerned that their children are not getting sufficient nutrients from their diet, I thought I should include a few guidelines. After the BSE and CJD debacle, more and more people are turning to a vegetarian diet, which basically means not eating any foods or products derived from the slaughter of animals. Generally, a vegetarian diet is a healthy diet and vegetarians tend to suffer less arthritis and inflammatory conditions than meat eaters. But many people, especially teenagers who call themselves vegetarians, often have a pretty unhealthy diet that includes lots of dairy foods, especially melted cheese, plus refined sugar and white flour-based foods. These people are at a higher risk of increased homocysteine levels, because they are more likely to have fewer B-vitamins and zinc in their diet. For full details of homocysteine, see under *High Blood Pressure*.

Vegetarians generally suffer less ill health, heart disease and cancer than meat-eaters, mainly because vegetarian diets tend to be higher in fibre and lower in saturated fats. Many parents worry that their children will become deficient in nutrients, especially vitamin B12, iron, zinc and vitamin D, but this tends to be more of a problem for vegans. Dr Shamin Daya, a nutritional physician based at the Wholistic Medical Centre in London, says: 'In clinical practice we often find that many people, including vegetarians and vegans who eat a highly refined diet, suffer from leaky gut syndrome. They should definitely investigate this possibility and take plenty of hemp seed protein-type powders. They should also make sure that they and their children eat as great a variety of foods as possible.'

See under *Leaky Gut Syndrome*.

Foods to Avoid
- Don't go overboard on full-fat cheeses, which are high in saturated fats.
- Products that are high in processed palm oil should be kept to a minimum, as they are also very high in saturated fats.
- Avoid too many starchy foods high in white flour, refined sugar and unsaturated fats (see *Fats You Need To Eat*).

Friendly Foods
- Green leafy vegetables, sesame seeds, low-fat yoghurts (organic soya) and Parmesan cheese are all high in calcium.
- For protein, eat lentils, quinoa, beans (especially soya beans), tempeh, miso, brown rice, peas, cereals, corn, organic almonds, Brazil nuts, peanuts, sunflower seeds and sesame seeds, which also contain good levels of zinc.
- For non-vegans, mozzarella, goat's or sheep's cheese (such as feta) are better absorbed by the body than cow's products.
- Eggs and dried skimmed milk are rich sources of vitamin B12. Alfalfa sprouts and spirulina also contain small amounts.
- For carbohydrates, eat low-sugar cereals, oats, wholemeal bread, brown rice and pasta, barley, amaranth, millet, buckwheat and rye. Quinoa is an excellent source of protein.
- Potatoes, sweet potatoes, parsnips, pumpkin, turnips and swedes are also good sources of carbohydrates.
- Red or yellow vegetables, carrots, tomatoes, pumpkin, sweet potatoes, dried apricots, and leafy green vegetables are all rich in vitamin A, as is liver.

- Nuts and seeds are high in essential fats.
- Wheat germ can be sprinkled onto cereals and desserts as a rich source of B-vitamins.
- Mushrooms and peas also contain the B-group vitamins.
- Use unrefined walnut, sunflower and olive oils for salad dressings.
- Iron is found in leafy green vegetables, wholemeal bread, black strap molasses, eggs, dried fruits (especially apricots), beans, seeds, pulses (peas and chickpeas), nuts, chocolate and cocoa.
- Eat plenty of fruits rich in vitamin C, such as kiwi and cherries, as vitamin C aids absorption of iron from foods.
- Use organic soya, rice, hemp- or pea-based protein powders in smoothies. See under *General Health Hints* for a basic smoothie recipe.
- For sugar use xylitol, stevia or organic agave syrup, which have a minimal impact on blood sugar levels.

Useful Remedies
- Take a high-strength vitamin B-complex daily with breakfast or lunch.
- Take a multi-vitamin and mineral that contains a full spectrum of B-vitamins, plus zinc (30mg) and selenium (100mcg), and is suitable for vegetarians. If your multi has good amounts of Bs, then you would not need to take it separately.
- If you have been found to be low in iron, take a formula such as Spatone – available worldwide from health stores.

Helpful Hints
- Most bookshops now sell a huge range of healthy vegetarian cookbooks. Treat yourself to a couple, and remember that the greater the variety of foods you eat, the more nutrients you will be ingesting.

VERRUCAS   *(see also Immune Function)*

Verrucas are 'plantar warts' that occur on the soles of the feet. They are extremely common, highly contagious and can be very painful. Verrucas are essentially a viral infection and you are more likely to contract them if you are really run down.

Foods to Avoid
- Reduce your intake of all foods and drinks containing refined sugar, which lowers immune function.
- Reduce caffeine, alcohol and all highly processed white-flour-based foods.
- See also dietary advice in *Immune Function*.

Friendly Foods
- Eat lots of garlic, asparagus, parsley, avocados, sea vegetables such as kelp and samphire, plus whey, hemp, pea or soya protein powders, apples, cucumbers, millet, rice bran and sprouts.
- See also *Immune Function* and *General Health Hints*.

Useful Remedies
- If you suffer from verrucas regularly, start taking a high-strength bee propolis tincture or capsules, which are highly anti-viral and greatly help to boost your immune system.
- To fight the virus take 20,000iu of vitamin A daily for 1 month only and then reduce to 5,000iu daily in a multi-vitamin and mineral complex. **NB If you are pregnant or are planning a pregnancy, take no more than 3,000iu of vitamin A daily. Or eat organic liver once a week.**
- After the month begin taking a natural-source carotene complex, which naturally converts to vitamin A in the body and is totally non-toxic. **SVHC**
- Take a garlic capsule daily for its anti-viral properties.
- Vitamin C is vital for boosting your immune system; take 2 grams daily with food in divided doses.
- Take 30mg of zinc daily for its immune-enhancing properties – this is found in most multi-vitamin/mineral complexes.
- See this section under *Immune Function*.

Helpful Hints
- Apply a tiny amount of crushed garlic or tea tree oil onto the affected area twice a day. **NB Garlic oil can cause burning, so make sure it is placed only directly on the verruca for several minutes at a time.**
- There is an enzyme in banana skin that can attack the verruca. Many people have written to say that, although this sounds somewhat bizarre, this remedy really does work! Apply the inside of the banana skin to the verruca and tape on. Change every 2 days until the verruca disappears.
- Homeopathic Thuja 6C can be helpful, as well as Thuja Mother tincture applied directly onto the warts and covered with a plaster.
- Place a tiny amount of fresh urine on a small cotton-wool ball and attach it over the verruca with a plaster. Change the dressing twice daily. Urine is a sterile liquid that contains anti-viral and anti-bacterial components and also softens the skin.

VERTIGO   *(see also Adrenal Exhaustion, Ménière's Syndrome and Stress)*

Around three in every ten adults over 65 suffer from vertigo – a very unpleasant sensation of moving or spinning or a feeling that you are losing your balance, even when you are standing or sitting still. It can be accompanied by nausea. Symptoms usually last for a few minutes, but can continue for hours, days or, in extreme cases, far longer.

Such symptoms may be triggered by impacted ear wax, blockage of the eustachian tube, or by a viral infection of the balancing mechanism of the inner ear (see also *Catarrh* and *Sinus Problems*). High blood pressure can also be a factor, as can iron deficiency (see *Anaemia*).

It is also linked to blood sugar problems (see under *Adrenal Exhaustion* and *Low and High Blood Sugar*) and poor circulation. Vertigo is also a symptom of Ménière's syndrome and may also be triggered by an injury to the head or neck. Beta blockers and some prescription drugs can trigger an attack – make sure you carefully note any contraindications with drugs. Nutritional physician Dr Shamin Daya adds: 'In practice, we have also found that some patients with vertigo are deficient in zinc.'

Extreme exhaustion and an overgrowth of the fungus candida may also be a contributing factor in vertigo (see also *Candida*), as can a misalignment of the neck and skull. If you suspect this is the cause, consult a cranial osteopath or chiropractor as soon as possible.

In Dutch research, doctors found that as many as 50% of people with chronic dizziness are actually suffering from some type of cardiovascular disease and over 60% of patients have two or more causes for their problem. Therefore, if you suffer from vertigo that continues for more than a couple of weeks, have a thorough check-up and possibly also X-rays via your doctor. See under *Heart Disease*.

Nutritionist Gareth Zeal says: 'We often see patients with this problem who may be low in iron, so this should also be tested and if people are extremely stressed it can trigger vertigo. And once they reduce their stress levels, symptoms can disappear.'

Naturopath Stephen Langley adds: 'Many people who are chronically stressed will not have been absorbing nutrients such as zinc or iron from their diet, possibly for quite some time. And once stress levels are reduced and the gut is working properly, then as absorption is restored – symptoms are often alleviated.' See under *Adrenal Exhaustion* and *Stress*.

Foods to Avoid
- Generally, you need to cut down on saturated fats found in full-fat animal-sourced milk and dairy produce, cheeses, meat, mass-produced high-fat chocolates, cakes, biscuits, pies, sausages and so on.
- Avoid caffeine, especially cappuccinos and chocolates, fizzy drinks, fried foods, alcohol and aspartame.
- Cut down your intake of sodium-based salts; there are now plenty of magnesium- and potassium-based salts available from health stores.

Friendly Foods
- If you have a specific ear problem, then Vitamin A and carotene-rich foods are needed for sensory cells in the inner ear to function normally. Eat more oily fish and fish oils, sweet potatoes, pumpkin, papaya, watercress, apricots and sweet potatoes.
- Liver is very high in vitamin A, but only eat it once a week.
- Eat more garlic, onions and ginger.
- Calves' or lambs' liver, eggs and leafy green vegetables are also a rich source of iron plus the vitamin A.
- Use organic rice, oat or almond milk instead of cow's milk.
- Eat more sunflower or pumpkin seeds and linseeds (flax seeds), which are rich in essential fats and zinc, and use their unrefined oils for salad dressings.
- Eat more bananas, dried fruit, fish and sunflower seeds, which are rich in potassium.
- See *General Health Hints*.

Useful Remedies

- Take vitamin A, 25,000iu per day for one week. The inner ear needs a high concentration of vitamin A and sensory cells are dependent upon vitamin A. **NB If you are pregnant or planning a pregnancy, only take 3000iu of Vitamin A daily.**
- A full-spectrum B-complex helps nourish the nerve endings in the inner ear.
- Take a multi-mineral that contains at least 100mg of calcium and 99mg of potassium. The potassium reduces the sodium (salt) levels in the body – high levels of sodium in the blood can make symptoms worse.
- Try Triple Zinc formula by Metabolics (call 01380 812799), which contains three types of zinc (picolinate, citrate and sulphate); these are easy to absorb and improve zinc levels quickly. Initially take 2 capsules daily for 6 weeks, then one a day for 6 weeks, and then just 1 capsule per week.
- The herb ginkgo biloba helps to improve circulation to the inner ear. Take 120–150mg of standardized extract twice daily until symptoms ease. **NB People taking anticoagulant drugs need to check with their GP before taking the ginkgo – take no more than 120mg daily.**
- Take a vitamin C and bioflavonoid complex – up to 2000mg daily in divided doses with meals.
- Ginger capsules can be taken 4–6 times daily during an attack to help reduce feelings of nausea.
- Co-enzyme Q10, a vitamin-like substance, helps to improve cellular function in the brain and may help to alleviate the vertigo. Take 100mg daily with either breakfast or lunch.
- As low vitamin D levels are associated with an increased risk of falling, take 1000iu of D3 daily. This also greatly boosts immune functioning.

Helpful Hints

- If you smoke, stop, as it thickens your blood and slows circulation to the head.
- Avoid rapid body movements, especially of the head. Avoid standing up quickly after lying down, especially first thing in the morning.
- Use two pillows at night and avoid sleeping on the affected side as much as possible.
- Reduce stress levels and make sure you are getting sufficient sleep.
- See a chiropractor or cranial osteopath to make sure your neck and spine are not misaligned, which can trigger problems in the ear. Hypnotherapy and acupuncture have helped in some cases (see *Useful Information*).
- If you have been taking prescription drugs for a long period of time, check with your GP, as high blood pressure and beta-blockers are a known factor.
- Ask your doctor to check if you have impacted ear wax, which can trigger vertigo-like symptoms (see under *Glue Ear*).

VIRAL INFECTIONS
(see Immune Function)

VITILIGO

This is a difficult multi-factorial condition that causes white patches to appear on the skin when the natural pigment production stops. The darker the skin colour, the more obvious and distressing the appearance of the skin. This condition has been linked to low stomach-acid levels, stress, low levels of the B-group of vitamins, pernicious anaemia, and an overactive thyroid gland. It could also be triggered by nutritional deficiencies or a fungal overgrowth.

Dr Shamin Daya, a nutritional physician based at the Wholistic Medical Centre in Harley Street, London, says: 'In patients with this autoimmune condition, we have found in clinical practice that certain parasites in the gut produce chemical toxins, which can have a 'bleaching' effect on the skin, therefore it's well worth patients have a Genova Test to find out if parasites are indeed a contributing factor.' (See details under *Allergies*.)

Foods to Avoid
- Alcohol, caffeine, processed foods, and refined sugar all deplete the body of B-vitamins.
- See *General Health Hints*.

Friendly Foods
- Papaya and pineapple contain enzymes that aid digestion and absorption of nutrients.
- Foods rich in B-vitamins include wheat germ, brewer's yeast, Bovril, calves' liver, eggs, whole grains such as brown rice, quinoa, nuts, fish, chicken, turkey, dates, oats, cereals, mushrooms, green vegetables (especially kale, watercress, broccoli and spinach), black strap molasses, fruits and apricots.
- As low zinc levels are linked to vitiligo, eat more fresh fish, nuts and sunflower and pumpkin seeds.
- Live, low-fat yoghurt also aids digestion.
- Drink plenty of water – at least 6–8 glasses daily.
- Eat more foods high in natural carotenes – apricots, cantaloupe melon, pumpkin, carrots, tomatoes, sweet potatoes, papaya, red and yellow peppers and mangoes.

Useful Remedies

- As lack of stomach acid is also linked to this problem, take betaine hydrochloride (HCl) for up to 2 years with main meals. If you have active stomach ulcers, just take a digestive enzyme without HCl with main meals instead. **BC**
- Take a high-strength B-complex, plus 400mcg of folic acid and 500mcg of vitamin B12.
- PABA is a B-vitamin – take 100mg 3 times daily, to help to re-pigment the skin.
- Include 1–2 grams of vitamin C daily – which is vital for collagen production. Take in divided doses with food.
- Copper – take 2mg per day. Copper is needed for certain enzymes that are required for skin pigmentation. Take 30–40mg of zinc at the same time. Both of these are usually found in most multi-vitamin and mineral formulas.
- The amino acid phenylalanine – 50mg per kilo of body weight, taken on an empty stomach in divided doses daily – with careful sun bathing, should help to re-pigment the skin. Take this suggested dose for one month and then reduce to half the dose until the desired effects are achieved. If no positive results are noted after three months, discontinue. Use a high-factor sunscreen and don't sit in the midday sun. Just take 15 minutes twice daily for a few days and gradually the skin should re-pigment.
- Natural-source carotenes are great for the skin. Take daily.
- The herb ashwagandha has been found to help prevent abnormalities in skin pigmentation if 1–2 grams are taken daily. Again, try this dose for 2 months, then reduce to 1 gram daily until no longer needed.

Helpful Hints
- Some people believe that small amounts of sun are beneficial for vitiligo. However, I believe that you should keep areas of vitiligo out of the sun, or at the very least use a strong sunscreen (see *Sunburn*). Never allow these areas to burn, as your skin has no natural protection.

VOMITING
(see also Food Poisoning)

Vomiting can have many causes, the most obvious being food poisoning, food intolerances and binge drinking, but it could also be prescription drugs that disagree with you. Morning sickness, migraines, bulimia, drinking too much alcohol, and eating a really high-fat, rich meal can all trigger nausea. If an infant vomits violently within a few minutes of being fed, you need to seek medical attention. If a child drinks a poison, such as bleach, or swallows an object and begins to vomit, urgent medical attention is needed.

Dehydration is the biggest concern with vomiting. If the person is small, also has diarrhoea, and cannot keep down any fluids, obviously the rate of dehydration will be much faster than in a tall, weighty person. If a baby or small child suffers frequent vomiting and diarrhoea, they are at a greater risk of dehydration and need immediate medical attention.

In some people when they vomit, low blood pressure can kick in, thus triggering loss of consciousness, in which case a saline drip is needed to bring the person around – seek urgent medical attention. If you suffer low blood pressure and begin vomiting frequently, call a doctor. If you have severe abdominal pain or begin vomiting any blood, have a fever and the vomiting has continued for more than 24 hours, seek urgent medical help. Nausea after fatty foods can be related to liver congestion, in which case you need to greatly reduce your intake of fats, coffee and alcohol. See *Liver Problems*.

Foods to Avoid
- See all dietary advice in *Food Poisoning*.

Friendly Foods
- Sip clear fluids, such as boiled water, fruit juices, or an electrolyte powdered drink, such as Re-hydrate, available from all chemists.
- If you can tolerate it, sip a little ginger ale or ginger tea.
- Don't drink more than a couple of tablespoonfuls of liquid at any one time until the nausea has stopped.
- Once vomiting has stopped, gently increase your fluid intake. Drink no coffee or black tea for 24 hours.
- Slowly begin eating again: dry toast, dry crackers, arrowroot, tapioca or semolina, fresh soups, a little poached fish with mashed potato, low-fat yoghurts or brown rice should be fine.
- To replace lost potassium – once you are feeling able to eat – include high-potassium foods, such as bananas and most fresh fruits, in your diet.

Useful Remedies
- Don't take these supplements until at least 24 hours after the vomiting has stopped.
- A small capful of pure aloe vera juice taken before foods will help soothe the gut. Aloe Pura make an excellent Stomach Formula. Available from all good health stores.
- Deglycerrhized liquorice – 15 drops twice daily – helps to soothe the digestive tract.
- Acidophilus/bifidus – take 2 capsules daily for a couple of weeks – to replenish healthy bacteria in the bowel. **BC**

Helpful Hints
- Place some essential oils of ginger and peppermint under your nose; this greatly helps to reduce the dreadful feeling of nausea.
- Homeopathic Nux Vomica 6x or Arsenicum Album 6x – take 1 dose every 30 minutes up to 10 doses daily until symptoms ease.

WARTS

(see also Immune Function)

Warts are caused by a varied assortment of viruses, which invade the skin, causing cells to multiply and rapidly form raised lumps. When your immune system is at a low ebb, you are more likely to pick up the virus. Warts are contagious, and touching warts can transfer viruses to new sites, and encourage new warts to develop. They are commonly found on the soles of the feet (see *Verrucas*) and on the hands or arms. They can also occur if your tissues become too acid – therefore see *Acid–Alkaline Balance*.

Foods to Avoid
- See *Foods to Avoid* under *Acid–Alkaline Balance* and *Immune Function*.

Friendly Foods
- As vitamin A and carotenes are vital for healing the skin, eat more leafy greens – especially spinach, watercress, cabbage, broccoli and kale – plus pumpkin, papaya, apricots, sweet potatoes, tomatoes, cantaloupe melon, oily fish and liver.
- Eat more sulphur-containing foods, such as onions, leeks, garlic, Brussels sprouts, cabbage, and broccoli.
- Eat more low-fat, bio yoghurt.
- See *Friendly Foods* under *Immune Function*.

Useful Remedies
- If you are not pregnant take 20,000iu of vitamin A daily for 1 month to help fight the virus. **NB If you are pregnant or planning a pregnancy, then take no more than 3000iu of pure vitamin A daily.** After the month, switch to natural-source carotene complex capsules; take 1 or 2 daily, which are safe and non-toxic. **SVHC, VN**
- Take 2 grams of vitamin C twice daily in divided doses with food to boost your immune system.
- Take a high-strength multi-vitamin and mineral that contains 200mcg of selenium and 30mg of zinc.
- Olive leaf extract is highly anti-viral – take 500mg twice daily for a month.

Helpful Hints
- Oregano oil or thyme therapeutic grade essential oils are very powerful – dab a small amount of neat oil onto the wart twice daily until it disappears. It will take about 2–3 weeks.
- Mix a little bicarbonate of soda dissolved in the palm of your hand with a drop or two of water to make a paste, apply it to the wart, cover with a sticking plaster and change daily. The wart should be gone within a week.
- Or crush half an aspirin, place this on the plaster and immediately place it over the wart. Change the plaster daily. It's the salicylic acid that helps to break the wart. The wart should disappear within 2 weeks.
- Dandelion tincture can be added to the wart through a small piece of card in which you have cut a small hole. Dab on the tincture for 3 days.
- Apply the following mixture twice daily for up to 10 days: add a little freshly crushed garlic to the contents of 1 vitamin E and 1 vitamin A capsule and mix with some zinc cream. Add only

to the site of the wart and cover with a dressing. If the skin surrounding the wart becomes inflamed, then eliminate the garlic.
- Homeopathic Thuja 6c or Causticum 6c can be taken twice daily – but you must stop this remedy as soon as you see an improvement.

WATER ON THE KNEE   *(see also Water Retention)*

This condition is triggered when the little fluid-filled sacks that surround the knee joint become inflamed. The problem is usually generated by a knock or a fall, or by a chronic condition such as arthritis.

Foods to Avoid
- Reduce or avoid red meat, salt, caffeine, black tea and all highly processed sugary, starchy foods – which can all exacerbate inflammation in the body.
- Any foods that are high in salt, such as crisps, olives, preserved meats and foods, will make the body retain more water.
- Avoid foods from the nightshade family – tomatoes, potatoes, eggplant and sweet peppers, especially if you suffer arthritis-type conditions.
- See *Foods to Avoid* under *Bursitis*.

Friendly Foods
- Eat foods high in magnesium, dark leafy greens, especially watercress, kale, spinach, cabbage, broccoli and pak choy, which all help to alkalize the body.
- Squash, fruits, vegetables and organic raw honey also help to alkalize the body, as an over-acid system can make this condition worse. For more help, see *Acid–Alkaline Balance*.
- Add a teaspoon of apple cider vinegar and a touch of raw, organic honey to cooled, boiled water and sip the mixture throughout the day. This is another way of helping to re-alkalize the body.
- Eat plenty of potassium-rich foods: bananas, papaya and celery plus most fruits, linseeds (flax seeds), sunflower and pumpkin seeds, and nuts.
- Eat more avocado and raw wheat germ, which are rich in vitamin E.
- Pineapple is a rich source of bromelain, which has anti-inflammatory properties. Cherries are also anti-inflammatory.
- Eat oily fish, such as mackerel, pilchards, salmon and sardines, twice a week.
- Drink plenty of water – for details as to why, see *Water Retention*.
- Use nori seaweed salt flakes or kelp flakes instead of sodium-based salts
- For sugar, use small amounts of xylitol, stevia or organic agave syrup, which have a low glycaemic effect on blood sugar.

Useful Remedies
- Silica helps to strengthen the tissues in the knees. Take 200mg daily, or drink more Fiji water, which is high in silica.
- Take 1 gram of vitamin C twice daily with bioflavonoids to help reduce the swelling.
- Bromelain from pineapples is highly anti-inflammatory – take 500mg twice daily while symptoms last.
- Take zinc – 30mg per day – which helps the body fight inflammation.
- Take 2 grams of omega-3 fish oils daily – which are highly anti-inflammatory.
- MSM is an organic form of sulphur that counteracts inflammation and pain. Start on 1 gram a day and then increase to 2 grams daily. It is great for your skin, too.

- Celery seed extract acts as a mild diuretic, which helps to flush the excess fluid from the body. Take 200mg twice daily with food.

Helpful Hints

- At the onset of inflammation, rest the affected area and avoid putting pressure on the joint for a few days. Keep your leg raised as much as possible.
- Alternating hot and cold compresses can help to disperse the swelling.
- Homeopathic Ruta 6c, taken twice daily for 3–5 days, really helps reduce knee problems. Also Apis 6c taken 3 times daily between meals helps to reduce the swelling.
- Perseverance with this regime is important, as knee problems can take some time to heal.
- Regular acupuncture can greatly reduce not only the pain but also the swelling (see *Useful Information*).
- Ask at your local health or sports shop for a knee support that contains magnets, as magnets help increase blood flow and therefore bring more oxygenated blood to the area, which speeds healing.

WATER RETENTION (OEDEMA)

(see also Allergies and Rheumatoid Arthritis)

Water retention can be seen throughout the body and, unlike water on the knee, general water retention is not caused by an injury. It can usually be seen in the hands, legs, ankles or feet, or around the eyes. The most common cause is excess sodium-based salt in the body, but it can also be triggered by food intolerances (the usual culprits being wheat and dairy produce from cows – see under *Allergies*). It can also occur during pregnancy, when taking the pill or HRT, and is very common in women, especially those over 60.

Another trigger can be standing for too long in hot weather. Occasionally, fluid retention can denote more serious problems that affect the heart, kidneys or liver. Therefore, if these suggestions do not work after 2–3 weeks, please have a thorough check-up with your doctor. Some people mistakenly think that if they cut back on their fluid intake, their water retention will disappear – but in fact the opposite is true. The problem is that, as we get older, water finds it harder to penetrate your cells, and therefore a person can be suffering from water retention but technically be dehydrated. The secret is getting the water into the cells that need them.

Foods to Avoid

- Cut down on high-salt foods and pre-packaged meals – and don't add salt to meals.
- Meat pies, cheese, sauces, pizza, olives, crisps, preserved meats and pickles can all be high in sodium.
- Some breakfast cereals contain more salt than an average bag of crisps.
- Don't add salt to cooking unless it's a potassium- or magnesium-based salt, such as powdered kelp or nori seaweed flakes.
- Even some chocolate drinks can be very high in salt.
- Alcoholic and caffeinated foods and drinks act as diuretics. They cause water to be leached out of the cells where it is needed, which increases dehydration.

Friendly Foods

- Eat lots of fresh fruit and vegetables, as they are very rich in potassium.
- Include more spinach, celery, kale, watercress, cabbage, bananas, almonds, sunflower seeds, apricots, sweet potatoes, raisins, blackberries, cherries, bilberries and blueberries in your diet.

- Drink at least 6–8 glasses of pure filtered water daily.
- Eat good-quality protein, such as fish, eggs, quinoa, chicken, turkey or tempeh, at least once a day.
- Otherwise, try a protein powder drink for breakfast – see recipe under *General Health Hints*.
- Ask at your local health shop for various seaweeds, such as kombu, arame, nori or kelp. Soak them for 5 minutes and then chop over meals. These seaweeds are high in potassium and can really help to remove any excess fluid from the body. They are also high in organic sodium, but this does not cause the body to hold water to the same extent as normal table salt does.
- Drink more green or white tea, which acts as a natural diuretic.

Useful Remedies
- Dandelion leaf tea or tincture – 1ml can be taken 3 times a day – is a gentle diuretic, which puts more potassium into the body than it takes out. **NC**
- Take 1–2 grams of vitamin C as potassium ascorbate with meals in divided doses, which can help lymph drainage. **BC**
- Take a vitamin B-complex that contains 100mg of B6, which is a natural diuretic.
- Take celery seed extract – 1 x 200mg capsule twice daily. Celery is a natural liver and kidney cleanser and helps to neutralize excess acid in the tissues. **BC**
- The herb gotu kola stimulates circulation in the lower limbs and improves lymph drainage. Take up to 500mg twice daily when symptoms are acute.
- Celloid sodium sulphate is known as the problem-fluid remover. Take 200mg 3 times daily. **BLK**; or ask at your local pharmacy for the tissue salts.

Helpful Hints
- Try to elevate your feet for at least 15 minutes every day. Lie on the floor and place your lower limbs higher than your waist. This really helps the excess fluids to drain via the lymphatic system.
- Rebounding on a mini-trampoline is particularly good for enhancing lymph drainage. Have regular lymph-drainage massage (see under *Useful Information* at back of book).
- The homeopathic drops Lymphomyosot made by Heel can be used to help lymph drainage. **OP**
- Take regular exercise, such as swimming, walking, skipping or jogging.
- Skin brushing is a great way to remove excess fluids from the body. Start at the feet and work towards the heart, and then go to your chest and shoulders and again work towards the heart area. When you brush your arms, work from the hands up towards the shoulders and throat areas.
- If you are overweight, try to lose weight.

WEIGHT PROBLEMS

(see also Allergies, Candida, Insulin Resistance, Low Blood Sugar, Stress and Thyroid Problems)

In 1993, only 16% of women and 13% of men were obese, whereas more recently more than 26% of the UK population is now clinically obese. Obesity in boys aged 2–15 has increased from 11% in 1995 to 19%, and in girls from 12% to around 18%. One in five children is either overweight or obese when they start school and that increases to one in three by the time they finish primary education. If this growth in obesity continues unabated then children and young people will undoubtedly have a shorter life expectancy than their parents.

This is shocking if you also consider that obesity contributes to more than 30,000 premature deaths, which could have been prevented, a year in the UK alone. It's time for us all to take greater responsibility for our health.

Research shows that women who gain more than 44 pounds above the weight they should be for their height and age after the age of 18 are 2.5 times more likely eventually to suffer a stroke. People who are significantly overweight are 5 times more likely to develop late-onset diabetes. More than 85% of people with type 2 diabetes are overweight when first diagnosed. Obese men are 33% more likely to die of cancer and this figure rises to 55% in women.

The basics of finding your perfect weight and then maintaining it are: controlling your blood sugar levels, eating a varied diet that contains plenty of fibre, and taking sufficient exercise. If you feel that you have truly tried every diet and you are still finding it hard to lose weight, then you may have an underactive thyroid or a chronic food intolerance that is causing water retention, or you may have developed insulin resistance (one of the major factors is weight gain, which contributes to an overloaded liver allowing toxins to accumulate, which your body then stores away in fat cells). Steroids are also well known to trigger weight gain.

The human body contains 30–40 million fat cells and any extra calories we eat are stored as fat. A lot of people now take regular exercise, but the majority still do not. Lack of regular exercise slows our metabolic rate and toxins begin to accumulate. The net result is 'middle-age spread' – which is happening to young and old alike.

How many overweight people do you know who regularly say: 'I really cannot imagine why I'm overweight, I hardly ever touch bread, cakes, chocolate', and so on, and when they think no one is looking they eat a chocolate croissant followed by a cappucino.

I realize that weight gain can have a multitude of causes – but **98% of people who are overweight are simply eating too much and taking insufficient exercise.** After all, if we are truly honest about obesity, I have yet to see anyone leave a prison-type camp looking overweight. This book is about living consciously – you can choose. Choose what you put in your mouth and you can choose your weight. And if you choose to lose weight, then do it for yourself, and if you are happy being 'overweight' then so be it.

Meanwhile, I believe it is important to stop thinking about the word 'diet' and start thinking 'eating more healthily for the rest of our lives'. There are cabbage diets, protein-only diets, carbohydrate-free diets, eat-a-twinkie-only-at-night diets – and so on. And almost half of women between 25 and 35 are on a diet, but in the long term **they don't work.**

Naturopath Stephen Langley says: 'The major problem today is blood-sugar problems; basically thanks to our increased love of refined sugary, starchy foods, our bodies are overproducing insulin to try to balance loss of sensitivity in our cells. Insulin causes excess sugar to be converted into fat and excess insulin then prevents that fat from being released by the body.'

If this is allowed to continue, not only does the person pile on weight, but also the insidious insulin resistance can eventually lead to full-blown diabetes.

If you are 20% or more over your ideal weight, you are technically obese. This extra weight puts undue stress on your back, legs, joints, circulation and internal organs. Obesity increases the body's susceptibility to infection, the risk of heart disease, high blood pressure, arthritis, late-onset type 2 diabetes, stroke and other serious health problems that can result in premature death.

So how do you know if, for your height, build, age and sex, you're 'normal', overweight or obese? There have been numerous charts produced, but the most recognized method that's easy to do is the Body Mass Index (BMI). Simply the ratio of your weight in kilograms to your height in metres squared, it's a good rough guide and is widely used. The 'normal' range is 20–25, over 25 is considered overweight, over 30 is moderately obese and over 40 is very obese. As an example, a man of 1.83 metres (6ft) weighing 80kg has a BMI of 24, which is 80 divided by (1.83 x 1.83 = 3.34), which is a normal weight. But a man of 1.52 metres (5ft) weighing 80kg has a BMI of 34 and is regarded as obese – his 'normal' weight should be no more than 58kg. Calculate your BMI and use it to determine what your target weight should be.

Many fad diets suggest high protein and few or no carbohydrates, such as rice or potatoes, as protein can be harder to digest and metabolize and therefore releases its energy more slowly. This diet isn't a good long-term weight-loss strategy, as too much protein makes the blood and tissues too acid, and can become a high-risk factor for osteoporosis in later life. Excess protein also places a great burden on the kidneys, metabolism becomes imbalanced, and the saturated fat that accompanies animal protein can increase the risk of heart disease. People do experience initial weight loss on this diet, perhaps due in large part to the exclusion of wheat and refined sugar (most people's main carbohydrate). A far better approach is to eat as great a variety of foods as possible and to make a life-long change to your diet, whilst cutting down on wheat-based, white starchy foods.

Many people find that on a trial 'exclusion diet' for food intolerances they lose weight easily, while eating heartily. The most common food intolerances are usually starchy or sugary in nature (wheat, corn, milk from cows, refined sugar and potatoes) and this is not unlike the low-carbohydrate diet mentioned above. But avoiding any food that is badly tolerated, whether it is 'fattening' or not, usually enables rapid weight loss. Also, naturopath Stephen Langley says: 'If people can eat according to their blood type, they will naturally lose weight. For example, people with Type A blood will tend to put on weight if they eat meat and dairy, whereas those with Type O will increase their weight by eating gluten and corn. Therefore, I suggest that people read Peter J. D'Adamo's books such as *Fatigue: Fight It with the Blood Type Diet* (Berkley Publishing Corporation) or *Eat Right For Your Type* (Century).'

Finally, don't be tempted to cut corners and use weight-loss pills that claim to be fat blockers. These types of products encourage you to eat a cheeseburger, then take a pill so you won't gain weight. This is definitely not the way to try to improve your health, and like low-fat diets, they can stop you absorbing essential fats (the healthy fats), plus other fat-soluble nutrients that depend on fats to be transported into the body, such as vitamins A, D, E and K. Weight loss is best done slowly and for the long haul if you want to improve not just your weight, but your health too.

At the end of the day you need to ask yourself honestly:

1 Am I exercising enough?
2 What foods do I tend to eat and crave the most? If the answer to this is wheat, flour, breads, pies, biscuits, colas, coffee and so on, then you may well have a leaky gut and fungal overgrowth problems, such as candida, as well as food intolerances (commonly to refined carbohydrates, wheat and possibly gluten, caffeine, sugar or alcohol), which is a huge factor in people who cannot lose weight. See under *Allergies* to organize a test.
3 Might my thyroid be underactive? This is incredibly common and to answer this question, see the *Thyroid* section.
4 Am I drinking 6–8 glasses of water a day?

Be honest about these answers. Face the truth!

Meanwhile, in a research study from The University of Buffalo in America, 40% of obese men were found to have low testosterone levels – therefore both men and women should have hormone levels checked by a doctor, as testosterone and other hormones such as DHEA and oestrogen are easily supplemented if needed. See under *Menopause*.

Foods to Avoid

- Cut down on the refined carbohydrates, white breads and rice, croissants, Danish pastries, meat pies, desserts, anything with pastry, burgers, pizzas and melted-cheese-type snacks. By all means have a treat, once a week or so, but once you start losing weight and stop eating these foods all the time, your need for them will gradually disappear.
- Gluten found in grains is very hard for the body to digest – eating gluten foods can trigger overeating because you are not absorbing the nutrients that you should be (such as zinc, magnesium, selenium, vitamin C and B vitamins) from the grains. You are getting the calories but not the corresponding energy, which makes you crave these foods even more. Try eliminating any foods containing gluten for a few weeks; all supermarkets sell alternatives.
- Artificial sweeteners, found in more than 3,000 foods and low-calorie drinks, place a strain on the liver and can slow weight loss. The worst offender is aspartame. Manufactured fructose, maltose, dextrose and so on should all be avoided.
- Cut down on fried, fast foods and high-fat take-aways and processed foods – Indian foods in sauces are among the worst offenders.
- Research has shown that many adults are consuming up to 46 teaspoons of sugar a day. Keep in mind that many low-fat labelled foods may be high in sugar or sweeteners; check labels. Reduce all foods high in refined and artificial sugars, which convert to fat inside the body if not used up during exercise. We all need a certain amount of fat and fat-free diets are dangerous (see *Fats You Need To Eat*).

- Chocolates are highly acid forming, and although dark chocolate is high in antioxidants and can often contain fewer calories than crisps, please remember it may still be high in saturated fats and sugar. The occasional piece of dark chocolate is fine, but keep in mind the word 'occasional'. Or look for sugar- and dairy-free chocolates such as Glamour Food – made with coconut oil, goji and acai berries. For details and stockists, call 0844 800 8399.
- Avoid salted nuts, crisps and preserved meats.
- Reduce sodium-based table salt.
- Avoid all hard margarines, full-fat milk and full-fat cheeses.
- Stop ordering desserts – or try the fruit salad or a low-fat yoghurt.
- In most cases, the weight is coming from foods that you tend to eat every day or crave the most. Keep a food diary and note what you eat and when – you will soon be able to identify the culprits!

Friendly Foods

- Eat more organic foods, which contain fewer pesticides – pesticides live in your fat tissue and are really hard to eliminate.
- In summer, eat nothing but fruit before midday – this is a great way to kick start a sluggish metabolism. See under *General Health Hints* for a great smoothie with added protein powder that keeps you well satisfied until lunchtime.
- In winter, try gluten-free porridge with a grated raw apple and a few raisins for breakfast, which helps reduce cravings mid-morning.
- Instead of white-flour-based foods, use wholemeal, stone-ground bread and experiment with various pastas and meals made from corn, rice, spelt, quinoa, buckwheat, millet, lentil, amaranth and potato flour.

- Instead of wheat-based breads, try amaranth crackers, rice or oatcakes, spread with a little humous or cottage cheese; add a tomato and cucumber for a quick, healthy snack.
- Eat far more brown rice, lentils, chickpeas, barley and dried (or tinned) beans.
- Eat plenty of fresh fruits and vegetables – the more fibre the better. Cabbage, broccoli and cauliflower are great healthy foods, but avoid cabbages and cauliflower if you have an underactive thyroid or have Type O blood (broccoli is okay). See *Thyroid*.
- Onions, ginger, spring greens, spinach, pak choy, celery, pineapple and apples are all great foods for assisting weight loss. Radicchio, chicory, fennel, celeriac and bitter foods help to cleanse the liver, which aids weight loss (see *Liver Problems*).
- Use organic rice milk, or skimmed milk (or skimmed goat's milk) instead of full-fat milk. Experiment with almond or coconut milks.
- Eat 1 portion of quality protein a day, such as fish, eggs, chicken or cooked tofu, as protein balances blood sugar for a longer period. Try to eat the protein at breakfast and/or lunchtime.
- A small jacket potato is fine (sweet potato would be even better), but fill it with low-fat bio yoghurt and chives instead of butter. Or use a spread such as Olivio, or hemp- or pumpkin-seed butters. Available from good health stores or call Higher Nature. **HN**
- Always eat breakfast – there are dozens of organic low-sugar cereals now available and a great breakfast is organic porridge made with half water and half rice milk. Use a few raisins and a chopped apple to sweeten.
- If you are desperate for sugar, try xylitol, stevia or organic agave syrup – plant-based natural sugars, which do not greatly impact your glycaemic level. For a larger list see *Low Blood Sugar* and *Insulin Resistance*.

- Drink lots of herbal teas and at least 6–8 glasses of water a day. Water suppresses appetite and helps prevent fat depositing in the body; it reduces water retention and encourages toxins to be flushed through the body.
- Essential fats are vital if you want to lose weight (see *Fats You Need To Eat*).
- Use rice or oat bran for extra fibre.
- Ask at your health shop for a magnesium- or potassium-based salt such as Himalayan Crystal Salt (sold at most health stores), or use powdered kelp or nori seaweed flakes as a salt substitute.
- Vegetarians tend to suffer less obesity, less heart disease and significantly less cancer. See *Vegetarianism*.
- Caffeine is an appetite suppressant, although a fairly toxic one. Use organic coffee.

Useful Remedies
- Refined foods deplete many vital minerals from the body and virtually everyone who eats them to excess is lacking in the mineral chromium. Begin taking 200mcg daily to help reduce your chance of developing late-onset diabetes and to reduce cravings for sweet and refined foods. Take 200mcg twice daily in between meals. It takes a while to kick in, but it really does help to reduce sugar cravings. Furthermore, scientific investigations show that during exercise chromium can help reduce body fat and increase muscle concentration.
- Take a high-strength B-complex to support your nerves and aid digestion.
- Include a good-quality multi-vitamin and mineral for your age and gender in your regimen. All the vitamin companies on pages 15–16 will be able to help you choose the right supplement.
- Co-enzyme Q10, a vitamin-like substance needed for the conversion of fat into energy within the cells. Research shows that as many as half of all obese people are deficient in CoQ10. Take 100mg per day with breakfast or lunch.
- The amino acid L-carnitine helps the body produce energy from fat – take 500mg twice daily 30 minutes before food.

- Soluble fibre, such as ready-cracked linseeds (flax seeds), aids fat elimination from the intestines and helps prevent the re-absorption of toxins by keeping you regular. Soak a tablespoon of linseeds overnight in cold water, drain and add to smoothies or porridge daily.
- The amino acid tyrosine helps you to maintain your chosen weight once you have reached it. Take 500mg twice daily before meals.
- Try Freecarb, made from white kidney bean extract, which helps prevent the digestion and absorption of approximately 60% of starches (such as pasta, rice, cereals, potatoes, bread) that you may consume. If you continue to eat lots of white-based cakes, biscuits and desserts this supplement would be less effective. HN

Helpful Hints

- Some people find it easier to lose weight by 'grazing' all day on healthy snacks, to balance their blood sugar. So regular nibbling is one of the simplest but most effective ways to start losing weight. Others says that if they eat 3 sensible meals a day – which includes a porridge-type breakfast, a good lunch (without dessert) and a light supper, with no snacks in between – they also lose weight. Listen to your body.
- Many people now consider food combining as being out of date – but naturopath Stephen Langley adds: 'There is no doubt that food combining aids better digestion and encourages weight loss. The basic rule is, if you are eating a protein food such as meat, eggs, cheese, fish or chicken – then avoid the major starches such as bread, pasta, rice or potatoes in the same meal. And if you are eating starches – then eat them without any of the major proteins.'
- Regular exercise increases your metabolic rate, decreases fat deposits and helps reduce food cravings. Regular exercise also increases muscle mass, which burns more energy just to keep the muscles functioning properly. The most important part of regular exercise is that it needs to be **regular,** and burning yourself out in the first week is the surest way to not continue. Aim for 30 minutes of exercise at least 5 times per week. The best way is simply to walk for 30 minutes or more every single day. I have a girlfriend who was 16 stone, and would not diet at all, but she agreed to start walking daily. At first she hated it, but as the pounds and then stones fell away over several months, she was delighted, and now feels irritable if she does not get her daily walk. She is 69. It's never too late to start!
- Gradually, build the intensity, and vary the style of exercise. Consider joining a local dance, aerobic exercise or swimming club. It really helps if you work with people who have the same goal in mind. For this reason join Weight Watchers. To find your nearest club, log on to www.weightwatchers.co.uk or call 0845 345 1500.
- Eat the majority of your food before 7.30pm if possible and try to make breakfast and lunch your larger meals of the day.
- An excess of oestrogen can cause weight gain and water retention if your body is low in progesterone (for details of natural progesterone cream, see *Menopause*).
- Try reading *Eat More, Weigh Less* by Dr Dean Ornish (Quill Press) or *The End of Overeating* by David A Kessler (Penguin).
- If you suffer from an eating disorder, get professional help. Contact The Eating Disorders Association via their helpline on 0845 634 1414. Website: www.b-eat.co.uk.

Author's note

After six months of intense research, hundreds of hours of typing, plus phone calls and interviews that I thought would never end, I am delighted to have reached the end of the Hints Section!

In updating this book I have learned huge amounts and I hope you will, too. I have added several new headings, but if your specific condition is not mentioned, I apologize. If I had tried to feature every illness, this book would be thousands of pages thick rather than an easy-to-read health reference guide. But without doubt Steve, Gareth and I have endeavoured in our own ways to give you a good basis to enable you to become your own health detective.

Due to my work schedule I can no longer answer individual letters, but there are plenty of names and addresses to turn to for more help. Alternatively, find me via my website: www.hazelcourteney.com.

Remember, you can still enjoy treats, but simply balance them out with plenty of healthy foods. It's never too late and always keep in mind that the right food is the best medicine! Your body is perfectly capable of healing itself, if given the right tools for the job. Above all, reduce the stress in your life, exercise regularly if you can and, as much as possible, enjoy your journey.

Good luck and good health.

Hazel Courteney, Stephen Langley and Gareth Zeal

USEFUL INFORMATION

ACUPUNCTURE
This practice goes back over 3,000 years. Basically, an acupuncturist inserts fine sterile needles into specific meridian energy points in the body, which encourage energy and blood to flow more freely around the body. Specialist scanners can now clearly see blocked energies within the human body (see *Electrical Pollution* and *Healing*). And when these blockages are released, the body's self-healing mechanisms become more effective. Acupuncture is medically and scientifically proven to reduce pain and can also help to alleviate inflammation, water retention, balance hormones and emotions, help infertility and pregnancy problems, nausea, sciatica, back and neck pain, migraines, and so on.
To find your nearest practitioner, send an SAE to:
British Acupuncture Council, BAcC,
63, Jeddo Road,
London W12 9HQ
Tel: 020 8735 0400
Website: www.acupuncture.org.uk

Stephen Langley, MBAc, my co-author, specializes in facial acupuncture at:
The Hale Clinic,
7, Park Crescent,
London W1B 1PF
Tel: 020 7631 0156

ADVANCED REFLEXOLOGY
Anthony Porter has been a reflexologist since 1972. During the 80s he went to China and the Far East to teach reflexology and found that their methods, when combined with his own, gave even better results. He has taught his advanced techniques to thousands of reflexologists internationally and says: 'With ART we can not only balance various parts of the body (which is what happens with normal reflexology), but we can also feel more subtle changes within the 7000 nerve endings or reflex areas of the feet, and, after working on them, this has a profound therapeutic affect.' Medical research with a leading gynaecologist has shown huge success with easing the pain and distress of many gynaecological conditions that might otherwise need surgery. He also has had great success with infertility, stress, and a host of health problems. To find details of Anthony's practice in central London or for an ART therapist in your area, log on to www.artreflex.com or call 020 8920 9555.

ALEXANDER TECHNIQUE
Teaches you how to use your body more efficiently and how to have balance and poise with minimum tension in order to avoid pain, strain and injury. To find your nearest practitioner, or list of affiliated societies worldwide, contact:
Society of Teachers of the Alexander Technique,
1st Floor, Linton House, 39-51 Highgate Road,
London NW5 1RS
Tel: 020 7482 5135
Website: www.stat.org.uk
Email: office@stat.org.uk

AROMATHERAPY
The use of essential oils to improve health and well-being, by massage, inhalation, compresses and baths. It is excellent for reducing muscle spasm, stress, and anxiety. For a register of practitioners, contact:
International Federation of Aromatherapists (IFA),
Suite 7B, Walpole Court, Ealing Green,
London W5 5ED
Tel: 020 8567 2243/020 8567 1923
Website: www.ifaroma.org

Or contact:
International Federation of Professional Aromatherapists (IFPA),
82 Ashby Road, Hinckley,
Leicestershire LE10 1SN
Tel: 01455 637987
Website: www.ifparoma.org
Email: admin@ifparoma.org

BACH FLOWER REMEDIES
A healing system used to treat emotional problems, such as fear and hopelessness. The liquid remedies are made from the flowers of wild plants, bushes and trees.
For further information, contact:
The Bach Centre,
Mount Vernon, Bakers Lane, Sotwell,
Oxfordshire OX10 0PZ
Tel: 01491 834678
Website: www.bachcentre.com

BOOKS
If you have difficulty finding any of the recommended books, or simply want to find a book on your condition, the Nutri Centre bookshop in London has an extensive library of self-help books and would be happy to order for you, or give assistance on specific subjects.

Tel: 020 7323 2382 or 0800 587 2290
Website: www.nutricentre.com

CHELATION

Chelation, an intravenous treatment using the synthetic amino acid EDTA, has been proven to improve blood flow in blocked arteries in heart, diabetic and stroke patients, by removing toxic metals from the body. When combined with antioxidants and other substances, the healing and anti-ageing effects are amplified. It is very useful if you have any of the above conditions, plus senile dementia, Alzheimer's disease, Parkinson's, ME, chronic fatigue, arthritis or multiple sclerosis, or you want to prevent cancers. It is also known as IVAT – Intravenous Antioxidant Therapy.

For further details, read *Detox With Oral Chelation* by David Jay Brown or *Everything You Should Know About Chelation Therapy* by Dr Morton Walker. To order, call 020 7323 2382.

In the UK there are several chelation clinics. Call the Arterial Disease Clinic on 01942 886644 for details, or Dr Wendy Denning on 020 7224 2423.

CHIROPRACTIC

This is a manipulation treatment for disorders of the joints and muscles and their effects on the nervous system. Chiropractors treat the entire body to bring it back into balance and restore health. Once a month I visit my chiropractor, who keeps my spine and neck mobile after an injury several years ago.

To find a practitioner in your local area, contact:
The British Chiropractic Association
59 Castle Street, Reading,
Berkshire RG1 7SN
Tel: 0118 950 5950
Website: www.chiropractic-uk.co.uk
Email: enquiries@chiropractic-uk.co.uk

McTimoney Chiropractic Association:
Crowmarsh Gifford, Wallingford,
Oxfordshire OX10 8DJ
Tel: 01491 829211
Website: www.mctimoney-chiropractic.org
Email: admin@mctimoney-chiropractic.org

COLONIC HYDROTHERAPY

A method of cleansing the colon to flush away toxic waste, gas, accumulated faeces and mucous deposits. This is a safe treatment when given by a qualified professional. Check with your GP before undertaking this therapy. Colonics are very useful if you are chronically constipated or have taken antibiotics or painkillers, which can cause constipation.
A list of practitioners is available online from:

Association and Register of Colon Hydrotherapists (ARCH)
Tel: 0870 241 6567
Website: www.colonic-association.org
Email: info@colonic-association.org

COUNSELLING

If you, or a member of your family, is in need of professional counselling, send an SAE to:
British Association for Counselling and Psychotherapy (BACP).
BACP House, 15 St John's Business Park,
Lutterworth LE17 4HB
Tel: 01455 883300
Website: www.bacp.co.uk
Email: bacp@bacp.co.uk

CRANIAL OSTEOPATHY

A gentle method of osteopathy that concentrates on nerves and bones in the head, neck and shoulders. Many readers have reported relief from ME (chronic fatigue syndrome), facial pain, jaw pain and arthritis from this therapy. It is also excellent for draining lymph from head and neck area.
To find your nearest practitioner, contact:
The Bio-Cranial Institute (Europe),
41–43 Castle Street, Comber,
Co. Down BT23 5DY
Tel: 028 9187 1334
Website: www.biocranial.com
Email: neil.perks@btinternet.com

GENERAL ORGANIZATIONS

If you want to know more about specific alternative therapies, you can contact the Institute for Complementary Medicine (ICM), who will be happy to give you advice and put you in touch with the practitioners and societies that now meet with their high standards of practice and therapy:
Institute for Complementary and Natural Medicine (ICNM),
Can-Mezzanine, 32–36 Loman Street,
London SE1 0EH
Tel: 020 7922 7980
Website: www.i-c-m.org.uk

HALE CLINIC

This clinic is the largest alternative treatment centre in Europe with more than 100 practitioners, some of whom are also qualified medical doctors.
The Hale Clinic,
7 Park Crescent,
London W1B 1PF
Tel: 020 7631 0156
Website: www.haleclinic.com
Email: info@haleclinic.com

HEALING

Healers channel healing energies through their bodies and out through their hands into the patient's energy field, which encourages the body to heal itself. It is especially good for chronic fatigue and for raising energy levels when you are under the weather or suffering any illness.

Although there are hundreds of good healers in the UK alone, there are three I would mention. The first is Seka Nikolic, who practices in London. Contact her on 0207 443 5544. Her books are well worth a read or log on to her website: www.sekanikolic.com. The second healer is her brother, Momo Kovacevic, also an exceptional healer. Contact him on 0845 234 0339. The third is Kelvin Heard, who specializes in chronic fatigue or ME and is based in France, but treats people in the UK once a month. His number is 020 7483 0099 and his website is: www.kelvinheardhealer.org.

There is now a wealth of scientific research to show how healing works. See under *Healing*. To find your nearest practitioner, send a SAE to:
The Healing Trust,
21 York Road,
Northampton, NN1 5QG
Tel: 01604 603247
Website: www.thehealingtrust.org.uk

HEALING, REIKI

A very popular form of hands-on healing.
For general enquiries, contact:
Sonia Thornton, The Reiki Association,
Westgate Court, Spittal,
Haverfordwest SA62 5QP
Tel: 07704 270727 (As this is a mobile number, Sonia will be happy to call you back.)
Website: www.reikiassociation.org.uk
Email: enquiries@reikiassociation.org.uk

HERBALISM

The practice of using plants to treat disease. Treatment may be given in the form of fluid extracts, tinctures, tablets or teas.
For further details and a register of qualified members, send a SAE to:
The National Institute of Medical Herbalists,
Clover House, James Court,
South Street, Exeter EX1 1EE
Tel: 01392 426022
Website: www.nimh.org.uk
Email: info@nimh.org.uk

HOMEOPATHY

Works in harmony with the body to stimulate the body's natural healing mechanisms. Homeopathy is the use of minute amounts of a particular substance (made from animal, vegetable or mineral matter) working under the concept that if you are exposed to minute amounts of the same bacteria or virus, or whatever ails you, this stimulates the body's natural defence mechanisms. It treats like with like. For example, a large amount of the 'poison nut' found in nature (which becomes homeopathic nux vomica) would make you feel very ill indeed – however a minute amount in homeopathic form can alleviate symptoms of vomiting and nausea in most cases very quickly.

For a register of professionally qualified homeopaths and general information about homeopathy, contact :

The Society of Homeopaths
11 Brookfield, Duncan Close, Moulton Park, Northampton NN3 6WL
Tel: 01604 817890
Website: www.homeopathy-soh.org
Email: info@homeopathy-soh.org

Homeopathic Medical Association (HMA),
7 Darnley Road, Gravesend
Kent DA11 0RU
Tel: 01474 560336
Website: www.the-hma.org
Email: info@the-hma.org

British Homeopathic Association (BHA)
Hahnemann House, 29 Park Street West
Luton LU1 3BE
Tel: 01582 408675
Website: www.trusthomeopathy.org
Email: info@britishhomeopathic.org

HYPNOTHERAPY

By allowing external distractions to fade, the therapy allows you to fully relax and understand the root cause of many of your problems, phobias and addictions.
To find your nearest practitioner, contact.
The National Council for Hypnotherapists
Tel: 08455 440788
Website: www.hypnotherapists.org.uk

Leila Hart is a highly qualified accredited clinical hypnotherapist who works with emotional and physical problems, phobias, weight loss and stress and can be contacted from 10am to 6pm on 020 7402 4311.

INSTITUTE FOR OPTIMUM NUTRITION

The Institute for Optimum Nutrition has a great on-line newsletter packed with the latest health news and they also train nutritionists. The Institute also holds seminars on health and it has in-house nutritionists. For details and to find

your nearest practitioner, contact:
Institute for Optimum Nutrition (ION),
Avalon House, 72 Lower Mortlake Road,
Richmond, Surrey TW9 2JY
Tel: 020 8614 7800
Website: www.ion.ac.uk
Email: ionreception@ion.ac.uk

IRIDOLOGY
A method of analysis rather than treatment,
based on the theory that the whole body is
reflected in the eyes. Using a magnifier, the
practitioner examines the visible parts of the
eyes to pinpoint physical and emotional
weaknesses or potential areas that might be
causing you problems, either currently or in the
years to come.
Send an SAE for a list of qualified practitioners to:
Guild of Naturopathic Iridologists Int.,
94 Grosvenor Road,
London SW1V 3LF
Tel: 020 7821 0255
Website: www.gni-international.org

KINESIOLOGY
The science of testing muscle response to
discover areas of impaired energy and function
in the body. Kinesiology is especially useful if you
think you have a sensitivity or negative reaction
either to a food or an external allergen. Can also
be used to test if the supplements you are taking
suit your unique physiology.
To find your nearest practitioner, contact:
Association for Systematic Kinesiology,
16 Iris Road, West Ewell, Epsom,
Surrey KT19 9NH
Tel: 020 8391 5988
Website: www.kinesiology.co.uk
Email: info@kinesiology.co.uk

MANUAL LYMPHATIC DRAINAGE
A very gentle pulsing massage, which helps to
drain the lymph nodes, thereby reducing
swelling and pain related to the lymph glands.
This is a very useful treatment for ladies who
have had breast and/or lymph surgery. It is also
great for reducing water retention anywhere in
the body.
To find your nearest practitioner, send an SAE to:
Manual Lymphatic Drainage UK,
PO Box 14491, Glenrothes,
Fife KY6 3YE
Tel: 0844 800 1988
Website: www.mlduk.org.uk
Email: admin@mlduk.org.uk

NATUROPATHY
Naturopaths treat the whole person, on a
spiritual, physical and emotional level, to

discover any underlying dysfunctions in a
patient's life. They then offer advice on dietary
changes, supplements and herbs to help improve
or alleviate your condition. Many naturopaths
are also qualified homeopaths and/or
acupuncturists. They help provide the right tools
for the body to heal itself naturally. Because
naturopaths treat the person not the ailment,
any treatments are tailored to each individual.
For more help, contact:
The College of Naturopathic Medicine
Tel: 01342 410505
Website: www.naturopathy-uk.com
They run college courses in London, Bristol,
Manchester, Edinburgh, Dublin and Cork.

The General Council and Register of Naturopaths
(GCRN)
Tel: 01458 840072
To find your nearest practitioner, log on to:
www.naturopathy.org.uk

NEURO-LINGUISTIC PROGRAMMING
This is a profound and yet simple way to re-
programme any negative thoughts or habits to
more positive ones. Great for phobias and panic
attacks, and for attaining your goals in life.
For further information on NLP, contact
The Association for Neuro Linguistic
Programming (ANLP)
Tel: 020 3051 6740
Website: www.anlp.org

NUTRI CENTRE, THE
The Nutri Centre, located on the lower ground
floor of the Hale Clinic at 7 Park Crescent,
London, is unique in being able to supply almost
every alternative product currently available from
any country, including specialized practitioner
products. The Nutri Centre offers an excellent
and reliable mail-order service worldwide for all
its products.
For supplements, tel: 0845 602 6744
For books, tel: 020 7323 2382
Website: www.nutricentre.com
Email: admin@nutricentre.com

NUTRITIONAL THERAPY
To find your nearest qualified nutritionist who
can help you to balance your diet and suggest
the correct vitamins and minerals, contact:
The British Association of Nutritional Therapists,
27 Old Gloucester Street,
London WC1N 3XX
Tel: 0870 606 1284
Website: www.bant.org.uk
Email: theadministrator@bant.org.uk

The Institute for Optimum Nutrition
Tel: 020 8614 7800
Website: www.ion.ac.uk
Email: info@ion.ac.uk
A directory of practitioners is available online.

ORGANIC PRODUCE

The Soil Association has published an Organic Directory, which is packed with information on where to buy organic produce throughout the country. This is available online for free on their website.
Soil Association,
South Plaza, Marlborough Street,
Bristol BS1 3NX
Tel: 0117 314 5000
Website: www.soilassociation.org

Soil Association Scotland,
18C Liberton Brae, Tower Mains,
Edinburgh, EH16 6AE
Tel: 0131 666 2474
Website: www.soilassociationscotland.org

OSTEOPATHY

A system of healing that works on the physical structure of the body. Practitioners use manipulation, massage and stretching techniques. If you suffer chronic or sudden back, hip, neck or shoulder displacement or injury, go to see an osteopath.
To find your nearest practitioner, contact:
General Osteopathic Council,
176 Tower Bridge Road,
London SE1 3LU
Tel: 020 7357 6655
Website: www.osteopathy.org.uk
Email: contactus@osteopathy.org.uk

PILATES

This is a highly effective, low-impact, isometric form of exercise, which you can practise even if you have suffered some kind of injury. Very powerful but gentle.
Pilates Foundation Administrator,
PO Box 58235,
London N1 5UY
Tel: 020 7033 0078
Website: www.pilatesfoundation.com
Email: admin@pilatesfoundation.com
I visit Pilates in Motion, in London W5. My teacher Anouska Boone is a miracle worker! Contact Anouska on 020 8810 7344.

QIGONG

An extremely gentle form of exercise (like t'ai chi), which helps people with impaired mobility, such as severe arthritis. Anyone can practise qigong and no special clothes are needed. For further information contact:
TSE Qigong Centre,
PO Box 918-A, Kingston-upon-Thames,
Surrey KT1 9PA
Tel: 020 8224 2306
Website: www.qimagazine.com
Email: tse@tseqigongcentre.com

REFLEXOLOGY

Gentle stimulation of the reflex/nerve-ending points on the hands and feet correspond to every part of the body. By working with pressure on these points, blockages in the energy pathways are released, which encourages the body to heal itself. This is a great way to boost circulation and is really relaxing.
To find your nearest practitioner, contact:
Association of Reflexologists,
5 Fore Street, Taunton,
Somerset TA1 1HX
Tel: 01823 351010
Web: www.aor.org.uk
AOR is a member of Reflexology in Europe Network and International Council of Reflexology.

The British Reflexology Association, Monks Orchard, Whitbourne, Worcester WR6 5RB
Tel: 01886 821207
Fax: 01886 822017
Website: www.britreflex.co.uk
Email: bra@britreflex.co.uk
See also Advanced Reflexology (page 423).

YOGA

The ancient principles of yoga are beneficial for staying healthy and supple well into one's 80s and beyond. Yoga teaches relaxation and breathing techniques, together with gentle stretching exercises, which help keep the 'whole' self fit for life. It is especially useful for keeping the spine strong. There is also a monthly YOGA magazine, especially for yoga enthusiasts.
To find your nearest class, contact:
The British Wheel of Yoga,
25 Jermyn Street, Sleaford,
Lincolnshire NG34 7RU
Tel: 01529 306851
Website: www.bwy.org.uk
Email: office@bwy.org.uk

Index